Pain in Dementia

Pain in Dementia

Stefan Lautenbacher, PhD
Professor
Physiological Psychology
University of Bamberg
Bamberg, Germany

Stephen J. Gibson, PhD
Professor
Deputy Director
National Ageing Research Institute
Royal Melbourne Hospital
Melbourne, Australia

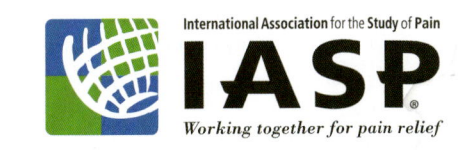

Wolters Kluwer
Philadelphia · Baltimore · New York · London
Buenos Aires · Hong Kong · Sydney · Tokyo

International Association for the Study of Pain
IASP
Working together for pain relief

Acquisitions Editor: Keith Donnellan
Product Development Editor: Lauren Pecarich
Senior Production Project Manager: Alicia Jackson
Design Coordinator: Holly McLaughlin
Manufacturing Coordinator: Beth Welsh
Marketing Manager: Dan Dressler
Prepress Vendor: S4Carlisle Publishing Services

Copyright © 2017 IASP Press®

International Association for the Study of Pain®

All rights reserved. This book is protected by copyright. No part of this book may be reproduced or transmitted in any form or by any means, including as photocopies or scanned-in or other electronic copies, or utilized by any information storage and retrieval system without written permission from the copyright owner, except for brief quotations embodied in critical articles and reviews. Materials appearing in this book prepared by individuals as part of their official duties as U.S. government employees are not covered by the above-mentioned copyright. To request permission, please contact Wolters Kluwer Health at Two Commerce Square, 2001 Market Street, Philadelphia, PA 19103, via email at permissions@lww.com, or via our website at lww.com (products and services).

9 8 7 6 5 4 3 2 1

Printed in China

Library of Congress Cataloging-in-Publication Data

Names: Lautenbacher, Stefan, 1956– editor. | Gibson, Stephen J., 1959– editor. | International Association for the Study of Pain, issuing body.
Title: Pain in dementia / [edited by] Stefan Lautenbacher, Stephen J. Gibson.
Description: Philadelphia : Wolters Kluwer Health, [2017] | Includes bibliographical references and index.
Identifiers: LCCN 2016051258 | ISBN 9781496332134
Subjects: | MESH: Pain—complications | Dementia—complications | Pain Measurement | Pain Management | Aged
Classification: LCC RC521 | NLM WL 704 | DDC 616.8/30472—dc23 LC record available at https://lccn.loc.gov/2016051258

This work is provided "as is," and the publisher disclaims any and all warranties, express or implied, including any warranties as to accuracy, comprehensiveness, or currency of the content of this work.

This work is no substitute for individual patient assessment based upon healthcare professionals' examination of each patient and consideration of, among other things, age, weight, gender, current or prior medical conditions, medication history, laboratory data and other factors unique to the patient. The publisher does not provide medical advice or guidance and this work is merely a reference tool. Healthcare professionals, and not the publisher, are solely responsible for the use of this work including all medical judgments and for any resulting diagnosis and treatments.

Given continuous, rapid advances in medical science and health information, independent professional verification of medical diagnoses, indications, appropriate pharmaceutical selections and dosages, and treatment options should be made and healthcare professionals should consult a variety of sources. When prescribing medication, healthcare professionals are advised to consult the product information sheet (the manufacturer's package insert) accompanying each drug to verify, among other things, conditions of use, warnings and side effects and identify any changes in dosage schedule or contradictions, particularly if the medication to be administered is new, infrequently used or has a narrow therapeutic range. To the maximum extent permitted under applicable law, no responsibility is assumed by the publisher for any injury and/or damage to persons or property, as a matter of products liability, negligence law or otherwise, or from any reference to or use by any person of this work.

LWW.com

DEDICATION

For those, who lost their voice to speak for themselves, and for those, who try to speak for these but often do not exactly know what to say. They all were reason for writing and editing this book and deserve our gratitude for their inspiration. May this book be a little help for them!

CONTRIBUTORS

Wilco P. Achterberg, MD, PhD
Professor of Institutional Care and Elderly Care Medicine
Department of Public Health and Primary Care
Leiden University Medical Center
Leiden, The Netherlands

Martina Amanzio, PhD
Associate Professor of Psychobiology
Department of Psychology
University of Turin
Turin, Italy

David Ames, BA, MD, FRCPsych, FRANZCP
Director
National Ageing Research Institute
Professor of Ageing and Health
The University of Melbourne
Victoria, Australia

Fabrizio Benedetti, MD
Professor of Physiology and Neuroscience
University of Turin
Turin, Italy

Rachel Bieu, PhD
Psychologist
Baptist Behavioral Health
Jacksonville, Florida

Terence Chong, MBBS, MP, MBA, FRANZCP
Research Fellow
Academic Unit for Psychiatry of Old Age
The University of Melbourne
Melbourne, Australia

Leonie J. Cole
Melbourne School of Psychological Sciences
The University of Melbourne
Melbourne, Australia

Anne Corbett, BSc (Hons), MReS, PhD
Lecturer in Dementia Research Communications
Wolfson Centre for Age-Related Diseases
King's College London
London, United Kingdom

Ruth Defrin, PhD
Associate Professor
Department of Physical Therapy
Sackler Faculty of Medicine
Tel-Aviv University
Tel-Aviv, Israel

Suzanne Delwel, MSc
Faculty of Psychology and Education
Department of Neuropsychology
Department of Oral Kinesiology
Academic Centre of Dentistry Amsterdam (ACTA)
University of Amsterdam and VU University Amsterdam
Amsterdam, The Netherlands

Margot W.M. de Waal, PhD
Leiden University Medical Centre
Leiden, The Netherlands

Leslie Dowson, BSc (Hons)
Research Officer
National Ageing Research Institute
Melbourne, Australia

Colleen Doyle, PhD, MAPS
Professor of Aged Care
School of Nursing, Paramedicine & Midwifery
Faculty of Health Sciences
Australian Catholic University in Partnership with Villa Maria Catholic Homes
Principal Research Fellow
National Ageing Research Institute
Victoria, Australia

Michael Farrell, PhD, MSc, BAppSc (Phy)
Associate Professor
Department of Medical Imaging and Radiation Sciences
Monash University
Melbourne, Australia

Elisabeth Flo, PhD
Associate Professor
Centre for Elderly and Nursing Home Medicine
Department of Global Public Health and Primary Care
University of Bergen
Bergen, Norway

Stephen J. Gibson, PhD
Professor
Deputy Director
National Ageing Research Institute
Royal Melbourne Hospital
Melbourne, Australia

Lydia Giménez-Llort, BSc, PhD
Professor
Department of Psychiatry and Forensic Medicine
School of Medicine
Universitat Autònoma de Barcelona
Bellaterra, Spain

Toni L. Glover, PhD, GNP-BC, FNP-BC, CPE
Assistant Professor
Department of Adult and Elderly Nursing
College of Nursing, University of Florida
Gerontological Nurse Practitioner
Pain Research and Intervention Center of Excellence (PRICE)
Gainesville, Florida

Marjolein Gysels, PhD
Senior Researcher
Centre for Social Science and Global Health
University of Amsterdam
Amsterdam, The Netherlands

Thomas Hadjistavropoulos, PhD, ABPP, FCAHS
Registered Doctoral Psychologist
Research Chair in Aging and Health
CACBT Certified in Cognitive Behaviour Therapy
Professor of Psychology
Director, Centre on Aging and Health
Regina, Saskatchewan, Canada

Keela A. Herr, PhD, RN, FAAN, AGSF
Professor and Chair, Adult and Gerontology
RWJ Executive Nurse Fellow
College of Nursing
The University of Iowa
Iowa City, Iowa

Ann L. Horgas, PhD, RN, FGSA, FAAN
Associate Professor
Department of Adult and Elderly Nursing
University of Florida, College of Nursing
Gainesville, Florida

Bettina S. Husebø, MD, PhD
Associate Professor
Centre for Elderly and Nursing Home Medicine
Department of Global Public Health and Primary Care
University of Bergen
Bergen, Norway

Stein B. Husebø, MD
Dignity Center: Care for the Frail Old
Bergen, Norway

Benny Katz, MBBS, FRACP, FFPMANZCA
Director of Geriatric Medicine
St. Vincent's Hospital Melbourne
Fitzroy, Australia
Honorary Clinical Associate Professor
The University of Melbourne
Adjunct Associate Professor, ACEBAC
LaTrobe University
Melbourne, Australia

Robert Kerns, PhD
Research Psychologist
Pain Research, Informatics, Multimorbidities and Education (PRIME) Center
VA Connecticut Healthcare System
Professor of Psychiatry, Neurology and Psychology
Yale University
New Haven, Connecticut

Joseph Kulas, PhD
Assistant Professor of Psychiatry
Yale School of Medicine
Yale University
New Haven, Connecticut

Miriam Kunz, PhD
Rosalind Franklin Fellow
Assistant Professor in the Department of General Practice
University Medical Center
Groningen, The Netherlands

Stefan Lautenbacher, PhD
Professor
Physiological Psychology
University of Bamberg
Bamberg, Germany

Frank Lobbezoo, DDS, PhD
Professor, Chair and Vice-Dean
Department of Oral Kinesiology
Academic Centre of Dentistry Amsterdam (ACTA)
University of Amsterdam and Vrije Universiteit University Amsterdam (VU)
Amsterdam, The Netherlands

Samantha Loi, MBBS, MPsych, FRANZCP
Senior Lecturer
Academic Unit for Psychiatry of Old Age
The University of Melbourne
Melbourne, Australia

Brian E. McGuire, BA, MClinPsych, DipCrim, DipHSc, PhD
Professor of Clinical Psychology & HRB Research Leader
Co-Director, Centre for Pain Research
School of Psychology
National University of Ireland
Galway, Ireland

Sophie Pautex, MD
Professor
Community Palliative Care Unit
Division of Primary Care
University Hospital Geneva
Geneva, Switzerland

C.G. Pick, PhD
Professor
Department of Anatomy and Anthropology
Sackler Faculty of Medicine and Sago School of Neuroscience
Tel-Aviv University
Tel-Aviv, Israel

Gisèle Pickering, MD, PhD, DPharm
Professor of Clinical Pharmacology
Director of the Clinical Research Centre
Clinical Pharmacology Department
University Hospital Clermont-Ferrand
Laboratory of Fundamental and Clinical Pharmacology of Pain
Clermont-Ferrand University
Clermont-Ferrand, France

Bart Plooij, PhD
Psychologist
Alrijne Zorggroep
Leiderdorp, Netherlands

Michael A. Rapp, MD, PhD
Professor
Social and Preventive Medicine
University of Potsdam
Potsdam, Germany

Bronagh Reynolds, MPsych
Assistant Psychologist
NHS Lothian
Edinburgh, Scotland

Gail Roberts, MA, RN
Research Officer
School of Nursing, Paramedicine & Midwifery
Faculty of Health Sciences
Australian Catholic University in Partnership with Villa Maria Catholic Homes
National Ageing Research Institute
Victoria, Australia

Elizabeth L. Sampson, MBChB, MD, MRCPsych
Senior Clinical Lecturer
Marie Curie Palliative Care Research Unit
Division of Psychiatry
University College Medical School London
London, United Kingdom

Steven M. Savvas, PhD
Researcher
National Ageing Research Institute
Parkville, Australia

Erik J.A. Scherder, PhD
Professor
Head of the Department of Clinical
    Neuropsychology
Vrije Universiteit Amsterdam
Amsterdam, The Netherlands

Kristen Swafford, RN, PhD, CNS
Affiliate Faculty
Oregon Health & Science University
School of Nursing
Portland, Oregon

Darragh Taheny, BA (Psych)
Research Assistant
Centre for Pain Research
National University of Ireland
Galway, Ireland

Nele van den Noortgate, MD, PhD
Professor
University Hospital Ghent
Ghent, Belgium

J.T. van der Steen, PhD
Associate Professor
VU University Medical Center, EMGO Institute
    for Health and Care Research
Department of General Practice & Elderly Care
    Medicine
Amsterdam, The Netherlands

Roxane A.F. Weijenberg, PhD
Faculty of Behavioral and Movement Sciences
Department of Clinical Neuropsychology
Vrije Universiteit Amsterdam (VU)
Assistant Professor
Department of Oral Kinesiology
Academic Centre for Dentistry Amsterdam
    (ACTA)
Amsterdam, The Netherlands

Sandra Zwakhalen, PhD
Assistant Professor
Department of Health Care and Nursing Science
CAPHRI School for Public Health and Primary
    Care
Faculty of Health, Medicine and Life Sciences
Maastricht University
Maastricht, The Netherlands

PREFACE

PAIN IN DEMENTIA: A DISTRESSING DOUBLE BURDEN ON MANY

Dementia has been called "the 21st century plague". There are many millions of people suffering from dementia worldwide and the number continues to rise. Up to 80% of people with dementia living in care homes regularly experience pain. Pain in dementia is usually related to musculoskeletal, gastrointestinal and cardiac conditions, genitourinary infections, pressure ulcers, and oral pain. Neuropathic pain, defined as pain caused by a lesion or dysfunction in the central nervous system, is common in dementia. Despite these numerous established causes of pain, international epidemiological research has reported that the use of pain medication is often inappropriate in this patient group. Consequences of untreated pain include mental and physical impairment, a higher frequency of neuropsychiatric symptoms such as agitation, depression and sleep problems, and adverse events like falls, hallucination, and even death.

Thorough assessment of pain is essential to ensure effective treatment and ongoing care. In most patient groups, the most effective method of identifying pain is through self-report. However, a key symptom of dementia is the loss of ability to communicate, particularly in the later stages of the condition, largely allowing only observers to identify and rate the pain. A further major problem in assessing pain in dementia is the difficulty to distinguish pain from other behavioral symptoms that commonly arise in people with dementia. The inaccuracy in diagnosis can in turn result in inappropriate treatment, even including the use of antipsychotic medications instead of analgesics. Treatment approaches are further hindered by a neglect of nonpharmacological options, too few multidisciplinary and palliative care programs, as well as an insufficient integration of treatment and care.

To overcome this distressing situation for patients, relatives, and societies, basic and applied research, which provide better diagnostic tools and treatment strategies, as well as education of a new generation of experts are urgently needed. As with many aspects of dementia research, the critical relevance of the troublesome combination of pain and dementia was overlooked until the latter part of the last century. **The present book is an attempt to stress the relevance of these topics and delineate the state of the art in the search for solutions.** A short outline of the book should give some evidence for the seriousness and comprehensiveness of this attempt.

- **Preserving the dignity** of those suffering both from pain and dementia is a major obligation for all being active in research, care, and treatment and should therefore be the ethical guideline for all our scientific and clinical considerations *(Chapter 1)*.
- **Basic knowledge and facts about pain in dementia** are always necessary as the basis for deeper understanding and scientific as well as clinical applications. Therefore, the nature of dementia *(Chapter 2)*, the specific characteristics *(Chapter 3)*, and the prevalence *(Chapter 4)* of pain in dementia are implemented as contents in the book.
- The **neurophysiological interaction between dementia and pain** is described from the perspective of neuroimaging *(Chapter 5)* as well as from the perspective of neuropathology and neuropsychology *(Chapter 6)*.
- The **neuropsychiatric consequences of pain in dementia** sometimes mask the classical symptoms of pain and therefore deserve extra attention *(Chapter 7)*.

- In **other forms of cognitive impairment** (e.g., mental retardation), similar problems regarding pain assessment and treatment may arise, making mutual exchanges of experience and knowledge between domains worthwhile *(Chapter 8)*.
- The proper **assessment of pain and associated problems of pain in dementia** is a scientific milestone of finding clinical solutions for this major health problem and requires various approaches, namely using self-report measures of pain *(Chapter 9)*, applying instruments for observer ratings *(Chapter 10)*, detailing analysis by psychophysical and behavioral tools of assessment *(Chapter 11)*, considering not only pain in general but also specific forms like orofacial pain *(Chapter 12)*, integrating the use of various instruments into informative guidelines *(Chapter 13)*, and finally widening the scope by seeing the pain-associated problems leading to mood and emotional disturbances *(Chapter 14)*, and cognitive *(Chapter 15)* and functional *(Chapter 16)* impairments.
- The **care and management of pain in dementia** are necessarily multidisciplinary and multiprofessional, including approaches developed by caregivers and academic nurses *(Chapter 17)*, pharmacological strategies of treatment *(Chapter 18)*, treatment attempts contributed by physiotherapists, ergotherapists, and others engaged in physical activity–related therapies *(Chapter 19)*, or by psychologists and psychotherapists *(Chapter 20)*. The proponents of all these therapeutic attempts have to bear in mind that the mind of patients with dementia can no longer heal as good as before and placebo action is reduced *(Chapter 21)*.
- **Special challenges and conditions of pain management in dementia** are given on the one hand when the complexity of caring and managing patients with both pain and dementia is further enhanced as soon as patients enter the end-of-life phase *(Chapter 22)* and may be unburdened when the potentially active treatments just mentioned are combined in multidisciplinary programs for the easy participation of aged patients with dementia *(Chapter 23)*.
- **Special ethical considerations** are necessary when patients with dementia become participants in clinical research and treatment trials *(Chapter 24)*.
- Cross-**cultural thinking** is required to see the stability and variability of the problem of pain in dementia across different societal settings *(Chapter 25)*.
- Whether **research on nonhuman animals** can improve our understanding of pain in dementia and may help to avoid frail patients being study subjects is worth discussing *(Chapter 26)*.
- A few thoughts about **future directions of research and clinical practice** regarding pain in dementia may round up the accumulation of facts and theories in the book *(Chapter 27)*.

We cordially thank the International Association for the Study of Pain (IASP), IASP Press, and Wolters Kluwer for their support in making this book with such a wide and comprehensive scope, which allows us to consider all relevant aspects of this pressing topic. We also thank our authors for their outstanding contributions.

Pain in dementia will unfortunately remain a problem for many more decades. We hope that this book may add a bit to the multidisciplinary and international approaches to educate clinicians, researchers, and caregivers in the presence and to form a new generation of experts better prepared to look for new scientific and clinical solutions as well as to inform a best-possible practice for the future.

Stefan Lautenbacher and Stephen J. Gibson
November 2016

CONTENTS

1. The Concept of Dignity, Suffering, and Pain in Frail Old Patients and Persons with Dementia 1
   Stein B. Husebø and Bettina S. Husebø

2. The Scope of Dementia: Variants, Symptoms, Stages, and Causes 11
   Anne Corbett

3. Pain Perception and Report in Persons with Dementia 31
   Stephen J. Gibson and Stefan Lautenbacher

4. The Epidemiology of Pain in Dementia 43
   Brian E. McGuire, Darragh Taheny, and Bronagh Reynolds

5. Central Pathophysiology of Dementia and Pain 55
   Michael J. Farrell and Leonie J. Cole

6. Pain in People with Dementia—Its Relationship to Neuropathology 71
   Erik J. A. Scherder

7. Neuropsychiatric Sequels of Pain in Dementia 85
   Bettina S. Husebø and Elisabeth Flo

8. Pain in Other Types of Cognitive Impairment with a Focus on Developmental Disability 99
   Ruth Defrin

9. Methods of Assessing Pain and Associated Conditions in Dementia: Self-report Pain Scales 119
   Sophie Pautex and Stefan Lautenbacher

10. Observational Pain Tools 133
    Sandra Zwakhalen, Keela A. Herr, and Kristen Swafford

11. Behavioral Approaches and Psychophysics 155
    Miriam Kunz and Stefan Lautenbacher

12. Assessment of Specific Forms of Pain in Dementia: Orofacial Pain 167
    Frank Lobbezoo, Suzanne Delwel, and Roxane A. F. Weijenberg

13. Guidelines and Practical Approaches for the Effective Pain Assessment of the Patient with Dementia 177
    Thomas Hadjistavropoulos

14. Assessment of Behavioral and Mood Symptoms in Dementia Patients Suffering from Pain 193
    Michael A. Rapp

15	**Cognitive Screening for Dementia**	209
	Samantha Loi, Terence Chong, and David Ames	
16	**Pain-Related Functional Impairment in Dementia**	219
	Wilco P. Achterberg, Bart Plooij, and Margot W. M. de Waal	
17	**Nursing Care of Pain in Persons with Dementia**	235
	Ann L. Horgas and Toni L. Glover	
18	**Pharmacological Treatment of Pain in Dementia**	245
	Gisèle Pickering	
19	**Pain, Exercise, and Dementia**	253
	Steven M. Savvas and Stephen J. Gibson	
20	**Psychological Approaches to Therapy**	267
	Rachel Bieu, Joseph Kulas, and Robert Kerns	
21	**Placebo Analgesia in Dementia**	285
	Martina Amanzio and Fabrizio Benedetti	
22	**Palliative Care of Patients with Dementia and Pain**	293
	Elizabeth L. Sampson, Nele van den Noortgate, and J. T. van der Steen	
23	**Multidisciplinary and Multiprofessional Treatments**	305
	Benny Katz	
24	**Ethical Issues in Research with Persons with Dementia: Potential and Restrictions**	317
	Colleen Doyle, Leslie Dowson, Gail Roberts, and Stephen J. Gibson	
25	**Pain in Dementia: Cross-Cultural Considerations**	331
	Wilco P. Achterberg and Marjolein Gysels	
26	**Pain Assessment in Cognitively Impaired Animals**	345
	Lydia Giménez-Llort and C. G. Pick	
27	**Future Direction of Research**	363
	Stefan Lautenbacher, Wilco P. Achterberg, Elizabeth L. Sampson, and Miriam Kunz	
	Index	373

CHAPTER 1

The Concept of Dignity, Suffering, and Pain in Frail Old Patients and Persons with Dementia

Stein B. Husebø and Bettina S. Husebø

> "A medical revolution has extended the lives of our elder citizens without providing the dignity and security those later years deserve."
>
> (John F. Kennedy, 1960)

In most developed countries most of the population will reach an age of 80 years or more. In their final frail years before death, they will increasingly need support of care services, and be more or less dependent on others. What are their needs? How can we establish and provide optimal care, security, pain, and symptom assessment and management? How can we identify and relieve suffering? How can we respect their dignity and relieve their suffering and pain in their final years before death [23]? This chapter will discuss the concepts and practical challenges of dignity, suffering and pain, both for the multiprofessional team, and for the frail old and their next of kin.

DIGNITY

United Nations Universal Declaration of Human Rights 1948 stated, "All human beings are born free and equal in dignity and rights," (www.humanrights.com). We also find the concept of and duty to protect dignity implemented in the basic laws and judicial decisions in many legal systems, as well as in international covenants and declarations on human rights. But no country has gone so far as Germany in integrating dignity in its legal system. As stated in the first sentences of the Basic Law (Grundgesetz, www.bundestag.de), the inviolable dignity of human being is a fundamental constitutional principle: "Human dignity is inviolable. To respect it and protect it is the duty of all state power. The German people therefore acknowledge inviolable and inalienable human rights as the basic of every community, of peace and justice of the world [27]." But, what is the meaning and content of dignity? Dignity as an idea has a long and important history in ethics, not denoted to a single essence. A central statement to dignity comes from Immanuel Kant, "In the kingdom of ends everything has either a price or a dignity. What has a price can be replaced by something equivalent; what on the other side is raised above all prices and therefore admits of no equivalent, has a dignity [35]."

Human dignity is complex, ambiguous, and multivalent, challenging us to look at the use of ideas in order to probe the depth of their meaning. On the one side all human beings have their inviolable, intrinsic dignity. On the other side their dignity can be violated or confirmed by others. Moody argues for the need to address, discuss, and understand basic words, specific ideas, and challenges of dignity in each specific patient, such as [27] follows:

Self-respect	vs.	Shame
Honor	vs.	Humiliation
Decorum	vs.	Inappropriate behavior
Privacy	vs.	Exposure
Power	vs.	Vulnerability
Equality	vs.	Favoritism
Adulthood	vs.	Infantilization
Ego integrity	vs.	Despair
Individuation	vs.	Objectification
Autonomy	vs.	Dependency

Whether by stroke, by dementia, by other severe or chronic disease, by loss of close relatives, by poverty, or by pain, we stand at risk of losing everything achieved over a lifetime. Each of us, however, dimly, carries this unspoken awareness during our lives. Life can end badly, filled with pain and suffering; fear of aging is rooted in this understanding.

Dignity in old age matters because every one of us carries this sense of future vulnerability and because we fear becoming dependent burdens to ourselves and others in our last stages of life. Contemporary debates about euthanasia, concern over mistreatment of the frail elderly, anxiety for isolation, pain and suffering, all revolve around a primal fare: loss of dignity in old age [10, 34].

Pain, suffering, and dignity are closely linked to each other, demonstrated by the research and publications of the psychologist H. Chochinov who provides practical guidelines for "dignity therapy" in end-of-life care, primarily with focus on cancer patients [5]. Recently, his model was tested on older persons in nursing homes [12, 13], also on patients with cognitive impairment [6], providing courage for practical dignity interventions in long-term care.

DIGNITY—WITH LACK OF AUTONOMY

Most philosophers connect dignity with autonomy. Max Frisch (1911–1991) probably has the shortest version: "Dignity means the freedom to choose" [11].

Among publications with regard to quality in long-term care, one of the earliest, Home Life introduces the principles of care as "Residents have a fundamental right to self-determination and individuality"—that is autonomy [4]. Although, most centers for elderly care have procedures in place to exercise choice, on information, or services provided and how to complain, only a few provide the opportunities to comment on policy and procedures, planned changes, and suggested treatment and care [2]. This is even more concerning in patients with dementia or without a supportive relative.

For the large and rapidly increasing number of patients with dementia, there will be a decline of autonomy. Their dependency on the choices of others will increase. Their ability to self-report diminishes. They lose ability to claim their human rights. They still have their basic, intrinsic dignity, but now dependent on the respectful and wise choices of care givers, based on their insight, attitude, and competence. Our approach caring for these patients with lack of autonomy must have main focus on "seeing" the individual with his/her biography and life project: which goals, preferences, and decisions will the patient have, and would have had, for the rest of their life? Respecting dignity, All care givers should be aware of the patient's biography, also including the patient's life project: which goals, preferences, and decisions will the patient have, and would have had, for the rest of their life?

A nurse's statement illustrates how vulnerable dignity and autonomy at old age can be: "If I suffer from dementia, no longer able to make competent decisions and somebody remove my breast holder, without reflection if I would have liked my breast holder to be removed, I would kill them..."

Nora, 92 years old, patient in our nursing home, expressed her view on dignity: "Well, they give me a pill to stop me from crying, because my husband died..."

The appeal to dignity, more strongly the insistent claim to dignity, points to something in us which is genuinely transcendent, something which reflects our freedom to call into question all social roles, to say out loud that I am something more than my frailty or my role performances or my buying power. At that moment, the passive witness rises up to say, "You can't treat me that way." The moment we speak these words, dialogue becomes possible and advocacy becomes inevitable. The outcome of this struggle is never certain, but this struggle for dignity emerges again and again through the course of history. It is a cry for justice as much as an affirmation of meaning.

SUFFERING

In a remarkable article in *New England Journal of Medicine* 1982, Cassell [3] discusses the question of suffering and its relation to organic illness, which has rarely been addressed in the medical literature before. His article offers a description of the nature and causes of suffering in patients undergoing medical treatment. A distinction based on clinical observations is made between suffering and physical distress. "Suffering is experienced by persons, not merely by bodies, and has its source in challenges that threaten the intactness of the person as a complex social and psychological entity. Suffering can include physical pain but is by no means limited to it. The relief of suffering and the cure of disease must be seen as twin obligations of a medical profession that is truly dedicated to the care of the sick. Physicians' failure to understand the nature of suffering can result in medical intervention that (though technically adequate) not only fails to relieve suffering but becomes a source of suffering itself."

THE CONCEPT OF PAIN

The concept of pain also needs to be addressed. In IASP (International Association for Study of Pain, www.iasp-pain.org) taxonomy, we find the following definition:

"Pain is an unpleasant sensory and emotional experience associated with actual or potential tissue damage, or described in terms of such damage."

Merskey and Bodguk [25] note that "the inability to communicate verbally does not negate the possibility that an individual is experiencing pain and is in need of appropriate pain-relieving treatment. Pain is always subjective. Each individual learns the application of the word through experiences related to injury in early life. It is unquestionably a sensation in a part or parts of the body, but it is also always unpleasant and therefore also an emotional experience. Many people report pain in the absence of tissue damage or any likely pathophysiological cause; usually this happens for psychological reasons. There is usually no way to distinguish their experience from that due to tissue damage if we take the subjective report. If they regard their experience as pain, and if they report it in the same ways as pain caused by tissue damage, it should be accepted as pain. This definition avoids tying pain to the stimulus. Activity induced in the nociceptor and a nociceptive pathway by a noxious stimulus is not pain, which is always a psychological state, even though we may well appreciate that pain most often has a proximate physical cause." Interestingly, in most articles, lectures, and clinical settings on pain, only the first part of this definition is presented and addressed, overlooking the very important included "Notes on Usage" as the second part, concluding with "Activity induced in the nociceptor and a nociceptive pathway by a noxious stimulus is not pain, which is always a psychological state."

Biologists like to tie pain to a bodily stimulus, then loosing that pain always is a psychological state experienced by persons. It is important to include reference to Cicelys Saunders' (the founder of palliative care) term "total pain" since it nicely encapsulates the foundational concept underlying all suffering and that is that all human experience is modified by the status of the whole person in each domain. The first reference for it appears to be in her paper "The Last Frontier" by Saunders [31]. In it, she quotes a patient describing her pain, "It began in my back, but now it seems that all of me is wrong." Cicely Saunders then explains, "This kind of 'total pain' has physical, mental, social and spiritual elements. Neither the patient in her words nor we in our approach and treatment can deal with any of these separately."

When persons state, "I suffer," or "I am in pain," we need to accept their statement. Our next task is to reflect on and analyze their statements, asking the questions: What do they express? What does that mean, for them, and for me? Is it a warning signal? Fracture of a hip, toothache, appendicitis, or cancer disease? My husband left me? I am depressed? I feel lonely?

Before we eagerly start with interventions, operations, analgesics, or exercise, we need to assess the details. But first of all we must read the patient's pain concept as a whole. Examinations, self-rapport, and systematic observation of behavior provide important information. In many situations in life, to listen with patience, to provide a plaster, and to provide a good explanation or rest will relieve the suffering and pain, depending on the underlying cause.

ADVANCE CARE PLANNING

Another central key to optimal treatment and care and end-of-life care is open, preparing communication, Advance Care Planning (ACP) with patient and relatives, addressing the closer-coming death and the practical challenges regarding ethics, site and quality of stay and care in good time before the situation and symptoms develops [8, 26].

The physician must take the initiative and role as conductor in this process. Without the physician, the communication will develop huge and unnecessary gaps and remain fragmental. The key questions all physicians caring for frail, dependent old patients with multimorbidity or dementia must consider are "How long the time frame my patient has left? Will she be alive in 6–12 months?" [24]. If the answer to the last question is no, he or she should take initiative to meetings with the patient (if possible), the relatives, and caring staff. Central issues should be addressed and discussed, for example, the physician's considerations regarding health, illness, treatment options, side effects and limitations, time perspective, goals, pain and symptom assessment and treatment, and palliative care.

A special attention should be on ethical questions like informed consent, presumed consent and advance directives, the written ethical decisions at the end of life. The physician's statements should be reflective and clear, especially regarding who is responsible for what, and invite to questions and discussion. A summary of the meeting must be documented in the patients chart and available for all. In the next weeks and months, follow-up meetings should be planned and organized, especially when life-threatening complications occur.

Patients suffering from progressing dementia represent a special challenge due to cognitive failure in their last years increasingly will lose their ability to understand and make qualified statements and choices. The optimal goal must be to openly discuss and document the developing of the disease, ethical and practical challenges with them and their relatives before cognitive failure becomes a problem.

"IS THERE HOPE, DOCTOR?"

The physician's hope is often connected to survival. Comments such as "My task as physician is to fight for survival and to support the patient hopes" are common [16].

The professionals in the health services have an education and focus on prevention and cure of illness, goals shared by the patients and their relatives. The central target of medical interventions is mainly to identify and treat diseases. As long as these goals of restoring health or prolonging life with quality seem reachable, we all will fight for this hope of more time of life, and accept all burdens of treatments side effects.

But earlier or later all of us, especially the frail old, reach a point where there no longer is hope of curation or a prolonged life with quality. This "point of no return" must be identified and communicated. It should be a "point of establishing maximal attention," a time for fundamental shift with new therapeutic and caring goals, now with main focus on all perspectives of palliative care [17–20].

Many physicians find this fundamental shift difficult [24]. Some hardly recognize its existence. But the disease-focused model often becomes a burden for dying old patients [15]. To focus on survival or life-prolonging interventions can destroy their hope. Their hope at end of life is huge, now connected to openness, preparing communication, pain and symptom relief, relations, meaning, grief, love, attitude, and farewell.

The largest violation of a dying person's dignity and hope we can imagine is that they in their last days and hours of life are transported and referred between home, nursing homes, emergency wards, hospital or intensive care units, without the necessary, open, preparatory communication that a human being is dying, and that time has come for farewell.

PATIENTS WITH COGNITIVE FAILURE

Oddvar was 82 years old. After a serious stroke, his vascular dementia was diagnosed 4 years ago. He had been in the nursing home the last 6 months. His cognitive failure was moderate with mini-mental-state examination score of 18. He did not complain or report on pain. Due to his degenerative arthritis he received acetaminophen 3 g daily. Benefit in mobility and activities of daily living were observed. Despite some improvements in his physical function, he was increasingly depressed, and attempts with antidepressants without positive response. Talking about his life story, we discovered his previous occupation; he had been carpenter for more than 40 years! We asked Oddvar for his help to repair at the ward, first a chair—then a cupboard. He immediately responded to the question, went out of bed, dressed, and asked for the tools. Within a week he patiently repaired all at his ward, and with good supervision, he was lent out to other wards. In the following weeks and months his motivation, mood, behavior, and mobility was excellent.

Ten months later his situation had changed suddenly. A new apoplexy changed his life. Oddvar was now bed-ridden with hemiparesis, swallowing difficulties, and reduced consciousness. Communication was no longer possible. His wife still visited him every day and cared for him. One day, in the late evening, a nurse called from his ward: "Oddvar's wife is here. She says he must have pneumonia."

In our nursing home, physicians are on call 24 hours every day, the whole year. I drove to the nursing home and examined Oddvar. Then we sat down in the ward room: his wife, the nurse, and I.

His wife looked at me and said, "He has pneumonia, right?"

"Yes," I replied: "You are a good doctor."

"Then we should give him penicillin, doctor, shouldn't we?"

"To give penicillin is one side. . ." I replied. "I have an important question for you. You know Oddvar better than anyone else. What would he have wanted in this situation?"

After some seconds she replied: "He was a very proud man, you know, a man with dignity. . . There is not much dignity left now, is there. . . He. . . would have wanted to be dead, months ago."

"That is the other side," I said.

"But doesn't it mean a lot of suffering to die from pneumonia?"

"Earlier we said pneumonia is the friend of old people," I answered. "And we can relieve his suffering sufficiently if problems develop."

"Doctor, then we should not give him penicillin. But you must know that I love him very deeply. And promise me. Relieve his pain."

Oddvar received palliative care and not penicillin. He died peaceful 4 days later, with his wife at his side.

Our question "What would he have wanted?" means "What is the presumed consent?"

Oddvar's wife openly stated that he in the last months would have seen death as a relief. On the other side, she loves him and is not quite ready to let him go. To ask her, "What do *you* want us to do?" probably would lead to therapeutic intervention and penicillin. He might have lived longer, for some more days or weeks. But who would gain?

Most old patients will earlier or later reach a point where death no longer is the enemy they should fight against with all measures. Prolonging of life is no longer the target. Death will provide the longed-for relief from a life that has become a-not-bearable strain, suffering, and burden. Many elderly patients, due to dementia, age, or illness, have lost their cognitive competence to take part in ethical discussions and decisions.

Our ethical task is then their presumed consent: "What would they have wanted?" The question and answer is not as difficult as many of us imagine. Most elderly people tell us, "When I lose my conscience and am bed ridden, when my strains are far beyond my quality of life, please, don't keep me alive; let me die in peace, but relieve the pain [1].

In these situations, the disease-orientated medicine can become a violation of the patient's dignity. Dying patients die due to complication of the disease. We, earlier or later, no longer should fight against these medical diseases and their complications. Reasonable indications for artificial nutrition or intravenous fluid substitution and other life-prolonging measures are no longer established. The final stroke, heart failure, renal failure, or pneumonia becomes the dying patient's friend, allowing the longed-for peaceful death. The therapeutic goal is optimal palliative care till life comes to an end and with the signal "You mean something for us, because you are, until the last moment of your life."

WHO SHALL DECIDE?—INFORMED CONSENT

As the responsible anesthetist, I met Liv, 84 years old, for preoperative preparation. Eight months before, she had been operated for colon cancer. She developed multiple bowel metastases. Now, she had fistula from the bowels, followed by thin feces delivery from the vagina and urinary tract. Surgery was planned for the next day.

Her general condition was extremely poor. I rapidly developed doubt for the success of this intervention and found the surgeon responsible for the operation.

"Will she survive the operation?" I asked.

"Well," he answered, "she will die soon, but my hope is that we can provide some relief... We have no choice."

"And, what's about the postoperative complications?"

"You are the intensive care specialist," he answered: "What do you think?"

"She probably will develop postoperative infections and die on a respirator," I responded.

"But we have no choice," he said.

Then we discussed the interesting question: "Who has choice?"

Together we went to Liv, sat down, and discussed her situation, as openly as we had discussed it together.

She listened. Then she asked some questions, before saying, "You tell me that I have a choice between an operation followed by high risk of complications, or going home. Regardless how I choose, I will die in the following weeks, perhaps a month or two. Did I get you right?"

"Yes."

"Thank you for your openness," she said. "I want to go home and die where I have lived."

"We will do our best to establish optimal care for you at home. What is most important for you now?"

"My family," she answered, "and a guarantee that you relieve my pain and suffering as best you can."

At home she received excellent home care and palliative care. She died peacefully 4 weeks later in their living room with husband, children, and grandchildren at her side.

Physicians are obliged to establish "informed consent" before all kinds of diagnostic or therapeutically interventions. This duty is the key task in medical ethics, especially facing severely ill patients with life-threatening conditions. We must show them their road map, open discuss the options, the benefit and side effects of the therapeutic options [14, 28].

We must speak a language which they are able to understand, listen to concerns and questions, and give them advice if they ask for it. We should not hide vital information of crucial importance for their decision-making. Informed consent means open, frank and truthful information and consent for the further steps of intervention and, when death is coming closer, also speaks openly about the expected life prognosis.

Before the second open information and discussion with Liv, her informed consent was not informed. It was based on half-truth and half openness. She needed that we directly addressed her poor prognosis and very limited life expectancy, before she finally could make her decision, refusing an operation with burden and strains, deciding to go home.

In the literature of fiction we find impressive statements concerning the developing loneliness and despair when persons are left alone, when ignorance and superficial information hinder the needed bridge of communication regarding the impending death, central among them are Leo Tolstoy's *The Death of Ivan Ilych* [33] and Henrik Ibsen's playwright *The Wild Duck* [22]. This is also a central issue in psychotherapy, theology, and philosophy.

In these so important ethical discussions with patients and relatives we at the end of the discussion should build in a control question to them: "Could you please repeat the major content of our discussion?" What they then tell us is often not what we said, but what they understood, different from what we thought was the essence of our information. It gives us an important possibility to improve the level of common agreement and to reach the optimal informed consent.

Liv was not cognitively impaired. It was possible to reach and establish informed consent.

Most dying patients will lose their conscience the last hours, days or weeks before they die. For them, and for the large number of patients with dementia and cognitive failure, communication and planning must take place before the cognitive failure, establishing a palliative plan and ACP before it is too late. The challenge is open, preparing communication, addressing the life before death, including patient and relatives, respecting the patient's values, good advanced care planning.

Oddvar's and Liv's examples set focus on an overwhelming challenge in long-term care for the frail old compared to younger cancer patients. Most patients with progressive, metastatic cancer have a life trajectory with high quality of life until the last months and weeks of their life [14, 28]. They have low level of dependency and high level of self-control, autonomy, and dignity until they die. They are met by attention, competence and resources, also in open, preparing communication, and have access to competent physicians and nurses, when they need them. They receive palliative care and morphine when needed. In the most challenging situations they have access to palliative care units with special competence 24 hours every day. To have cancer means high status and high priority. They often live and die on first class.

For the vast number of frail, old patients needing long-term care, especially patients suffering from dementia, their situation is contrary. They do not have high status and high priority. In their life trajectory quality of life, self-control, autonomy, and dignity become increasingly low during their last years. Their dependency is high. Access to competence, physicians, and caring resources are limited. They suffer from a combination of chronic illnesses, followed by challenging polypharmacy with multiple, sometimes life-threatening, side effects. Palliative care units are not open to them. A central goal in end-of-life care and long-term care is to establish competence in palliative care for all patients when they need it, regardless of site of stay, diagnosis, and age.

In a remarkable editorial in the *British Medical Journal* titled "Why are doctors providing life-prolonging treatment to dying patients?" [9], the authors focus on the central challenges in end-of-life-care for the elderly. They state that the physicians learned behavior and attitude in these situations is "Don't just stand there. Do something!" But facing and treating ill and dying old patients, this approach violates the dignity of the dying; therefore, they state that the approach often should be changed to "Don't just do something. Sit down!"

How a person dies remains in the memory of the family—disturbing, hindering, and destroying the process of grief; or relieving it, as a highlight of dignity and a caring farewell [30]. When we in the last time of a person's life succeed with open, preparing communication, good and skilled ethics respecting informed or presumed consent, relief of troublesome symptoms, and provide excellent palliative care, we often, after the death of the patient, will receive the optimal feedback from the relatives: "We could not imagine that we would lose her. We were filled with fear and denial. But these last weeks and days of her life has been a highlight for all of us..."

Still attention and competence is needed. Pain can be a crucial warning for underlying serious illness, demanding imminent assessment and intervention. Chronic pain can cause severe suffering and unrepairable damage to body and soul.

Most patients with severe life-threatening illnesses choose "relive my pain" on the first place of their priority list. Relieve my suffering and respect my dignity. Pain, suffering, and dignity need to be addressed and assessed with competence. If you do not understand the suffering and pain, you cannot sufficiently relieve the suffering and pain. These tasks are increasingly challenging caring for patients with cognitive failure.

BASIC HUMAN RIGHTS

On top of the hierarchy is dignity, connected to basic human rights. Kant pleads that we all have "a moral duty" to preserve, represent, and protect dignity [35]. He also goes a step further asking first how we have to act in order to treat our dignity, our inner kernel of intrinsic value, with the proper respect. We have a moral duty to our self.

Kant hereby also addresses our personal dignity, as caring physicians, nurses, psychologists, etc. Our moral duty is to preserve the dignity of humankind through our own person. When patients due to treatments or progression of illnesses experience unrelieved and not addressed pain and suffering, our negligence make us guilty that we are violating dignity and basic human rights.

These challenges become more severe, if the patient due to cognitive failure, loses his or her ability to express and protect himself. In the last decades, numerous articles state that pain and suffering is poorly assessed and treated in patients with cognitive failure [7, 21]. Our moral duty is to change this, to establish tools for assessment and treatments, and to implement our knowledge everywhere in the care for the elderly, especially for patients with cognitive failure.

One of the key ways in which human dignity is violated is by preventing human beings, patients, relatives, caring staff, and physicians from behaving in ways that are dignified. When working with patients who are incompetent due to physical or mental illness, staff should discover past preferences, interests, priorities, experience and capabilities, and aim to provide for these, as soon as, and as far as possible [32].

At the vulnerable side of human existence, our preferences, values, and solidarity are tested. Do we care and provide caring services with security and competence for the old who due to frailty and cognitive impairment no longer can protect their dignity and human rights or speak for themselves? Do we discover, understand, assess, and relieve their suffering and pain? The carpenter Oddvar was discovered. His suffering and pain was assessed and relieved. His dignity was respected for the rest of his life.

REFERENCES

1. Allen RS, DeLaine SR, Chaplin WF, Marson DC, Bourgeois MS, Dijkstra K, Burgio LD. Advance care planning in nursing homes: correlates of capacity and possession of advance directives. Gerontologist 2003;43:309–17.
2. Brocklehurst J, Dickinson E. Cause for concern—autonomy for elderly people in long-term care. Age Ageing 1996;25:329–32.
3. Cassell EJ. The nature of suffering and the goals of medicine. N Engl J Med 1982;306:639–45.

4. Centre for Policy and Ageing. Home life: a code of practice for residential care. London: Centre for Policy and Ageing; 1984.
5. Chochinov HM, Hack T, Hassard T, Kristjanson LJ, McClement S, Harlos M. Dignity in the terminally ill: a cross-sectional, cohort study. Lancet 2002;360:2026–30.
6. Chochinov HM, Cann B, Cullihall K, Kristjanson L, Harlos M, McClement SE, Hack TF, Hassard T. Dignity therapy: a feasibility study of elders in long-term care. Palliat Support Care 2012;10:3–15.
7. Corbett A, Husebo BS, Malcangio M, Cohen-Mansfield J, Aarsland D, Ballard C. Assessment, diagnosis and treatment of pain in people with dementia. Nat Rev Neurol 2012;8:264–74.
8. Dening KH, Jones L, Sampson EL. Advance care planning for people with dementia: a review. Int Psychogeriatr 2011;23:1535–51.
9. Doust J, Del Mar C. Why do doctors use treatments that do not work? For many reasons - including their inability to stand idle and do nothing. BMJ 2004;328:474–5.
10. Finlay IG, George R. Legal physician-assisted suicide in Oregon and The Netherlands: evidence concerning the impact on patients in vulnerable groups-another perspective on Oregon's data. J Med Ethics 2011;37:171–4.
11. Frisch M. Tagebuch 1966–1971. Frankfurt am Main: Suhrkamp Verlag; 1972.
12. Goddard C, Speck P, Martin P, Hall S. Dignity therapy for older people in care homes: a qualitative study of the views of residents and recipients of 'generativity' documents. J Adv Nurs 2013;69:122–32.
13. Hall S, Goddard C, Opio D, Speck P, Higginson IJ. Feasibility, acceptability and potential effectiveness of dignity therapy for older people in care homes: a phase II randomized controlled trial of a brief palliative care psychotherapy. Palliat Med 2012;26:703–12.
14. Harris D. Forget me not: palliative care for people with dementia. Postgrad Med J 2007;83:362–6.
15. Hertogh CMPM, Ribbe MW. Ethical aspects of medical decision-making in demented patients: a report from the Netherlands. Alzheimer Dis Assoc Dis 1996; 10:11–9.
16. Husebo SB. Is there hope, doctor? J Palliat Care 1998;14:43–8.
17. Husebo BS, Husebo SB. Palliative care—also in geriatrics? Schmerz 2001; 15:350–5.
18. Husebo BS, Husebo SB. Ethical end-of-life decision making in nursing homes [in Norwegian]. Tidsskr Nor Laegeforen 2004;124:2926–7.
19. Husebo BS, Husebo SB. Nursing homes as arenas of terminal care--how do we do in practice? [in Norwegian]. Tidsskr Nor Laegeforen 2005;125:1352–4.
20. Husebo SB, Husebo BS. Palliativ plan—eldreomsorg. Nord Tidsskr Palliat Med 2011;28:43–50.
21. Husebo BS, Strand LI, Moe-Nilssen R, Husebo SB, Aarsland D, Ljunggren AE. Who suffers most? Dementia and pain in nursing home patients. J Am Med Dir Assoc 2008;9:427–33.
22. Ibsen H. The wild duck; trans. Stephen Mulrine. London: Nick Hern Books; 2006.
23. Lothian K, Philp I. Care of older people—maintaining the dignity and autonomy of older people in the healthcare setting. BMJ 2001;322:668–70.
24. Lynn J. Serving patients who may die soon and their families—the role of hospice and other services. JAMA 2001;285:925–32.
25. Merskey H, Bogduk N. Classification of chronic pain: descriptions of chronic pain syndromes and definitions of pain terms. Seattle: International Association for the Study of Pain; 1994.
26. Molloy DW, Guyatt GH, Russo R, Goeree R, O'Brien BJ, Bedard M, Willan A, Watson J, Patterson C, Harrison C, et al. Systematic implementation of an advance directive program in nursing homes—a randomized controlled trial. JAMA 2000;283:1437–44.
27. Moody HR. Why dignity in old age matters. In: Disch R, Dobrof R, Moody HR, editors. Dignity and old age. New York: Routledge; 1998.
28. Murray SA, Kendall M, Boyd K, Sheikh A. Illness trajectories and palliative care. BMJ 2005;330:1007–11.
29. Rosen M. Dignity—its history and meaning. London: Harvard University press; 2012.
30. Saunders C. Pain and impending death. Textbook of Pain. London: Churchill Livingstone; 1994.
31. Saunders C. 'The Last Frontier', autumn 1966. In: Selected writings 1958–2004. Oxford: Oxford University Press; 2006.
32. Seedhouse D, Gallagher A. Undignifying institutions. J Med Ethics 2002;28:368–72.
33. Tolstoy L. The death of Ivan Ilyich. New York: Melville House; 1886.
34. van Deijck RHPD, Krijnsen PJC, Hasselaar JGJ, Verhagen SCAH, Vissers KCP, Koopmans RTCM. The practice of continuous palliative sedation in elderly patients: A nationwide explorative study among Dutch nursing home physicians. J Am Geriatr Soc 2010;58:1671–8.
35. Wood AW. Immanuel Kant 1724–1804. In: Groundwork to metaphysics and moral. New Haven and London: Yale University Press; 2002.

CHAPTER 2

The Scope of Dementia: Variants, Symptoms, Stages, and Causes

Anne Corbett

The term "dementia" is used as an umbrella to describe a broad set of symptoms caused by neurodegeneration in the brain. Dementia is characterized by the progressive loss of neuronal function and brain volume, leading to gradual cognitive and functional impairment. Symptoms of dementia are dictated by the precise nature and cause of the underlying pathology and damage to the brain, resulting in an enormous range of symptoms, prognoses, and treatment needs. Broadly, however, dementia is characterized by the progressive and terminal loss of cognition and function, leading to complete loss of capacity and eventual death. While old age is closely associated with the condition, dementia is not a natural part of the aging process. It can be caused by over 100 different diseases and conditions which often dictate the type of symptoms a person will experience.

Dementia is a devastating condition that affects 35.6 million people worldwide. Recent systematic reviews of epidemiological studies have been important in providing a comprehensive world view of dementia. A World Health Organization (WHO) report estimated that dementia contributed 11.2% of years spent living with a disability in people over 60, more than stroke, cardiovascular disease, and cancer [95]. These prevalence numbers are expected to rise rapidly, reaching an estimated 65.7 million in 2030 and 115.4 million in 2050 as Western populations age and life expectancy lengthens in countries around the world. The most substantial growth is expected to occur in low- and middle-income countries. As a result, the cost of dementia worldwide is considerable. Care and treatment of people with the condition costs $604 billion a year worldwide [95]. The varied and complex needs of people with dementia place substantial pressure on health-care services in all countries. As the numbers of people affected continue to rise, dementia is becoming a serious public health concern, which affects all aspects of medical and care services. For example, in the United Kingdom 80% of older residents in long-term care such as nursing homes have a diagnosis or suspected diagnosis of dementia.

The most accurate estimation of prevalence and cost of dementia was achieved through the Alzheimer's Disease International reports carried out in 2009 and 2010, using exhaustive meta-analysis and evaluation of study quality to provide a comprehensive view of the global situation and to predict the growth in dementia worldwide over the next 40 years. Table 2-1 shows the key findings of this important work, highlighting the discrepancies in cost and prevalence between regions of the world and the potential implications of increased prevalence in low- and middle-income countries [4]. The quality of available data varies between different regions, so questions remain about whether differences in prevalence are real or reflections of different methods.

TABLE 2-1 Worldwide Epidemiology of Dementia

Region/Country	Estimated Point Prevalence of Dementia (%) (2010)	Number of People with Dementia in 2010 (Millions)	Predicted Number of People with Dementia in 2050 (Millions)	Estimated Cost of Dementia per Annum (Billions $US)
ASIA	3.9	15.94	60.92	123.67
Australasia	6.4	0.31	0.79	10.08
Asia Pacific	6.1	2.83	7.03	82.13
Oceania	4.0	0.02	0.10	0.10
Asia, Central	4.6	0.33	1.19	0.94
Asia, East	3.2	5.49	22.54	22.41
Asia, South	3.6	4.48	18.12	4.04
Asia, Southeast	4.8	2.48	11.13	3.97
EUROPE	6.2	9.95	18.65	238.64
Europe, Western	7.2	6.98	13.44	210.12
Europe, Central	4.7	1.10	2.10	14.19
Europe, East	4.8	1.87	3.10	14.33
THE AMERICAS	6.5	7.82	27.08	235.84
North America	6.9	4.38	11.01	213.04
Caribbean	6.5	0.33	1.04	2.98
Latin America, Andean	5.6	0.25	1.29	0.93
Latin America, Central	6.1	1.19	6.37	6.56
Latin America, Southern	7.0	0.61	1.83	5.07
Latin America, Tropical	5.5	1.05	5.54	7.26
AFRICA	2.6	1.86	8.74	5.84
North Africa/Middle East	3.7	1.15	6.19	4.50
Sub-Saharan Africa, Central	1.8	0.07	0.24	0.07
Sub-Saharan Africa, East	2.3	0.36	1.38	0.40
Sub-Saharan Africa, Southern	2.1	0.10	0.20	0.69
Sub-Saharan Africa, West	1.2	0.18	0.72	0.18
WORLD	4.7	35.56	115.38	603.99

In addition to this financial burden dementia exerts an enormous personal and emotional cost on the people affected, as well as their families. Caring for a person with dementia can be a distressing experience, and informal care, in which the families or close friends care for the person, accounts for a large proportion of people with dementia who live in the community. The impact on these informal carers is difficult to quantify, often affecting quality of life and well-being beyond the direct impact of the condition on the individual themselves.

SYMPTOMS AND PROGRESSION OF DEMENTIA

The symptoms experienced by a person with dementia are dictated by the area of the brain affected, and by the underlying cause of the condition. The broad functions of the brain and likely symptoms that would result if they were to be affected are shown in Fig 2-1.

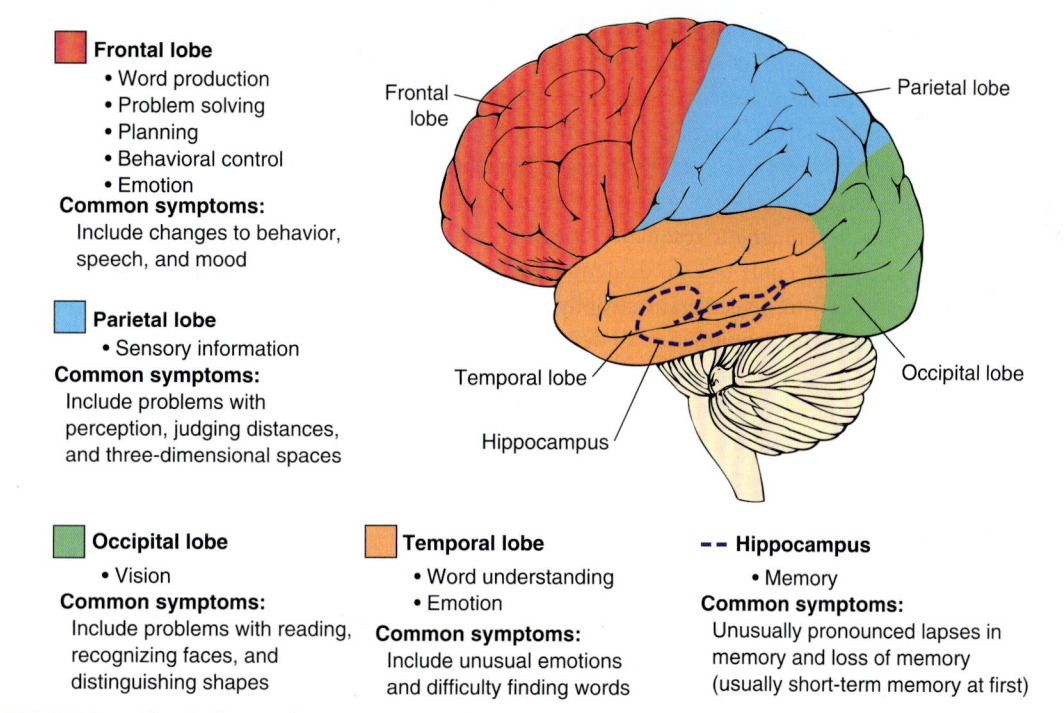

Frontal lobe
- Word production
- Problem solving
- Planning
- Behavioral control
- Emotion

Common symptoms:
Include changes to behavior, speech, and mood

Parietal lobe
- Sensory information

Common symptoms:
Include problems with perception, judging distances, and three-dimensional spaces

Occipital lobe
- Vision

Common symptoms:
Include problems with reading, recognizing faces, and distinguishing shapes

Temporal lobe
- Word understanding
- Emotion

Common symptoms:
Include unusual emotions and difficulty finding words

-- Hippocampus
- Memory

Common symptoms:
Unusually pronounced lapses in memory and loss of memory (usually short-term memory at first)

FIGURE 2-1 The challenge of concurrent pathology. One of the biggest challenges for biomarker research is the substantial overlap of major brain pathologies. For example,
- 90% of people with dementia with Lewy bodies have significant concurrent Alzheimer's disease (AD) pathology.
- Almost all patients with significant cerebrovascular disease also have substantial amyloid pathology, particularly in people over the age of 80.
- 40% of patients with AD have significant cerebrovascular disease.

Early symptoms of cognitive and functional impairment that occurs in dementia may include, but are not limited to, the following:

- Memory loss or uncharacteristic lapses in memory, particularly in short-term memory. While memory loss is very commonly associated with the early signs of dementia, particularly Alzheimer's disease (AD), this is not true for all patients, some of which show no memory dysfunction until much later in their condition.
- Difficulties in language and communication. Although a person was previously articulate, he or she may show a loss of vocabulary or difficulty in forming sentences.
- Changes to personality or behavior. This is particularly common in frontotemporal dementia (FTD) and may result in a misdiagnosis of depression.
- Difficulties in coordination and motor control. This symptom is often difficult to distinguish from Parkinson's disease, which can also be associated with a form of dementia.
- Difficulties with vision, for example, in the ability to read or recognize faces and shapes
- Difficulties in performing everyday activities that were previously easy to manage, such as household accounts or shopping

The breadth and scope of symptoms is often a critical obstacle to achieving a diagnosis, and dementia is commonly misdiagnosed and remain undetected over long periods. Diagnosis of dementia is achieved initially through psychological testing in combination with consultation with the individual and a close family member or friend to identify signs of impairment. Many assessment tools are available for clinicians to detect cognitive impairment, most of which focus on assessing memory, reasoning, and processing as measures of cognition. Where there is an indication of cognitive impairment a diagnosis will be gained through further in-depth psychological testing. Different neuropsychological tests are available, and are recommended for use in specific settings. Based on the outcome of these tests dementia is usually categorized as mild, moderate, or severe, although the distinction between these stages is frequently blurred. Currently available, recommended tests are summarized in Table 2-2. Diagnosis of dementia may involve neuroimaging in an attempt to discover the underlying cause of the dementia. The use of computed tomography (CT) or structural magnetic resonance imaging (MRI) is recommended to identify key pathologies that may contribute to dementia, such as a tumor, hydrocephalus, or cerebrovascular disease, and to detect brain atrophy [91]. Loss of brain volume in the medial temporal lobe is a particular signature of dementia, and studies indicate that this hallmark may be detected in people with mild cognitive impairment (MCI) before they develop dementia [8]. In some cases diagnosis may also be enhanced through the sampling of cerebrospinal fluid (CSF) through a lumbar puncture to detect specific peptide biomarkers of causative diseases [73]. An accurate dementia diagnosis allows the detection of potentially treatable disorders, facilitating planning of future life and finances, including advance directives, and optimal treatment and care.

Progression of symptoms will similarly be dictated by the progressive underlying pathology that is present in each case of dementia. Cognitive impairment frequently affects one cognitive or functional domain in the early stages, spreading to more pervasive impairment over time. The speed and pattern of decline is often indicative of the underlying cause. For example, AD usually progresses through a steady decline, while vascular dementia (VaD) is characterized by sudden decline in stepwise increments. Neuropsychological testing and neuroimaging is also used to monitor the progression of dementia. This is essential as it informs decision-making about treatment choice and judgments relating to an individuals' capacity, particularly in making decisions about their future care and treatment.

A common and distressing set of symptoms are behavioral and psychological symptoms of dementia (BPSD) such as agitation, aggression, psychosis (hallucinations and delusions), apathy, and depression. These symptoms are particularly frequent in people with frontotemporal dementia but will affect 90% of people with dementia at some point in their condition [24]. BPSD present a particular challenge for carers, and are often a trigger for people moving to a care home setting [34]. In addition to arising as a result of dementia pathologies, BPSD are frequently caused by underlying issues such as untreated pain and discomfort or environmental factors within the care setting. Early detection and management of BPSD is vital in order to address any causative factors and to inform treatment decisions.

TREATMENT OF DEMENTIA

Treatment of dementia relies on rapid clinical response following diagnosis and on effective communication with person and their families. Although there is no long-term effective treatment, early intervention provides the best opportunity to maximize a person's cognition in the earlier stages of the condition. This is particularly valuable as it enables people to plan their future treatment and care while they have the capacity, and to take an active role in decision-making. However, few pharmacological options are available for treatment for people with dementia. Four medications, rivastigmine, donepezil, galanthamine, and memantine, are currently licensed for treatment of the symptoms of AD, but currently no

TABLE 2-2 Available Cognitive Assessment Tools

Scale	Overview of Scale	Duration of Application (min)	Cutoff Point for Dementia	References
Abbreviated Mental Test Score (AMTS)	A 10-item scale validated in wards but used in UK primary care	<5	6–8/10	[44, 46]
Six-item Cognitive Impairment Test (6-CIT)	Three orientation items, count backward from 20, months of the year in reverse order, and learn an address. Validated in primary care	<5	8/24	[17, 20]
MiniCog	Three-item word memory and clock drawing. Validated in primary care. Low sensitivity	2–4	5/8	[14, 19]
GPCog	Developed for primary care and includes a carer's interview	5		[16]
Montreal Cognitive Assessment Scale (MoCA)	Tasks are executive function and attention, with some language, memory, and visuospatial skills. Validated in MCI in memory clinics and Parkinson's disease dementia	10	26/30	[27, 62, 83]
Addenbrooke's Cognitive Examination-III (ACE)	ACE-R is well-validated, longer test in secondary care and this test developed form it has similar characteristics	10–20	82–88/100	[26]
Mini Mental State Examination (MMSE)	This 11-item measure of cognitive functioning and its change is extensively studied and has good validity. Less good for Lewy body dementia and frontotemporal dementia due to its focus on memory. Cut point not valid in different cultures and, in particular highly educated or uneducated participants.	≤10	24/30	[32, 64, 87]
Hopkins Verbal Learning Test (HVLT)	HVLT assesses only verbal recall and recognition. It has six equivalent forms. It does not have ceiling effects and is not sensitive to educational levels.	<10	14/36	[15, 33, 48]
Test for the Early Detection of Dementia (TE4D cog)	An eight-item test with recall, clock drawing, category fluency, orientation to time and ideomotor praxis. Sensitive and specific and age, gender, and education independent but is not widely validated	4–6	35/45	[53]
Test Your Memory Test (TYM)	10-item test, self-administered but requires the doctor to be present. It includes orientation, copying, memory, calculation, verbal fluency, similarities, object naming, visuospatial, and executive function. Specific and sensitive for the diagnosis of AD in memory clinic patients with higher levels of education. Not widely validated	10	45/50	[18, 39]
Consortium to Establish a Registry for Alzheimer's Disease (CERAD) Neuropsychological Test Battery	Verbal fluency (animal naming), Boston naming (15 items), mini mental state examination (serial sevens omitted), word list learning, constructional praxis, word list recall, word list recognition (10 original words, 10 foils), constructional praxis recall	>40	77/100	[31]

licensed drugs are available for other types of dementia. People with dementia frequently have diagnoses of comorbidities such as cardiovascular disease, cancer, and infections. Therefore, the potential cognitive impact of concomitant medications should be considered. Nonpharmacological treatments such as cognitive training, stimulation, and rehabilitation may be helpful in reducing cognitive decline [96].

A particular treatment challenge for clinicians is the management of BPSD. In the absence of effective alternatives, these symptoms have frequently been treated with antipsychotic medications despite the very limited license available for this practice. Evidence to support the use of the antipsychotic risperidone for short-time periods up to 6 weeks is available, but very little benefit is seen with other antipsychotics or with long-term prescriptions [7]. Furthermore, antipsychotics are associated with considerable severe side effects, which include worsening of cognitive decline, falls, sedation, stroke, and increased mortality. Following numerous initiatives to reduce antipsychotics in people with dementia there has been a substantial drop in their use. However, a culture of antipsychotic prescribing continues to exist despite guidance for their judicious use. This issue is exacerbated by the lack of effective pharmacological treatments. However, a growing body of evidence supports the use of nondrug psychosocial approaches to prevent and manage BPSD [24]. The most promising of these are embedded within the principles of person-centered care, the gold standard for dementia care which promoted a personalized, tailored approach to care. Studies have shown that simple structured approaches to provide personalized activities and social interaction can improve BPSD such as agitation and aggression [86]. These approaches are key elements in best practice for dementia care, although a lack of standardized training for health-care professionals is a barrier to their implementation.

CAUSES OF DEMENTIA

Over 100 conditions and diseases that can cause dementia through neurodegeneration exist. The majority affect older adults and relate to the development of specific pathologies in the brain, although rarer causes can occur in younger individuals as a result of specific events or lifestyle factors, for example, as a result of a brain injury or excessive alcohol consumption. In addition to the numerous established causes there is evidence of general risk factors for dementia which increase the likelihood of dementia later in life when considered on a population basis. These include midlife hypertension and hypercholesterolemia, diabetes, obesity, and stroke [8]. This evidence supports the view that from a public health perspective prevention of dementia could be achieved through management of risk factors in order to reduce the risk of development of underlying diseases and conditions that lead to dementia. The various causes of dementia are complicated by the considerable overlap in underlying pathologies, which result in a blurring of boundaries between different types. The most common causes of dementia are discussed in detail in the subsequent sections.

ALZHEIMER'S DISEASE

AD is the primary cause of dementia worldwide, affecting up to 80% of people with the condition [4]. AD is most common in people with dementia over 65 (late-onset AD), although AD can develop during midlife (early-onset AD), usually due to rare genetic factors. Cognitive decline in AD usually follows a steady trajectory, frequently commencing with impairment in memory as AD commonly develops in the hippocampus.

Pathology

The two core pathological hallmarks are amyloid plaques and neurofibrillary tangles that develop in the brain of a person with AD. This accumulation of proteins is central to the "amyloid cascade hypothesis," in which amyloid-β peptides are thought to trigger neuronal dysfunction [61]. This in turn is thought to influence the processing of the tau protein, resulting in intracellular "tangles" that contribute to cell death. The sequence of pathological events and causal relationship of AD pathology remains unclear, and the precise relationship between amyloid-β and tau has not been established [82]. More recent evidence challenging the established hypothesis and suggesting that amyloid pathology is the result, rather than the cause, of dysfunction [11].

Genetic Risk Factors

A number of genes have been identified as playing a role in the development and risk of AD. These include dominant mutations of the genes encoding amyloid precursor protein (*APP*) and presenilins (*PSEN1* and *PSEN2*) [35, 49, 79]. These genes account for only 5% of people with AD, and result in early-onset AD. These genes hold significant risk for AD, and usually manifest in a clear hereditary link.

In late-onset AD the genetic causes are less clear-cut. There are several risk genes, including *ApoE4*, which confers a sevenfold increased risk, although this translates to only a very small overall increased risk, particularly when viewed from a population perspective [25]. More recently, research has identified additional genes such as *TOMM40*, *CLU*, and *PICALM*, but large cohort studies are needed to confirm their role [42, 78, 81]. The gene *SORL1* has been highlighted as an important genetic cause of late-onset AD, and at least one further familial AD gene has not yet been identified [12, 74].

These late-onset genes do not significantly assist in predicting AD risk, but perhaps have more important roles in indicating the pathways involved and in identifying potential drug target [68]. Most of the confirmed risk genes act within the amyloid processing pathway. With the exception of *APOE*, most of the best candidate genes confer a very small relative risk of 1.2–1.5 [3]. Mutations in genes related to tau also result in dementias, but do not play a role in AD [72].

Diagnosis

Currently the most accurate way to diagnose AD is postmortem, through detection of pathology through immunohistochemical analysis of tissue samples. At best, clinical diagnosis can provide a probable diagnosis of AD. In addition to the standard neuropsychological testing, published diagnostic criteria are available for specifically detecting AD, such as those developed in 1984 by the National Institute of Neurological and Communicative Disorders and Stroke and the Alzheimer's Disease and Related Disorders Association (NINCDS-ARDA) [57]. The NINCDS-ARDA criteria have over 80% sensitivity and specificity for distinguishing people with AD from those without dementia, although differentiating between AD and other dementias is less accurate (23–88% specificity) [10]. The accuracy can be increased through clinical judgment and medical examination to rule out other underlying conditions.

> **Biomarkers**
> 1. A panel of CSF biomarkers to be used in combination to provide an Alzheimer's disease (AD) profile, for example, $A\beta_{1-42}$, total tau and phosphorylated tau with novel markers. Potential additional candidates include $A\beta_{1-38}$, inflammatory and oxidative stress markers [60, 61]
> 2. Studies into blood biomarkers have been inconsistent, but the most promising include complement factor H, A2M, and clusterin [49, 63]
> 3. Researchers have postulated that early changes in $A\beta$ occur before onset of dementia symptoms, supporting new work to identify suitable biomarkers and models for testing in older adults.
>
> **Neuroimaging**
> 1. Functional neuroimaging shows promise in differentiating dementia types, particularly *Single-Photon Emission Computed Tomography* (SPECT). Progress has been made in the use of ^{99m}Tc-HMPAO SPECT to distinguish AD from frontotemporal dementia (FTD) and FP-CIT (123I-N-3-fluoropropyl-2beta-carbomethoxy-3beta-4-iodophenyl tropane) (DAT scan) to differentiate DLB and PAD from AD [71].
> 2. Positron emission tomography (PET) enhanced through use of amyloid-β ligands to visualize amyloid pathology. This technique has shown high levels of accuracy in predicting conversion to AD [75].

FIGURE 2-2 Promising diagnostic approaches currently in development.

A diagnosis of AD may also be strengthened through neuroimaging, of which the most commonly used and most accurate technique is Positron Emission Tomography (PET). PET is used to distinguish AD from other dementias, including early stage AD, through detection of reduced glucose metabolism in the brain [67]. Promising new neuroimaging techniques are currently undergoing testing in large clinical cohorts, including PET markers for AD pathology such as amyloid-β, and structural methods including volumetric calculation, measurement of cortical thickness, and three-dimensional brain mapping [70, 80, 89].

Both amyloid-β and tau are detectable as markers of AD in CSF and may be used in diagnosing AD. Analysis of CSF can be used to differentiate AD from other dementias, with a hallmark profile of reduced $A\beta_{1-42}$ and higher levels of total tau or hyperphosphorylated tau [41, 54]. However, sampling of CSF is considered to be controversial in many countries due to its perceived risk and the discomfort associated with the procedure.

Diagnosis of AD therefore relies on a combination of different assessment methods, and a clear guidance on specific diagnostic criteria is needed. There is a large body of research currently ongoing to refine novel combinations of neuropsychological tests, neuroimaging, and biomarkers for AD, described in more detail in Fig. 2-2. In 2012 new diagnostic criteria for use in research were published with the aim of identifying people in different stages of AD, particularly for recruitment in clinical trials [28]. This is the first-time biomarkers have been included as part of operationalized clinical criteria for AD. The key items in the DuBois criteria are summarized in Fig. 2-3. Ongoing research will inform future decisions for guidance on diagnosis in clinical practice.

Treatment

Four pharmacological agents are available for the treatment of symptoms of AD. Three acetylcholinesterase inhibitors (AChEI), donepezil, rivastigmine, and galanthamine, are licensed for mild to moderate AD. These drugs enhance the levels of acetylcholine in the brain in order to protect cognitive pathways. Memantine, which is licensed for use in moderate to severe AD, acts to block NMDA receptors in the brain and prevents neuronal excitotoxicity, which is a hallmark of AD. While these medications provide some improvement in cognition, their efficacy is limited. Clinical trial data shows a modest benefit to cognition for 6–12 months with AChEI or memantine, and some improvement in mood and function

Item A: Core diagnostic criteria
Presence of an early and significant episodic memory impairment that includes the following features:
1. Gradual and progressive change in memory function reported by patients or informants over more than 6 months
2. Objective evidence of significantly impaired episodic memory on testing: this generally consists of recall deficit that does not improve significantly or does not normalize with cueing or recognition testing and after effective encoding of information has been previously controlled
3. The episodic memory impairment can be isolated or associated with other cognitive changes at the onset of AD or as AD advances

Item B: Presence of medial temporal lobe atrophy
1. Volume loss of hippocampus/entorhinal cortex/amygdala evidenced on MRI with qualitative ratings using visual scoring (referenced to well-characterized population with age norms)
Or
2. Quantitative volumetry of regions of interest (referenced to well-characterized population with age norms)

Item C: Abnormal cerebrospinal fluid biomarker
1. Low amyloid β_{1-42} concentrations, increased total tau concentrations, or increased phospho–tau concentrations, or combinations of the three
Or
2. Other well-validated markers to be discovered in the future

Item D: Specific pattern on functional neuroimaging with PET
1. Reduced glucose metabolism in bilateral temporal parietal regions
Or
2. Change in other well-validated ligands, for example, Pittsburg compound B or FDDNP

Item E: Proven AD autosomal-dominant mutation within the immediate family

FIGURE 2-3 DuBois diagnostic criteria for Alzheimer's disease (AD) in research. Probable AD is present where an individual fulfills the criteria in item A, plus one or more supportive features from criteria in items B, C, D, or E.

of people with AD treated with AChEI [13, 51, 58, 93]. All of the current licensed treatments target the symptoms, rather than the underlying disease, in AD.

A number of novel disease-modifying drugs have been developed but are still in clinical trials. Most of these have focused on the amyloid cascade, including a number of immunotherapies designed to promote amyloid clearance. Despite promising indications in animal studies, early immunotherapies were disappointing, showing little impact on cognition and with some associated with severe side effects and encephalitis [38]. Following evidence of potential efficacy earlier in AD, modified immunotherapies with better safety profiles have now entered trials in people with early AD, and the findings are eagerly awaited. Other potential avenues for novel AD drugs include agents to selectively inhibit amyloid processing enzymes, prevent tau phosphorylation, for example, through glycogen synthase-kinase 3β inhibition, and target specific transcriptional factors involved in AD [85, 94]. However, most of these compounds are still in very preliminary testing.

A promising and complementary approach to drug development for AD is drug repositioning, a process involving the identification of existing treatments that could be repurposed for use in AD. A number of candidate drugs have been identified, including antibiotics, antihypertensives, and retinoids, which already have safety data and evidence to support a potential mechanism for treating AD [23]. A number of treatments entered phase III clinical trials in 2014, highlighting the value of this approach in accelerating drug discovery for AD.

VASCULAR DEMENTIA

VaD is the second most common cause of dementia affecting approximately 20% of people, and accounting for over 7 million people with dementia worldwide. The condition affects up to 4 of every 100 individuals over 65, and up to 16 of every 100 people over 80 [76]. VaD commonly arises in people with preexisting cardiovascular or cerebrovascular conditions as they are closely linked. As such, VaD is a highly heterogeneous condition. Carers of individuals with VaD are known to experience a greater caregiver burden compared to those caring for people with AD [5, 88], and this is in part due to the lack of treatment options available for this type of dementia.

Pathology

The most common types of VaD are infarct dementia and subcortical ischemic VaD (SIVD). Infarct dementia can result from single large strokes, smaller infarcts in strategically important brain areas and multiple infarcts. SIVD involves extensive damage to the subcortical microvasculature, most commonly as a result of untreated or undertreated hypertension. Importantly, VaD pathology is extremely common in people with AD, and may sometimes be referred to as mixed dementia, emphasizing the impact of cerebrovascular pathologies in dementia as a whole [84].

Risk Factors

The most important risk factors for VaD relate to cardiovascular and cerebrovascular health. Clear evidence exists for the role of hypertension, diabetes, and obesity as critical risk factors for VaD, and this is supported by a number of epidemiological studies in large populations. Stroke is a key factor, with 25% of people developing dementia within 1 year of having a first stroke [8]. Interestingly, no clear evidence is available to prove that elevated cholesterol is a risk factor [6]. Lifestyle factors, most importantly smoking, play a critical role in the risk of VaD. There is also considerable ethnic variation in the prevalence of VaD, with a higher-than-usual proportion of people with Indian, Bengali, Pakistani, Sri Lankan, and African-Caribbean background developing the condition. This is thought to be linked to the considerable level of vascular risk factors present in these communities.

Many underlying risks for VaD indicate the potential for prevention of the condition, particularly since they relate to cardiovascular health and weight. In addition to heart disease, stroke, diabetes, and cancer, public health messaging for healthy living, particularly in midlife, is also directly applicable to reducing risk of dementia. The best evidence for prevention of VaD is through exercise.

Diagnosis

Diagnosis of VaD relies on a physician observing the pattern of cognitive decline in an individual. Cognitive decline usually commences following a stroke or transient ischaemic attack. Cognition commonly remains stable for long periods in people with VaD, followed by a sudden worsening of symptoms and a rapid drop in cognitive function as a result of subsequent cerebrovascular events. Importantly, individuals with VaD often experience extensive medical comorbidity, with physical disability commonly compounding the impact of their cognitive impairment. These factors must be taken into account when diagnosing VaD, emphasizing the importance of a full medical history and review in cases of suspected dementia. In order to confirm a diagnosis of VaD neuroimaging techniques may be used. MRI scanning is used to detect lesions and vascular pathology in the brain, and this may be supported by the use of SPECT, which can detect specific alterations in blood flow indicative of VaD. The specific criteria for diagnosing VaD through neuroimaging vary considerably, with the strictest guidance laid out by the NINDS/AIREN criteria (National Institute of Neurological Disorders and Stroke and the Association Internationale pour la Recherche et l'Enseignement Neurosciences) [77]. According to these guidelines, probable VaD is indicated by multiple infarcts or strategic single infarcts as well as multiple subcortical or white matter lesions. Importantly, if no cerebrovascular lesions are detected by CT or MRI the diagnosis can only be probable and not certain VaD. These techniques, in combination with neuropsychological assessment, are increasingly used to monitor the progression of VaD pathology over time.

Treatment

VaD represents a major source of frustration and distress for clinicians, carers, and patients alike due to the massive impact, high prevalence, and lack of effective treatment options. Currently no licensed treatments for VaD are available. Although research has raised a number of potential candidates, there are no drugs with clear evidence of benefit. AChEI have shown some benefits to cognition in people with VaD, but this does not extend to improvements in function, and the benefit is not large enough to support a license [47]. The findings of some small studies indicate that people with established mixed dementia respond better to this treatment than those with VaD alone, although this distinction is difficult to make [30]. Other potential treatments such as memantine, oxypentofylline, and cerebrolysin have shown little or no benefit.

The most promising treatment trials of VaD relate to the management of cardiovascular factors through established pharmacological routes. Treatment with aspirin, which is routinely used as a preventative treatment for stroke and cardiovascular disease, has shown benefit to cognition [60]. The antihypertensive calcium channel blockers have also shown some modest benefit, which is most promising in people with SIVD [65]. There is also some initial evidence supporting the value of risk factor management in order to prevent both VaD and AD, although trials are very limited. Even in the absence of direct evidence to support it, management of vascular risk factors plays a key role in treatment of VaD in practice, and many people with VaD receive regular prescriptions of antihypertensives, statins, or aspirin.

PARKINSON'S DISEASE DEMENTIA AND LEWY BODY DEMENTIA

The third most common cause of dementia is Parkinson's Disease Dementia (PDD) and Lewy Body Dementia (LBD), which affect 3% and 15–20% of people with dementia respectively. PDD develops in most of the people with Parkinson's disease. Both are associated with a specific synuclein pathology and distinct pattern of symptoms.

Pathology

Both LBD and PDD are characterized by the presence of Lewy bodies and Lewy neurites in the brain. These are distinct aggregates of ubiquitin and other misfolded proteins that combine with the α-synuclein protein and lead to neuronal death [50]. This synucleinopathy is particularly found in discrete areas of the brain stem, diencephalon, basal ganglia, and neocortex, leading to loss of neurons that commences in the medulla and gradually progresses to affect cholinergic cells [90]. The pattern of progressive neurodegeneration is similar in nature to AD. Indeed, in LBD in particular, AD pathology may also develop, including accumulation of both amyloid and tau [2, 45].

Genetic Risk Factors

Risk factors associated with LBD and PDD are unclear. Two main groups of genes have been highlighted by genetic studies, which report considerable overlap with genes linked to AD and PD. These include mutations in the glucocerebrosidase gene (*GBA*), gene which is associated with PD, which appear to specifically increase the risk of LBD. In addition, the AD risk gene *ApoE4* is overrepresented in people with LBD, indicating its importance as a risk factor [59].

Diagnosis

In addition to symptoms of progressive cognitive decline, people with LBD and PDD are more likely to experience symptoms related to vision, motor control, and attention, including visual hallucinations and parkinsonism. In addition, these individuals often show fluctuating levels of cognition, particularly attention [9]. These specific symptoms reflect the underlying pathology of the conditions. LBD and PDD are distinguished by the sequence of symptom development. In LBD, parkinsonism arises concurrently with or after dementia, while in PDD develops after the onset of Parkinson's disease [56].

The diagnosis of PDD is usually straight forward and aligns with ongoing monitoring of PD. Specific tools for detecting cognitive decline in PD do exist, although they are primarily used in research and not practice. LBD is also usually fairly simple to diagnose through the detection of the hallmark symptoms by neuropsychological testing. However, diagnosis may be complicated in small groups of people with the condition, for example, in those who do not develop parkinsonism. Confirmation of a LBD diagnosis is therefore often achieved through neuroimaging to detect LBD pathology. SPECT or PET using a validated marker, FP-CIT, is recommended to differentiate LBD and PDD from AD, and this technique is now included as part of the diagnostic criteria for LBD [55, 56]. Other markers and diagnostic methods such as measurement of medial temporal atrophy by MRI, amyloid binding by PET, or levels of amyloid and tau in CSF are less useful in diagnosing LBD and PDD due to the similarity with AD [1]. Despite the characteristic symptomatology, LBD is commonly misdiagnosed due to a lack of understanding and familiarity in physicians.

Treatment

Currently only one licensed therapy for PDD exists, the cholinesterase inhibitor rivastigmine, which has been shown to improve cognition and overall clinical outcome in this group. People with PDD also usually receive the Parkinson's therapy, levodopa, to address their motor symptoms. No licensed treatments for LBD are available [75], although initial evidence shows that AChEI may be effective. The use of levodopa is rarely beneficial in LBD and is associated with worsening of behavioral and psychological symptoms such as psychosis [36].

A small number of drugs are proposed as candidate treatments for LBD and PDD, including memantine and atomexatine, which have initial supporting evidence. Very few disease-modifying drugs are available in the pipeline, although initial studies have suggested the potential value of targeting mitochondrial dysfunction, immunotherapies, and treatment to target pathological processes through heavy metal chelators and enzyme inhibition. Many of the proposed strategies are similar to those currently under investigation in AD, although they are in very preliminary stages for LBD and PDD.

Antipsychotics are particularly contraindicated for people with LBD due to established sensitivity in these individuals leading to a higher risk of physical and cognitive decline and increased mortality [43].

FRONTOTEMPORAL DEMENTIA

Also known as Pick's disease, FTD is a term for a fairly rare group of dementias that specifically affect the frontal and temporal lobes in the brain. FTD can arise in people as young as 30, and the three specific types of FTD are determined by the symptoms experienced by the person.

Pathology

FTD is characterized by accumulation of three key proteins within neurons in the frontal and temporal lobes. The most common pathologies involve phosphorylated tau or a DNA-binding protein TDP-43, with fewer cases involving the "fused in sarcoma" (FUS) protein. Pathology is specific to this area of the brain until much later in the condition, when it progresses to include more general neurodegeneration [63].

Genetic Risk Factors

A strong genetic link for FTD is seen, and this is often reflected in a person's family history. Up to 20% of people with FTD carry a known risk gene. Most people with a clear hereditary link to the condition have detectable mutations in genes that code for tau-related protein MAPT or progranulin protein GRN, both of which are disrupted and play a role in the development of pathology [52].

Diagnosis

The defining symptoms of FTD are changes in behavior, language, and semantic memory as a result of the pathology in the frontal and temporal lobes. As FTD progresses common dementia-related symptoms begin to develop, such as memory impairment, parkinsonism, and BPSD. The early detection of FTD is therefore critical in order to distinguish it from other causes. Identification of the hallmark symptoms is central to the diagnosis of FTD. Although FTD is of three distinct types, considerable overlap in symptoms are noted, leading to a blurring in diagnosis and often leading to a general diagnosis of FTD rather than a specific diagnosis of the subtype. These subtypes are as follows:

- Behavioral variant frontotemporal dementia (bvFTD)—characterized by behavioral changes, affecting half of people with FTD

- Progressive nonfluent aphasia—language decline characterized by impaired speech
- Progressive aphasia with semantic dementia—language decline characterized by impaired word comprehension and semantic memory (memory for meaning) [71]

BvFTD is primarily diagnosed by clinical assessment through identification of the hallmark symptoms of FTD which distinguish the condition from AD. These include apathy, unusual social conduct, and changes in eating habits in the notable absence of memory impairment or changes in visuospatial ability [71]. A diagnosis may be strengthened through neuroimaging to detect hallmarks specific to FTD. MRI may be used to detect the selective pattern of brain atrophy, although this is often not detectable in the early stages. A more accurate technique is to use fluorodeoxyglucose-PET imaging to specifically detect hypometabolism in the frontal, cingulate, and temporal regions of the brain [69].

Progressive aphasias are distinguishable from BvFTD and other dementias through the development of specific language deficit prior to any other cognitive impairment. Neuropsychological assessments are used to detect difficulty in naming objects, producing words and understanding words, in the absence of any other impact on cognition or activities of daily living [37]. Fluent and nonfluent forms of this type of dementia are identified through a detailed assessment of the person's speech by a specialist. Neuroimaging through MRI and PET to confirm the specific patterns of atrophy or dysfunction can also be used to strengthen the outcomes of a clinical assessment [22].

Treatment

No pharmacological treatments are licensed for use in FTD. Trials of AChEI have not shown any significant benefit, and it is generally accepted that side effects associated with other proposed drugs such as memantine and lithium, outweigh the minimal and inconsistent effect they might confer. Serotonin selective reuptake inhibitors may be effective in the treatment of certain symptoms including eating disorders, disinhibition, and impulsivity, and studies have shown that trazodone may provide benefit in agitation and aggression [92]. However, these findings await further validation. Current best practice to treatment of FTD is to adopt a person-centered approach to nondrug interventions to address symptoms and support the person in maintaining independence through their condition. This includes the use of psychological therapies and social interaction to manage behavioral symptoms, speech therapy, exercise, and physical therapy [69]. Caring for a person with FTD is particularly challenging, and so is to ensure the caregiver also receives support and psychological therapy where appropriate to enable them to cope with their caring role.

DOWN'S SYNDROME DEMENTIA

Down's syndrome (DS) affects 5.8 million people worldwide [21]. Dementia is highly prevalent in people with DS, representing the most common form of dementia in people under 50. This form of dementia is not well understood, and diagnosis is often complicated by the underlying learning disability.

Pathology

Significant AD-like pathology, including extensive accumulation of amyloid peptides and hyperphosphorylated tau, develops in all people with DS by the age of 40 [29]. This is driven by the trisomy of chromosome 21 in people with DS, which results in triplicate copies of AD-risk genes including *ApoE4* [66]. However, key differences present between this form of dementia and AD. People with DS show overproduction of amyloid pathology throughout their lives as opposed to its emergence later in life, and this is compounded by altered expression of several genes, many of which are not associated with AD [40].

Risk Factors

DS is a key risk factor for dementia in its own right. People with the condition share heightened genetic risk factors with AD, most importantly the triplicate copies of genes located on chromosome 21.

Diagnosis

Cognitive impairment is a core symptom of DS. It can therefore be challenging to detect cognitive decline despite its inclusion as a core element of DS prognosis. The use of standard neuropsychological tests such as the Mini Mental State Examination (MMSE) is not appropriate for this patient group, and this has led to the development of specific scales for use in DS. The Down syndrome Attention, Memory, and Executive function Scales (DAMES) was developed for use in clinical trials in dementia in DS to enable researchers to detect changes in cognition over time [40]. Dementia in DS is not frequently diagnosed. However, with the growing life expectancy of people with the condition, it will become more important for clinicians to consider dementia in people with DS as they grow older.

Treatment

No pharmacological treatments are available for dementia in DS. Several AD treatments have been proposed due to the similarity in underlying pathology. However, large-trial memantine showed no improvement in symptoms, highlighting the caution that must be taken when inferring benefit of treatment across different dementias [40]. The complex, unique pattern of amyloid and tau pathology seen in DS dementia alters the treatment response, emphasizing the need for clinical trials specifically in this group of individuals.

SUMMARY

- Over 100 causes of dementia, of which the most common is Alzheimer's disease, are present.
- Diagnosis of dementia and the underlying cause should be achieved through a combination of neuropsychological testing, neuroimaging, and biomarker analysis where possible.
- No licensed treatments for any forms of dementia apart from Alzheimer's disease (rivastigmine, donepezil, galanthamine, memantine) are available. However, consideration of underlying pathology and comorbidity may highlight treatments that will confer benefit. For example, an individual with vascular dementia may benefit from treatment with licensed cardiovascular medications.
- Antipsychotics should be used for up to 12 weeks only in cases of severe, intractable symptoms that have not responded to alternative approaches. Monitoring of

prescriptions is essential. These drugs should not be prescribed to people with LBD due to heightened sensitivity.
- Involve family carers in diagnosis and treatment decisions.

REFERENCES

1. Aarsland D, Andersen K, Larsen JP, Lolk A, Kragh-Sorensen P. Prevalence and characteristics of dementia in Parkinson disease: an 8-year prospective study. Arch Neurol 2003;60:387–92.
2. Aarsland D, Ballard C, Rongve A, Broadstock M, Svenningsson P. Clinical trials of dementia with Lewy bodies and Parkinson's disease dementia. Curr Neurol Neurosci Rep 2012;12:492–501.
3. Alzforum. Alzgene—field synopsis of genetic association studies in AD, Vol. 2014. Cambridge, MA: Alzforum; 2011.a
4. Alzheimer's Disease International. World Alzheimer Report, Vol. 2013. 2009. Accessed at http://www.alz.co.uk/research/files/WorldAlzheimerReport.pdf
5. Annerstedt L, Elmstahl S, Ingvad B, Samuelsson SM. Family caregiving in dementia—an analysis of the caregiver's burden and the "breaking-point" when home care becomes inadequate. Scand J Public Health 2000;28:23–31.
6. Anstey KJ, Lipnicki DM, Low LF. Cholesterol as a risk factor for dementia and cognitive decline: a systematic review of prospective studies with meta-analysis. Am J Geriatr Psychiatry 2008;16:343–54.
7. Ballard C, Creese B, Corbett A, Aarsland D. Atypical antipsychotics for the treatment of behavioral and psychological symptoms in dementia, with a particular focus on longer term outcomes and mortality. Exp Opin Drug Saf 2011;10:35–43.
8. Ballard C, Gauthier S, Corbett A, Brayne C, Aarsland D, Jones E. Alzheimer's disease. Lancet 2011;377:1019–31.
9. Ballard C, Kahn Z, Corbett A. Treatment of dementia with Lewy bodies and Parkinson's disease dementia. Drugs Aging 2011;28:769–77.
10. Ballard CG, Bannister C. Criteria in the diagnosis of dementia. In: O'Brein J, Burns A, Ames D, editors. Dementia, Vol. 3. London: Hodder; 2005.
11. Bandiera T, Lansen J, Post C, Varasi M. Inhibitors of Ab peptide aggregation as potential anti-Alzheimer agents. In: Atta-ur-Rahman, editor. Current Medicinal Chemistry, Vol. 4. Hilversum, Netherlands: Bentham Science; 1997.
12. Bertram L, Blacker D, Mullin K, Keeney D, Jones J, Basu S, Yhu S, McInnis MG, Go RC, Vekrellis K, et al. Evidence for genetic linkage of Alzheimer's disease to chromosome 10q. Science 2000;290:2302–3.
13. Birks J, Grimley Evans J, Iakovidou V, Tsolaki M, Holt FE. Rivastigmine for Alzheimer's disease. Cochrane Database Syst Rev 2009;2:CD001191.
14. Borson S, Scanlan JM, Watanabe J, Tu SP, Lessig M. Simplifying detection of cognitive impairment: comparison of the Mini-Cog and Mini-Mental State Examination in a multiethnic sample. J Am Geriatr Soc 2005;53(5):871–4.
15. Brandt J. The Hopkins Verbal Learning Test: Development of a new memory test with six equivalent forms. Clin Neuropsychol 1991;5(2):125–42.
16. Brodaty H, Pond D, Kemp NM, Luscombe G, Harding L, Berman K, Huppert FA. The GPCOG: a new screening test for dementia designed for general practice. J Am Geriatr Soc 2002;50(3):530–4.
17. Brooke P, Bullock R. Validation of a 6 item cognitive impairment test with a view to primary care usage. Int J Geriatr Psychiatry 1999;14(11):936–40.
18. Brown J, Pengas G, Dawson K, Brown LA, Clatworthy P. Self administered cognitive screening test (TYM) for detection of Alzheimer's disease: cross sectional study. BMJ. 2009 Jun 10;338:b2030.
19. Buschke H, Kuslansky G, Katz M, Stewart WF, Sliwinski MJ, Eckholdt HM, Lipton RB. Screening for dementia with the memory impairment screen. Neurology 1999;52(2):231–8.
20. Callahan CM, Unverzagt FW, Hui SL, Perkins AJ, Hendrie HC. Six-item screener to identify cognitive impairment among potential subjects for clinical research. Med Care 2002;40(9):771–81.
21. CDC. Improved National Prevalence Estimates for 18 Selected Major Birth Defects, United States, 1999–2001. Morb Mortal Wkly Rep 2006;54:1301–5.
22. Chare L, Hodges JR, Leyton CE, McGinley C, Tan RH, Kril JJ, Halliday GM. New criteria for frontotemporal dementia syndromes: clinical and pathological diagnostic implications. J Neurol Neurosurg Psychiatry 2014;85:865–70.
23. Corbett A, Pickett J, Burns A, Corcoran J, Dunnett SB, Edison P, Hagan JJ, Holmes C, Jones E, Katona C, et al. Drug repositioning for Alzheimer's disease. Nat Rev Drug Discov 2012;11:833–46.

24. Corbett A, Smith J, Creese B, Ballard C. Treatment of behavioral and psychological symptoms of Alzheimer's disease. Curr Treat Options Neurol 2012;14:113–25.
25. Corder EH, Saunders AM, Strittmatter WJ, Schmechel DE, Gaskell PC, Small GW, Roses AD, Haines JL, Pericak-Vance MA. Gene dose of apolipoprotein E type 4 allele and the risk of Alzheimer's disease in late onset families. Science 1993;261:921–3.
26. Crawford S, Whitnall L, Robertson J, Evans JJ. A systematic review of the accuracy and clinical utility of the Addenbrooke's cognitive examination and the Addenbrooke's cognitive examination—revised in the diagnosis of dementia. Int J Geriatr Psychiatry 2012;27(7):659–69.
27. Dalrymple-Alford JC, MacAskill MR, Nakas CT, Livingston L, Graham C, Crucian GP, Melzer TR, Kirwan J, Keenan R, Wells S, et al. The MoCA well-suited screen for cognitive impairment in Parkinson disease. Neurology 2010;75(19):1717–25.
28. Dubois B, Gauthier S, Cummings J. The utility of the new research diagnostic criteria for Alzheimer's disease. Int Psychogeriatr 2013;25:175–7.
29. Epstein CJ. Down's syndrome: critical genes in a critical region. Nature 2006;441:582–3.
30. Erkinjuntti T, Kurz A, Gauthier S, Bullock R, Lilienfeld S, Damaraju CV. Efficacy of galantamine in probable vascular dementia and Alzheimer's disease combined with cerebrovascular disease: a randomised trial. Lancet 2002;359:1283–90.
31. Fillenbaum GG, van Belle G, Morris JC, Mohs RC, Mirra SS, Davis PC, Tariot PN, Silverman JM, Clark CM, Welsh-Bohmer KA, et al. Consortium to Establish a Registry for Alzheimer's Disease (CERAD): the first twenty years. Alzheimer's Dement 2008;4(2):96–109.
32. Folstein MF, Folstein SE, McHugh PR. "Mini-mental state": a practical method for grading the cognitive state of patients for the clinician. J Psychiatr Res 1975;12(3):189–98.
33. Frank RM, Byrne GJ. The clinical utility of the Hopkins Verbal Learning Test as a screening test for mild dementia. Int J Geriatr Psychiatry 2000;15(4):317–24.
34. Gaugler JE, Yu F, Krichbaum K, Wyman JF. Predictors of nursing home admission for persons with dementia. Med Care 2009;47:191–8.
35. Goate A, Chartier-Harlin MC, Mullan M, Brown J, Crawford F, Fidani L, Giuffra L, Haynes A, Irving N, James L, et al. Segregation of a missense mutation in the amyloid precursor protein gene with familial Alzheimer's disease. Nature 1991;349:704–6.
36. Goldman JG, Goetz CG, Brandabur M, Sanfilippo M, Stebbins GT. Effects of dopaminergic medications on psychosis and motor function in dementia with Lewy bodies. Mov Disord 2008;23(15):2248–50.
37. Gorno-Tempini ML, Hillis AE, Weintraub S, Kertesz A, Mendez M, Cappa SF, Ogar JM, Rohrer JD, Black S, Boeve BF, et al. Classification of primary progressive aphasia and its variants. Neurology 2011;76:1006–14.
38. Gupta VB, Gupta VK, Martins R. Semagacestat for treatment of Alzheimer's disease. N Engl J Med 2013;369:1660–1.
39. Hancock P, Larner AJ. Test Your Memory test: diagnostic utility in a memory clinic population. Int J Geriatr Psychiatry 2011;26(9):976–80.
40. Hanney M, Prasher V, Williams N, Jones EL, Aarsland D, Corbett A, Lawrence D, Yu LM, Tyrer S, Francis PT, et al. Memantine for dementia in adults older than 40 years with Down's syndrome (MEADOWS): a randomised, double-blind, placebo-controlled trial. Lancet 2012;379:528–36.
41. Hansson O, Zetterberg H, Buchhave P, Londos E, Blennow K, Minthon L. Association between CSF biomarkers and incipient Alzheimer's disease in patients with mild cognitive impairment: a follow-up study. Lancet Neurol 2006;5:228–34.
42. Harold D, Abraham R, Hollingworth P, Sims R, Gerrish A, Hamshere ML, Pahwa JS, Moskvina V, Dowzell K, Williams A, et al. Genome-wide association study identifies variants at CLU and PICALM associated with Alzheimer's disease. Nat Genet 2009;41:1088–93.
43. Henriksen AL, St Dennis C, Setter SM, Tran JT. Dementia with lewy bodies: therapeutic opportunities and pitfalls. Consult Pharm 2006;21:563–75.
44. Hodkinson HM. Evaluation of a mental test score for assessment of mental impairment in the elderly. Age Ageing 1972;1(4):233–8.
45. Jellinger KA, Wenning GK, Seppi K. Predictors of survival in dementia with lewy bodies and Parkinson dementia. Neuro-degener Dis 2007;4:428–30.
46. Jitapunkul S, Pillay I, Ebrahim S. The abbreviated mental test: its use and validity. Age Ageing 1991;20(5):332–6.
47. Kavirajan H, Schneider LS. Efficacy and adverse effects of cholinesterase inhibitors and memantine in vascular dementia: a meta-analysis of randomised controlled trials. Lancet Neurol 2007;6:782–92.

48. Kuslansky G, Katz M, Verghese J, Hall CB, Lapuerta P, LaRuffa G, Lipton RB. Detecting dementia with the Hopkins verbal learning test and the mini-mental state examination. Arch Clin Neuropsychol 2004;19(1):89–104.
49. Levy-Lahad E, Wasco W, Poorkaj P, Romano DM, Oshima J, Pettingell WH, Yu CE, Jondro PD, Schmidt SD, Wang K, et al. Candidate gene for the chromosome 1 familial Alzheimer's disease locus. Science 1995;269:973–7.
50. Lippa CF. Synaptophysin immunoreactivity in Pick's disease: comparison with Alzheimer's disease and dementia with Lewy bodies. Am J Alzheimer's Dis Other Dement 2004;19:341–4.
51. Loy C, Schneider L. Galantamine for Alzheimer's disease and mild cognitive impairment. Cochrane Database Syst Rev 2006;1:CD001747.
52. Loy CT, Schofield PR, Turner AM, Kwok JB. Genetics of dementia. Lancet 2014;383:828–40.
53. Mahoney R, Johnston K, Katona C, Maxmin K, Livingston G. The TE4D-Cog: a new test for detecting early dementia in English-speaking populations. Int J Geriatr Psychiatry 2005;20(12):1172–9.
54. Mattsson N, Zetterberg H. Alzheimer's disease and CSF biomarkers: key challenges for broad clinical applications. Biomark Med 2009;3:735–7.
55. McKeith I, O'Brien J, Walker Z, Tatsch K, Booij J, Darcourt J, Padovani A, Giubbini R, Bonuccelli U, Volterrani D, et al. Sensitivity and specificity of dopamine transporter imaging with 123I-FP-CIT SPECT in dementia with Lewy bodies: a phase III, multicentre study. Lancet Neurol 2007;6:305–13.
56. McKeith IG, Dickson DW, Lowe J, Emre M, O'Brien JT, Feldman H, Cummings J, Duda JE, Lippa C, Perry EK, et al. Diagnosis and management of dementia with Lewy bodies: third report of the LBD Consortium. Neurology 2005;65:1863–72.
57. McKhann G, Drachman D, Folstein M, Katzman R, Price D, Stadlan EM. Clinical diagnosis of Alzheimer's disease: report of the NINCDS-ADRDA Work Group under the auspices of Department of Health and Human Services Task Force on Alzheimer's Disease. Neurology 1984;34:939–44.
58. McShane R, Areora Sastre A, Minakaran N. Memantine for dementia. Cochrane Database Syst Rev 2009;1:CD007657.
59. Meeus B, Theuns J, Van Broeckhoven C. The genetics of dementia with Lewy bodies: what are we missing? Arch Neurol 2012;69:1113–8.
60. Meyer JS, Rogers RL, McClintic K, Mortel KF, Lotfi J. Randomized clinical trial of daily aspirin therapy in multi-infarct dementia. A pilot study. J Am Geriatr Soc 1989;37:549–55.
61. Morris R, Mucke L. Alzheimer's disease: a needle from the haystack. Nature 2006;440:284–5.
62. Nasreddine ZS, Phillips NA, Bédirian V, Charbonneau S, Whitehead V, Collin I, Cummings JL, Chertkow H. The Montreal Cognitive Assessment, MoCA: a brief screening tool for mild cognitive impairment. J Am Geriatr Soc 2005;53(4):695–9.
63. Neary D, Snowden J. Fronto-temporal dementia: nosology, neuropsychology, and neuropathology. Brain Cogn 1996;31:176–87.
64. Nilsson FM. Mini mental state examination (MMSE)–probably one of the most cited papers in health science. Acta Psychiatr Scand 2007;116(2):156–7.
65. Pantoni L, Rossi R, Inzitari D, Bianchi C, Beneke M, Erkinjuntti T, Wallin A. Efficacy and safety of nimodipine in subcortical vascular dementia: a subgroup analysis of the Scandinavian multi-infarct dementia trial. J Neurol Sci 2000;175:124–34.
66. Park J, Yang EJ, Yoon JH, Chung KC. Dyrk1A overexpression in immortalized hippocampal cells produces the neuropathological features of Down syndrome. Mol Cell Neurosci 2007;36:270–9.
67. Patwardhan MB, McCrory DC, Matchar DB, Samsa GP, Rutschmann OT. Alzheimer disease: operating characteristics of PET—a meta-analysis. Radiology 2004;231:73–80.
68. Pedersen NL. Reaching the limits of genome-wide significance in Alzheimer disease: back to the environment. JAMA 2010;303:1864–5.
69. Pressman PS, Miller BL. Diagnosis and management of behavioral variant frontotemporal dementia. Biol Psychiatry 2014;75:574–81.
70. Querbes O, Aubry F, Pariente J, Lotterie JA, Demonet JF, Duret V, Puel M, Berry I, Fort JC, Celsis P. Early diagnosis of Alzheimer's disease using cortical thickness: impact of cognitive reserve. Brain 2009;132:2036–47.
71. Rascovsky K, Hodges JR, Knopman D, Mendez MF, Kramer JH, Neuhaus J, van Swieten JC, Seelaar H, Dopper EG, Onyike CU, et al. Sensitivity of revised diagnostic criteria for the behavioural variant of frontotemporal dementia. Brain 2011;134:2456–77.
72. Reiman EM, Chen K, Liu X, Bandy D, Yu M, Lee W, Ayutyanont N, Keppler J, Reeder SA, Langbaum JB, et al. Fibrillar amyloid-beta burden in cognitively normal people at 3 levels of genetic risk for Alzheimer's disease. Proc Natl Acad Sci USA 2009;106:6820–5.

73. Ritchie C, Smailagic N, Noel-Storr AH, Takwoingi Y, Flicker L, Mason SE, McShane R. Plasma and cerebrospinal fluid amyloid beta for the diagnosis of Alzheimer's disease dementia and other dementias in people with mild cognitive impairment (MCI). Cochrane Database Syst Rev 2014;6:CD008782.
74. Rogaeva E, Meng Y, Lee JH, Gu Y, Kawarai T, Zou F, Katayama T, Baldwin CT, Cheng R, Hasegawa H, et al. The neuronal sortilin-related receptor SORL1 is genetically associated with Alzheimer disease. Nat Genet 2007;39:168–77.
75. Rolinski M, Fox C, Maidment I, McShane R. Cholinesterase inhibitors for dementia with Lewy bodies, Parkinson's disease dementia and cognitive impairment in Parkinson's disease. Cochrane Database Syst Rev 2012;3:CD006504.
76. Roman GC. Vascular dementia may be the most common form of dementia in the elderly. J Neurol Sci 2002;203/204:7–10.
77. Roman GC. Vascular dementia: distinguishing characteristics, treatment, and prevention. J Am Geriatr Soc 2003;51:S296–304.
78. Roses AD. An inherited variable poly-T repeat genotype in TOMM40 in Alzheimer disease. Arch Neurol 2010;67:536–41.
79. Schellenberg GD, Bird TD, Wijsman EM, Orr HT, Anderson L, Nemens E, White JA, Bonnycastle L, Weber JL, Alonso ME, et al. Genetic linkage evidence for a familial Alzheimer's disease locus on chromosome 14. Science 1992;258:668–71.
80. Scheltens P, Fox N, Barkhof F, De Carli C. Structural magnetic resonance imaging in the practical assessment of dementia: beyond exclusion. Lancet Neurol 2002;1:13–21.
81. Seshadri S, Fitzpatrick AL, Ikram MA, DeStefano AL, Gudnason V, Boada M, Bis JC, Smith AV, Carassquillo MM, Lambert JC, et al. Genome-wide analysis of genetic loci associated with Alzheimer disease. JAMA 2010;303:1832–40.
82. Small SA, Duff K. Linking Abeta and tau in late-onset Alzheimer's disease: a dual pathway hypothesis. Neuron 2008;60:534–42.
83. Smith T, Gildeh N, Holmes C. The Montreal Cognitive Assessment: validity and utility in a memory clinic setting. Can J Psychiatry 2007;52(5):329.
84. Snowdon DA, Greiner LH, Mortimer JA, Riley KP, Greiner PA, Markesbery WR. Brain infarction and the clinical expression of Alzheimer disease. The Nun Study. JAMA 1997;277:813–7.
85. Straten G, Saur R, Laske C, Gasser T, Annas P, Basun H, Leyhe T. Influence of lithium treatment on GDNF serum and CSF concentrations in patients with early Alzheimer's disease. Curr Alzheimer Res 2011;8:853–9.
86. Testad I, Corbett A, Aarsland D, Lexow KO, Fossey J, Woods B, Ballard C. The value of personalized psychosocial interventions to address behavioral and psychological symptoms in people with dementia living in care home settings: a systematic review. Int Psychogeriatr 2014;26:1083–98.
87. Tombaugh TN, McIntyre NJ. The mini-mental state examination: a comprehensive review. J Am Geriatr Soc 1992;40(9):922–35.
88. Vetter PH, Krauss S, Steiner O, Kropp P, Moller WD, Moises HW, Koller O. Vascular dementia versus dementia of Alzheimer's type: do they have differential effects on caregivers' burden? J Gerontol Ser B Psychol Sci Soc Sci 1999;54:S93–8.
89. Wahlund LO, Julin P, Johansson SE, Scheltens P. Visual rating and volumetry of the medial temporal lobe on magnetic resonance imaging in dementia: a comparative study. J Neurol Neurosurg Psychiatry 2000;69:630–5.
90. Wakabayashi K, Tanji K, Odagiri S, Miki Y, Mori F, Takahashi H. The Lewy body in Parkinson's disease and related neurodegenerative disorders. Mol Neurobiol 2013;47:495–508.
91. Waldemar G, Dubois B, Emre M, Georges J, McKeith IG, Rossor M, Scheltens P, Tariska P, Winblad B. Recommendations for the diagnosis and management of Alzheimer's disease and other disorders associated with dementia: EFNS guideline. Eur J Neurol 2007;14:e1–26.
92. Warren JD, Rohrer JD, Rossor MN. Clinical review. Frontotemporal dementia. BMJ 2013;347:f4827.
93. Wilkinson D, Schindler R, Schwam E, Waldemar G, Jones RW, Gauthier S, Lopez OL, Cummings J, Xu Y, Feldman HH. Effectiveness of donepezil in reducing clinical worsening in patients with mild-to-moderate alzheimer's disease. Dement Geriatr Cogn Disord 2009;28:244–51.
94. Wischik CM, Harrington CR, Storey JM. Tau-aggregation inhibitor therapy for Alzheimer's disease. Biochem Pharmacol 2014;88:529–39.
95. World Health Organization. World Health Report 2003—Shaping the future. Book World Health Organization. Geneva: WHO; 2003.
96. Yu F, Rose KM, Burgener SC, Cunningham C, Buettner LL, Beattie E, Bossen AL, Buckwalter KC, Fick DM, Fitzsimmons S, et al. Cognitive training for early-stage Alzheimer's disease and dementia. J Gerontol Nurs 2009;35:23–29.

CHAPTER 3

Pain Perception and Report in Persons with Dementia

Stephen J. Gibson and Stefan Lautenbacher

Pain is a major health problem for all older persons, and the recent studies indicate that more than 50% of community-dwelling older adults and up to 80% of Nursing Home residents suffer from some persistent pain complaint. Given that dementia is predominately a disease of old age, one might expect that bothersome pain would also be a particularly common problem for people with dementia or cognitive impairment. Considerable evidence exists to show that older adults with dementia or cognitive impairment may receive fewer analgesic medications than cognitively intact persons despite having similar levels of painful disease and medical morbidity [17, 39, 41, 43, 52]. For instance, approximately 64% of older adults were shown to receive appropriate analgesic treatments for pain compared with only 33% of patients with Alzheimer disease (AD) [54]. This was true for simple analgesics, such as acetaminophen or NSAIDs, as well as stronger analgesics, such as opioids, even though the treating physician had judged the need for pain relief as equivalent in both groups [54]. Several other studies have reported similar levels of apparent undertreatment [7, 25, 46, 61], regardless of the health-care setting (community, acute hospitalization, long-term care). A study of people in postoperative recovery from hip fracture surgery showed that persons with dementia received one-third the amount of morphine equivalents when compared with cognitively intact adults [18, 41] and over three-fourth of patients with dementia had no routinely scheduled order for postoperative analgesia [41]. Although some more recent reports have raised questions about the extent of undertreatment of pain in persons with dementia [22, 29, 51], others continue to confirm the extensive early data on reduced analgesic prescription and administration in persons with cognitive impairment or dementia [15, 24, 61].

The most widely accepted explanation for this apparent undertreatment is that pain in persons with dementia remains largely undetected because of deterioration in verbal communication skills and/or an inability to accurately identify pain in this group. In fact, there has been growing international concern over the apparent inadequacy of pain assessment techniques for this group, and this has prompted the development of multiple new observational pain assessment tools (see Chapter 10 for summary). However, another explanation has been proposed to account for the observed undertreatment, namely, that dementia may directly interfere with the perceptual experience of pain and alter the sensitivity to incoming noxious sensation. This view suggests that persons with dementia or cognitive impairment might actually experience pain to a lesser extent and so do not require the same levels of analgesia as cognitively intact older adults.

When considering potential alterations in pain processing in persons with dementia, it is important to recognize that dementia is a generic term indicating a loss of intellectual functions, including memory, significant deterioration in the ability to carry out day-to-day activities, and, often, changes in emotional control and social behavior. Many different diseases can result in dementia, of which AD is the most prevalent, accounting for 70–80% of cases [2, 59]. Modern conceptualizations of pain note that it is a complex and subjective perceptual experience that incorporates sensory, emotional, and cognitive components. The context in which noxious information is processed, the cognitive beliefs of the individual, and the meaning attributed to pain symptoms are known to be important factors in shaping the overall pain experience. A disturbance of multiple higher cortical functions (e.g., memory, judgment, comprehension, emotional control, perceptual skills), as typically seen in adults with AD, would be expected to have a profound influence on the cognitive aspects of pain. Unfortunately, pain beliefs have yet to be examined in adults with cognitive impairment or dementia, and so it remains unclear the extent to which cognitive factors might alter the perceptual pain experience in this group. The neuropathology of dementia may also directly interfere with the transmission and central nervous system (CNS) processing of noxious input (see Chapters 5 and 6 for a detailed description). Pain is transmitted to supraspinal regions via two major pathways. One projection ascends through the lateral thalamus and onto the somatosensory cortex and other cerebral regions involved with sensory discriminative aspects of sensation (e.g., location, intensity) [3]. These CNS regions are relatively well preserved from the neurodegenerative changes commonly seen in AD. The second major pathway branches at the level of the medulla and ascends via the medial thalamus, hypothalamic nuclei, insula, anterior cingulate, and other limbic regions and then onto orbitofrontal areas, all of which are known to be involved in the control of emotion, arousal, and attention. Marked changes in hypothalamic and limbic regions have been previously noted in AD [9]. Other regions of the cerebral cortex are thought to contribute toward the cognitive integration of pain-related sensory information, such as stimulus meaning and reference to past experience. These regions also show progressive degeneration in patients with AD. Based on the underlying pathophysiology of AD, it seems possible that pain-related CNS processing may be potentially compromised. The cognitive and affective components of pain rather than intensity might be most affected in persons with AD. Nonetheless, pain sensitivity represents a combination of all three components and so would be expected to change even if only one dimension is affected. The study of possible alterations in pain perception in other types of dementia is still in its infancy, although given the differences in underlying neuropathology between different types of dementia, any changes in pain perception might be expected to differ from those typically seen in AD.

To date, there have been very few studies to examine the pain experience of older persons with dementia. Much speculation exists over the nature and extent of change in pain sensitivity associated with AD and other dementing syndromes, but relatively few empirical studies. This chapter seeks to review the empirical studies on possible alterations in the quality and intensity of clinical pain in persons with cognitive impairment or dementia. One potential limitation with most studies of clinical pain states is that you can seldom control for the severity of pain-inducing disease. Any observed difference could, therefore, be due to some difference in the type or severity of disease rather than an actual change in the pain experience. As a result, some investigators have turned to psychophysical studies and use experimentally controlled levels of noxious input to anchor the subjective experience against a stimulus of known intensity, thereby providing a quantitative comparison of pain sensitivity between those with and without dementia or cognitive impairment. For this reason, this chapter will also consider the growing body of evidence on potential alterations in pain sensitivity and pain perception seen in response to laboratory-based investigations using experimentally controlled levels of noxious stimulation.

CLINICAL PAIN IN PERSONS WITH COGNITIVE IMPAIRMENT OR DEMENTIA

Based on the available literature, it appears that there is some evidence for a lower prevalence of pain in persons with cognitive impairment or dementia (see Chapter 4 for detailed discussion of pain prevalence), particularly when using observer-rated pain assessment tools. The findings on pain prevalence when using self-report measures are more equivocal and suggest no change in the frequency of reported pain. Fewer studies are available on any dementia-related changes in the severity or quality of clinical pain (see Fig. 3-1). Only, three out of nine studies suggested an increase of pain severity in more severe forms of cognitive impairment, whereas one study even provided some evidence for the opposite. Whether it is a stable trend or rather a chance finding that the observations of an increase of pain severity related to more advanced forms of cognitive impairment stem from the most recent investigations is a question to be answered in future studies. In summary, neither epidemiological investigations nor cross-sectional correlational studies using observer-ratings or self-report measures could provide clear evidence, indicating that with advanced severity and progress of dementia, clinical pain undergoes major changes. However, it is definitely clear that the available data do not justify an undertreatment of pain. The equivocal

- Parmelee et al. [43]: Self-reported pain severity (over last 2 weeks, $n = 758$): Found a small but significant negative correlation ($r = -0.106$) between cognition and pain, suggestive of a *decrease* in pain severity. Marked impaired ($\mu = 1.47$) < mild impaired ($\mu = 1.75$) < intact ($\mu = 1.8$).
- Ferrell et al. [19]: No significant correlation between self-reported MPQ score and cognitive function ($n = 134$).
- Cipher et al. [11]: No significant correlation between pain severity and cognitive function ($n = 234$).
- Schuler et al. [57]: In a hospital sample persons with cognitive impairment reported no difference in pain severity compared with cognitively intact age-matched controls ($n = 91$).
- Wu et al. [63]: Using the MDS (staff proxy ratings), authors report no difference in pain intensity between those with mild, moderate, severe, or no cognitive impairment ($n = 3736$).
- Leong et al. [37]: Examined a NH sample and showed that self-reported pain severity was *increased* in those with severe cognitive impairment (76% with moderate+ pain) compared with intact adults (39.5% with moderate + pain) ($n = 358$).
- Husebo et al. [27]: In a nursing home sample, proxy-rated pain severity (MOBID) was not different between intact ($\mu = 2.5$), mild impaired ($\mu = 2.2$), and moderate-severe impaired ($\mu = 2.9$) ($n = 181$).
- Monroe et al. [40]: Noted a significant *increase* in self-rated pain between those with a diagnosis of dementia ($\mu = 8.0$) compared with cognitively intact adults ($\mu = 6.0$) ($n = 52$).
- Patel and Turk [45]: Report significantly *greater* self-rated pain (NRS) in a community sample of persons with dementia ($n = 215$) compared with age-matched controls ($n = 1552$).

FIGURE 3-1 Studies examining intensity of clinical pain in persons with cognitive impairment or dementia.

MPQ = McGill Pain Questionnaire; MDS = Minimum Data Set scale; MOBID = Mobilization-Observation-Behavior-Intensity-Dementia pain scale; NRS = Numerical Rating Scale.

findings as regards clinical pain, which likely cannot be resolved in the near future because of the huge methodological barriers, upvalue alternative approaches using psychophysical studies as well as other behavioral and CNS indicators of pain sensitivity.

PSYCHOPHYSICAL STUDIES OF PAIN PERCEPTION IN PERSONS WITH DEMENTIA

The most salient characteristic of dementia, regardless of pathogenic etiology, is an irreversible decline in multiple cognitive abilities, including thinking, memory, language, perceptual skills, judgment, emotional control, and thinking [2]. These types of cognitive impairment will impact on the ability to communicate pain, but it is also worth considering whether such deficits might also affect the fundamental experience of pain itself. For instance, given severe memory loss, can pain ever be persistent or is the current experience the total lived experience? Would a disturbance of multiple higher cortical functions impair an individual's ability to discriminate potentially damaging from innocuous sensations? How can one make sense and meaning of pain symptoms when lacking cognitive functions? Would deterioration in emotional control preclude the integration of noxious sensations into an appropriate emotional context? Could errors of judgment interfere with the capacity to evaluate the sensory-discriminative aspects of painful symptoms (i.e., location, intensity, quality)? Thus, a disturbance of multiple higher cognitive functions could be sufficient, in itself, to impair the complex, subjective perceptual experience of pain.

Another viable explanation for the apparent undertreatment of pain in persons with dementia is that the neuropathology of disease might directly interfere with the CNS structures underlying the perceptual experience of pain and alter the sensitivity to incoming noxious sensations [17, 52, 53, 56] (see Chapters 5 and 6 for a full description). This might diminish the pain experience and lead to a reduction in the number of pain complaints. Given the widely distributed pain network and the knowledge that the neuropathologic damage of dementia varies between the common subtypes (AD, vascular, mixed, Lewy body dementia, frontotemporal dementia, and others), each specific type of dementia may need to be considered as its own distinct entity. Furthermore, both excitatory and inhibitory acting CNS structures might be affected by the neuropathology of dementia, leading to varying effects on the overall experience of pain.

Pain Processing in Alzheimer Disease

The vast majority of empirical studies examining the potential interaction between pain processing and dementia have focused on AD. Psychophysical studies using experimental pain stimuli as well as most studies of other behavioral and physiologic indicators of pain (facial expressions, autonomic measures, flexion withdrawal reflexes) and neuroimaging studies have nearly all been undertaken in persons with AD. On the basis of the known specific neuropathology of AD and its interaction with the pain processing network, Scherder and colleagues have proposed a selective impairment in the affective and cognitive dimensions of pain [54]. The lateral pain pathway responsible for sensory discriminative aspects of pain is relatively well preserved from the neurodegenerative changes commonly seen in AD, until very advanced stages [17, 60]. Conversely, intralaminar thalamic nuclei assigned to the medial pain system are subject to neurofibrillary pathology at the earliest preclinical stage of AD [50]. The early loss of limbic structures, hippocampus and prefrontal cortical structures of the medial pain pathway, suggest a potentially selective impairment in the unpleasantness and cognitive dimensions of pain [56].

A summary of studies on pain threshold or the minimum level of noxious stimulation required to elicit a self-report of just noticeable pain in persons with dementia is shown in Fig. 3-2. This work has consistently shown no apparent change in pain threshold in persons with AD when compared with age-matched controls (see recent review by Defrin et al. [16]). The observed lack of change in pain threshold occurs regardless of stimulus type, including electricity [5, 6, 32, 49], heat [20, 31], cold [31], ischemia [6], and, with one exception [12], mechanical pressure [30, 34]. Pain threshold requires ratings of the sensory-discriminative properties of experimental noxious stimuli and so can be seen to support the notion of an unaffected lateral pain pathway in persons with AD. By necessity, all participants in pain threshold studies had only mild levels of cognitive impairment. Nonetheless, the ability to provide self-report ratings has been shown to decline with a greater severity of cognitive impairment in these studies [32], and ratings of pain intensity appear to be negatively correlated with Mini-Mental State Examination (MMSE) score [5, 49]. This might suggest that alterations in pain processing are very much dependent on the stage of AD even in the mild-moderate range.

Pain tolerance or the maximum intensity of noxious stimulation that can be endured before voluntary withdrawal has been examined less often in empirical studies (see Fig. 3-2). Benedetti and colleagues showed a significant increase in pain tolerance to electrical and ischemic stimuli in persons with AD [6, 49], and the magnitude of this increase was associated with the severity of cognitive impairment. Given the lack of change in pain threshold, these findings were taken to suggest a dissociation between the sensory

Study	Type of Dementia	MMSE	Stimulus	Results
Benedetti et al. [6]	AD	10–19	Electrical, ischemia	Threshold: → Tolerance: ↑
Rainero et al. [49]	AD	10–22	Electrical, ischemia	Threshold: → Tolerance: ↑
Gibson et al. [20]	AD	12.7	Laser	Threshold: →
Cole et al. [12]	AD	19.4	Mechanical	Threshold: ↑ Rating—moderate: →
Kunz et al. [34]	Mixed	16.3	Mechanical	Rating—weak: → Rating—moderate: →
Kunz et al. [32]	Mixed	16.4	Electrical	Rating—moderate: →
Carlino et al. [10]	FTD	21.7	Mechanical, electrical	Threshold: ↑ Tolerance: →
Jensen-Dahm et al. [31]	AD	22.4	Cold, heat, mechanical	Threshold: → Tolerance (cold, heat): → Tolerance (mechanical): ↓

FIGURE 3-2 Summary of self-report psychophysical studies in persons with dementia. AD, Alzheimer disease; Mixed, mainly AD but also other types of dementia; FTP, frontotemporal dementia; ↑, increase; →, no change; ↓, decrease.

and affective aspects of the pain experience in AD [6]. A more recent study has, however, failed to replicate these findings, with no reported change in pain tolerance to ice water and an even decreased pain tolerance to mechanical pressure [30]. This may indicate a modality-specific change in pain tolerance and does raise some questions about the ubiquity of impaired affective pain processing in persons with AD. Further studies are needed to help resolve this disparity.

PAIN SENSITIVITY IN PERSONS WITH AD AS MONITORED BY NONVERBAL PSYCHOPHYSIOLOGICAL AND CNS MEASURES

One might expect that the more severe the level of cognitive impairment, the greater the likely change in pain perception. However, the capacity of self-report also declines with increasing severity of dementia, and so other measures of pain are needed to isolate the true effects. A summary of experimental studies using nonverbal psychophysiological measures of pain in persons with dementia is shown in Fig. 3-3. Studies monitoring facial expressions in response to controlled levels of noxious stimulation reveal either a significantly increased response in those with AD in two studies [32, 34] or no change in one study [38]. The facial expressions were able to differentiate non-noxious and noxious stimulus intensities as well as different levels of noxious stimulation in both controls and AD, suggesting specific nonverbal behaviors signaling pain still in early dementia [34, 38]. Facial expressions were shown to be unchanged in AD immediately following a uniform clinical pain stimulus, such as venipuncture or injection in three studies [23, 26, 48]. The tendency toward increased facial expressions in response to pain could suggest an increased sensitivity to pain in persons with AD or that facial actions represent a different aspect of the pain experience—a more reflexive, automatic response that may be disinhibited in persons with cognitive impairment (see recent review about this matter by Lautenbacher and Kunz [35]).

Study	Type of Dementia	MMSE	Results
Vreeling et al. [63]	AD	–	RIII: ↑
Porter et al. [48]	AD	–	FACS: →
			HR: ↓
Rainero et al. [49]	AD	10–12	HR: ↓
Benedetti et al. [5]	AD	10–19	HR: ↓
Lints-Martindale et al. [38]	AD	19.4	FACS: →
Kunz et al. [34]	Mixed	16.3	FACS: ↑
Hsu et al. [26]	AD	–	FACS: →
			HR: →
Hadjistavropoulos et al. [23]	AD	–	FACS: →
Kunz et al. [32]	Mixed	16.4	FACS: ↑
			RIII: ↑
			HR: →
			SSR: ↓

FIGURE 3-3 Summary of studies using nonverbal measures of pain perception in persons with dementia. AD, Alzheimer disease; Mixed, mainly AD but also other types of dementia; RIII, nocifensive reflex; FACS, facial action coding system; HR, heart rate; SSR, sympathetic skin response; ↑, increase; →, no change; ↓, decrease.

In support of this conclusion, persons with AD have also been found to display enhanced nociceptive flexion withdrawal reflexes (RIII) in response to experimental pain [33, 34, 36, 62]. However, autonomic responses typically associated with the onset of acute pain (i.e., increased heart rate, blood pressure, galvanic skin resistance, breathing) appear to be blunted in persons with AD [47].

Much of the elevation in autonomic indices typically occurs during anticipation of an impending painful stimulus, yet this anticipatory response is lacking in those with AD [5, 48, 49]. Group differences in the poststimulus autonomic response, particularly in heart rate change, are less obvious [48] or unchanged [26, 32]. The poststimulus autonomic response to stronger intensity pain is also unchanged in those with AD [49], indicating that autonomic responses are still present in older people with AD [47]. The autonomic responses to noxious stimulation have been interpreted as evidence of impaired medial pain pathways processing and as such as indicators of disturbed emotional pain control [5, 49]. However, such measures are very indirect markers of the functional integrity of medial pain pathways, and a known dysfunction in sympathetic and parasympathetic nervous system with AD [21, 28] could also explain the blunted response as a generalized phenomenon, rather than a pain-specific deficit.

Given the CNS neuropathology of AD, the most profound effects on pain would be expected to occur in the CNS processing of noxious information. Neurophysiological and neuroimaging studies have been undertaken using both EEG and fMRI. An early study by Cornu [14] employed a nonquantitative methodology to examine EEG power spectra following painful electrical stimulation. Those with dementia and controls exhibited a block in the EEG alpha rhythm in response to painful stimulation, and this was interpreted as evidence of comparable levels of nociceptive processing in both groups. Benedetti et al. reported that the increase in pain tolerance observed in those with AD was most noticeable in persons with EEG alpha and high delta peaks and that blunted autonomic responses to pain were also associated with these EEG changes [5]. A disruption of expectation and placebo-related analgesia has also been shown in AD, and this was particularly marked in those with a reduced connectivity of the prefrontal cortex as measured by EEG responses, thereby highlighting the importance of integrated cortical processing in shaping the pain experience and the impairment in such processes in those with AD [4].

Consistent with a previous study in patients with any type of dementia [64], in persons with AD, the amplitude of pain-related evoked potentials (stimulus-locked EEG changes) was unchanged, suggesting a comparable amplitude of brain response to noxious heat, although a slower latency might indicate a slower cortical processing of nociceptive input [20]. In perhaps the most definitive study of CNS processing to date, persons with mild AD were shown to have significantly enhanced fMRI pain-related activation across the entire lateral and medial pain networks [12]. This included the mid anterior cingulate, medial thalamus, somatosensory cortex, dorsolateral prefrontal cortex, and supplementary motor areas. The increased activation was apparently due to a prolonged processing of noxious input, rather than higher amplitude of brain activation. These findings suggest that pain processing in sensory and affective CNS regions is not diminished in those with mild AD, possibly reflecting a prolonged attention to, and appraisal of noxious stimulation. A connectivity analysis of fMRI data was undertaken to examine the integrated functioning of CNS regions mediating the sensory, emotional, and cognitive aspects of pain [13]. The findings showed enhanced functional connectivity between the dorsolateral prefrontal cortex and the anterior cingulate, thalamus, hypothalamus, and motor regions. Three main nodes—the dorsolateral prefrontal cortex, hypothalamus, and periaqueductal gray—were thought to drive the prolonged CNS activation following noxious input. Once again, these findings emphasize a heightened processing of pain in persons with mild AD, possibly reflecting a more distressing experience due to an inability to ascribe adequate meaning and future implications of the experienced pain sensation [13]. It is worth noting that these findings are limited to those with mild-moderate AD and that alterations in pain processing may be quite different in those with more advanced disease. Further studies in those with severe AD or longitudinal studies of CNS pain processing across the entire course of AD are required to answer this question.

Pain Processing in Other Types of Dementia

More than 100 different diseases result in dementia, including AD, vascular dementias, Lewy body dementia, frontotemporal dementia, Creutzfeldt–Jakob disease, and a range of less common metabolic, infectious, and neurodegenerative disorders. If the neuropathology of dementia, rather than the generalized cognitive impairment, is most critical for determining alterations in pain perception, then different types of dementia might be expected to lead to different types of deficits. As discussed earlier, it has been argued that AD should selectively impair the cognitive affective dimension of pain mediated by the medial pain pathways, and there is partial empirical support for this view. Vascular dementia, the second most common type, is characterized by cerebrovascular infarcts and is a highly heterogeneous condition. Cerebrovascular disease can lead to infarcts and consequent white matter lesions at any site within the CNS, although sites within the frontocortical region are most commonly seen in those with impaired cognition or dementia [8]. Deafferentation in cortico-subcortical networks could also result in disruption or disconnection between various neural substrates within the pain pathways [56] and potentially lead to the well-recognized clinical entity of central poststroke pain [58]. An increase in pain is one possible outcome in vascular dementia [17, 56], although given that the location of infarcts and white matter lesions will vary from person to person, any component of the pain pathways could be affected with presumably different impacts on pain perception. To date, there have been no experimental studies to examine pain processing in persons with vascular dementia.

In frontotemporal dementia, the major loci of neuropathology reside in the prefrontal cortex and lateral temporal lobe, with additional atrophy often seen in parietal regions [8]. Involvement of the prefrontal cortex, anterior cingulate, insular, and orbitofrontal regions [56] would imply an impaired medial pain system with a likely reduction in the motivational-affective and cognitive aspects of pain. A study of pain threshold and tolerance in persons with frontotemporal dementia revealed a significant increase in pain threshold but no change in pain tolerance [10]. A subgroup analysis of those with clear neuropsychological evidence of frontal lobe dysfunction confirmed the same result, although frontotemporal dementia patients with radiological evidence of frontal and temporal lobe hypoperfusion (under activity) demonstrated significant changes in both pain threshold and pain tolerance. The consistent reported change in pain threshold would suggest a greater degree of impairment in the lateral pain pathways and is seemingly at odds with the interaction hypothesized by Scherder and colleagues. The temporal lobe is functionally connected to the somatosensory cortex [44], and patients with the amyotrophic lateral sclerosis variant of frontotemporal dementia are known to exhibit significant cortical atrophy in the somatosensory regions as well as adjacent frontal and parietal areas. This may help explain the observed increase in sensory-discriminative threshold, although functional neuroimaging studies of pain processing in persons with frontotemporal dementia would be required to confirm this view.

Such considerations may also upvalue the meaning of neuropsychological results because it is widely accepted that certain neuropsychological functions are predominantly implemented in certain brain regions. Thus, prefrontal regions have appeared to be responsible for executive functions and the medial temporal region for declarative memory. In line with this reasoning, preliminary evidence suggests that especially deterioration of processes based in prefrontal regions indicated by neuropsychological tests of executive functions is associated with pathological changes in pain processing [33, 42, 55]. It may be appropriate to screen for executive dysfunction in order to help identify those patients with dementia who are especially vulnerable for the development of pain problems.

The interaction between pain processing and neuropathology of other types of dementia has received scant attention [1]. The possible impacts of multiple sclerosis and Parkinson disease have been mentioned [53], but not in conjunction with cases of dementia in these conditions. The field is still very much in its infancy, and it remains somewhat unclear the extent to which dementia etiology might impact differentially on various components of the pain experience. Indeed, pain by definition is a sensory and emotional experience, and so a selective change in any one aspect will still impair pain and the overall integrated perceptual experience. Moreover, it is worth noting that many patients with dementia have mixed pathologies [1], with combinations of AD, vascular, and/or Lewy body neurodegenerative changes often being present in the one individual. This type of mixed neuropathogical etiology makes it difficult to use the diagnostic type of dementia as a major demarcation point for considering alterations in pain processing. Instead, it may be necessary to characterize the specific CNS neuropathology of each individual to accurately understand the precise nature of deficits in pain processing that are typically seen in clinical practice.

SUMMARY

Key points related to the experience of pain with respect to studies of clinical pain, psychophysical studies, and psychophysiological as well as CNS indicators of experimental pain in persons with dementia have been discussed in this chapter. Over the past decade, considerable advances have occurred in knowledge and approaches to addressing the many challenges faced by clinicians caring for persons with dementia. The overall findings on altered pain perception (pointing most likely to hyperalgesic changes) in persons with dementia suggest that it is unjustified to assume that dementia is a natural form of analgesic, which makes further pain management dispensable. Instead, more and more evidence emerges that pain strongly impacts on these frail individuals in ways different from those of cognitively healthy people. Given the many variants and different stages of dementia, it is necessary that pain research and management will be based on more personalized approaches in the future, which make better use of nonverbal pain-indicative tools for pain diagnosis and assessment. The better we can care and treat these individuals with limited abilities as regards cognition and language, the longer they communicate their suffering aside from the usual verbal routes. As the population of persons with dementia rapidly grows in the next 30 years, targeted research that follows these lines of reasoning is essential.

REFERENCES

1. Achterberg WP, Pieper MJ, van Dalen-Kok AH, de Waal MW, Husebo BS, Lautenbacher S, Kunz M, Scherder EJ, Corbett A. Pain management in patients with dementia. Clin Interv Aging 2013;8:1471–82.
2. American Psychiatric Association. Practice guideline for the treatment of patients with Alzheimer's disease and other dementias of late life. Am J Psychiatry 1997;154:1–39.
3. Apkarian AV, Bushnell MC, Treede RD, Zubieta JK. Human brain mechanisms of pain perception and regulation in health and disease. Eur J Pain 2005;9:463–84.
4. Benedetti F, Arduino C, Costa S, Vighetti S, Tarenzi L, Rainero I, Asteggiano G. Loss of expectation-related mechanisms in Alzheimer's disease makes analgesic therapies less effective. Pain 2006;121:133–44.
5. Benedetti F, Arduino C, Vighetti S, Asteggiano G, Tarenzi L, Rainero I. Pain reactivity in Alzheimer patients with different degrees of cognitive impairment and brain electrical activity deterioration. Pain 2004;111:22–9.
6. Benedetti F, Vighetti S, Ricco C, Lagna E, Bergamasco B, Pinessi L, Rainero I. Pain threshold and tolerance in Alzheimer's disease. Pain 1999;80:377–82.
7. Bernabei R, Gambassi G, Lapane K, Landi F, Gatsonis C, Dunlop R, Lipsitz L, Steel K, Mor V. Management of pain in elderly patients with cancer. SAGE study group. Systematic assessment of geriatric drug use via epidemiology. JAMA 1998;279:1877–82.
8. Bertelson JA, Ajtai B. Neuroimaging of dementia. Neurol Clin 2014;32:59–93.
9. Braak H, Braak E. Staging of Alzheimer-related cortical destruction. Int Psychogeriatr 1997;9:257–61; discussion 269–72.
10. Carlino E, Benedetti F, Rainero I, Asteggiano G, Cappa G, Tarenzi L, Vighetti S, Pollo A. Pain perception and tolerance in patients with frontotemporal dementia. Pain 2010;151:783–9.
11. Cipher DJ, Clifford PA. Dementia, pain, depression, behavioral disturbances, and ADLs: Toward a comprehensive conceptualization of quality of life in long-term care. Int J Geriatr Psychiatry 2004;19:741–8.
12. Cole LJ, Farrell MJ, Duff EP, Barber JB, Egan GF, Gibson SJ. Pain sensitivity and fMRI pain-related brain activity in Alzheimer's disease. Brain 2006;129:2957–65.
13. Cole LJ, Gavrilescu M, Johnston LA, Gibson SJ, Farrell MJ, Egan GF. The impact of Alzheimer's disease on the functional connectivity between brain regions underlying pain perception. Eur J Pain 2011;15:568.e1–e11.
14. Cornu F. Perturbations de la perception de la doleur chez les dements degeneratifs. J Physiol Norm Patholog 1975;72:81–96.
15. de Souto Barreto P, Lapeyre-Mestre M, Vellas B, Rolland Y. Potential underuse of analgesics for recognized pain in nursing home residents with dementia: a cross-sectional study. Pain 2013;154:2427–31.
16. Defrin R, Amanzio M, de Tommaso M, Dimova V, Filipovic S, Finn DP, Gimenez-Llort L, Invitto S, Jensen-Dahm C, Lautenbacher S, et al. Experimental pain processing in individuals with cognitive impairment: current state of the science. Pain 2015;156:1396–408.
17. Farrell MJ, Katz B, Helme RD. The impact of dementia on the pain experience. Pain 1996;67:7–15.
18. Feldt KS, Ryden MB, Miles S. Treatment of pain in cognitively impaired compared with cognitively intact older patients with hip-fracture. J Am Geriatr Soc 1998;46:1079–85.
19. Ferrell BA, Ferrell BR, Rivera L. Pain in cognitively impaired nursing home patients. J Pain Symptom Manag 1995;10:591–8.
20. Gibson SJ, Voukelatos X, Ames D, Flicker L, Helme RD. An examination of pain perception and cerebral event-related potentials following carbon dioxide laser stimulation in patients with Alzheimer's disease and age-matched control volunteers. Pain Res Manag 2001;6:126–32.
21. Giubilei F, Strano S, Imbimbo BP, Tisei P, Calcagnini G, Lino S, Frontoni M, Santini M, Fieschi C. Cardiac autonomic dysfunction in patients with Alzheimer disease: possible pathogenetic mechanisms. Alzheimer Dis Assoc Disord 1998;12:356–61.
22. Haasum Y, Fastbom J, Fratiglioni L, Kareholt I, Johnell K. Pain treatment in elderly persons with and without dementia: a population-based study of institutionalized and home dwelling elderly. Drugs Aging 2011;28:283–93.
23. Hadjistavropoulos T, Voyer P, Sharpe D, Verreault R, Aubin M. Assessing pain in dementia patients with comorbid delirium and/or depression. Pain Manag Nurs 2008; 9:48–54.
24. Hoffmann F, van den Bussche H, Wiese B, Glaeske G, Kaduszkiewicz H. Diagnoses indicating pain and analgesic drug prescription in patients with dementia: a comparison to age- and sex-matched controls. BMC Geriatr 2014;14:20.
25. Horgas AL, Tsai PF. Analgesic drug prescription and use in cognitively impaired nursing home residents. Nurs Res 1998;47:235–42.
26. Hsu KT, Shuman SK, Hamamoto DT, Hodges JS, Feldt KS. The application of facial expressions to the assessment of orofacial pain in cognitively impaired older adults. J Am Dent Assoc 2007;138:963–69.

27. Husebo BS, Strand LI, Moe-Nilssen R, Borgehusebo S, Aarsland D, Ljunggren AE. Who suffers most? Dementia and pain in nursing home patients: a cross-sectional study. J Am Med Dir Assoc 2008;9:427–33.
28. Idiaquez J, Roman GC. Autonomic dysfunction in neurodegenerative dementias. J Neurol Sci 2011;305:22–7.
29. Jensen-Dahm C, Gasse C, Astrup A, Mortensen PB, Waldemar G. Frequent use of opioids in patients with dementia and nursing home residents: a study of the entire elderly population of Denmark. Alzheimers Dement 2015;11:691–9.
30. Jensen-Dahm C, Werner MU, Dahl JB, Jensen TS, Ballegaard M, Hejl AM, Waldemar G. Quantitative sensory testing and pain tolerance in patients with mild to moderate Alzheimer disease compared to healthy control subjects. Pain 2014;155:1439–45.
31. Jensen-Dahm C, Werner MU, Jensen TS, Ballegaard M, Andersen BB, Høgh P, Waldemar G. Discrepancy between stimulus response and tolerance of pain in Alzheimer disease. Neurology 2015;84:1575–81.
32. Kunz M, Mylius V, Scharmann S, Schepelmann K, Lautenbacher S. Influence of dementia on multiple components of pain. Eur J Pain 2009;13:317–25.
33. Kunz M, Mylius V, Schepelmann K, Lautenbacher S. Loss in executive functioning best explains changes in pain responsiveness in patients with dementia-related cognitive decline. Behav Neurol 2015;2015:878157.
34. Kunz M, Scharmann S, Hemmeter U, Schepelmann K, Lautenbacher S. The facial expression of pain in patients with dementia. Pain 2007;133:221–8
35. Lautenbacher S, Kunz M. Facial pain expression in dementia: a review of the experimental and clinical evidence. Curr Alzheimer Res 2016; Epub June 2.
36. Lautenbacher S, Kunz M, Mylius V, Scharmann S, Hemmeter U, Schepelmann K. "Multidimensional pain assessment in patients with dementia" [in German]. Schmerz 2007;21:529–38.
37. Leong IY, Nuo TH. Prevalence of pain in nursing home residents with different cognitive and communicative abilities. Clin J Pain 2007;23:119–27.
38. Lints-Martindale AC, Hadjistavropoulos T, Barber B, Gibson SJ. A psychophysical investigation of the facial action coding system as an index of pain variability among older adults with and without Alzheimer's disease. Pain Med 2007;8: 678–89.
39. Marzinski LR. The tragedy of dementia: clinically assessing pain in the confused nonverbal elderly. J Gerontol Nurs 1991;17:25–8.
40. Monroe TB, Misra SK, Habermann RC, Dietrich MS, Cowan RL, Simmons SF. Pain reports and pain medication treatment in nursing home residents with and without dementia. Geriatr Gerontol Int 2014;14:541–8.
41. Morrison RS, Siu AL. A comparison of pain and its treatment in advanced dementia and cognitively intact patients with hip fracture. J Pain Symptom Manag 2000;19:240–8.
42. Oosterman JM, Traxler J, Kunz M. The influence of executive functioning on facial and subjective pain responses in older adults. Behav Neurol 2016;2016:1984827.
43. Parmelee, PA, Smith B, Katz IR. Pain complaints and cognitive status among elderly institution residents. J Am Geriatr Soc 1993;41:517–22.
44. Pascual B, Masdeu JC, Hollenbeck M, Makris N, Insausti R, Ding SL, Dickerson BC. Large-scale brain networks of the human left temporal pole: a functional connectivity MRI study. Cereb Cortex 2015;25:680–702.
45. Patel K, Turk D. Evaluation of pain intensity ratings among older adults with and without dementia: findings from the national health and aging trends study. J Pain 2016;17:S8.
46. Pickering G, Jourdan D, Dubray C. Acute versus chronic pain treatment in Alzheimer's disease. Eur J Pain 2006;10:379–84.
47. Plooij B, Swaab D, Scherder E. Autonomic responses to pain in aging and dementia. Rev Neurosci 2011;22:583–9.
48. Porter FL, Malhotra KM, Wolf CM, Morris JC, Miller JP, Smith MC. Dementia and response to pain in the alderly. Pain 1996;68:413–21.
49. Rainero I, Vighetti S, Bergamasco B, Pinessi L, Benedetti F. Autonomic responses and pain perception in Alzheimer's disease. Eur J Pain 2000;4:267–74.
50. Rüb U, Del Tredici K, Del Turco D, Braak H. The intralaminar nuclei assigned to the medial pain system and other components of this system are early and progressively affected by the Alzheimer's disease-related cytoskeletal pathology. J Chem Neuroanat 2002;23:279–90.
51. Sandvik R, Selbaek G, Kirkevold O, Aarsland D, Husebo BS. Analgesic prescribing patterns in Norwegian nursing homes from 2000 to 2011: trend analyses of four data samples. Age Ageing 2016;45:54–60.
52. Scherder E, Herr K, Pickering G, Gibson S, Benedetti F, Lautenbacher S. Pain in dementia. Pain 2009;145:276–8.
53. Scherder E, Oosterman J, Swaab D, Herr K, Ooms M, Ribbe M, Sergeant J, Pickering G, Benedetti F. Recent developments in pain in dementia. BMJ 2005;330:461–4.
54. Scherder EJ, Bouma A. Is decreased use of analgesics in Alzheimer disease due to a change in the affective component of pain? Alzheimer Dis Assoc Disord 1997;11:171–4.

55. Scherder EJ, Eggermont L, Plooij B, Oudshoorn J, Vuijk PJ, Pickering G, Lautenbacher S, Achterberg W, Oosterman J. Relationship between chronic pain and cognition in cognitively intact older persons and in patients with Alzheimer's disease. The need to control for mood. Gerontology 2008;54:50–8.
56. Scherder EJ, Sergeant JA, Swaab DF. Pain processing in dementia and its relation to neuropathology. Lancet Neurol 2003;2:677–86.
57. Schuler M, Njoo N, Hestermann M, Oster P, Hauer K. Acute and chronic pain in geriatrics: clinical characteristics of pain and the influence of cognition. Pain Med 2004;5:253–62.
58. Siniscalchi A, Gallelli L, De Sarro G, Malferrari G, Santangelo E. Antiepileptic drugs for central post-stroke pain management. Pharmacol Res 2012;65:171–5.
59. Small GW, Rabins PV, Barry PP, Buckholtz NS, DeKosky ST, Ferris SH, Finkel SI, Gwyther LP, Khachaturian ZS, Lebowitz BD, et al. Diagnosis and treatment of Alzheimer disease and related disorders. Consensus statement of the American Association for Geriatric Psychiatry, the Alzheimer's Association, and the American Geriatrics Society. JAMA 1997;278:1363–71.
60. Thompson PM, Hayashi KM, de Zubicaray G, Janke AL, Rose SE, Semple J, Herman D, Hong MS, Dittmer SS, Doddrell DM, Toga AW. Dynamics of gray matter loss in Alzheimer's disease. J Neurosci 2003;23:994–1005.
61. Veal FC, Bereznicki LR, Thompson AJ, Peterson GM. Pharmacological management of pain in australian aged care facilities. Age Ageing 2014;43:851–6.
62. Vreeling FW, Jolles J, Verhey FR, Houx PJ. Primitive reflexes in healthy, adult volunteers and neurological patients: methodological issues. J Neurol 1993;240:495–504.
63. Wu N, Miller SC, Lapane K, Roy J, Mor V. Impact of cognitive function on assessments of nursing home residents' pain. Med Care 2005;43:934–9.
64. Yamamoto M, Kachi T, Igata A. Pain-related somatosensory evoked potentials in dementia. J Neurol Sci 1996;137:117–9.

CHAPTER 4

The Epidemiology of Pain in Dementia

Brian E. McGuire, Darragh Taheny, and Bronagh Reynolds

WHAT IS EPIDEMIOLOGY?

Epidemiology is the study of the rates of disease in a population and the causes and risk factors for that disease. The number of new cases of the disease in a given time period, such as a year, is known as the incidence of the disease. In contrast, the total number of people in the population having the disease at a particular point in time is known as the prevalence. The prevalence estimate of the disease includes incident cases and can be considered as the total burden of disease in a population. Prevalence data is typically either (a) point prevalence, which is the total number of people in the population with the disease at a point in time, or (b) lifetime prevalence, which is the risk of developing a disease across the life span.

Epidemiological data is very important for a number of reasons. For example, when one knows the total number of people in the population with a particular disease (prevalence), resources can then be allocated on the basis of need. Knowing the lifetime prevalence of the disease enables health service providers to plan for service provision based on the likely number of people to develop a disease in the future, relative to the size of the overall population (e.g., if the lifetime prevalence of a disease is 1% and the population is 10 million, health service planners can estimate that approximately 100,000 people in the population will have the disease in their lifetime). Although epidemiological research is typically focused on disease rate estimation and disease monitoring at a population level, it also provides important statistical data about risk estimation for individuals. While this is not likely to be a fine-tuned estimation based on an individual patient's particular characteristics, one can nevertheless provide a gross estimation based on the prevalence of the disease in the population, especially for subpopulations with a specific risk profile (e.g., people with genetic predisposition to develop a disease). This may then assist clinicians and patients in making decisions regarding treatment options and future care needs, and with epidemiological studies providing disease prevalence information, it also guides health policy makers in making decisions on screening, immunization, insurance rebates, and so on. Finally, epidemiology can shed light on the etiology of a disease through comparisons of its disease rates across different groups, which may point to the pathophysiological mechanisms that play a role. In the context of pain in dementia, if we know the prevalence of pain in an age cohort but identify a smaller prevalence in that same age group and where dementia is also present, we can hypothesize either that dementia disrupts pain experience or that the expression of pain is more difficult to measure. For further reading on epidemiology, refer to *Epidemiology: An Introduction* [46].

WHY STUDY PAIN AND DEMENTIA?

The study of the epidemiology of pain in people with dementia is important for a number of reasons. It has been well established in several studies that pain is experienced by people with dementia, and in that context, it is necessary to know how frequently pain presents in the population. Pain may also be a significant problem because people with dementia, by virtue of their impaired cognition, may (i) be at increased risk of having accidents, (ii) have increased likelihood of prolonged immobility, (iii) have greater risk of development of painful conditions associated with the dementing disease process itself and associated complications (e.g., musculoskeletal problems, problems with swallow, infections), (iv) have possible altered sensory perception arising from the disease, which may confer increased risk to perceive pain in response to nonpainful stimuli, and (v) show exacerbation of pain associated with noncommunication and nonidentification of painful conditions requiring pain relief.

THE EPIDEMIOLOGY OF DEMENTIA

General cognitive decline is strongly associated with age progression. Indeed, the prevalence of dementia rises drastically from about 1% in individuals aged 65 years to over 25% in those aged over 85 years [9]. In the United States, dementia is the most common cause of disability among the elderly, with Alzheimer disease (AD) accounting for the bulk of those suffering from dementia [16]. Drawing on selected studies, Table 4-1 summarizes the population prevalence of dementia with reference to dementia as a generic construct. Although dementia can occur in early adulthood, it is relatively rare—most patients develop the disease from their 60's onward. As is evident from the estimates provided, there is a high level of consistency regarding the population-level burden of disease, with rates rising exponentially from the seventh decade.

Several kinds of primary progressive dementia (where the dementia itself is the primary illness) exist, including AD, frontotemporal dementia, vascular dementia, dementia with Lewy bodies (DLBs). Dementia may also occur secondary to other recognizable illnesses such as Parkinson disease, multiple sclerosis, and Huntington disease. In addition, dementia can be nonprogressive (e.g., in traumatic brain injury) and can be temporary and transient (e.g., in people with delirium). It is worth noting that delirium is commonly present in people with dementia and adds an additional challenge to assessment. Although

TABLE 4-1 Prevalence of Dementia from Age 60 Years (Age-Categorized)

Author	Age Group (Range of Years) and Point Prevalence (%) of Dementia						
Ferri et al. [9]	60–64 0.9%	65–69 1.5%	70–74 3.6%	75–79 6.0%	80–84 12.2%	≥85 24.8%	
World Health Organization [56]	60–64 1.6%	65–69 2.6%	70–74 4.3%	75–79 7.4%	80–84 12.9%	85–89 21.7%	>90 43.1%
Hebert et al. [15]	65–74 3.0%			75–84 17.6%		≥85 32.3%	

TABLE 4-2 Population Point Prevalence (%) of Different Forms of Primary Progressive Dementia

Dementia Type	Prevalence	Sample Characteristics
Alzheimer disease	3.0% (65–74 y) 17.6% (75–84 y) 32.3% (85+ y) (Hebert et al. [16])	USA Age: >65, N = 10,800
	2.0% (Dong et al. [7])	China Age: >65, N = 87,761
	2.7% (Kalaria et al. [26])	Brazil Age: >65, N = 7513
Vascular dementia	1.0% (Ott et al. [38])	USA Age: >65, N = 7528
	0.9% (Dong et al. [7])	China Age: >65, N = 87,761
	0.9% (Kalaria et al. [26])	Brazil Age: >65, N = 7513
Frontotemporal dementia	0.02% (Ratnavalli et al. [44]) Early onset study	UK Age: <65, N = 32,6019
	1.7% (Zhang et al. [58])	China Age: >65, N = 29,454
	0.02–0.022% (Onyike and Diehl-Schmid [37])	Review
Dementia with Lewy bodies	0.1% (Herrera et al. [17])	Brazil Age: >65, N = 1656
	3.8% (Yamada et al. [57])	Japan Age: >65, N = 3715

we are focused on primary dementia, similar issues arise for identification of pain in the broad range of conditions in which dementia is a central component. Table 4-2 summarizes the estimates of different kinds of dementia in the general population from the medical literature. By far, AD is the most common form of progressive primary dementia, usually accounting for 60% of dementia patients [56].

Different types of progressive dementia have varying average age of onset and varying course. For example, frontotemporal dementia is more likely to have an early onset (before 65 years in 75% of patients), whereas AD is much more a feature of advancing age, and thus considerably more prevalent in those over 65 years.

THE EPIDEMIOLOGY OF PAIN

Pain is also a prevalent problem across the life span and increases in prevalence among older individuals [3], irrespective of level of cognitive ability [48]. Although pain is a near-universal experience, the personal, economic, and social burden of pain is most obvious for chronic pain.

Chronic pain is defined by the International Association for the Study of Pain (IASP) as persistent or recurrent pain that lasts for more than 3 months [23]. Although recognition and management of short-lasting pain is very important, much of the research literature in dementia has focused on the impact of chronic pain since chronic pain can have a significant deleterious effect on capacity to partake in activities, sleep, mood, behavior, and overall quality of life. Table 4-3 shows a sample of prevalence studies that highlight the enormous prevalence of chronic pain. These studies indicate that the prevalence of chronic pain in people over 65 years is substantial, affecting at least 14% of the population, but most studies suggest that the prevalence is around 30%. Note that the prevalence of chronic pain in the large cross-European study [3] in Table 4-3 showed a declining prevalence of chronic pain in older age groups, but the study did not attempt to recruit people in nursing homes and so may have missed a portion of the population that is most likely to have significant health problems [3].

As it is clear from the data presented in these studies, dementia and pain are independently highly prevalent across the life span. Without taking into consideration the possibility of one condition actually being a risk factor for the other, we can infer that dementia and pain are commonly comorbid; thus, it may be a growing problem as our population lives longer. Recognition of the prevalence rates of pain in people with dementia is a necessary first step in alerting caregivers to this problem to ensure adequate pain management.

PAIN IN DEMENTIA: AN EPIDEMIOLOGICAL CHALLENGE

Up to 80% of people living in nursing homes report pain [19]. However, the literature is also quite clear that patients with dementia are actually undertreated for pain [12, 34] (see also Chapter 3). The undertreatment of pain in patients with dementia may arise from the difficulty in assessing and detecting acute or chronic pain in populations with progressive cognitive decline. Zwakhalen [59] found that those with dementia report pain less often and at a lower intensity than those without cognitive impairment. As pain is a subjective experience, it is difficult to identify pain in those who are essentially unable to verbally communicate their discomfort or distress [12]; (see also Chapters 9 and 10).

Table 4-4 summarizes a number of studies that examined the prevalence of chronic pain in people with dementia. The varied prevalence rates are indicative of the host of different methods used in assessing pain, some of which are not suited to accurately detect pain in those with dementia. For acute and chronic pain assessments, verbal communication is commonly a core requirement on the part of the patient. However, the ability to accurately self-report reduces with the severity of dementia [35], and the ability to remember pain and to describe pain diminishes [51] (see also Chapter 10). Although people with AD report pain less often and tend to show blunted autonomic reactions to procedures such as injections, many experimental studies have found that pain thresholds reduce with age [15] so that increased pain perception may actually occur. Furthermore, patients with AD are frequently found to display increased facial expressions of pain and to have enhanced withdrawal reactions [28, 29] (see also Chapter 11).

These difficulties in reliably identifying pain can lead to a situation where pain is poorly managed or undertreated. Observational methods of assessment are no doubt more appropriate in situations where there is impairment in the patient's ability to communicate (see Chapter 10). Consequently, when observational methods are employed over other methods to detect pain, the prevalence rates of pain in dementia rise [48].

TABLE 4-3 Point Prevalence of Chronic Pain Across the Life Span

Author	Sample Characteristics	Age Groups (Range of Years) and Prevalence (%) of Chronic Pain
Johannes et al. [25]	USA (N = 27,035)	18–24 12.4%	25–34 21%	35–44 29.7%	45–54 35.7%	55–64 38.2%	≥65 38.5%
Wong and Fielding [55]	Hong Kong (N = 5001)	18–29 22.7%	30–39 33.8%	40–49 41.7%	50–59 40%	≥60 37.1%	
Blyth et al. [2]	Australia (N = 3596)	15–29 F: 12.5% M: 10%	30–39 F: 14.5% M: 15.5%	40–49 F: 19% M: 20%	50–59 F: 28.5% M: 22.5%	60–69 F: 28.5% M: 25%	70–79 F: 27% M: 21%	80–84 F: 31% M: 18.5%
Breivik et al. [3]	Europe (N = 46,394)	18–30 16%	31–40 18%	41–50 21%	51–60 15%	61–70 14%	71–80 10%	≥81 4%
Reitsma et al. [45]	Canada (N = 13,1061)	20–44 13%			45–64 25%		≥65 31%	
Tsang et al. [52]	17 countries (USA, Europe, Middle East, Asia, New Zealand) (N = 85,052)	18–35 (a) Developing countries F: 35.2% M: 22% (b) Developed countries F: 30.4% M: 20.9%	36–50 (a) Developing countries F: 47.2% M: 30.8% (b) Developed countries F: 42.6% M: 31.5%		51–65 (a) Developing countries F: 59.4% M: 43.8% (b) Developed countries F: 55% M: 42.5%		>66 (a) Developing countries F: 73.3% M: 59.8% (b) Developed countries F: 63.1% M: 47.2%	

TABLE 4-4 Prevalence of Pain in Dementia

Author	Pain Type	Patient Characteristics	Measure(s) Used	Pain Prevalence	Setting
Zwakhalen et al. [60]	Unspecified	Average age 82.8 y, 80% women	PACSLAC-D	Mean 47% (41–52%)	3 nursing homes Netherlands
Mäntyselk et al. [33]	Unspecified	Average age 80.3 y, 73.3% women Dementia severity: Mild, N = 43 Moderate, N = 27 Severe, N = 5	Interview and medical examination	Any pain: 42.7% Any daily pain: 22.7% Daily pain interfering with activities: 18.7% Daily pain at rest: 4%	Home-dwelling Finland
Ferrell et al. [3]	Musculoskeletal: 83% Neuropathy: 10% Other: 7%	Average age 84.9 y, 85% women. MMSE: 12.1 ± 7.9 Dementia and delirium	McGill pain questionnaire and 4 unidimensional scales	62%	Community-skilled nursing homes N = 217
Shega et al. [51]	Unspecified	Average age 84.1 y, 75.7% women	PEACE-Interview (VDS)	Pain: 32% Slight: 21% Moderate: 8% Severe pain: 3%	Community-dwelling USA
Leong and Nuo [30]	Chronic pain	No cognitive impairment, N = 39 Mild cognitive impairment, N = 46 Severe cognitive impairment, N = 54	Verbal report of pain PAIN-AD	No cognitive impairment, 48.7% Mildly impaired cognition, 46.5% Severely impaired cognition, 42.9%	3 nursing homes Singapore

Williams et al. [54]	Unspecified	Average age 84.4 y, 82% women	PGC-PIS NRS	Pain: PGC-PIS ≥2 Supervisor report: 20%/23% Residents report: 39%/25% Any pain: Supervisor report: 62% Resident report: 76%	10 nursing homes 35 RC/AL facilities USA
Pautex et al. [39]	Unspecified	Average age 83.7 y, 69% women	Pain Self-report (direct question) McGill questionnaire	44%	Hospitalized patients Switzerland
Husebo et al. [22]	Head, mouth, neck: 24.7% Abdomen: 27.3% Pelvis, genitals: 29.9% Skin: 22.1%	Average age 84.1 y, 79% women Severe dementia	MOBID-2 Part 1	Any pain: 80.5%	Various care facilities Norway
Kamel et al. [27]	Unspecified	(a) Average age 81 y, 67% women (b) Average age 83, 84% women	(Direct question) Do you have pain? VAS B(F)S PDS	(a) 15% (b) 30%	2 academic nursing homes

Abbreviations: PACSLAC-D, pain assessment checklist for seniors with limited ability to communicate (Dutch language); MMSE, mini-mental state examination; RC/AL, residential care/assisted living; PEACE, palliative excellence in Alzheimer care efforts; VDS, verbal descriptor scale—pain; PAIN-AD, pain assessment in advanced dementia scale; PGC-PIS, Philadelphia geriatric center—pain intensity scale; NRS, numeric rating scale; MOBID-2, mobilization–observation–behavior-intensity-dementia; VAS, visual analog scale; B(F)S, behavior (faces) scale; PDS, pain descriptive scale.

IMPACT OF UNDETECTED PAIN

The difficulty in identifying pain in dementia patients must be considered carefully as the undertreatment of pain can have a major impact on those with limited expressive capacities. Dementia patients are consistently treated with less pain medication than patients with no communicative disabilities [32] (see also Chapter 18). Decreased life expectancy, increased risks of falls, sleep disorders, and appetite disturbance are linked with the undertreatment of pain over and above that due to deterioration of cognitive and physical abilities [6] (see also Chapter 3).

Pain contributes to aggressive behaviors; instances of verbal and physical aggression rise with persistent pain [20] (see also Chapter 7). Verbally agitated behaviors such as negativity, repetitive questions, and complaining are common [6]. Other nonaggressive behaviors such as repetitive mannerisms or persistent, restless pacing may be other manifestations of untreated pain. These are often treated with antipsychotics instead of with appropriate pain management, despite the many potential adverse side effects of psychotropic drugs [31, 40]. This highlights further the need for accurate pain assessment methods in dementia patients to avoid risks associated with inappropriate treatments.

A recent systematic review found that interventions conducted on people with dementia who exhibited these behaviors were effective in reducing the behavioral symptoms when the employed interventions targeted pain [40]. Behavioral symptoms of pain such as depression, aggression, and anxiety are all appropriate targets for intervention.

RISK FACTORS FOR PAIN IN DEMENTIA

Gender differences have been observed in many studies of pain perception involving healthy adults, with women commonly having a lower pain tolerance and threshold than do men and an increased prevalence of chronic pain [11, 43, 53]. However, little is known about gender as a risk factor for pain in dementia. A recent study conducted in Northern Ireland among 75 dementia patients did find an effect of gender on reports of pain "right now" [1]. Among the 42 women in the study, 63% expressed that they had pain at the time of assessment compared with 37% of male dementia patients. However, this relationship was not significant; only analgesic use was predictive of pain "right now."

Similar findings were observed in a Dutch nursing home study involving 23 male and 94 female dementia patients [60]. Multiple linear regression analysis revealed that gender was a significant predictor of pain, which was assessed using the pain assessment checklist for seniors with limited ability to communicate (PACSLAC-D) [13]. Women were found to be at higher risk of suffering from pain than their male counterparts, although this effect was weak in comparison to the predictive value of analgesic use and comorbidities. Other studies have not reported a link between gender and pain in dementia, for example, in a study on a sample of dementia patients admitted to general hospital [47]. Thus, there is some evidence that women with dementia may be at risk for pain, but this is far from conclusive.

Severity of dementia also suggests a possible risk factor for increased likelihood of having pain. Cross-sectional studies have found decreased pain prevalence among those with moderate and severe dementia in comparison with individuals with mild dementia [28, 40]. However, rather than reflecting a true reduction in risk, it may be the case that patients with severe dementia may be uncommunicative, with existing pain assessment scales proving inadequate for appropriate assessment of this population [12].

Evidence emerging from the literature appears to suggest that pain perception is affected in those with dementia, and the ability to process pain can be significantly altered in severe cases. One study that induced acute pain in the form of a venipuncture revealed that with increasing severity of dementia, physiological response (heart rate) became blunted, despite increased facial expressions [41]. Similarly, a longitudinal study revealed that increased severity of dementia was associated with lower incidence of headache after a lumbar puncture procedure, compared with those in the mild stage of dementia [18]. A recent review suggests that pain perception is decreased in those with severe dementia, but an experimental study conducted with mild to moderate AD showed no increase in pain tolerance to ice and a decrease in pain tolerance when mechanical pressure was applied [24] (see also Chapter 11).

In AD, the most common form of dementia, it has been suggested that limbic neuropathology affects areas of the brain important for pain processing [49]. These areas are responsible for the qualitative or motivational-affective aspect of the pain experience, while somatosensory cortical areas are relatively unaffected, meaning that acute painful stimuli can still be processed. This disruption is significant, as motivational-affective pain responding is likely to alert caregivers to pain that requires treatment [50]. A study of pain processes within the brain with fMRI technology [4] (see also Chapter 5) examined brain responses of younger and older adults, with and without AD. The study found increased rather than decreased pain-related activation in the regions responsible for affective and cognitive aspects of the pain experience. The authors noted that it is mostly individuals in the mild and moderate stages of dementia who are included in experimental research [15] and that qualitative pain processing regions may be better preserved in the early stages of dementia, and so pain perception is not overly distorted.

Appropriate, reliable, and valid assessment is essential then, if the relationship between severity of dementia and pain response is to be better understood, so that pain can be recognized and treated in individuals with dementia. Continuing research has put more emphasis on comprehensive and individual measurement, which may serve to increase our ability to recognize pain in the later stages of dementia [21].

Overall, the results from these studies suggest that degeneration in areas requiring motivational-affective pain processing leaves the individual unable to adequately process or prepare for painful events [48] but that this should not be interpreted as insensitivity to pain.

DIRECTIONS FOR FUTURE RESEARCH

Although there has been a relative abundance of research addressing the epidemiology of dementia and the epidemiology of chronic pain, there still remains a number of unanswered questions about the prevalence of these conditions among (a) people in developing countries, (b) people in minority populations, and (c) people in earlier stages of life. Furthermore, relatively little is known about risk factors and protective factors at a population level—for example, much remains to be understood about the relative importance of dietary factors, the role of environmental pollutants in disease onset, and the role of population-level interventions (whether biological or psychosocial) to prevent disease onset or to vary disease severity or course. These research questions are challenging because population-level research, because of its scale, is inherently expensive and complex—especially when translating findings from the population level to the individual level, and vice versa.

These challenges are magnified when considering pain and dementia as comorbid conditions. As a starting point, taking assessment as the first challenge, there is as yet no agreed tool for the identification of pain in dementia [42], although this is now the subject of a concerted international effort [5]. Then, having agreed a valid, reliable, and usable method for identifying pain in people with dementia, more research is needed regarding the most appropriate clinical management strategies [36]. Ideally, this should involve a stepped approach, beginning with relatively simple interventions (environmental and pharmacological) and progressing to more potent and/or multimodal interventions. The methods used to assess pain must then be evaluated to ascertain that they are suitably sensitive to detect and monitor responsiveness to interventions.

Considerable scope exists to evaluate either new technologies that will facilitate people with dementia to communicate their pain experience or automated systems that will alert caregivers to the likelihood of pain being present based on physiological indicators and facial expression analysis. Of course, this requires a better understanding of the variability in physiological and facial expression of pain in people with altered brain processing consequent to the dementia process. Registry research also serves as an additional tool to enhance the epidemiological information available regarding pain in dementia.

In conclusion, it is now well established that pain is a prevalent condition in the general population and that the chance of developing chronic pain increases with advancing age. Aging also brings a higher likelihood of developing dementia. Despite this double risk, the identification of pain in people with dementia remains quite challenging—especially when the dementia progresses and the capacity for meaningful verbal communication is lost. Further advances are needed in developing and evaluating pain detection tools, based on a range of approaches such as proxy reports, client self-report, and physiological indicators.

REFERENCES

1. Barry HE, Parsons C, Passmore AP, Hughes CM. Exploring the prevalence of and factors associated with pain: a cross-sectional study of community-dwelling people with dementia. Health Soc Care Community 2015;24:270–82. doi:10.1111/hsc.12204
2. Blyth FM, March LM, Barnabic AJ, Jorm LR, Williamson M, Cousins MJ. Chronic pain in Australia: a prevalence study. Pain 2001;89:127–34.
3. Breivik H, Collett B, Ventafridda V, Cohen R, Gallacher D. Survey of chronic pain in Europe: prevalence, impact on daily life, and treatment. Eur J Pain 2006;10:287–333.
4. Cole LJ, Farrell MJ, Duff EP, Barber JB, Egan GF, Gibson SJ. Pain sensitivity and fMRI pain-related brain activity in Alzheimer's disease. Brain. 2006;129:2957–65.
5. Corbett A, Achterberg W, Husebo B, Lobbezoo F, de Vet H, Kunz M, Strand L, Constantinou M, Tudose C, et al. An international road map to improve pain assessment in people with impaired cognition: the development of the Pain Assessment in Impaired Cognition (PAIC) tool. BMC Neurol 2014;14:229. doi:10.1186/s12883-014-0229-5
6. Corbett A, Husebo BS, Achterberg WP, Aarsland D, Erdal A, Flo E. The importance of pain management in older people with dementia. Br Med Bull 2014;111:139–48. doi:10.1093/bmb/ldu023
7. Dong MJ, Peng B, Lin XT, Zhao J, Zhou YR, Wang RH. The prevalence of dementia in the People's Republic of China: a systematic analysis of 1980–2004 studies. Age Ageing 2007;36:619–24. doi:10.1093/ageing/afm128
8. Ferrell BA, Ferrell BR, Rivera L. Pain in cognitively impaired nursing home patients. J Pain Symptom Manage 1995;10:591–8. doi:10.1016/0885-3924(95)00121-2
9. Farrell MJ, Katz B, Helme RD. The impact of dementia on the pain experience. Pain 1996;67:7–15. doi:10.1016/0304-3959(96)03041-2
10. Ferri CP, Prince M, Brayne C, Brodaty H, Fratiglioni L, Ganguli M, Hall K, Hasegawa K, Hendrie H, Huang Y, et al. Global prevalence of dementia: a Delphi consensus study. Lancet 2005;366:2112–7. doi:10.1016%2FS0140-6736(05)67889-0
11. Fillingim R. Sex, gender, and pain: women and men really are different. Curr Rev Pain 2000;4:24–30. doi:10.1007/s11916-000-0006-6
12. Frampton M. Experience assessment and management of pain in people with dementia. Age Ageing 2003;32:248–51.

13. Fuchs-Lacelle S, Hadjistavropoulos T. Development and preliminary validation of the pain assessment checklist for seniors with limited ability to communicate (PACSLAC). Pain Manage Nurs 2004;5:37–49.
14. Gibson SJ. IASP global year against pain in older persons: highlighting the current status and future perspectives in geriatric pain. Expert Rev Neurother 2007;7:627–35. doi:10.1586/14737175.7.6.627
15. Hadjistavropoulos T, Herr K, Prkachin, KM, Craig KD, Gibson SJ, Lukas A, Smith JH. Pain assessment in elderly adults with dementia. Lancet Neurol 2014;13:1216–27. doi:10.1016/S1474-4422(14)70103-6
16. Hebert LE, Weuve J, Scherr PA, Evans DA. Alzheimer disease in the United States (2010–2050) estimated using the 2010 census. Neurology 2013;80:1778–83. doi:10.1212/WNL.0b013e31828726f5
17. Herrera E Jr, Caramelli P, Silveira ASB, Nitrini R. Epidemiologic survey of dementia in a community-dwelling Brazilian population. Alzheimer Dis Assoc Disord 2002:16:103–8.
18. Hindley NJ, Jobst KA, King E, Barnetson L, Smith A, Haigh AM. High acceptability and low morbidity of diagnostic lumbar puncture in elderly subjects of mixed cognitive status. Acta Neurol Scand 1995;91:405–11. doi:10.1111/j.1600-0404.1995.tb07029.x
19. Horgas AL, Nichols AL, Schapson, CA, Vietes K. Assessing pain in persons with dementia: relationships among the non-communicative patient's pain assessment instrument, self-report, and behavioral observations. Pain Manag Nurs 2007;8:77–85. doi:10.1016/j.pmn.2007.03.003
20. Husebo BS, Ballard C, Sandvik R, Nilsen OB, Aarsland D. Efficacy of treating pain to reduce behavioural disturbances in residents of nursing homes with dementia: cluster randomised clinical trial. BMJ (Clin Res Ed) 2011;343:193. doi:10.1136/bmj.d4065
21. Husebo BS, Strand LI, Moe-Nilssen R, BorgeHusebo, S, Aarsland D, Ljunggren AE. Who suffers most? Dementia and pain in nursing home patients: a cross-sectional study. J Am Med Dir Assoc 2008;9:427–33. doi:10.1016/j.jamda.2008.03.001
22. Husebo BS, Strand LI, Moe-Nilssen R, Husebo SB, Ljunggren AE. Pain in older persons with severe dementia. Psychometric properties of the Mobilization-Observation-Behaviour-Intensity-Dementia (MOBID-2) pain scale in clinical setting. Scand J Caring Sci 2010;24:380–91.
23. International Association for the Study of Pain. Classification of chronic pain: descriptions of chronic pain syndromes and definitions of pain terms. Seattle: IASP Press; 1996.
24. Jensen-Dahm C, Werner MU, Dahl JB, Jensen TS, Ballegaard M, Hejl AM, Waldemar G. Quantitative sensory testing and pain tolerance in patients with mild to moderate Alzheimer disease compared to healthy control subjects. PAIN® 2014;155:1439–45.
25. Johannes CB, Kim Le T, Zhou X, Johnston JA, Dworkin RH. The prevalence of chronic pain in United States adults: results of an internet-based survey. J Pain 2010;11:1230–9. doi:10.1016/j.jpain.2010.07.002
26. Kalaria RN, Maestre GE, Arizaga R, Friedland RP, Galasko D, Hall K, Luchsinger A, Ogunniyi A, Perry E, Potocnik F, et al. Alzheimer's disease and vascular dementia in developing countries: prevalence, management, and risk factors. Lancet Neurol 2008;7:812–826. doi:10.1016/S1474-4422(08)70169-8
27. Kamel HK, Phlavan M, Malekgoudarzi B, Gogel P, Morley JE. Utilizing pain assessment scales increases the frequency of diagnosing pain among elderly nursing home residents. J Pain Symptom Manage 2001;21:450–5. doi:10.1016/S0885-3924(01)00287-1
28. Kunz M, Mylius V, Scharmann S, Karsten Schepelman SL. Influence of dementia on multiple components of pain. Eur J Pain 2009;13:317–25.
29. Kunz M, Scharmann S, Hemmeter U, Karsten Schepelmann SL. The facial expression of pain in patients with dementia. Pain 2007;133:221–8.
30. Leong IY, Nuo TH. Prevalence of pain in nursing home residents with different cognitive and communicative abilities. Clin J Pain 2007;23:119–27.
31. Locca JF, Büla CJ, Zumbach S, Bugnon O. Pharmacological treatment of Behavioral and Psychological Symptoms of Dementia (BPSD) in nursing homes: development of practice recommendations in a Swiss Canton. J Am Med Dir Assoc 2008;9:439–48. doi:10.1016/j.jamda.2008.04.003
32. Lukas A, Schuler M, Fischer TW, Gibson SJ, Savvas SM, Nikolaus T, Denkinger M. Pain and dementia: a diagnostic challenge. Z Gerontol Geriatr 2012;45:45–9. doi:10.1007/s00391-011-0272-4
33. Mäntyselkä P, Äntyselkä PEM, Artikainen SIH, Aako KILO, Ulkava RAS. Effects of dementia on perceived daily pain in home-dwelling elderly people : a population-based study. Age Ageing 2004;33:496–9. doi:10.1093/ageing/afh165
34. Markey G, Rabbani W, Kelly P. 022: association of dementia with delayed ED analgesia in patients over 70 with acute musculoskeletal injury. Emerg Med J 2013;30:875.
35. McAuliffe L, Brown D, Fetherstonhaugh D. Pain and dementia: an overview of the literature. Int J Older People Nurs 2012;7:219–26. doi:10.1111/j.1748-3743.2012.00331.x

36. McGuire BE, Nicholas MK, Asghari A, Wood BM, Main CJ. Psychological interventions for pain in older adults: Cautious optimism and an agenda for research. Curr Opin Psych 2014:27;380–84.
37. Onyike CU, Diehl-Schmid J. The epidemiology of frontotemporal dementia. Int Rev Psychiatry 2013;25:130–7. doi:10.3109/09540261.2013.776523.
38. Ott A, Breteler MM, van Harskamp F, Claus JJ, van der Cammen TJ, Grobbee DE, Hofman A. Prevalence of Alzheimer's disease and vascular dementia: association with education. The Rotterdam study. BMJ (Clin Res Ed) 1995;310:970–3. doi:10.1136/bmj.310.6985.970
39. Pautex S, Michon A, Guedira M, Emond H, Le Lous P, Samaras D, Michel JP, Herrmann F, Giannakopoulos P, Gold G. Pain in severe dementia: self-assessment or observational scale. J Am Geriatric Soc 2006;54:1040–45. doi:10.1111/j.1532-5415.2006.00766.x
40. Pieper MJC, van Dalen-Kok AH, Francke AL, van der Steen JT, Scherder EJ, Husebø BS, Achterberg WP. Interventions targeting pain or behaviour in dementia: a systematic review. Ageing Res Rev 2013;12:1042–55. doi:10.1016/j.arr.2013.05.002
41. Porter FL, Malhotra K, Wolf CM, Morris JC, Miller JP, Smith MC. Dementia and response to pain in the elderly. Pain 1996;68:413–21.
42. Proctor WR, Hirdes JP. Pain and cognitive status among nursing home residents in Canada. Pain Res Manag 2001;6:119–25.
43. Racine M, Tousignant-Laflamme Y, Kloda L. A systematic literature review of 10 years of research on sex/gender and pain perception—Part 2: do biopsychosocial factors alter pain sensitivity differently in women. Pain 2012;153:602–18. doi:10.1016/j.pain.2011.11.025
44. Ratnavalli E, Brayne C, Dawson K, Hodges JR. The prevalence of frontotemporal dementia. Neurol 2002;58:1615–21.
45. Reitsma ML, Tranmer JE, Buchanan DM, Vandenkerkhof EG. Prevalence of chronic pain and pain-related interference in the Canadian population from 1994 to 2008. Chronic Dis Inj Can 2011;31:157–164.
46. Rothman KJ. Epidemiology: an introduction. Oxford: Oxford University Press; 2012.
47. Sampson E, White N, Lord K, Leurent B. Pain, agitation, and behavioural problems in people with dementia admitted to general hospital wards: a longitudinal cohort study. Pain 2015;156:675–83. doi: 10.1097/j.pain.0000000000000095
48. Scherder EJ, Oosterman J, Swaab D, Herr K, Ooms M, Ribbe M, Sergeant J, Pickering G, Benedetti F. Recent developments in pain in dementia. BMJ 2005;330:461–64. doi:10.1136/bmj.330.7489.461
49. Scherder EJ, Sergeant JA, Swaab DF. Pain processing in dementia and its relation to neuropathology. The Lancet Neurology. 2003;2:677–86. doi:10.1016/S1474-4422(03)00556-8
50. Sewards TV, Sewards MA. The medial pain system: neural representations of the motivational aspect of pain. Brain Res Bull 2002;59:163–80. doi:10.1016/S0361-9230(02)00864-X
51. Shega JW, Hougham GW, Stocking CB, Cox-Hayley D, Sachs G. Pain in community-dwelling persons with dementia: frequency, intensity, and congruence between patient and caregiver report. J Pain Symptom Manage 2004;28:585–92. doi:10.1016/j.jpainsymman.2004.04.012
52. Tsang A, Von Korff M, Lee S, Alonso J, Karam E, Angermeyer MC, Borges G, Bromet EJ, de Girolamo G, de Graaf R, et al. Common persistent pain conditions in developed and developing countries: gender and age differences and comorbidity with depression-anxiety disorders. J Pain 2008;9:883–91.
53. Wiesenfeld-Hallin Z. Sex differences in pain perception. Gend Med 2005;2:137–45. doi:10.1016/S1550-8579(05)80042-7
54. Williams CS, Zimmerman S, Sloane PD, Reed P. Characteristics associated with pain in long-term care residents with dementia. Gerontologist 2005;45:68–73. doi:10.1093/geront/45.suppl_1.96
55. Wong WS, Fielding R. Prevalence and characteristics of chronic pain in the general population of Hong Kong. J Pain 2011;12:236–45. doi:10.1016/j.jpain.2010.07.004
56. World Health Organization. Dementia: a public health priority. Geneva: World Health Organization; 2012.
57. Yamada T, Hattori H, Miura A, Tanabe M, Yamori Y. Prevalence of Alzheimer's disease, vascular dementia and dementia with Lewy bodies in a Japanese population. Psychiatry Clin Neurosci 2001;55:21–5. doi:10.1046/j.1440-1819.2001.00779.x
58. Zhang Z, Roman GC, Hong Z, Wu CB, Qu QM, Huang JB, Zhou B, Geng ZP, Wu JX, Wen HB, et al. Parkinson's disease in China: prevalence in Beijing, Xian, and Shanghai. Lancet 2005;365:595–7. doi:10.1016/S0140-6736(05)17909-4
59. Zwakhalen SMG, Hamers JPH, Berger MPF. The psychometric quality and clinical usefulness of three pain assessment tools for elderly people with dementia. Pain 2006;126:210–20.
60. Zwakhalen SMG, Koopmans R, Geels P, Berger M, Hamers J. The prevalence of pain in nursing home residents with dementia measured using an observational pain scale. Eur J Pain 2009;13:89–93. doi:10.1016/j.ejpain.2008.02.009

CHAPTER 5

Central Pathophysiology of Dementia and Pain

Michael J. Farrell and Leonie J. Cole

The experience of pain is a function of the brain. Dementia occurs as a result of brain dysfunction, which has the potential to interact with pain processing. It is feasible to make inferences about the likely impact of dementia on pain processing by comparing the functional neuroanatomy of pain with the regional expression of pathology in those diseases that cause cognitive impairment, and other chapters touch on these issues. The primary objective of this chapter is to review the literature of neuroimaging as it relates to pain and dementia. The first part of this chapter will focus on studies involving neuroimaging techniques that have a bearing on interactions between dementia and regional brain responses associated with pain. The second part of the chapter will discuss the possibility that neuroimaging techniques could be used to identify pain in nonverbal people with dementia.

INTERACTIONS BETWEEN DEMENTIA AND REGIONAL BRAIN RESPONSES TO PAINFUL STIMULATION

Other chapters in this book address the dementia syndrome, dementia-related disorders, neuropsychological features of dementia, the functional neuroanatomy of pain processing, and hypothesized interactions between dementia-related disorders and the experience of pain. A general conclusion from these discussions is that the multifactorial nature of dementia and the multiple dimensions of pain are unlikely to intersect in a unitary manner. Indeed, it is possible to hypothesize exacerbation of pain, attenuation of pain, or no change in pain experience among people with dementia depending on contingencies such as dementia-related pathology and environmental factors. It is important to investigate the complexities of dementia and pain because the implications for management could be profoundly different depending on the nature of putative interactions. Neuroimaging techniques are a viable way to gather empirical information about the impact of dementia-related disorders on the brain, the representation of pain in the brain, and how dementia influences central pain processing. This section of the chapter will discuss findings from neuroimaging techniques that relate to these issues. The focus will be on Alzheimer disease (AD) because this disorder, the single most common cause of dementia [22], has been the subject of extensive neuroimaging research [36], whereas the literature pertaining to other dementia-related disorders is less mature.

Neuroimaging of Alzheimer Disease

The last two decades have seen substantial developments in the application of neuroimaging techniques to the investigation of AD. Both positron emission tomography (PET) and magnetic resonance imaging (MRI) have contributed to these advances [1]. The spatial resolutions of the techniques makes it possible to characterize the regional distribution of pathological changes in the brains of people with dementia, which may suggest possible intersections with pain processing regions.

The staging of AD has a major bearing on the outcomes of neuroimaging studies [36]. For instance, contrasts between images of AD-related pathology and healthy brains have fidelity for case identification even before cognitive impairment has been detected. PET images using Pittsburgh compound-B (PiB) to identify beta-amyloid deposits in the brain reveal differences between people at increased risk of AD and controls many years before the onset of cognitive impairment would be expected to occur [50]. Measures of brain hypometabolism made with [^{18}F]-fluorodeoxyglucose–PET and regional decreases in gray matter density measured with MRI are also apparent in preclinical patients of AD, albeit at later times compared to the earliest differences seen with PiB imaging [10]. People with mild cognitive impairment (MCI) show decreased levels of connectivity between brain regions measured with functional MRI (fMRI) suggesting decrements of processing capacity are also apparent before a diagnosis of dementia has been made [26, 68]. Ultimately, dementia and accompanying deficits of cognition lead to changes in regional brain activations during the performance of cognitive tasks, most notably involving memory [64]. However, these changes cannot be characterized simply as decreases. Networks of activation related to cognition in patients with AD often include novel regional responses that have been interpreted as compensation for decrements of processing elsewhere in the brain [13, 64].

Of primary interest for this chapter in the context of dementia neuroimaging are the regional expressions of brain changes associated with dementia-related pathologies in clinical patients. Different imaging methods are more or less likely to be informative when considering the potential for dementia-related pathologies to interact with regions processing pain.

Levels of PiB throughout the brains of people with AD are so pronounced as to have questionable utility as a marker of regional disease expression. The amyloid hypothesis suggests that accumulation of the compound is the earliest step in a series of detrimental effects that eventually lead to cognitive impairment, at which time amyloid levels are very high, but of lesser relevance to subsequent neurodegeneration [37, 38]. Indeed, PiB measures do not show substantial changes in longitudinal or cross sectional comparisons among AD patients with varied levels of cognitive impairment [39]. While the evidence implicating amyloid in AD is undeniable, drawing inferences about regional decrements of brain function on the basis of PiB levels in AD patients may not be applicable when considering pain processing.

Ultimately, it is the loss of functional, interconnected neurons that leads to failing capacity in the brains of people with dementia. Decreased density of neurons is likely to result in atrophy of the gray matter and reduced levels of metabolic activity, both of which can be assessed with neuroimaging. Studies using MRI to compare brain morphology between AD patients and controls have been reported by many independent groups. The volume of this literature has now reached a level where meta-analyses of morphological studies can be undertaken using empirical methods such as anatomical likelihood estimation. A recent meta-analysis of voxel-based comparisons between patients and controls was able to draw upon data collected from 2394 participants from 35 separate studies to characterize the regional distribution of gray matter loss in people with AD [77]. The results of the analysis revealed

AD-related atrophy bilaterally in the hippocampii, parahippocampii, amgdalae, medial thalami, caudate, ventromedial prefrontal cortex, precuneus/posterior cingulate, posterior parietal cortices and inferior frontal gyri. This distribution of atrophy is very similar to the regions implicated in AD-related hypometabolism by studies using glucose-PET. The most consistent findings across all studies, irrespective of imaging method are AD-related changes in medial temporal structures, of which the hippocampus is the most prominent.

Outcomes of fMRI studies of memory-related tasks in AD patients and controls have been subject to meta-analysis using activity likelihood estimation [13, 64]. The general conclusion from these analyses is that medial temporal regions show consistent decrements of memory-related function in people with AD, which is wholly compatible with the morphological and metabolic changes seen in this clinical group. Increased levels of task-related activation are also a feature of AD, and are consistently seen bilaterally in the prefrontal cortices [13, 64]. This increase of regional activation is presumably related to compensatory processes. Importantly, the probability and location of such compensatory responses would not be predicted on the basis of AD-related pathology in the brain. The implications of this observation are that pain processing could feasibly incorporate activation in unexpected regions in people with AD if these putative compensatory effects generalize beyond memory tasks.

Additional effects of AD on brain function could have implications for pain processing. Specifically, AD is associated with decrements of inter-regional connectivity. fMRI measures collected from participants lying in a scanner at rest show low frequency fluctuations that reliably occur in distributed networks. There are multiple resting state networks [67], of which the default mode network (DMN) has received the most empirical attention. The DMN is notable for deactivating during tasks and activating during rest [58]. The network includes mesial structures (ventromedial prefrontal cortex, posterior cingulate cortex, precuneus) and the lateral posterior parietal cortices. The functional role of spontaneous signal fluctuations in the DMN is not clear [44], but current views hold that the correlated activity represents introspection and mind wandering [47, 69]. It is notable that memory retrieval tasks activate the same regions [73]. The prefrontal and posterior elements of the DMN are among the regions that show morphological and metabolic decrements in AD, and consequently it is not surprising that regions within the DMN show decreased levels of functional connectivity at rest in people with AD compared to controls [28]. However, AD is not the only disorder that is associated with decreased DMN activity. People with other neurological disorders, such as multiple sclerosis [60], as well as psychiatric disorders [14] and other illnesses [51] have shown impairment of the DMN. Importantly, clinical pain is also associated with decreased activity in the DMN [5].

The overarching conclusion from a synthesis of neuroimaging outcomes in AD is that the regional expression of the disease is most pronounced in the medial temporal lobes, medial thalamus, medial frontal and parietal cortices, and the lateral posterior parietal cortices.

Brain Regions Implicated in Pain Processing

There is a wealth of neuroimaging studies examining pain processing in the human brain, and excellent reviews have been written on varied aspects of this literature [3, 72]. Of critical interest for this chapter is the location of brain regions implicated in pain processing because this information can be integrated with outcomes from dementia neuroimaging to identify points of intersection. An important distinction to be made when considering neuroimaging studies of pain is the difference between experimental and clinical contexts.

Studies involving functional brain imaging of responses to noxious experimental stimuli predominate the literature and provide a rich source of information about the location of regional brain responses under the circumstances of relatively short duration pain. Neuroimaging outcomes that implicate brain regions in processes related to the experience of spontaneous, ongoing clinical pain are much less frequently reported in the literature.

Regional Brain Responses to Experimental Pain

Functional brain imaging studies of experimental pain have identified a widely distributed network of brain regions that show responses to noxious stimulation. The components of the pain network that have support from meta-analyses of activation studies are the thalamus, anterior midcingulate cortex (aMCC), insula, primary and secondary somatosensory cortex, right inferior parietal cortex, premotor cortex, prefrontal cortex, lentiform nuclei and cerebellum [18, 21, 23, 31, 45, 62].

Components of the pain network appear more or less frequently in simple contrasts of activity between noxious stimulation and an innocuous or no-stimulus control. For instance, the insula and aMCC are almost invariably reported in pain activation studies, whereas the primary somatosensory cortex activates less reliably. Many factors can modulate responses to noxious stimulation, a discussion of which extends beyond the scope of this chapter. However, modulation of pain responses can be contingent on activation in brain regions that are not principle components of the pain network. These modulation-related regions include the dorsolateral prefrontal cortex, the pregenual cingulate cortex and brainstem regions such as the periaqueductal gray (PAG) and the rostroventral medulla [12, 40]. It is important to consider these regions when assessing the possible impact of dementia-related disorders because impairments of modulation could influence the expression of endogenous analgesia or hyperalgesia.

Recently reported investigations have expanded the list of brain regions implicated in pain processing. Perhaps counter intuitively, regions that deactivate during pain and show activity in non-pain periods have an influence on the experience of pain and levels of activation in the pain network during stimulation. This complex example of network dynamics warrants explanation in the current context because the regions involved are the DMN, which is adversely affected by AD. Independent groups have noted that regions in the DMN deactivate during pain, which is also the case during most tasks or stimuli. However, a recent study reported that the levels of activation in the DMN prior to painful stimulation predicts subsequent levels of pain intensity and regional brain responses [48]. A second study has found that the DMN becomes more active (less deactivated) during noxious stimulation when participants' minds wander away from the pain, and that functional connectivity between the DMN and the PAG is enhanced when attention is focused elsewhere [41]. The implication of these findings is that coordinated activity in brain regions independent of the pain network can influence the perceptual significance of stimuli and consequently shape the experience of pain. It is possible to speculate that failure of these network dynamics could lead to an impairment of the ability to disengage from noxious events.

Representation of Clinical Pain in the Brain

Functional brain imaging studies of clinical pain appear very rarely in the literature. The paucity of published studies relates to a mismatch between the execution of neuroimaging techniques and the behavior of spontaneous pain. Functional brain imaging is dependent on contrasts between different states that highlight regions where signals increase during a task or stimulus of interest compared to an alternative control period. Spontaneous pain may not conveniently turn on and off nor vary in predictable ways that permit meaningful tests of signal changes measured with functional brain imaging techniques such as fMRI and PET. However, there are some contingencies where clinical pain can be manipulated or varies naturally in ways that can be exploited with functional brain imaging. It is important to consider the outcomes of these studies because the brain regions implicated in clinical pain are not a simple recapitulation of regions identified in studies of experimental pain.

Functional brain imaging studies of clinical pain have included patients with neuropathic and musculoskeletal conditions [4, 6, 24, 29, 34, 42, 56, 76]. Activation has been identified in these groups by modeling spontaneous fluctuations in pain or by contrasting states before and after a manipulation to relieve or exacerbate pain. Differences are apparent between studies, but the outcomes have generally identified a medial/prefrontal network including the ventromedial prefrontal/pregenual cingulate cortices, amygdala, hippocampus, nucleus accumbens and orbitofrontal cortex. These regions are typically ascribed with a role in cognitive/emotional states and reward processing. It is notable that regions including the amygdala and hippocampus are also implicated in animal studies of persistent nociceptive and neuropathic pain [52, 53]. The distinction between outcomes in clinical pain states versus experimental pain models suggests that pain can change over time such that an early emphasis on discriminative aspects is replaced by an experience with emotional overtones, and that these changes stem from processes related to conditioning and learning. A very recent report of cross sectional and longitudinal changes in pain activation involving large cohorts of healthy controls, and subacute and chronic low back pain patients lends support to the evolution of clinical pain processing over time [29]. Furthermore, when compared to controls, brain morphology in chronic pain patients shows regional differences that are compatible with a medial/frontal shift in pain processing [66].

Intersections between Dementia-Related Brain Changes and Pain Processing Regions

Neuroimaging has identified the regional distribution of pathology and related functional changes in AD, as well as characterizing the networks of activation associated with experimental and clinical pain. Comparisons of the respective neuroanatomies of AD and pain networks highlights several points of intersection that allow for tentative hypotheses about the likely impact of dementia on central pain processing during experimental and clinical pain.

Experimental Pain and Dementia-Related Changes in the Brain

The first strain of information that has a bearing on speculative interactions between pain and dementia is the outcome of studies involving PET imaging with PiB. Intuitively, a neuroimaging index of amyloid load would be expected to provide insights into the development and regional expression of AD-related pathology with important implications for understanding how dementia might interact with pain. However, while amyloid levels may be especially useful for understanding the early, preclinical course of AD, PiB signal from clinical patients has less utility. The amyloid cascade hypothesis suggests that the adverse consequences of the substance are expressed early in the disease, and that subsequent accumulation of amyloid is not necessarily a good index of the later stages of pathology that drive decrements of brain function [36]. There are significant implications of this theory for the formulation of putative intersections between AD and pain processing. The widespread distribution of PiB levels in the brains of people with AD, and the lack of correlation between these levels and brain function would suggest that hypotheses about AD-related effects on pain processing based on amyloid plaque distributions could over-estimate intersections between the regional effects of AD and pain processing regions.

There is good correspondence between regional distributions of morphological changes in the brains of people with AD, evidence of hypometabolism and decrements of functional activation. The most parsimonious explanation for these consistent outcomes is that the neuroimaging modalities are sensitive to a common factor: AD-related neuronal loss. AD-related structural changes in the brain measured with MRI have been most frequently replicated and the amalgamation of these studies provides acceptable spatial information that can be compared with similarly reproducible experimental pain activation studies. The overwhelming impression of such a comparison is that almost all the regions activated during experimental pain are not involved in AD-related pathology. The single exception to this general observation is the medial thalamus.

The medial thalamus is mutually connected to pain processing regions including the aMCC and the anterior insula. Studies involving hypnosis and psychophysical procedures to create independent variance in the intensity and unpleasantness of pain have implicated the aMCC in pain unpleasantness [59, 70]. However, other studies also highlight the role of the aMCC in autonomic and skeletal motor responses to stimuli akin to, and including pain [7, 49, 57]. It is feasible that activation in the aMCC during experimental pain could represent processes related to both afferent and efferent functions, which conforms to the notions that this brain region plays an integrative role in motivated action [74]. The other pain region with medial thalamic connections is the anterior insula, as distinct to the posterior regions of the insula that receive inputs from the ventral posterior thalamus and likely play a role in somatosensory processing. The anterior insula often co-activates with the aMCC and it has been suggested that the region contributes to bodily awareness, or interoception [17]. The implications of AD-related atrophy of the medial thalamus is that relays of nociceptive inputs to the aMCC and anterior insula are likely to be impaired, which could lead to a failure of pain-related autonomic/skeletal motor responses, distorted awareness of threats to bodily integrity and impairment of affective responses [63]. However, it is important to note that the aMCC and anterior insula are not among the regions showing consistent AD-related changes in morphology and metabolism despite putative reductions in thalamic inputs.

The influence of AD on the morphology, metabolism and levels of inter-regional connectivity in the DMN has implications for pain processing, albeit in ways that could both increase and decrease pain-related activation in response to experimental stimuli. Higher levels of activation in the DMN at the moment of stimulus presentation are associated with increased pain compared to times when stimuli are preceded by relatively lower levels of DMN activation [48]. Consequently, an impairment of DMN functional connectivity in AD patients would be expected to reduce variability in pain reports to repeated stimuli and possibly lead to lower peak levels of evoked pain compared to healthy people. In contradistinction, enhanced levels of DMN activity during the course of painful stimulation is associated with recruitment of pain modulation regions and decreased pain report [41]. This apparent benefit of the mind wandering away during painful events may be impaired in AD patients. On balance, the impairment of intrinsic processes that permit disengagement from pain and down-regulate nociceptive inputs may have more functional consequences than impairments that are likely to constrain variability of responses.

Functional brain imaging studies of cognition have consistently noted activations in novel regions among people with AD [13, 64]. Interpreted as compensatory responses, it is possible to speculate that novel activations could also be a feature of the pain network in people with AD. However, this speculation does not readily suggest testable hypotheses about differences in regional brain responses to pain in people with AD.

Clinical Pain and Dementia-Related Changes in the Brain

The integration of neuroimaging outcomes from investigations of AD and clinical pain suggest that there is substantial overlap in the regions implicated in AD pathology and clinical pain processing. Of special note are reports of clinical pain activation in those medial temporal regions including the hippocampus and amygdala that are most adversely affected in AD. Additionally, clinical pain and AD intersect in the ventromedial prefrontal cortex.

Hypotheses about the consequences of medial temporal and prefrontal neuronal loss for the experience of clinical pain in patients with AD are difficult to formulate because the role of these mesial structures in pain processing are not well described. Classic views hold that the hippocampus is the principle brain region involved in memory [65], that the amygdala is important for the formation of memories associated with emotional events [46], and that the ventromedial prefrontal cortex links episodic memory with affective qualities of sensory events [61]. Prevailing theories of clinical pain emphasize a developmental role for the medial temporal and prefrontal regions in the transition from acute to chronic pain that involves associative learning [2]. It has been argued that pain after an injury or onset of a disease contributes to a state of continuous learning, in which aversive emotional associations are continuously made with incidental events simply due to the persistent presence of pain. In other words, pain is experienced during everyday activities and consequently associations are formed between the activities and the emotional states accompanying pain. The associations are repeatedly reinforced so long as pain persists, thus affording scant opportunity to extinguish links between pain-related emotions and daily life. Activations in mesolimbic regions during clinical pain presumably represent persistent associative processes contributing to an emotional state that characterizes pain in the chronic pain patient.

Extrapolating theories of clinical pain as an associative state to the experience of people with AD would suggest that dementia could interfere with the development of chronic pain. Failing memory capacity is accompanied by a loss of conditioned learning in people with AD [33], and this loss of function could impair the formation of associative links between pain and other behaviors or environments. A lack of pain association would presumably reduce the likelihood of pain persisting after recovery from injury or disease, or lead to the experience of persistent pain as a prolonged acute condition in the context of chronic disease (e.g., postherpetic neuralgia, osteoarthritis) in people with AD.

Neuroimaging of Pain in People with AD

The preceding discussions have integrated findings from the neuroimaging of AD and pain to generate hypotheses about how dementia could impact on the experience of pain. Neuroimaging also has the potential to test these hypotheses by contrasting pain activations between healthy people and AD patients. However, despite a strong rationale to investigate pain processing in AD patients using neuroimaging, examples of this approach have rarely appeared in the scientific literature.

Neuroimaging studies of pain processing in AD are confined to experimental pain. Electroencephalography (EEG) has been measured in studies involving painful stimuli and AD patients. Most of these studies used EEG recordings to estimate dementia-related effects on brain function, as opposed to measuring pain-related brain activation [8, 9]. There is one reported study that compared pain ratings and evoked responses measured with EEG (nociceptive evoked responses, NER) to brief laser stimuli applied to the dorsum of the hand in healthy older people and AD patients [25]. The two groups of participants had comparable pain thresholds and gave similar pain ratings to a fixed, supra-threshold stimulus. The peak of the NER at approximately 450 milliseconds post stimulus had a significantly longer latency in the AD participants compared to the healthy controls, but was of a similar magnitude in the two groups. This peak is thought to represent the earliest cognitive processes involved in the appraisal of nociceptive inputs. The authors proposed that the delay in the peak represented a slowing of cortical processing in participants with AD, but the possibility also exists that the increased latency could reflect sustained attention associated with impaired ability to disengage from a novel stimulus.

Two reports of a single fMRI study involving blood oxygen level-dependent (BOLD) contrast images acquired during experimental pain in AD patients and older healthy controls have appeared in the scientific literature [15, 16]. Hypothesized decrements of pain-related activation in the medial thalamus and connected cortical regions in the AD group were not apparent. Indeed, the medial thalamus, aMCC and insula all showed levels of pain activation in the AD group that exceed responses in the healthy participants [15]. Increased pain activation in the AD group was also seen in other regions not notable for being affected by dementia-related pathology including the dorsolateral prefrontal cortex, premotor regions, primary somatosensory/motor cortex, lentiform nuclei and cerebellum. Hemodynamic responses from regions showing group differences revealed two distinct temporal patterns of response during the 30-second stimulus blocks. BOLD signal increases in the healthy participants occurred with an expected delay to peak approximately 6 seconds after stimulus onset and then returned toward baseline levels well before stimulus offset, which is a temporal pattern that characterizes pain-related activation in younger samples [35, 43]. In contradistinction to the healthy older controls, hemodynamic responses in the AD group showed sustained levels of BOLD signal increase during stimulation blocks. A further analysis of BOLD signal correlations between activated regions in the two groups revealed that the pain network had higher levels of functional connectivity in the AD group compared to the healthy controls [16]. The authors interpreted the differences between the groups as probably due to sustained attention to the noxious stimulation among the participants with AD. Earlier discussions herein, based on more recently published pain neuroimaging studies would suggest that this inability to disengage from the painful stimuli could be due to decrements of function of the DMN in AD patients.

CONCLUSION

Neuroimaging of pain and the neuroimaging of AD have both developed substantially over the last decade. However, this development has occurred almost exclusively in parallel, with very few reports of pain neuroimaging performed in people with dementia. Synthesizing the literatures of pain and AD neuroimaging suggest intersections between the two that could have implications for acute and clinical pain processing in people with dementia.

In particular, it is possible to hypothesize that people with dementia could have difficulty disengaging from experimental pain, may show impairments in interoceptive awareness, and could fail to demonstrate associative learning in the development of chronic pain. At present, there is some empirical support for sustained attention to experimental pain in AD. Future studies will be required to test other hypotheses that arise from the integration of pain and AD neuroimaging.

MEASURING PAIN WITH NEUROIMAGING

Pain is a latent experience known only to the sufferer. Language can convey personal experience, and verbal report is the gold standard for pain measurement. However, language impairment in people with dementia precludes verbal report as a method to identify and characterize pain. Strategies to detect and quantify pain in nonverbal dementia patients using behavioral measures and career reports have been developed, although testing the validity of the strategies is confounded by the absence of self-report as a benchmark [27, 32]. An alternative approach might be to use neuroimaging techniques to identify pain in nonverbal dementia patients. The second section of this chapter will briefly review recent developments in neuroimaging and discuss the viability of the technique for identifying endogenous pain experiences.

Reframing the Neuroimaging Question

Neuroimaging techniques with applicability to the pain experience, such as fMRI and PET, are primarily used to investigate brain function. The usual objective of experiments involving neuroimaging is to ascribe function to brain regions. This objective is achieved by manipulating participants' behavior through the application of stimuli or imposition of tasks, and concurrently measuring signals from participants' brains. Analyses of the measured signals focus on changes that would be expected to occur in association with the stimulus or task. If the signal from a brain region reliably increases whenever a stimulus is applied or a task is performed then the region has shown stimulus-related or task-related activation, and this activation is interpreted as evidence for a functional role of the region in the behaviors implicated by the experimental paradigm.

The identification of pain activation can be readily appreciated. Measures of brain signals are made from participants at times when the experimenter is applying a painful stimulus and at times when the painful stimulus is not applied. The brain signals are measured from many small volumes, or voxels, that vary in size according to imaging technique, and are in the range of 15–50 mm^3. The signals from each voxel are analyzed separately to find regions where the average signal intensities measured during painful stimulation are significantly greater than the average signals measured during periods when painful stimulation wasn't applied. A threshold of significance is applied to decide which voxels are showing sufficient changes in signals to constitute "pain activation". This experimental rationale can be summarized by the following statement and question:

> You have pain.
> Where is the pain activation in your brain?

Using neuroimaging to identify clinical pain in a patient with dementia is not equivalent to the methods used in experimental studies of brain function. Experimental studies start with behavior (e.g., apply painful stimulation) to infer brain activation. Scanning a person to determine the presence or absence of clinical pain would involve reverse engineering of the experimental paradigm. In other words, the objective is to identify pain activation and then infer the behavior. Here is the rationale summarized in two statements:

There is pain activation in your brain.
You have pain.

At face value, it appears that the identification of pain in nonverbal people using neuroimaging should be possible by simply reversing the order of procedures that are typically used in functional brain imaging experiments. In reality, there are idiosyncrasies and constraints of neuroimaging that make reverse engineering difficult to achieve. At this juncture the problem has not been solved, but progress is being made. The following discussions will provide more detail of the nature of the problem and the methods being developed to make pain measurement with neuroimaging possible.

Activation is Relative and Non-exclusive

Signals measured from a voxel during neuroimaging do not imply activity or inactivity per se. Indeed, signal intensities using some methods (e.g., BOLD contrast images acquired for fMRI) have no measurement unit. Other methods can be used to estimate quantifiable units [e.g., mL/100 g/min of regional cerebral blood flow (rCBF) measured with PET H_2O^{15}] but activity or inactivity cannot be inferred from the intensity level of these measures. Activation, in the parlance of neuroimaging, is a statistical procedure that involves modeling variance in signals across time. Thus, it is how a signal changes from measurement to measurement, rather than the intensity of the signal at any single measurement that determines if activation has occurred. Furthermore, signals from a voxel can show more than one type of activation at the same time. A notional experiment demonstrates how activations can occur concurrently. A participant is scanned for 10 minutes during alternating 30 second blocks of painful stimulation and no-stimulation. Electrodermal responses are also measured to identify the onset of sweating events. Pain activation under the conditions of this experiment would be defined as increased signal intensity during stimulus periods compared to no-stimulus periods. Sweating activation would be defined as signal increases that occur whenever the participant sweats compared to all other time points. It is entirely possible that signals measured from a single voxel could incorporate variance that was consistent with both pain and sweating activation, and that the voxel would consequently be ascribed with a role in both functions. Voxels are likely to contain many neurons with heterogeneous functions that can variously contribute to the processes that give rise to the signals measured with neuroimaging. Consequently, the observation of signal increases measured from a single voxel cannot be used to imply a particular function because multiple functional processes could feasibly produce the signal changes. In other words, fluctuations of signal intensity have no intrinsic meaning, and only become informative when an explanation for the fluctuations are provided by additional information such as the timing of extrinsic stimuli and task performance.

Beyond Voxel-Wise Analyses

The preceding discussion highlighted the fact that variance in signals measured from a voxel in the brain could be due to multiple functional processes, which precludes inferences being drawn about any single function, such as pain processing. However, identifying a pain signature becomes feasible when signals from voxels are assessed collectively, rather than individually. The approach involves a search among many voxels for patterns of relative signal change that are unique to a particular functional process. The technique has been popularly described as "brain reading" or "mind reading," but is more accurately referred to as multivoxel pattern analysis (MVPA) [54].

The development of MVPA, like many other innovations in functional brain imaging, occurred in the field of visual neuroscience. In these experiments, participants view varied visual stimuli on many occasions during the acquisition of fMRI data. The experimenters then search for reproducible patterns of signal intensities across multiple voxels for each of the visual stimuli. The absolute intensity of any given voxel is not important for this process. Instead, it is the consistency of relative signal intensities among an identified grouping of voxels time locked to a specific stimulus that is required. The utilities of the multivoxel patterns are tested by presenting the visual stimuli to participants in a second scanning session and then predicting which visual stimulus was being presented at any given time. Early demonstrations of the method provided impressive levels of accuracy [30].

MVPA has been applied to brain functions other than visual processing including attentional processing, imagery, working memory, decision-making, and language [71]. The approach has also been used to decode responses to experimental pain. The earliest application of MVPA to pain involved near threshold laser stimuli with the objective of finding response patterns that distinguished painful from nonpainful experiences [11]. The accuracy of prediction was only modest, and certainly not sufficient to have clinical utility. However, the most recent application of MVPA to pain decoding has achieved levels of prediction in individual patients that rival the accuracy of visual stimuli [75]. These outcomes are very positive, but further issues will need to be addressed before the method can be applied in clinical settings.

Outstanding Issues with Pain Identification

The success of MVPA as a method to accurately identify the experience of pain in response to an experimental stimulus provides considerable impetus to explore the capacity of the method to identify clinical pain. However, there are aspects of clinical pain that are not ideal for the application of pattern recognition. It is likely that further developments will be required to identify a pain signature that can be reliably applied in the clinical situation. The following paragraphs discuss some of the issues that confront development of a clinical pain decoder.

MVPA is an example of machine learning, whereby early contingencies provide inputs to train algorithms that are subsequently applied to related contingencies in a novel situation. Experimental pain is well suited to this process because the events can be manipulated in the first instance to train the MVPA. Clinical pain is much more difficult to manipulate than experimental pain. Indeed, clinical pain can be present constantly, which precludes any opportunity to make critical contrasts between pain and its absence necessary for the training of a pain-decoding algorithm. The brief duration of experimental stimuli is another attribute that suits MPVA, but is unlike the experience of most people with clinical pain. A brief perturbation is very likely to evoke a signature response pattern in the distributed brain regions that code experimental pain, whereas signals measured at any given time point during the ongoing experience of clinical pain are likely to show many other sources of variance unrelated to the experience of interest. MVPA typically use BOLD contrast images acquired with fMRI, and it may be that alternative images would be more suited to the decoding of clinical pain. Regional cerebral blood flow levels estimated from arterial spin labeling images and averaged over minutes are more suited to the measurement of stable brain states [20], and this type of data were used with MVPA to identify postoperative pain [55].

A successful MVPA trained on one group of participants can be applied accurately to an independent group to identify pain [75]. This success is predicated on the assumption that patterns of voxel responses to a particular stimulus are consistently expressed in the healthy human brain. It is not known at present to what extent a signature for experimental pain evoked with one type of stimulus would be applicable for the identification of pain evoked by a different stimulus modality, but it seems likely that pain decoding would require optimization for particular types of experimental pain. The same situation is also likely to apply in the context of clinical pain, and pains arising from different clinical conditions are represented in discernibly different brain networks [19]. While not insurmountable, the complexity of clinical pain experience is a problem that would require sustained effort if accurate identification of pain in nonverbal groups is the objective.

CONCLUSION

Neuroimaging continues to provide new insights into pain processing and dementia-related pathology. This expanding literature has suggested several prospective points of intersection between AD-related pathology and the central representation of experimental and clinical pain. Generally, the implications of dementia for pain processing relate to the cognitive/emotional aspects of the experience. Neuroimaging holds considerable promise as a method that can directly test hypothesized effects of dementia on pain processing, but studies of this nature are rare. Nevertheless, the limited outcomes from pain activation studies of people with dementia are consistent with expectations based on other neuroimaging data. Recent developments in neuroimaging also hold promise for the identification of pain in nonverbal dementia patients, although achieving this objective will require further advances in imaging techniques and analyses.

REFERENCES

1. Agosta F, Caso F, Filippi M. Dementia and neuroimaging. J Neurol 2013;260:685–91.
2. Apkarian AV, Baliki MN, Geha PY. Towards a theory of chronic pain. Prog Neurobiol 2009;87:81–97.
3. Apkarian AV, Bushnell MC, Treede RD, Zubieta JK. Human brain mechanisms of pain perception and regulation in health and disease. Eur J Pain 2005;9:463–84.
4. Apkarian AV, Krauss BR, Fredrickson BE, Szeverenyi NM. Imaging the pain of low back pain: functional magnetic resonance imaging in combination with monitoring subjective pain perception allows the study of clinical pain states. Neurosci Lett 2001;299:57–60.
5. Baliki MN, Geha PY, Apkarian AV, Chialvo DR. Beyond feeling: chronic pain hurts the brain, disrupting the default-mode network dynamics. J Neurosci 2008;28:1398–403.
6. Baliki MN, Geha PY, Jabakhanji R, Harden N, Schnitzer TJ, Apkarian AV. A preliminary fMRI study of analgesic treatment in chronic back pain and knee osteoarthritis. Mol Pain 2008;4:47.
7. Beissner F, Meissner K, Bar KJ, Napadow V. The autonomic brain: an activation likelihood estimation meta-analysis for central processing of autonomic function. J Neurosci 2013;33:10503–11.
8. Benedetti F, Arduino C, Vighetti S, Asteggiano G, Tarenzi L, Rainero I. Pain reactivity in Alzheimer patients with different degrees of cognitive impairment and brain electrical activity deterioration. Pain 2004;111:22–9.
9. Benedetti F, Vighetti S, Ricco C, Lagna E, Bergamasco B, Pinessi L, Rainero I. Pain threshold and tolerance in Alzheimer's disease. Pain 1999;80:377–82.

10. Benzinger TL, Blazey T, Jack CR Jr, Koeppe RA, Su Y, Xiong C, Raichle ME, Snyder AZ, Ances BM, Bateman RJ, et al. Regional variability of imaging biomarkers in autosomal dominant Alzheimer's disease. Proc Natl Acad Sci USA 2013;110:E4502-9.
11. Brodersen KH, Wiech K, Lomakina EI, Lin CS, Buhmann JM, Bingel U, Ploner M, Stephan KE, Tracey I. Decoding the perception of pain from fMRI using multivariate pattern analysis. Neuroimage 2012;63:1162-70.
12. Brooks J, Tracey I. From nociception to pain perception: imaging the spinal and supraspinal pathways. J Anat 2005;207:19-33.
13. Browndyke JN, Giovanello K, Petrella J, Hayden K, Chiba-Falek O, Tucker KA, Burke JR, Welsh-Bohmer KA. Phenotypic regional functional imaging patterns during memory encoding in mild cognitive impairment and Alzheimer's disease. Alzheimers Dement 2013;9:284-94.
14. Broyd SJ, Demanuele C, Debener S, Helps SK, James CJ, Sonuga-Barke EJ. Default-mode brain dysfunction in mental disorders: a systematic review. Neurosci Biobehav Rev 2009;33:279-96.
15. Cole LJ, Farrell MJ, Duff EP, Barber JB, Egan GF, Gibson SJ. Pain sensitivity and fMRI pain-related brain activity in Alzheimer's disease. Brain 2006;129:2957-65.
16. Cole LJ, Gavrilescu M, Johnston LA, Gibson SJ, Farrell MJ, Egan GF. The impact of Alzheimer's disease on the functional connectivity between brain regions underlying pain perception. Eur J Pain 2011;15:568 e1-11.
17. Craig AD. How do you feel—now? The anterior insula and human awareness. Nat Rev Neurosci 2009;10:59-70.
18. Duerden EG, Albanese MC. Localization of pain-related brain activation: a meta-analysis of neuroimaging data. Hum Brain Mapp 2013;34:109-49.
19. Farmer MA, Baliki MN, Apkarian AV. A dynamic network perspective of chronic pain. Neurosci Lett 2012;520:197-203.
20. Farrell MJ, Bowala TK, Gavrilescu M, Phillips PA, McKinley MJ, McAllen RM, Denton DA, Egan GF. Cortical activation and lamina terminalis functional connectivity during thirst and drinking in humans. Am J Physiol Regul Integr Comp Physiol 2011;301:R623-31.
21. Farrell MJ, Laird AR, Egan GF. Brain activity associated with painfully hot stimuli applied to the upper limb: a meta-analysis. Hum Brain Mapp 2005;25:129-39.
22. Fratiglioni L, De Ronchi D, Aguero-Torres H. Worldwide prevalence and incidence of dementia. Drugs Aging 1999;15:365-75.
23. Friebel U, Eickhoff SB, Lotze M. Coordinate-based meta-analysis of experimentally induced and chronic persistent neuropathic pain. Neuroimage 2011;58:1070-80.
24. Geha PY, Baliki MN, Chialvo DR, Harden RN, Paice JA, Apkarian AV. Brain activity for spontaneous pain of postherpetic neuralgia and its modulation by lidocaine patch therapy. Pain 2007;128:88-100.
25. Gibson SJ, Voukelatos X, Ames D, Flicker L, Helme RD. An examination of pain perception and cerebral event-related potentials following carbon dioxide laser stimulation in patients with Alzheimer's disease and age-matched control volunteers. Pain Res Manag 2001;6:126-32.
26. Greicius MD, Kimmel DL. Neuroimaging insights into network-based neurodegeneration. Curr Opin Neurol 2012;25:727-34.
27. Hadjistavropoulos T, Herr K, Turk DC, Fine PG, Dworkin RH, Helme R, Jackson K, Parmelee PA, Rudy TE, Lynn Beattie B, et al. An interdisciplinary expert consensus statement on assessment of pain in older persons. Clin J Pain 2007;23:S1-43.
28. Hafkemeijer A, van der Grond J, Rombouts SA. Imaging the default mode network in aging and dementia. Biochim Biophys Acta 2012;1822:431-41.
29. Hashmi JA, Baliki MN, Huang L, Baria AT, Torbey S, Hermann KM, Schnitzer TJ, Apkarian AV. Shape shifting pain: chronification of back pain shifts brain representation from nociceptive to emotional circuits. Brain 2013;136:2751-68.
30. Haxby JV, Gobbini MI, Furey ML, Ishai A, Schouten JL, Pietrini P. Distributed and overlapping representations of faces and objects in ventral temporal cortex. Science 2001;293:2425-30.
31. Hayes DJ, Northoff G. Common brain activations for painful and non-painful aversive stimuli. BMC Neurosci 2012;13:60.
32. Herr K, Bjoro K, Decker S. Tools for assessment of pain in nonverbal older adults with dementia: a state-of-the-science review. J Pain Symptom Manag 2006;31:170-92.
33. Hoefer M, Allison SC, Schauer GF, Neuhaus JM, Hall J, Dang JN, Weiner MW, Miller BL, Rosen HJ. Fear conditioning in frontotemporal lobar degeneration and Alzheimer's disease. Brain 2008;131:1646-57.
34. Howard MA, Sanders D, Krause K, O'Muircheartaigh J, Fotopoulou A, Zelaya F, Thacker M, Massat N, Huggins JP, Vennart W, et al. Alterations in resting-state regional cerebral blood flow demonstrate ongoing pain in osteoarthritis: an arterial spin-labeled magnetic resonance imaging study. Arthritis Rheum 2012;64:3936-46.

35. Ibinson JW, Small RH, Algaze A, Roberts CJ, Clark DL, Schmalbrock P. Functional magnetic resonance imaging studies of pain: an investigation of signal decay during and across sessions. Anesthesiology 2004;101:960–9.
36. Jack CR Jr, Holtzman DM. Biomarker modeling of Alzheimer's disease. Neuron. 2013;80:1347–58.
37. Jack CR Jr, Knopman DS, Jagust WJ, Petersen RC, Weiner MW, Aisen PS, Shaw LM, Vemuri P, Wiste HJ, Weigand SD, et al. Tracking pathophysiological processes in Alzheimer's disease: an updated hypothetical model of dynamic biomarkers. Lancet Neurol 2013;12:207–16.
38. Jack CR Jr, Knopman DS, Jagust WJ, Shaw LM, Aisen PS, Weiner MW, Petersen RC, Trojanowski JQ. Hypothetical model of dynamic biomarkers of the Alzheimer's pathological cascade. Lancet Neurol 2010;9:119–28.
39. Jack CR Jr, Lowe VJ, Weigand SD, Wiste HJ, Senjem ML, Knopman DS, Shiung MM, Gunter JL, Boeve BF, Kemp BJ, et al. Serial PIB and MRI in normal, mild cognitive impairment and Alzheimer's disease: implications for sequence of pathological events in Alzheimer's disease. Brain 2009;132:1355–65.
40. Krummenacher P, Candia V, Folkers G, Schedlowski M, Schonbachler G. Prefrontal cortex modulates placebo analgesia. Pain 2010;148:368–74.
41. Kucyi A, Salomons TV, Davis KD. Mind wandering away from pain dynamically engages antinociceptive and default mode brain networks. Proc Natl Acad Sci USA 2013;110:18692–7.
42. Kulkarni B, Bentley DE, Elliott R, Julyan PJ, Boger E, Watson A, Boyle Y, El-Deredy W, Jones AK. Arthritic pain is processed in brain areas concerned with emotions and fear. Arthritis Rheum 2007;56:1345–54.
43. Kurata J, Thulborn KR, Gyulai FE, Firestone LL. Early decay of pain-related cerebral activation in functional magnetic resonance imaging: comparison with visual and motor tasks. Anesthesiology 2002;96:35–44.
44. Laird AR, Fox PM, Eickhoff SB, Turner JA, Ray KL, McKay DR, Glahn DC, Beckmann CF, Smith SM, Fox PT. Behavioral interpretations of intrinsic connectivity networks. J Cogn Neurosci 2011;23:4022–37.
45. Lanz S, Seifert F, Maihofner C. Brain activity associated with pain, hyperalgesia and allodynia: an ALE meta-analysis. J Neural Transm 2011;118:1139–54.
46. LeDoux J. The emotional brain, fear, and the amygdala. Cell Mol Neurobiol 2003;23:727–38.
47. Mason MF, Norton MI, Van Horn JD, Wegner DM, Grafton ST, Macrae CN. Wandering minds: the default network and stimulus-independent thought. Science 2007;315:393–5.
48. Mayhew SD, Hylands-White N, Porcaro C, Derbyshire SW, Bagshaw AP. Intrinsic variability in the human response to pain is assembled from multiple, dynamic brain processes. Neuroimage 2013;75:68–78.
49. Misra G, Coombes SA. Neuroimaging evidence of motor control and pain processing in the human midcingulate cortex. Cereb Cortex 2015;25(7):1906–19.
50. Morris JC, Roe CM, Xiong C, Fagan AM, Goate AM, Holtzman DM, Mintun MA. APOE predicts amyloid-beta but not tau Alzheimer pathology in cognitively normal aging. Ann Neurol 2010;67:122–31.
51. Musen G, Jacobson AM, Bolo NR, Simonson DC, Shenton ME, McCartney RL, Flores VL, Hoogenboom WS. Resting-state brain functional connectivity is altered in type 2 diabetes. Diabetes 2012;61:2375–9.
52. Mutso AA, Radzicki D, Baliki MN, Huang L, Banisadr G, Centeno MV, Radulovic J, Martina M, Miller RJ, Apkarian AV. Abnormalities in hippocampal functioning with persistent pain. J Neurosci 2012;32:5747–56.
53. Neugebauer V, Li W. Differential sensitization of amygdala neurons to afferent inputs in a model of arthritic pain. J Neurophysiol 2003;89:716–27.
54. Norman KA, Polyn SM, Detre GJ, Haxby JV. Beyond mind-reading: multi-voxel pattern analysis of fMRI data. Trends Cogn Sci 2006;10:424–30.
55. O'Muircheartaigh J, Marquand A, Hodkinson DJ, Krause K, Khawaja N, Renton TF, Huggins JP, Vennart W, Williams SC, Howard MA. Multivariate decoding of cerebral blood flow measures in a clinical model of on-going postsurgical pain. Hum Brain Mapp 2015;36:633–42.
56. Parks EL, Geha PY, Baliki MN, Katz J, Schnitzer TJ, Apkarian AV. Brain activity for chronic knee osteoarthritis: dissociating evoked pain from spontaneous pain. Eur J Pain 2011;15:843 e1–14.
57. Perini I, Bergstrand S, Morrison I. Where pain meets action in the human brain. J Neurosci 2013;33:15930–9.
58. Raichle ME, Snyder AZ. A default mode of brain function: a brief history of an evolving idea. Neuroimage 2007;37:1083–90; discussion 97–9.
59. Rainville P, Duncan GH, Price DD, Carrier B, Bushnell MC. Pain affect encoded in human anterior cingulate but not somatosensory cortex. Science 1997;277:968–71.
60. Rocca MA, Valsasina P, Absinta M, Riccitelli G, Rodegher ME, Misci P, Rossi P, Falini A, Comi G, Filippi M. Default-mode network dysfunction and cognitive impairment in progressive MS. Neurology 2010;74:1252–9.
61. Roy M, Shohamy D, Wager TD. Ventromedial prefrontal-subcortical systems and the generation of affective meaning. Trends Cogn Sci 2012;16:147–56.

62. Salimi-Khorshidi G, Smith SM, Keltner JR, Wager TD, Nichols TE. Meta-analysis of neuroimaging data: a comparison of image-based and coordinate-based pooling of studies. Neuroimage 2009;45:810–23.
63. Scherder EJ, Sergeant JA, Swaab DF. Pain processing in dementia and its relation to neuropathology. Lancet Neurol 2003;2:677–86.
64. Schwindt GC, Black SE. Functional imaging studies of episodic memory in Alzheimer's disease: a quantitative meta-analysis. Neuroimage 2009;45:181–90.
65. Scoville WB, Milner B. Loss of recent memory after bilateral hippocampal lesions. J Neurol Neurosurg Psychiatry 1957;20:11–21.
66. Smallwood RF, Laird AR, Ramage AE, Parkinson AL, Lewis J, Clauw DJ, Williams DA, Schmidt-Wilcke T, Farrell MJ, Eickhoff SB, Robin DA. Structural brain anomalies and chronic pain: a quantitative meta-analysis of gray matter volume. J Pain 2013;14:663–75.
67. Smith SM, Fox PT, Miller KL, Glahn DC, Fox PM, Mackay CE, Filippini N, Watkins KE, Toro R, Laird AR, Beckmann CF. Correspondence of the brain's functional architecture during activation and rest. Proc Natl Acad Sci USA 2009;106:13040–5.
68. Sperling R. Potential of functional MRI as a biomarker in early Alzheimer's disease. Neurobiol Aging 2011;32:S37–43.
69. Stawarczyk D, Majerus S, Maquet P, D'Argembeau A. Neural correlates of ongoing conscious experience: both task-unrelatedness and stimulus-independence are related to default network activity. PLoS One 2011;6:e16997.
70. Tolle TR, Kaufmann T, Siessmeier T, Lautenbacher S, Berthele A, Munz F, Zieglgansberger W, Willoch F, Schwaiger M, Conrad B, Bartenstein P. Region-specific encoding of sensory and affective components of pain in the human brain: a positron emission tomography correlation analysis. Ann Neurol 1999;45:40–7.
71. Tong F, Pratte MS. Decoding patterns of human brain activity. Annu Rev Psychol 2012;63:483–509.
72. Tracey I, Mantyh PW. The cerebral signature for pain perception and its modulation. Neuron 2007;55:377–91.
73. Vannini P, O'Brien J, O'Keefe K, Pihlajamaki M, Laviolette P, Sperling RA. What goes down must come up: role of the posteromedial cortices in encoding and retrieval. Cereb Cortex 2011;21:22–34.
74. Vogt BA. Pain and emotion interactions in subregions of the cingulate gyrus. Nat Rev Neurosci 2005;6:533–44.
75. Wager TD, Atlas LY, Lindquist MA, Roy M, Woo CW, Kross E. An fMRI-based neurologic signature of physical pain. N Engl J Med 2013;368:1388–97.
76. Wasan AD, Loggia ML, Chen LQ, Napadow V, Kong J, Gollub RL. Neural correlates of chronic low back pain measured by arterial spin labeling. Anesthesiology 2011;115:364–74.
77. Yang J, Pan P, Song W, Huang R, Li J, Chen K, Gong Q, Zhong J, Shi H, Shang H. Voxelwise meta-analysis of gray matter anomalies in Alzheimer's disease and mild cognitive impairment using anatomic likelihood estimation. J Neurol Sci 2012;316:21–9.

CHAPTER 6

Pain in People with Dementia— Its Relationship to Neuropathology

Erik J. A. Scherder

Population of seniors above the age of 65 will increase substantially in the next decades. As aging itself poses the greatest risk for dementia [104], an increase in the number of demented patients suffering from pain is expected because aging also coincides with an increase in the frequency of pain complaints, irrespective of the cognitive status [51]. As patients become less communicative during the course of dementia, assessing pain becomes more difficult. We argue that insight into the neuropathology that affects the neuronal systems in the brain that are involved in pain processing will strengthen the reliability of pain assessment in this vulnerable population, and may reduce or prevent undertreatment of pain in this group of patients.

Therefore, the main goal of this chapter is to highlight that the neuropathology affecting the pain processing systems differs between the various subtypes of dementia, that is, Alzheimer disease (AD), subcortical vascular dementia (sVaD), and frontotemporal dementia (FTD), but also between these subtypes of dementia and Parkinson disease (PD) and multiple sclerosis (MS) [93, 95]. Consequently, the alterations in pain processing may differ between these neurodegenerative diseases.

OUTLINE

First, the medial and lateral pain systems will be described, followed by the way these are affected in the various subtypes of dementia, in PD, and in MS. Subsequently, based on the neuropathology, the extent to which autonomic responses to pain are still possible in the various subtypes of dementia will be addressed. Finally, we discuss that the medial pain system is the same neuronal circuit that is also responsible for behavioral disturbances often seen in dementia, supporting the view that pain may provoke behavior disturbances such as agitation and vice versa.

MEDIAL AND LATERAL PAIN SYSTEM

The anatomical complexity of the medial and lateral pain systems is reflections of the multifaceted nature of pain. The focus of this chapter will be on those areas of the medial and lateral pain systems that constitute the main framework of both systems (see Fig. 6-1)

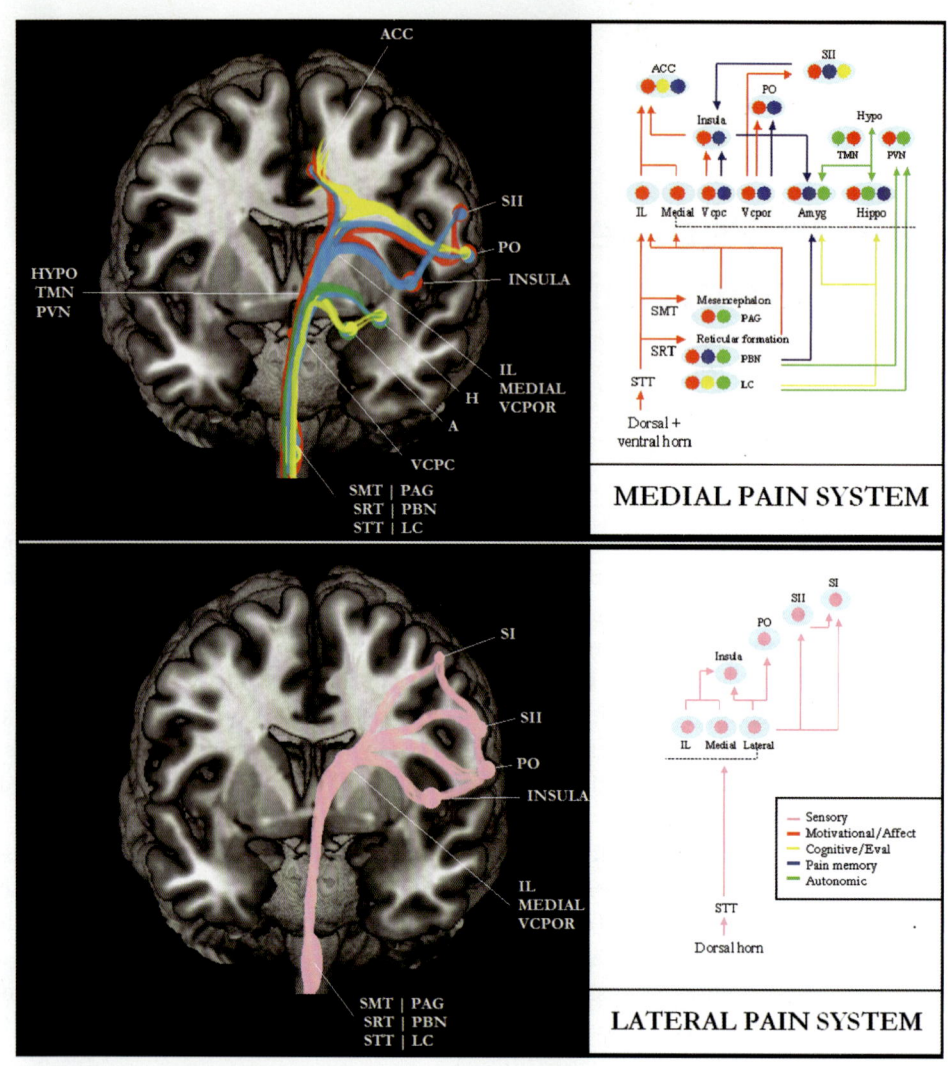

FIGURE 6-1 Sub/cortical area and pathways belonging to the medial and lateral pain systems in cognitively unimapired individuals. Note that most of the presented brain areas contribute to more than one pain modality. STT, spinothalamic tract; SRT, spinoreticular tract; SMT, spinomesencephalic tract; LC, locus coeruleus; PBN, parabrachial nucleus; PAG, periaqueductal gray; IL, intralaminar thalamic nuclei; Medial, medial thalamic nuclei; VCPC, ventral caudal parvocellular nucleus; VCPOR, ventral caudal portae nucleus; A, amygdala; H, hippocampus; HYPO, hypothalamus; TMN, tubermamillary nucleus; PVN, paraventricular nucleus; PO, parietal operculum; ACC, anterior cingulate cortex; S1, primary somatosensory area; S2, secondary somatosensory area.

and of which the most is affected in one or more subtypes of dementia, PD, and MS (see Figs. 6-2 to 6-8). For a comprehensive description of ascending pathways and connections between the areas that belong to the two pain systems, see Willis and Westlund [117]. It is worth noting that although the medial and lateral pain systems are anatomically distinct and mediate different aspects of the pain experience, they are not independent. Indeed, there is a lot of cross-talk between these systems, and both are required for the overall, integrated, multidimensional perceptual experience commonly identified as pain.

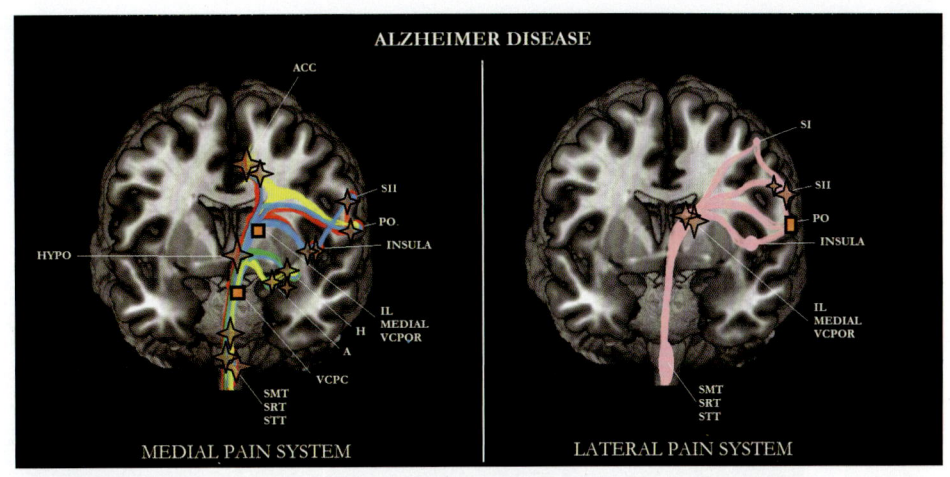

FIGURE 6-2 Sub/cortical area and pathways belonging to the medial and lateral pain systems in Alzheimer disease (AD). Note that most of the areas belonging to the medial pain system are particularly affected in AD. Aspects of pain: sensory/discriminative (*pink*); motivational/affective (*red*); cognitive/evaluative (*yellow*); pain memory (*blue*); autonomic responses (*green*). ◆, degeneration; ■ no studies.

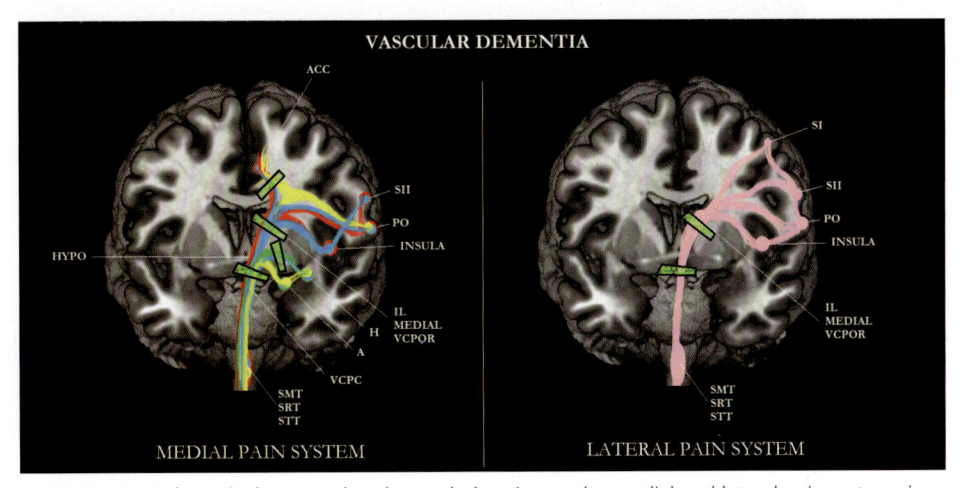

FIGURE 6-3 Sub/cortical area and pathways belonging to the medial and lateral pain systems in vascular dementia (VD). Note the disconnections between the various brain areas.

Medial Pain System

The medial pain system is involved in the motivational/affective aspects, cognitive/evaluative aspects, memory for pain, and autonomic aspects of pain [101, 114].

Thalamic nuclei, including medial and intralaminar nuclei, receive nociceptive information either directly through the spinothalamic tract (STT) or indirectly through the spinoreticular and spinomesencephalic tract (SRT and SMT, respectively). Subsequently, the thalamus transmits information to the anterior cingulate cortex (ACC), insula, parietal operculum (PO), and the secondary somatosensory cortex (S2). Areas of the reticular formation such as the locus coeruleus (LC) and parabrachial nucleus (PBN) convey nociceptive information to the amygdala, hippocampus, and the hypothalamic nuclei including the paraventricular nucleus (PVN) [89, 101, 114]. In the PVN, oxytocin and arginine

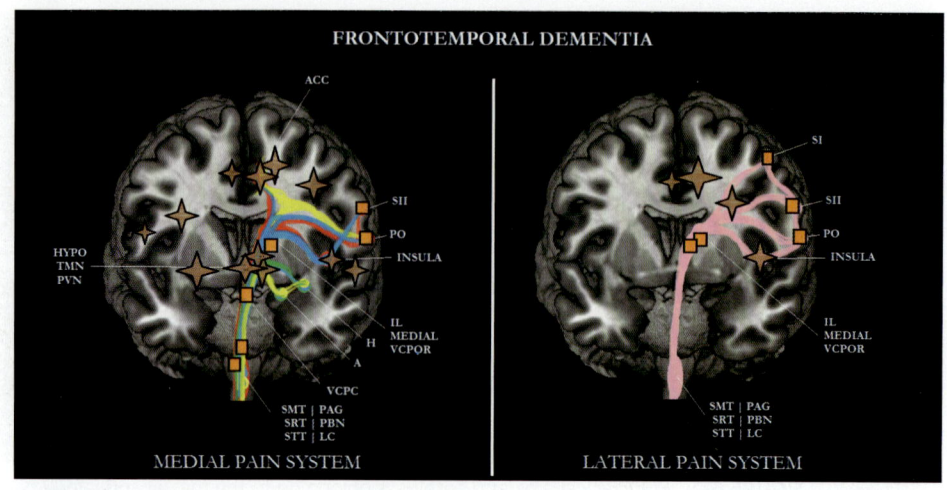

FIGURE 6-4 Sub/cortical area and pathways belonging to the medial and lateral pain systems in frontotemporal dementia (FTD). Note that the prefrontal cortex is more affected in FTD than in Alzheimer disease (AD). Aspects of pain: sensory/discriminative (*pink*); motivational/affective (*red*); cognitive/evaluative (*yellow*); pain memory (*blue*); autonomic responses (*green*). ✦, degeneration; ■ no studies.

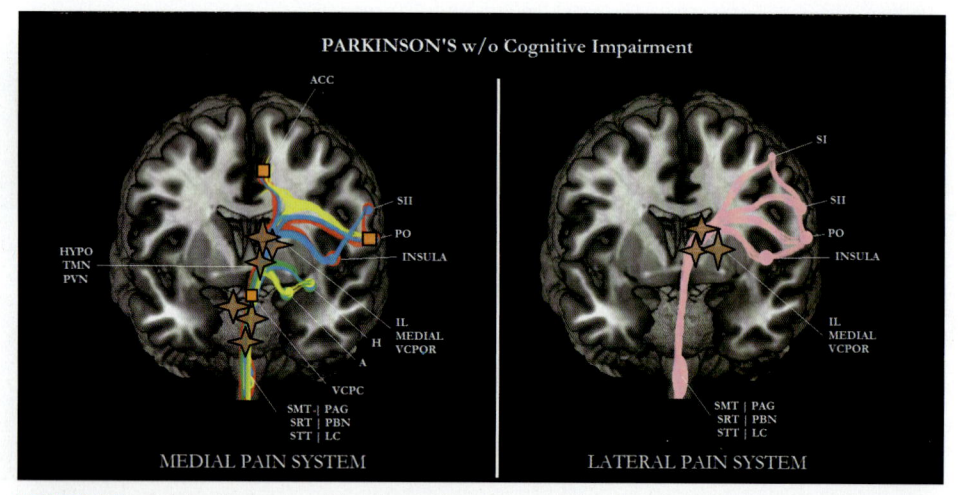

FIGURE 6-5 Sub/cortical area and pathways belonging to the medial and lateral pain systems in Parkinson disease (PD) without cognitive impairment. Aspects of pain: sensory/discriminative (*pink*); motivational/affective (*red*); cognitive/evaluative (*yellow*); pain memory (*blue*); autonomic responses (*green*). ✦, degeneration; ■ no studies.

vasopressin are produced; the latter is co-localized with corticotrophin-releasing hormone (CRH) [54, 84, 110]. The tuberomammillary nucleus (TMN) is the only histaminergic nucleus of the brain [54, 84, 110]. Histamine, oxytocin, arginine vasopressin, and CRH are neuroactive compounds with an antinociceptive effect [111].

Lateral Pain System

The STT also conveys information to the lateral thalamus, which projects to the insula, PO, S2, and the primary somatosensory cortex (S1). The lateral pain system is known to play a crucial role in the sensory/discriminative aspects of pain [101, 114].

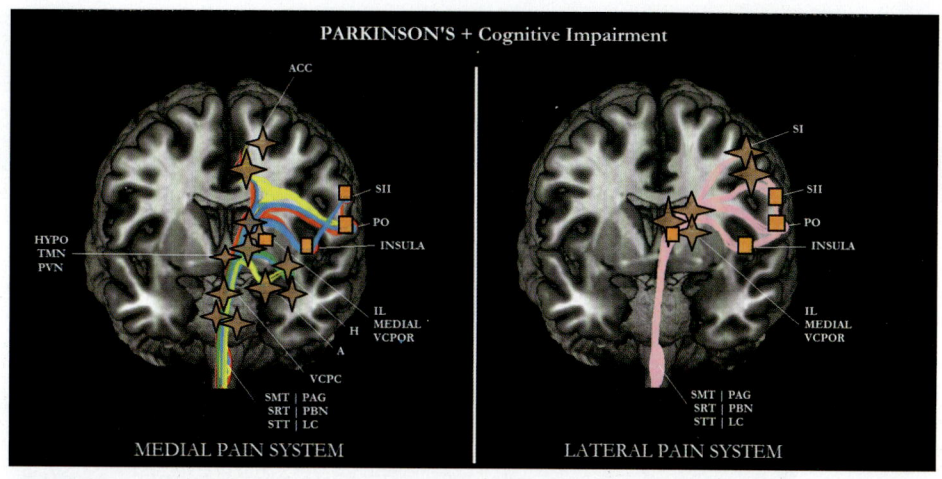

FIGURE 6-6 Sub/cortical area and pathways belonging to the medial and lateral pain systems in Parkinson disease (PD) with cognitive impairment. Aspects of pain: sensory/discriminative (*pink*); motivational/affective (*red*); cognitive/evaluative (*yellow*); pain memory (*blue*); autonomic responses (*green*). ✦, degeneration; ■ no studies.

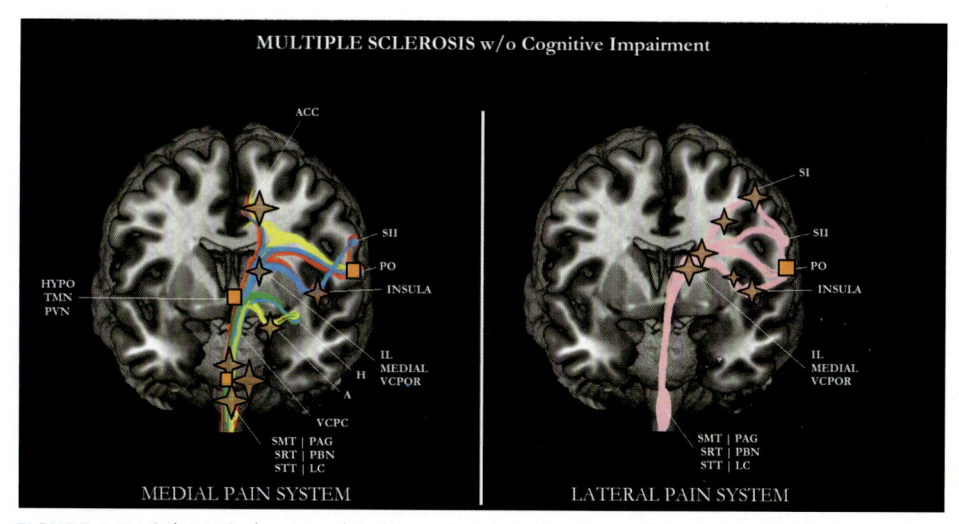

FIGURE 6-7 Sub/cortical area and pathways belonging to the medial and lateral pain systems in multiple sclerosis (MS) without cognitive impairment. Aspects of pain: sensory/discriminative (*pink*); motivational/affective (*red*); cognitive/evaluative (*yellow*); pain memory (*blue*); autonomic responses (*green*). ✦, degeneration; ■ no studies.

THE MEDIAL AND LATERAL PAIN SYSTEM IN DEMENTIAS

Alzheimer Disease

AD is characterized by degeneration in most of the areas of the medial pain system (see Fig. 6-2). More specifically, the degeneration of the amygdala and hippocampus [20, 40] might be responsible for a decline in memory for pain and, together with the TMN [109], for the blunting of the autonomic responses. Furthermore, one could hypothesize that because of atrophy of the amygdala, hippocampus, LC, ACC, and S2, cognitive/evaluative aspects of pain are likely to deteriorate as well, particularly in persistent pain, a type of pain

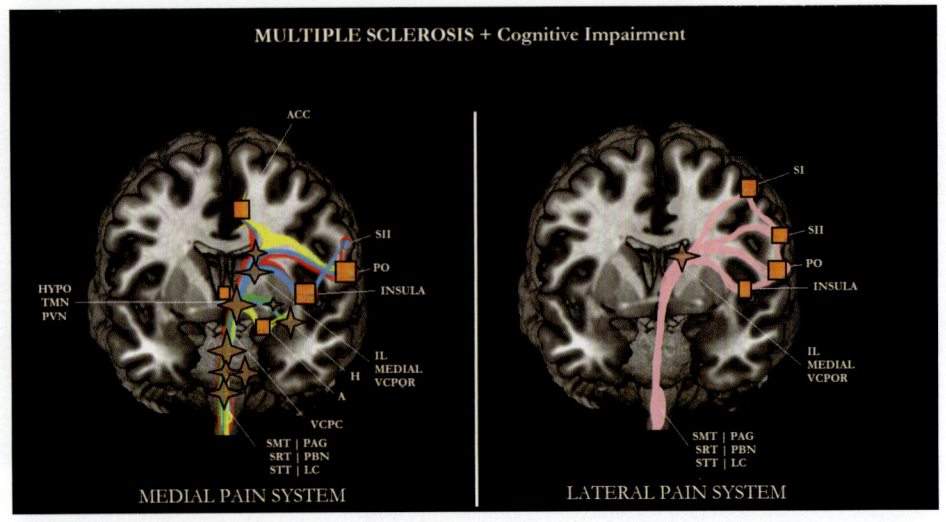

FIGURE 6-8 Sub/cortical area and pathways belonging to the medial and lateral pain systems in multiple sclerosis (MS) with cognitive impairment. Aspects of pain: sensory/discriminative (*pink*); motivational/affective (*red*); cognitive/evaluative (*yellow*); pain memory (*blue*); autonomic responses (*green*). ♦, degeneration; ■ no studies.

that is most prevalent in elderly persons in a nursing home setting [47]; cognitive processes such as anticipation of the future and behavioral responses to pain are most important [83]. As can be seen in Fig. 6-2, nociceptive information can still be transmitted to S1, which might explain that the pain threshold (lateral pain system; sensory-discriminative aspects of pain) in AD is not different from the pain threshold in elderly persons without dementia (see Defrin et al. 2015 for review and Chapter 4). The lateral pain system does show some functional decline in AD though; compared with elderly persons without dementia, the sensory threshold was elevated in AD [42].

Based on the above-mentioned findings, one might conclude that patients with AD may show a decrease in the motivational/affective aspects of pain, and hence may suffer from less pain than those without AD. Two important issues plead against this suggestion. In the first place, an experimental study applying mechanical stimuli as painful stimuli to patients with AD performed by Cole and coworkers [27] suggested that the activity in the medial and lateral pain systems was unaffected. Patients were in a moderate to mild stage of dementia. In the second place, white matter lesions are characteristic not only for vascular dementia but also for AD [80, Varma et al., 2002b].

Vascular Dementia

In one study, pain was assessed in patients with possible vascular dementia [96]. In that study, the prevalence of osteoporosis was higher in the elderly persons without dementia, whereas diabetes neuropathy occurred more frequently in elderly with vascular dementia. Various pain scales (also used in pain assessment for AD) indicated that elderly persons with vascular dementia communicated to suffer more from pain (motivational/affective aspects) than elderly persons without dementia. In a second recent study, patients with probable vascular dementia participated [92]. This diagnosis was possible because brain imaging data of these patients were available, indicating subcortical white matter lesions. These findings support the results of the first study, that is, more affective pain experience in this group of patients, compared with older persons without dementia. Moreover, we found a significant negative relationship between pain affect and global cognitive functioning, measured by the Mini-Mental State Examination. This latter finding implies that the lower the patient's global cognitive functioning, the more the patient suffers from pain. Further studies using experimental pain stimuli are required to substantiate this view.

An explanation for this finding is that subcortical white matter lesions, a neuropathological hallmark of vascular dementia [4], cause a disconnection between cortical areas and between cortical and subcortical areas [77], resulting in a so-called deafferentation pain [34]. For instance, white matter lesions may disrupt connections between the intralaminar thalamic nuclei and somatosensory areas (S1, S2), resulting in abnormal sensations (dysesthesia) [98]. A possible decline in the other four dimensions of pain will likely depend on exactly where in the brain that the infarctions have occurred.

Frontotemporal Dementia

In only one clinical study, pain experience was assessed in patients with frontal variant frontotemporal dementia and compared to the pain experience of those with AD and vascular dementia [6]. A remarkable finding was that in comparison with the latter two groups, elderly people with frontal FTD indicated to experience significantly less pain. A more recent experimental pain study [21], applying electrical stimuli as painful stimuli, observed a higher pain threshold and a higher pain tolerance in FTD patients compared with those without FTD. The findings of both studies strengthen each other; that is, patients with FTD may suffer from less pain than older persons without dementia and even less than those suffering from other subtypes of dementia.

One possible explanation for this finding might be the severe metabolic decline seen in frontal FTD, indicated by a marked decrease in cerebral blood flow to the prefrontal cortex and ACC (see Figs. 6-3 and 6-4) [113]. These cortical areas play an important role in the processing of motivational/affective aspects of pain. Although the amygdala and hippocampus are less affected in FTD than in AD (see Fig. 6-4) [12, 65], when assessing pain in patients with FTD, one should take into consideration a decline in the cognitive/evaluative aspects, the autonomic responses evoked by pain, and the memory for pain.

THE MEDIAL AND LATERAL PAIN SYSTEM IN PD AND MS

As a possible change in pain experience has not been examined in cognitively impaired patients with PD or MS, only studies in which pain was assessed in cognitively intact PD and MS patients will be discussed. Some caution is therefore required before simply extrapolating the findings from cognitively intact adults to those with disease-related dementia.

Parkinson Disease

Pain was one of the dependent variables in several studies that investigated the influence of PD on a patient's quality of life. In one study, a significant association between the progression of PD and an increase in pain was observed over a period of 4 years [59]. Importantly, the patients were not cognitively impaired (average Mini-Mental State Examination score after 4 years: 26.2). Similar findings were reported in another longitudinal study, in which pain was assessed over a 3-year period [90]. In two reviews, a considerable number of somatic pain syndromes including musculoskeletal disorders such as limb rigidity, radicular-neuropathic disorders such as restless legs syndrome, dystonia, akathisia, neck pain, and headache have been described in relation to PD [39, 116]. One nonsomatically-based pain syndrome with a less clear etiology comprises primary sensory symptoms [24] and is considered a type of *central pain* [39, 99, 116].

Based on the location of the neuropathology, Lewy bodies and Lewy neurites in areas such as the coeruleus–subcoeruleus region, the nucleus gigantocellularis, and the bulbar nuclei normally inhibit nociceptive transmission at the spinal dorsal horn malfunction in PD [58, 120] and are responsible for the clinically observed increase in motivational-affective aspects of pain (see Figs. 6-5 and 6-6). As can be seen in these figures, the other aspects of pain can still be processed. Although there is ample evidence that inpatients with PD may suffer from more pain than controls, it is also known that levodopa may attenuate the increased pain experience [37]. According to these authors, dopamine may exert its analgesic effect through serotonin.

Multiple Sclerosis

Evidence of pain experience in MS emerges from various reviews of the most frequently occurring pain syndromes in MS. These pain syndromes include trigeminal neuralgia, somatic pain such as back pain and pain related to spasticity, visceral pain most frequently caused by spasms of the bladder, and a variety of other painful conditions such as optic neuritis and an acute radicular syndrome [60, 78, 106].

In addition, dysesthesia, a type of central pain that consists of unpleasant sensations as a reaction to touch, has been described in patients with MS [3, 60, 106]. Others confirmed the presence of central pain in MS [79], which might also be reflected in the etiology of severe acute headaches [43] and painful tonic seizures [102]. The results of a clinical study show that MS patients (1) experienced a higher pain intensity than a reference group; (2) needed more pain treatment (drugs, physiotherapy); and (3) experienced pain in more locations [3].

Similar to vascular dementia, white matter lesions are probably the cause of an increase in motivational-affective aspects of pain in MS, by disrupting cortical and subcortical–cortical connections (deafferentation). Since areas of the medial pain system (e.g., insula, see Figs. 6-7 and 6-8) are affected but still show enhanced activation as a response to sensorimotor activity [87], these areas are still able to process sensory information.

EXPRESSION OF PAIN IN AUTONOMIC RESPONSES AND BEHAVIOR

Autonomic Responses to Pain

Taking the degeneration of the hypothalamic TMN in AD [109] into consideration, the question arises whether autonomic responses to pain (e.g., changes in skin conductance, changes in blood pressure, or changes in heart rate) are still present and, if so, whether these responses are present in older people with dementia, independent of the stage of dementia [81]. A limited number of studies on this topic are available. In one study, heart rate responses in reaction to a venipuncture were similar in both patients with AD and older persons without dementia [82]. However, the autonomic responses showed a positive relationship with the level of cognitive functioning (i.e., The lower the cognitive functioning, the lower the autonomic responses [82]). For example, in MCI the sympathetic skin response was lower than in cognitively unimpaired older persons [64]. Similar findings were observed in patients with dementia [63]. More specifically, in patients with AD, Benedetti and coworkers [8] observed a negative correlation between heart rate responses and degree of cognitive impairment in the presence of normal tactile and pain threshold. These findings imply that autonomic responses to pain deteriorate in dementia, whereas the processing of tactile and painful stimuli is still possible. Of note is that the *intensity* of a painful stimulus determines the presence/absence of autonomic responses to pain in AD [85]. More specifically, a strong (twice the pain threshold) electrical stimulus provoked a more profound heart rate increase in patients with AD, albeit less than in those without dementia; the increase in blood pressure during this stimulation was even similar to that of people without dementia. One should bear in mind that an increase in blood pressure and heart rate may only be indicative of (severe) pain when the patient is, in general, familiar with lower values. It is of clinical relevance to realize that the absence of an increase in heart rate and blood pressure may not be indicative of the absence of pain. For example, cardiovascular medication might prevent the occurrence of autonomic responses to pain [81]. Furthermore, it is known that β-adrenoceptor antagonists and calcium channel antagonists, medication frequently used by older people, lower blood pressure and heart rate [5, 86].

Pain in Dementia—Its Relationship to Agitation

Neuropathology

One of the pain-suppressing pathways in the brain originates from the prefrontal cortex. Consequently, lesions of the frontal-subcortical pathways may cause an increase in pain experience in dementia. In addition, disinhibited impulse aggression may result from lesions of the ventromedial and orbitofrontal prefrontal cortex [15, 103, 118]. Support for such a process emerges from neuroimaging studies, using, for example, positron emission tomography (PET), that show a relationship between aggression and prefrontal cortex dysfunction (i.e., anterior frontal, orbitofrontal, and ventromedial areas [15, 100]). Lesions of the ventromedial and orbitofrontal cortex causing disinhibition, and, consequently, agitation/aggression, may occur in neurodegenerative disorders such as dementia [103]. On the basis of this evidence and considering the role of the descending pathways with its origin in the prefrontal cortex in pain suppression, lesions of these pathways in dementia may not only cause agitation/aggression, but may also contribute to an increase in pain experience. Consequently, in dementia, agitation/aggression could be related to pain.

Clinical studies

The above-mentioned studies suggest that lesions of the prefrontal cortex may cause agitation and pain in patients with dementia. The question arises whether these two symptoms always occur simultaneously in dementia and whether a causal relationship exists between them, that is, does an increase in pain provoke agitation in patients with dementia?

Indeed, in one study, a significant proportion of the variance in discomfort of patients with moderate to severe dementia (14%) was explained by agitation [17]. In other words, the presence of a painful condition may contribute to agitation in patients with dementia [17]. The relationship between agitation and pain has also been observed in older patients visiting a day care center [26]. In that study, pain was a significant predictor of verbally nonaggressive agitation. In patients with dementia who received end-of-life care in a hospice, fewer complaints of pain coincided with a decreased prevalence of restlessness, sleep problems, agitation, and aggressiveness, compared with those who were not enrolled in a hospice [7]. Moreover, evidence for a causal relationship emerges from a study that administered opioids to patients with dementia [70]. In that study, a long-acting opioid (oxycodone, 10 mg every 12 hours, or 20 mg morphine a day for those with problems in swallowing pills), administered over the course of 4 weeks, significantly reduced the level of agitation only in the oldest patients (i.e., 85 years of age) who were in an advanced stage of dementia. Similar findings were observed after applying a stepwise protocol with paracetamol (acetaminophen), morphine, buprenorphine transdermal patch, or pregabalin to patients with moderate to severe dementia [53].

CONCLUSIONS

- Undoubtedly, clinical and experimental pain studies on the influence of the various *subtypes* of dementia on pain are desperately needed.
- Dependent on the neuropathology, patients with dementia may suffer either from a decrease or from an increase in pain or an alteration in pain experience may occur during the course of the disease (e.g., a progressive increase in pain due to a progressive deterioration of the white matter).
- Considering the overlap between brain regions that are involved in both cognitive functions and pain (e.g., hippocampus), a decline in cognitive functions (e.g. memory) may coincide with a decline in pain experience (gray matter), or a decline in cognitive functions (e.g., memory) may coincide with an increase in pain experience (white matter).
- Pain assessment instruments should focus on both the sensory-discriminative (among which the intensity of pain) and the motivational-affective aspects of pain (suffering from pain).
- Absence of autonomic responses to pain does not imply that the patient is not in pain; autonomic responses to pain may only occur in case of intense pain.
- Agitated behavior in patients with dementia should not automatically be interpreted as a consequence of dementia itself but could also be an expression of pain.
- Studies on disorders such as PD and MS are especially necessary, particularly longitudinal investigations of how pain experience changes as patients become increasingly cognitively impaired and less able to communicate their pain themselves.

REFERENCES

1. Aarsland D, Ballard C, McKeith I, Perry RH, Larsen JP. Comparison of extrapyramidal signs in dementia with Lewy bodies and Parkinson's disease. J Neuropsychiatry Clin Neurosci 2001;13:374–9.
2. Adriani W, Ognibene E, Heuland E, Ghirardi O, Caprioli A, Laviola G. Motor impulsivity in APP-SWE mice: a model of Alzheimer's disease. Behav Pharmacol 2006;17:525–33.
3. Bacher Svendsen K, Staehelin Jensen T, Overvad K, Hansen HJ, Koch-Henriksen N, Bach FW. Pain in patients with multiple sclerosis. A population-based study. Arch Neurol 2003;60:1089–94.
4. Barber R, Scheltens P, Gholkar A, Ballard C, MvKeith I, Ince P, Perry R, O'Brien J. White matter lesions on magnetic resonance imaging in dementia with Lewy bodies, Alzheimer's disease, vascular dementia, and normal aging. J Neurol Neurosurg Psychiatry 1999;67:66–72.
5. Basile J. The role of existing and newer calcium channel blockers in the treatment of hypertension. J Clin Hypertens 2004;6:621–31.

6. Bathgate D, Snowden JS, Varma A, Blackshaw A, Neary D. Behaviour in frontotemporal dementia, Alzheimer's disease and vascular dementia. Acta Neurol Scand 2001;103:367–78.
7. Bekelman DB, Black BS, Shore AD, Kasper JD, Rabins PV. Hospice care in a cohort of elders with dementia and mild cognitive impairment. J Pain Symptom Manag 2005;30:208–14.
8. Benedetti F, Arduino C, Vighetti S, Asteggiano G, Tarenzi L, Rainero I. Pain reactivity in Alzheimer patients with different degrees of cognitive impairment and brain electrical activity deterioration. Pain 2004;111:22–9.
9. Benedetti F, Vighetti S, Ricco C, Lagna E, Bergamasco B, Pinessi L, Rainero L. Pain threshold and pain tolerance in Alzheimer's disease. Pain 1999;80:377–82.
10. Bernabei R, Gambassi G, Lapane K, Landi F, Gatsoni C, Dunlop R, Lipsitz L, Mor V. Management of pain in elderly patients with cancer. JAMA 1998;279:1877–82.
11. Bieri D, Reeve RA, Champion GD, Addicoat L, Ziegler JB. The Face Pain Scale for the self-assessment of the severity of pain experienced by children: development, initial validation, and preliminary investigation for ratio scale properties. Pain 1990;41:139–50.
12. Boccardi M, Pennanen C, Laakso MP, Testa C, Geroldi C, Soininen H, Frisoni GB. Amygdaloid atrophy in frontotemporal dementia and Alzheimer's disease. Neurosci Lett 2002;335:139–43.
13. Borckardt JJ, Smith AR, Reeves ST, Weinstein M, Kozel FA, Nahas Z, Shelley N, Branham RK, Thomas KJ, George MS. Fifteen minutes of left prefrontal repetitive transcranial magnetic stimulation acutely increases thermal pain thresholds in healthy adults. Pain Res Manag 2007;12:287–90.
14. Braak H, Braak E. Neuropathological staging of Alzheimer-related changes. Act Neuropathol 1991;82:239–59.
15. Brower MC, Price BH. Neuropsychiatry of frontal lobe dysfunction in violent and criminal behaviour: a critical review. J Neurol Neurosurg Psychiatry 2001;71:720–6.
16. Bruen PD, McGeown WJ, Shanks MF, Venneri A. Neuroanatomical correlates of neuropsychiatric symptoms in Alzheimer's disease. Brain 2008;131:2455–63.
17. Buffum MD, Miaskowski C, Sands L. A pilot study of the relationship between discomfort and agitation in patients with dementia. Geriatr Nurs 2001;22:80–5.
18. Buffum MD, Sands L, Miaskowski C, Brod M, Washburn A. A clinical trial of the effectiveness of regularly scheduled versus as-needed administration of acetaminophen in the management of discomfort in older adults with dementia. J Am Geriatr Soc 2004;52:1093–97.
19. Caligiuri MP, Peavy G, Galasko DR. Extrapyramidal signs and cognitive abilities in Alzheimer's disease. Int J Geriatr Psychiatry 2001;16:907–11.
20. Callen DJA, Black SE, Gao F, Caldwell CB. Limbic system perfusion in Alzheimer's disease measured by MRI-coregistered HMPAO SPET. Eur J Nucl Med 2002;29:899–906.
21. Carlino E, Benedetti F, Rainero I, Asteggiano G, Cappa G, Tarenzi L, Vighetti S, Pollo A. Pain perception and tolerance in patients with frontotemporal dementia. Pain 2010 Dec;151:783–9.
22. Casey KL, Lorenz J, Minoshima S. Insights into the pathophysiology of neuropathic pain through functional brain imaging. Exp Neurol 2003;184:S80–8.
23. Chibnall JT, Tait RC. Pain assessment in cognitively impaired and unimpaired older adults: a comparison of four scales. Pain 2001;92:173–86.
24. Chudler EH, Dong WK. The role of the basal ganglia in nociception and pain. Pain 1995;60:3–38.
25. Closs SJ, Barr B, Briggs M, Cash K, Seers K. A comparison of five pain assessment scales for nursing home residents with varying degrees of cognitive impairment. J Pain Symptom Manag 2004;27:196–205.
26. Cohen-Mansfield J, Werner P. Longitudinal predictors of non-aggressive agitated behaviors in the elderly. Int J Geriatr Psychiatry 1999;14:831–44.
27. Cole LJ, Farrell MJ, Duff EP, Barber JB, Egan GF, Gibson SJ. Pain sensitivity and fMRI pain-related brain activity in Alzheimer's disease 2006;129:2957–65.
28. Cummings JL, Back C. The cholinergic hypothesis of neuropsychiatric symptoms in Alzheimer's disease. Am J Geriatr Psychiatry 1998;6:S64–78.
29. Dastoor D, Schwartz G, Kurzman D. Clock-drawing: an assessment technique in dementia. J Clin Exp Gerontol 1991;13:69–85.
30. de Knegt N, Scherder E. Pain in adults with intellectual disabilities. Pain 2011;152:971–4
31. Edwards-Lee T, Miller BL, Benson DF, Cummings JL, Russell GL, Boone K, Mena I. The temporal variant of frontotemporal dementia. Brain 1997;120:1027–40.
32. Ekman P, Friesen W. Investigator's guide to facial action coding system. Palo Alto: Consulting Psychologists Press; 1978.
33. Emre M. Dementia associated with Parkinson's disease. Lancet (Neurol) 2003;2:229–37.
34. Farrell MJ, Katz B, Helme RD. The impact of dementia on the pain experience. Pain 1996;67:7–15.

35. Feldt K. Checklist for non-verbal pain indicators. Pain Manag Nurs 2001;1:13–21.
36. Ferrell BA, Ferrell BR, Rivera L. Pain in cognitively impaired nursing home patients. J Pain Symptom Manag 1995;10:591–8.
37. Fil A, Cano-de-la-Cuerda R, Muñoz-Hellín E, Vela L, Ramiro-González M, Fernández-de-Las-Peñas C. Pain in Parkinson disease: a review of the literature. Parkinsonism Relat Disord 2013;19:285–94.
38. Fisher-Morris M, Gellatly A. The experience and expression of pain in Alzheimer patients. Age Ageing 1997;26:497–500.
39. Ford B. Pain in Parkinson's disease. Clin Neurosci 1998;5:63–72.
40. Foundas AL, Leonard CM, Mahoney SM, Agee OF, Heilman KM. Atrophy of the hippocampus, parietal cortex, and insula in Alzheimer's disease: a volumetric magnetic resonance imaging study. Neuropsychiatry Neuropsychol Behav Neurol 1997;10:81–9.
41. Fuchs-Lacelle S, Hadjistavropoulos T. Development and preliminary validation of the pain assessment checklist for seniors with limited ability to communicate (PACSLAC). Pain Manag Nurs 2004;5:37–49.
42. Gibson SJ, Voukelatos X, Ames D, Flicker L, Helme RD. An examination of pain perception and cerebral event-related potentials following carbon dioxide laser stimulation in patients with Alzheimer's disease and age-matched control volunteers. Pain Res Manag 2001;6:126–32.
43. Haas DC, Kent PF, Friedman DI. Headache caused by a single lesion of multiple sclerosis in the periaqueductal gray area. Headache 1993;33:452–55.
44. Hadjistovropoulos T, LaChapelle DL, Hadjistavropoulos HD, Green S, Asmundson GJG. Using facial expressions to assess musculoskeletal pain in older persons. Eur J Pain 2002;6:179–87.
45. Halper J, Kennedy P, Miller CM, Morgante L, Namey M, Ross AP. Rethinking cognitive function in multiple sclerosis: a nursing perspective. J Neurosci Nurs 2003;35:70–81.
46. Hanlon JT, Landerman LR, Wall WE, Horner RD, Fillenbaum GG, Dawson DV, Schmader KE, Cohen HJ, Blazer DG. Is medication use by community-dwelling elderly people influenced by cognitive function? Age Ageing 1996;25:190–6.
47. Helme RD, Gibson SJ. The epidemiology of pain in elderly people. Clin Geriatr Med 2001;17:417–31.
48. Herr K, Decker S. Assessment of pain in older adults with severe cognitive impairment. Ann Long-Term Care: Clin Care Aging 2004;12:46–52.
49. Herr KA, Spratt K, Mobily PR, Richardson G. Pain intensity assessment in older adults. Use of experimental pain to compare psychometric properties and usability of selected pain scales with younger adults. Clin J Pain 2004;20:207–19.
50. Hirono N, Mega MS, Dinov ID, Mishkin F, Cummings JL. Left frontotemporal hypoperfusion is associated with aggression in patients with dementia. Arch Neurol 2000;57:861–6.
51. Horgas AL, Elliott AF. Pain assessment and management in persons with dementia. Nurs Clin N Am 2004;39:593–606.
52. Hurley AC, Volicer BJ, Hanrahan PA, Houde S, Volicer L. Assessment of discomfort in advanced Alzheimer patients. Res Nurs Health 1992;15:369–77.
53. Husebo BS, Ballard C, Sandvik R, Nilsen OB, Aarsland D. Efficacy of treating pain to reduce behavioural disturbances in residents of nursing homes with dementia: cluster randomised clinical trial. BMJ 2011;343:d4065
54. Ishunina TA, Swaab DF. Neurohypophyseal peptides in aging and Alzheimer's disease. Ageing Res Rev 2002;1:537–558.
55. Jacobs J, Bernhard M, Delgado A, Strain JJ. Screening for organic mental syndromes in the medically ill. Ann Intern Med 1977;8:40–6.
56. Jellinger KA. α-Synuclein pathology in Parkinson's and Alzheimer's disease brain: incidence and topographic distribution—a pilot study. Acta Neuropathol 2003;106:191–201.
57. Jensen MP, Miller L, Fisher LD. Assessment of pain during medical procedures: a comparison of three scales. Clin J Pain 1998;14:343–9.
58. Jones SL. Descending noradrenergic influences on pain. In: Barnes CD, Pompeiano O, editors. Progress in brain research, Vol. 88. Amsterdam: Elsevier Science; 1991, p. 381–94.
59. Karlsen KH, Tandberg E, Årsland D, Larsen JP. Health related quality of life in Parkinson's disease: a prospective longitudinal study. J Neurol Neurosurg Psychiatry 2000;69:584–9.
60. Kerns RD, Kassirer M, Otis J. Pain in multiple sclerosis: a biopsychosocial perspective. J Rehabil Res Dev 2002;39:225–32.
61. Kovach CR, Weissman DE, Griffie J, Matson S, Muchka S. Assessment and treatment of discomfort for people with late-stage dementia. J Pain Symptom Manag 1999;18:412–9.
62. Krueger CE, Bird AC, Growdon ME, Jang JY, Miller BL, Kramer JH. Conflict monitoring in early frontotemporal dementia. Neurology 2009;73:349–55.

63. Kunz M, Mylius V, Scharmann S, Schepelman K, Lautenbacher S. Influence of dementia on multiple components of pain. Eur J Pain 2009;13:317–25.
64. Kunz M, Mylius V, Schepelmann K, Lautenbacher S. Effects of age and mild cognitive impairment on the pain response system. Gerontology 2009;55:674–82.
65. Laakso MP, Frisoni GB, Kononen M, Mikkonen M, Beltramello A, Geroldi C, Bianchetti A, Trabucchi M, Soininen H, Aronen HJ. Hippocampus and entorhinal cortex in frontotemporal dementia and Alzheimer's disease: a morphometric MRI study. Biol Psychiatry 2000;47:1056–63.
66. Lorenz J, Minoshima S, Casey KL. Keeping pain out of mind: the role of the dorsolateral prefrontal cortex in pain modulation. Brain 2003;126:1079–91.
67. Lucca U, Tettamanti M, Forloni G, Spagnoli A. Nonsteroidal antiinflammatory drug use in Alzheimer's disease. Biol Psychiatry 1994;36:854–6.
68. Luciani A, Balducci L. Multiple primary malignancies. Semin Oncol 2004;31:264–73.
69. Manfredi PL, Breuer B, Meier DE, Libow L. Pain assessment in elderly patients with severe dementia. J Pain Symptom Manag 2003;25:48–52.
70. Manfredi PL, Breuer B, Wallenstein S, Stegmann M, Bottomley G, Libow L. Opioid treatment for agitation in patients with advanced dementia. Int J Geriatr Psychiatry 2003;18:700–5.
71. Marzinski LR. The tragedy of dementia: clinically assessing pain in the confused, nonverbal elderly. J Gerontol Nurs 1991;17:25–8.
72. Massimo L, Powers C, Moore P, Vesely L, Avants B, Gee J, Libon DJ, Grossman M. Neuroanatomy of apathy and disinhibition in frontotemporal lobar degeneration. Dement Geriatr Cogn Disord 2009;27:96–104.
73. McCormick WC, Kukull WA, van Belle G, Bowen JD, Teri L, Larson EB. Symptom patterns and comorbidity in the early stages of Alzheimer's disease. J Am Geriatr Soc 1994;42:517–21.
74. McGrath PA, Seifert CE, Speechley KN, Booth JC, Stitt L, Gibson MC. A new analogue scale for assessing children's pain: an initial validation study. Pain 1996;64:435–43.
75. Melzack R. The McGill Pain Questionnaire: major properties and scoring methods. Pain 1975;1:275–95.
76. Mohr C, Leyendecker S, Mangels I, Machner B, Sander T, Helmchen C. Central representation of cold-evokedpain r elief in capsaicin induced pain: an event-related fMRI study. Pain 2008;139:416–30.
77. Mori E. Impact of subcortical ischemic lesions on behavior and cognition. Ann NY Acad Sci 2002;977:141–8.
78. Moulin DE. Pain in multiple sclerosis. Neurol Clin 1989;7:321–31.
79. Nurmikko TJ. Mechanisms of central pain. Clin J Pain 2000;16: S21–5.
80. O'Brien JT. Role of imaging techniques in the diagnosis of dementia. Br J Radiol 2007;80:S71–7.
81. Plooij B, Swaab D, Scherder E. Autonomic responses to pain in aging and dementia. Rev Neurosci. 2011;22: 583–9.
82. Porter FL, Malhotra KM, Wolf CM, Morris JC, Miller JP, Smith MC. Dementia and response to pain in the elderly. Pain 1996;68:413–21.
83. Price D. Psychological and neural mechanisms of the affective dimension of pain. Science 2000;288:1769–72.
84. Raadsheer FC, Tilders FJ, Swaab DF. Similar age related increase of vasopressin colocalization in paraventricular corticotropin-releasing hormone neurons in controls and Alzheimer patients. J Neuroendocrinol 1994;6:131–3.
85. Rainero I, Vighetti S, Bergamasco B, Pinessi L, Benedetti F. Autonomic responses and pain perception in Alzheimer's disease. Eur J Pain 2000;4:267–74.
86. Ram CV. Beta-blockers in hypertension. Am J Cardiol 2010;106:1819–25.
87. Rocca MA, Matthews PM, Caputo D, Ghezzi A, Falini A, Scotti G, Comi G, Filippi M. Evidence for widespread movement-associated functional MRI changes in patients with PPMS. Neurology 2002;58:866–72.
88. Rosen HJ, Allison SC, Schauer GF, Gorno-Tempini M-L, Weiner MW, Miller BL. Neuroanatomical correlates of behavioural disorders in dementia. Brain 2005;128:2612–25.
89. Rüb U, Del Tredici K, Schultz C, Ghebremedhin E, de Vos RA, Jansen Steur E, Braak H. Parkinson's disease: the thalamic components of the limbic loop are severely impaired by α-synuclein immunopositive inclusion body pathology. Neurobiol Aging 2002;23:245–54.
90. Schenkman M, Wei Zhu C, Cutson TM, Whetten-Goldstein K. Longitudinal evaluation of economic and physical impact of Parkinson's disease. Parkinsonism Relat Disord 2001;8:41–50.
91. Scherder E, Bouma A, Slaets J, Ooms M, Ribbe M, Blok A, Sergeant J. Repeated pain assessment in Alzheimer's disease. Dementia Geriatr Cogn Disord 2001;12:400–7.
92. Scherder E, Plooij B, Achterberg WP, Pieper M, Wiegersma M, Lobbezoo F, Oosterman J. Chronic pain in 'probable' subcortical vascular dementia. Pain Med 2015;16:442–50.
93. Scherder E, Wolters E, Chris Polman C, Sergeant J, Swaab D. Pain in Parkinson's disease and multiple sclerosis: Its relation to the medial and lateral pain systems. Neurosci Biobehav Rev 2005;29:1047–56.

94. Scherder EJ, Bouma A. Visual analogue scales for pain assessment in Alzheimer's disease. Gerontology 2000;46:47–53.
95. Scherder EJ, Sergeant JA, Swaab DF. Pain processing in dementia and its relation to neuropathology. Lancet Neurol 2003;2:677–86.
96. Scherder EJ, Slaets J, Deijen J-B, Gorter Y, Ooms ME, Ribbe M, Vuijk PJ, Feldt K, van de Valk M, Bouma A, Sergeant JA. Pain assessment in patients with possible vascular dementia. Psychiatry 2003;66:133–45.
97. Schmader KE, Hanlon JT, Fillen-Baum GG, Huber M, Pieper C, Horner R. Medication use patterns among demented, cognitively impaired and cognitively intact community-dwelling elderly people. Age Ageing 1998;27:493–501.
98. Schmahmann JD, Leifer D. Parietal pseudothalamic pain syndrome. Arch Neurol 1992;490:1032–37.
99. Schott GD. Pain in Parkinson's disease. Pain 1985;22:407–11.
100. Seo D, Patrick CJ. Role of serotonin and dopamine system interactions in the neurobiology of impulsive aggression and its comorbidity with other clinical disorders. Aggress Violent Behav 2008;13:383–95.
101. Sewards TV, Sewards MA. The medial pain system: neural representations of the motivational aspect of pain. Brain Res Bull 2002;59:163–80.
102. Shibasaki H, Kuroiwa Y. Painful tonic seizure in multiple sclerosis. Arch Neurol 1974;30:47–51.
103. Siever LJ. Neurobiology of aggression and violence. Am J Psychiatry 2008;165:429–42.
104. Skoog I. Psychiatric epidemiology of old age: the H70 study—the NAPE Lecture 2003. Acta Psychiatr Scand 2004;109:4–18.
105. Snow AL, Weber JB, O'Malley KJ, Cody M, Beck C, Bruera E, Ashton C, Kunik ME. NOPPAIN: a nursing assistant-administered pain assessment instrument for use in dementia. Dement Geriatr Cogn Disord 2004;17:240–6.
106. Solaro C, Lunardi GL, Mancardi GL. Pain and MS. Int MS J 2003;10:14–19.
107. Sperling RA, Guttmann CR, Hohol MJ, Warfield SK, Jakab M, Parente M, Diamond EL, Daffner KR, Olek MJ, Orav EJ, et al. Regional magnetic resonance imaging lesion burden and cognitive function in multiple sclerosis. A longitudinal study. Arch Neurol 2001;58:115–21.
108. Sultzer DL, Mahler ME, Mandelkern MA, Cummings JL, Van Gorp WG, Hinkin CH, Berisford MA. The relationship between psychiatric symptoms and regional cortical metabolism in Alzheimer's disease. J Neuropsychiatry Clin Neurosci 1995;7:476–84.
109. Swaab DF. Neurobiology and neuropathology of the human hypothalamus. In: Bloom FE, Björklund A, Hökfelt T, editors. Handbook of chemical neuroanatomy. The primate nervous system, Part I, Vol. 13. Amsterdam: Elsevier Science; 1997. p. 39–137.
110. Swaab DF. Nuclei of the human hypothalamus. Part 1. In: Aminoss MJ, Boller S, Swaab DF, editors. Handbook of clinical neurology, Vol. 79. Amsterdam: Elsevier Science; 2003.
111. Swaab DF. Neuropathology of the human hypothalamus and adjacent structures. Part 2. In: Aminoss MJ, Boller S, Swaab DF, editors. Handbook of clinical neurology, Vol. 80. Amsterdam: Elsevier Science; 2004.
112. Taylor LJ, Herr K. Pain intensity assessment: a comparison of selected pain intensity scales for use in cognitively intact and cognitively impaired African American older adults. Pain Manag Nurs 2003;4:87–95.
113. Varrone A, Pappatà S, Caracò C, Soricelli A, Milan G, Quarantelli M, Alfano B, Postiglione A, Salvatore M. Voxel-based comparison of rCBF SPET images in frontotemporal dementia and Alzheimer's disease highlights the involvement of different cortical networks. Eur J Nucl Med 2002;29:1447–54.
114. Vogt BA, Sikes RW. The medial pain system, cingulate cortex, and parallel processing of nociceptive information. In: Mayer EA, Saper CB, editors. Progress in brain research, Vol. 122. Amsterdam: Elsevier Science; 2000. p. 223–35.
115. Warden V, Hurley AC, Volicer L. Development and psychometric evaluation of the Pain Assessment in Advanced Dementia (PAINAD) scale. J Am Med Dir Assoc 2003;4:9–15.
116. Waseem S, Gwinn-Hardy K. Pain in Parkinson's disease. Common yet seldom recognized symptom is treatable. Postgrad Med 2001;110:33–46.
117. Willis WD, Westlund KN. Neuroanatomy of the pain system and the pathways that modulate pain. J Clin Neurophysiol 1997;14:2–31.
118. Witte AV, Flöel A, Stein P, Savli M, Mien L-K, Wadsak W, Spindelegger C, Moser U, Fink M, Hahn A, et al. Aggression is related to frontal serotonin-1A receptor distribution as revealed by PET in healthy subjects. Hum Brain Mapp 2009;30:2558–70.
119. Wolf-Klein GP, Silverstone FA, Brod MS, Levy A, Foley CJ, Termotto V, Breuer J. Are Alzheimer patients healthier? J Am Geriatr Soc 1988;36:219–24.
120. Zhuo M, Gebhart GF. Spinal serotonin receptors mediate descending faciliation of a nociceptive reflex from the nuclei reticularis gigantocellularis and gigantocellularis pars alpha in the rat. Brain Res 1991;550:35–48.

CHAPTER 7

Neuropsychiatric Sequels of Pain in Dementia

Bettina S. Husebø and Elisabeth Flo

Pain, especially in its chronic form, may exacerbate cognitive, emotional, and behavioral problems. The additional presence of dementia complicates a pain condition even more. Both dementia and pain may yield similar behavioral and psychological symptoms, often referred to as neuropsychiatric symptoms (NPSs). This chapter provides an overview of the most common NPSs and the conditions in which these symptoms are more or less likely to occur. A better understanding of neuropsychiatric symptoms in dementia and related to pain helps to establish a clear therapeutic rationale in the evaluation and treatment of pain in this vulnerable group.

A century ago, the life expectancy in Europe was 49 years and over half of the population died before the age of 20. Today, in the industrialized world, fewer children are being born while more than half of us will become at least 80 years old—humankind is getting radically older [42]. As a result, dementia is becoming increasingly prevalent. In nursing homes (NHs), 80% of the patients have dementia. Dementia is described as a progressive irreversible syndrome characterized by cognitive and functional decline and the presence of NPSs [9]. The nature of NPSs is poorly understood, but the cause is multifactorial, including physiological, psychological, and social antecedents [38].

Advancing age is also associated with high prevalence of pain, estimated to be as much as four times higher than in younger adults [28]. Many elderly individuals living at home and in NHs experience both dementia and pain. Patients with moderate or severe dementia are not able to express their suffering, and they express their pain in ways that are different from those without dementia. Thereby, pain and discomfort may trigger behavioral disturbances such as agitation and depression [30]. Probably, instead of pain treatment, almost 25% of the demented patients receive antipsychotic medications and restraints, despite all the adverse events of this treatment (e.g., drowsiness, falls, and depressed mood) [11]. Specialized dementia care services have increased worldwide, and guidelines recommend approaches for appropriate dementia care. However, proper pain management remains a considerable challenge.

Elsa B. is 88 years old and representative for nursing home residents. She is old and frail and suffers from dementia in combination with several diseases such as heart failure, behavioral disturbances (agitation, anxiety, and restlessness), and gait impairment caused by serious osteoporosis with old fractures. In addition, she is in pain.

What are her chances for receiving skilled pain assessment and pain management? Do family and staff have the skill and knowledge necessary for managing her increasing suffering? Or, will she receive psychotropic drugs to regulate her inappropriate behavior? Can we accept that old patients in need of high-quality dementia care and pain management have good reasons to fear their last stage of life?

During the last decades, different research areas have helped to shed light on the covert suffering in patients with dementia. This chapter provides an evidence-based understanding of the interactive relationship of pain and NPSs in people with dementia with the following themes:

- Definitions of NPSs
- Clinical differential assessment of pain versus NPSs in advanced dementia
- Correlation between pain and NPSs
- Intervention studies showing the efficacy of treating pain on NPSs

NEUROPSYCHIATRIC SYMPTOMS IN DEMENTIA

Classification

In neurocognitive disorders, including dementia disorders, patients usually show symptoms beyond that of cognitive decline. Apart from changes in social cognition (recognition of emotions, theory of mind), several behavioral and psychological symptoms are frequently present [47, 54].

Among patients with dementia, approximately 90% will have one or more NPS throughout the course of their disease [56]. Identifying NPSs is an elementary part of the diagnostic and clinical evaluation of patients with dementia. Meanwhile, the diverse terminology used to describe the types of dementia and these accompanying NPSs can be confusing.

The fifth version of the *Diagnostic and Statistical Manual of Mental Disorders (DSM-5)* describes relevant patient groups in the diagnostic category "neurocognitive disorders" [7]. The *DSM-5* differentiates between a major and a mild neurocognitive disorder and between etiological subtypes. Importantly, even in cases of mild cognitive decline, dementia may be disruptive if accompanied by disturbing NPSs.

The importance of these noncognitive symptoms started to receive full attention in the 1980s. The noncognitive symptoms are of clinical significance, as they are detrimental for both patients and family or caregivers [47], and are frequently the primary reason that health and care services are needed [58]. These symptoms are often referred to as neuropsychiatric symptoms (in dementia), which overlaps in large with the term *behavioral and psychological symptoms of dementia (BPSD)*. BPSD was coined by the International Psychogeriatric Association in the 1990s, comprising the following symptoms: apathy, depressive symptoms, anxiety, hallucinations, delusions, lack of inhibition, agitation, yelling, and pacing [38]. Meanwhile, the *DSM-5* manual has labeled these symptoms *behavioral disturbances in neurocognitive disorders* [7]. The grouping of these symptoms has effectively highlighted core issues of behavioral disturbances and psychiatric symptoms in dementia among researchers, health personnel, and industries. Meanwhile, it is doubtful that all symptoms share common etiology or approaches to treatment. For continuity, we will use the abbreviation NPSs in this chapter.

Studies have suggested a linear relationship between cognitive decline and risk of NPSs, with the lowest symptoms incidence in those with no cognitive impairment, intermediary incidence in those with Mild Cognitive Impairment (MCI), and highest incidence in patients with dementia [47]. However, the incidence of the different NPSs also varies according to the type of dementia and stages of dementia. Mood symptoms occur more frequently in the earlier stages of the illness. Agitation and psychotic symptoms become more pronounced in relation to moderate cognitive impairment, while they subsequently recede with the further progression of the dementia [38]. Much remains to be done to obtain a better understanding of the etiology of NPSs. The current multifactorial etiological model includes (1) psychological (e.g., response to pain/discomfort or stress, premorbid disposition); (2) social (e.g., environmental change and social relations); and (3) physiological (genetic and neurobiological) factors.

Although terminology and definitions vary considerably, the NPSs are commonly categorized in three main syndromes: agitation, psychosis, and mood [9].

The agitation syndrome includes symptoms of aggression, irritability, restlessness, and pacing and represents a complex challenge in patients with dementia. Approximately 20% of patients receiving clinical health services show aggression and nonaggressive agitation [10]. The symptoms are reckoned as highly disruptive and burdensome to caregivers/staff, and thus not surprisingly a common cause of admittance to long-term-care facilities, where 40–60% show these symptoms [9]. The etiology is considered to be multifactorial, including brain changes, genetics, pain, unmet needs, and illnesses with and without central nervous system affection such as stroke, cardiovascular disease, and infections [10, 12].

The concept of agitation lacks a universally accepted definition and often includes different behaviors (e.g., wandering, hyperactivity, and negativity) with different etiologies, treatment, and prognosis [45]. No unanimously accepted definition of what constitutes aggression in elderly persons exists either [22]. Various symptoms are called agitation without consideration of the setting in which they occur [8], and overlapping symptoms may thus be interpreted as agitation, irritability, aggression, or resistance to care.

Cohen-Mansfield and Libin [20] have suggested four factor groups in which behavioral disturbances are present: (1) aggressive behavior (e.g., hitting, kicking, pushing, scratching, biting, grabbing, throwing things, cursing or verbal aggression, spitting, tearing things/destroying property, hurting self or others, and screaming); (2) physical nonaggressive behavior (e.g., pacing, trying to get to a different place, general restlessness, inappropriate dressing or disrobing, handling things inappropriately, and performing repetitious mannerisms); (3) verbally agitated behavior (e.g., complaining, constant requests for attention, repetitive questions, and negativism); and (4) hiding and hoarding. These symptoms may be burdensome for the people close to the patient and often leads to social and family dysfunction, as well as institutionalization [14, 49].

The psychosis syndrome can be experienced as dramatic to the patients, their family, and the nursing staff. The most frequent psychotic symptoms include visual hallucinations, auditory hallucinations, and persecutory/paranoid delusions [9]. Depending on the definition of dementia, delusions have been found in 10–73% and hallucinations in 12–49% [38].

The mood syndrome comprises depression, anxiety, and apathy, as well as changes in sleep and appetite [1, 25]. Studies show that depressive symptoms are quite common in patients with dementia, whereas major depressions are found in approximately 20% of the population. Depression may represent a symptom of dementia, but it may also represent a comorbid condition, which may even cause or exacerbate cognitive decline [4]. As the dementia progresses, depression can be increasingly difficult to detect. This may be due to the loss of language and due to the occurrence of other symptoms such as apathy, weight loss, and sleep disturbances, which may be related both to dementia and depression [13, 26, 48].

The overlap of symptoms of depression and of the mood syndrome related to dementia can make a differential diagnosis difficult.

The mood symptoms such as apathy and anxiety are also quite prevalent in dementia. Apathy is found in up to 50% of patients in the early and intermediate dementia stages [38]. The prevalence of anxiety disorders in dementia has ranged from 17% to 38%, while up to 70% of patients with dementia show symptoms of anxiety (e.g., pronounced concern/worry, anxiousness, nervousness, and tension) [55]. The prevalence of anxiety symptoms may vary according to the dementia diagnosis (more common in vascular dementia than in Alzheimer disease) and severity of the dementia (decreases with the progression of the disease).

Changes in sleep and appetite may represent mood-related symptoms but may also have a different cause. For example, sleep may also be negatively affected by advancing age, chronic disease (e.g., heart disease, obesity, arthritis, diabetes, lung diseases, stroke, and osteoporosis), pain, and neurodegeneration [29]. Insomnia has been found in 25–35% of patients with Alzheimer disease and 54–60% of patients with Parkinson disease [51]. Disrupted sleep may set in motion a vicious cycle in which sleep fragmentation in turn leads to nocturnal wandering, increased daytime sleepiness, napping, further cognitive decline and confusion [24, 51], and potentially more perceived pain [46].

Changes in appetite and eating behavior entail increased/decreased appetite and weight, and new food preference and eating habits [25]. Changes in appetite and eating behavior vary according to type of dementia, and as a result, the incidence of this symptom varies across studies depending on the study population [16]. Changes in sleep and appetite may represent mood-related symptoms but may also have a different cause. For example, sleep may also be negatively affected by advancing age, chronic disease, pain, and neurodegeneration.

The mood cluster symptoms are prevalent in patients with dementia [25] and lead to considerable caregiver stress and institutionalization [57].

Assessment of Neuropsychiatric Symptoms in Dementia

The assessment of NPSs is a crucial part of a dementia evaluation and differential diagnostics. Since the late 1980s, numerous scales have been developed and tested to evaluate NPSs [see also chapter 14]. Some of these scales are symptom specific, such as the Cohen-Mansfield Agitation Inventory (CMAI) and the Cornell Scale for Depression in Dementia (CSDD) [4]. Other scales have a more broad focus and allow clinicians to rate the full range of NPSs, as is the case with the widely recognized Neuropsychiatric Inventory (NPI) [26].

The NPI addresses the following domains: (1) delusions; (2) hallucinations; (3) agitation; (4) depression/dysphoric; (5) anxiety; (6) euphoria/elation; (7) apathy/indifference; (8) disinhibition; (9) irritability/lability; (10) aberrant motor behavior; (11) nighttime disturbances; and (12) change in appetite/eating. The NPI has been shown to be responsive to behavioral changes in patients with Alzheimer disease and other disorders, and provides distinctive profiles of NPSs in a variety of neurological disorders [63]. The NPI is available in a nursing home edition (NPI-NH) [63].

The extensively used CMAI was developed in the 1980s to measure the prevalence and type of agitation in NHs [19]. The CMAI represents an important step in recognizing the presence of NPS in the NH, but it does not address other common NPSs (e.g., delusions, anxiety, and depression).

The CSDD is a screening tool for symptoms of depression in patients with dementia. Importantly, the CSDD includes nonverbal symptoms that could indicate depression in dementia patients with impaired communication. The CSDD covers a wide range of symptoms related to disrupted mood, behavior (agitation, retardation), and physical signs (changes in appetite, weight, and energy).

The overlap of symptom items in these different assessment tools illustrates the interconnection of symptoms. For example, apathy may be interpreted not only as a symptom of dementia, but also as a symptom of depression. The numerous potential sources of similar symptoms require staff trained in considering symptoms in context and with specific knowledge of the patients. The context to be considered might also be pain, which is prevalent in these patients.

Delirium—An Important Differential Diagnostic

Delirium is a frequent and imminent challenge in patients with dementia. Dementia is considered to be an important risk factor for developing delirium, which may be caused by medications, untreated pain, terminal illness, iatrogenic event, sepsis, infections, or alcohol/drug abuse. About 50% of the cases are reversible, but differentiation between delirium, dementia, depression, and psychosis is a prerequisite for appropriate treatment [62].

Importantly, patients in a state of delirium may show the behavioral and psychological symptoms typically seen in dementia. When a person already has dementia, detecting delirium is often difficult, because existing disordered thought and confusion can mask the delirium. Although challenging, it is possible to differentiate between delirium and dementia. Delirium usually entails subacute to acute symptoms' onset with changes in attention (heightened/reduced) or prominent fluctuations in symptoms in patients with dementia, visual hallucinations, agitation, and altered psychomotor activity.

Summary: Neuropsychiatric Symptoms in Dementia

- NPSs occur in virtually every patient with dementia.
- Symptoms have a crucial impact on disease progression.
- Disruptive symptoms increase risk of institutionalization.
- Differentiation between NPSs in dementia and delirium and adverse effects of medications is important.

NEUROPSYCHIATRIC SYMPTOMS AND PAIN-RELATED BEHAVIOR IN PATIENTS WITH DEMENTIA

To understand the relationship between NPSs and pain, several researchers have explored the characteristics of these issues and found that pain can be expressed as, for instance, agitation or aggression in people with dementia and that pain treatment may reduce pain, pain behavior, and NPSs [54].

NPS items such as agitation/aggression, depression, anxiety, apathy, irritability, aberrant motor behavior, disturbed sleep, and appetite are frequently included in pain assessment tools for patients with impaired cognition/dementia. Meanwhile, anxiety and irritability have been found to be unrelated to pain treatment, while aberrant motor

TABLE 7-1 Overview of the Overlap between Items Mentioned in Tools Assessing Neuropsychiatric Symptoms or Pain in Patients with Dementia and Being Either Responsive or Not to Pain Treatment

Delusions	÷	Apathy/indifference	+ √
Hallucinations	÷	Disinhibition	÷
Agitation/aggression	+ √	Irritability/lability	+ ×
Depression/dysphoria	+ √	Aberrant motor behavior	+ ÷
Anxiety	+ ×	Sleep and nighttime behavior disorders	+ √
Elation/euphoria	÷	Appetite and eating changes	+ √

Abbreviations: +, behavior symptom groups also listed in pain assessment tools; √, symptoms found to be related to pain treatment [31, 32, 34]; ×, symptoms found to be unrelated to pain treatment [31, 32, 34]; ÷, symptoms not yet investigated in randomized intervention studies.

behavior, delusion, hallucination, elation/euphoria, and disinhibition have not been investigated in any relevant RCT [31, 32, 34] (Table 7-1).

However, there are no standard procedures to assess or evaluate the impact of pain on NPSs, but at least two approaches are relevant [33]:

a. The straightforward approach that investigates the correlation between pain and NPSs at baseline
b. A more indirect approach where intervention studies investigate the effect of pain management and, in so doing, also assess the impact on NPSs

Although the idea that pain behavior overlaps or exacerbates dementia-related behavior has been suggested for decades, few clinical studies have investigated this assumption and results are equivocal.

Correlation between Pain and Neuropsychiatric Symptoms

With the straightforward approach, pain has been shown to correlate with agitation, aggression, depression, wandering behavior, inappropriate behavior, resistance to care, abnormal thought processes, delusions, aggression, and depression. Noticeably, some of the findings in these studies are contradictory.

To investigate the effect of pain on NPS in NH patients with dementia, Ahn and colleagues [3] used data from the Minimum Data Set (MDS 2.0) ($N = 56,577$) and examined the association between pain, wandering, aggression, agitation, and cognitive impairment. They found that more severe pain is less likely to display wandering behaviors but more likely to display aggressive and agitated behaviors. This supports earlier results that patients in pain may express a *pain avoidance effect*, which means that they do not move or pace when they experience severe pain [37].

Another cross-sectional study (SHELTER project) investigated the association between pain and wandering, verbally and physically abusive, socially inappropriate behavior, and resistance to care in patients with cognitive impairment [60]. Only 19% of 2822 patients from eight European countries were found to be in pain, as assessed by *self-report*. Although agitation, aggression, or depression was not investigated, the presence of pain was associated with inappropriate behavior, resistance to care, abnormal thought processes, and delusion but not with wandering.

Another study by Black et al. [15] included 123 NH patients with advanced dementia in order to investigate health problems and comorbid illnesses and correlates of staff-identified pain. Eighty-five percent of the residents had psychiatric/behavioral disturbances, and 63% had recognized pain, of whom 95% received pain medications. Pain was associated with aspiration, peripheral vascular disease, musculoskeletal disorders, and use of pain medications, but not NPSs.

The identification of factors predicting the development of aggression was investigated in a longitudinal study design of nonaggressive patients with newly diagnosed dementia [45]. Of 215 patients, 89 (41%) developed aggression. In individual models, high baseline mutuality decreased risk of aggression; high burden and pain increased risk. Increases in depression and pain and declines in total mutuality also increased risk. The prevalence of pain did not differ between participants who developed aggression in the course of the disease compared with nonaggressive persons. However, results suggested that the relationship between depression and aggression may be mediated by pain.

The modifiable effect of depression, psychosis, and pain on agitation was investigated in 2032 Dutch NH patients with dementia, using longitudinal Minimum Data Set (MDS) information [61]. Three quarters of the participants had at least one symptom of agitation at the beginning of the study, and almost half of the subjects experienced some level of pain. Correlations between agitation and pain were found, but pain scores did not change when agitation changed. This may be explained by the fact that pain and discomfort scales do not capture only pain but also other behaviors such as agitation, aggression, and resistance to care.

Summary: The Association between Pain and Neuropsychiatric Symptoms

- Pain can be idiosyncratic and present as agitation or aggression in people with dementia, and pain treatment may affect both the pain and the behavior.
- Although the suggestion that pain behavior overlaps with or exacerbates dementia-related behavior has existed over several decades, only few clinical studies are available, which have tested this assumption and results are still equivocal.
- Standard procedures are not available to assess or evaluate the impact of pain on agitation, aggression, and other NPSs.

The Effect of Pain Treatment on Neuropsychiatric Symptoms

More recently, the scope of research has extended from the assessment of pain to the treatment of pain and assessment of the treatment effect on pain and NPSs in patients with dementia [2, 23, 32, 54]. Now, long-term effects of untreated pain on NPSs such as agitation, depression, and apathy receive due attention [30]. To date, seven studies have explored whether analgesics would influence agitation using a retrospective or observational design without a comparison group.

One of the first studies addressing this research question included 10 NH patients with difficult behavior and standard treatment of psychotropic drugs [27]. This study found that behavioral symptoms decreased during pain treatment (acetaminophen). Another study included 143 patients with severe dementia who followed a systematic assessment and treatment plan for discomfort [44]. Part of the patients ($N = 91$) received acetaminophen, propoxyphene, or Darvocet, treatments, which effectively reduced discomfort and behavioral symptoms that might have been related to pain. It was concluded that psychotropic drug use masks typical signs of pain and contributed to undertreatment of discomfort.

In a third retrospective study, 154 patients with moderate dementia and nondemented controls were included in an All-inclusive Care Program investigating changes in pain intensity, use of pain medication, psychotropic drug use and NPSs, or mortality [17]. It was concluded that the level of pain was independent from the level of dementia and NPSs, use of pain medication, and use of psychotropic medication. In yet another study, the association between prescription patterns and self-reported pain, conversational ability, cognitive status, and activity levels were studied in 64 participants [5]. Significant association was not found between conversational ability and analgesic prescription and dosage. Interestingly, patients who were prescribed opioids spent more time being active than those not prescribed analgesics.

The first placebo-controlled, double-blinded trial that used opioids to treat pain and agitation in 47 patients with severe dementia [50] found no significant differences in agitation in the placebo and opioid condition. However, a subgroup of very old participants ($N = 13$) (>85 years) demonstrated significantly lower agitation level at the end of the opioid phase, without sedation. Another trial explored the effect of acetaminophen on behavior, emotional well-being, and use of as-needed psychotropic medications in 25 NH patients with moderate or severe dementia, without finding any effect on agitated behavior [18]. Interestingly, when participants received acetaminophen treatment, they were more active and engaged in social interaction and required less personal care. A third controlled trial used a stepwise clinical protocol for assessment and treatment of unmet needs of patients with advanced dementia (ranging from nonpharmacological to pharmacological pain/discomfort management) [43]. The pain intervention group including 26 patients had less discomfort than the controls. However, no difference in behavioral problems was found between the groups.

In a cluster randomized clinical trial to evaluate a stepwise protocol for the treatment of pain, 352 patients with moderate to severe dementia and significant NPSs were randomly assigned to receive either usual treatment (control group) or an 8-week stepwise administration of analgesics, where medication depended on prior treatment and assessment of pain [32]. The intervention group showed improvement in agitation and aggression (CMAI) and pain (Mobilization-Observation-Behavior-Intensity-Dementia-2 [MOBID-2]), compared with controls [31, 32]. Results demonstrated that verbally agitated behaviors, followed by physically nonaggressive behaviors, and aggressive behaviors were significantly improved after 8 weeks. In addition, restlessness and pacing were responsive to analgesics. It was concluded that such NPSs—typically also related to pain—should lead to both the assessment of pain and dementia-related behavioral symptoms. Further analyses showed significant improvements in the mood cluster, depression, apathy, nighttime behaviors, and appetite, while irritability and anxiety were not affected [34].

Pain Behavior versus Dementia Behavior—Assessment Is Key

In clinical studies on people with dementia, associations between pain and NPSs such as agitation [30], depression, and sleep disturbances [34] have been suggested.

A key challenge we face today is that behavior items used in most of the available pain observation tools may indicate behavior related to pain, or dementia, or both (Table 7-1).

Thus, pain items must be interpreted with being aware that they are also present in established instruments measuring NPSs (NPI) [25, 63], depression (CDDS) [4], and agitation (CMAI) [20]. Importantly, if the staff members also have pain diagnostics in mind, they judge the situation differently compared to staff with competence in and focus mainly on dementia care. This may reduce the validity of pain observation tools that include behavior typically defined as NPSs instead of keeping a specific focus on behavior typically related to pain [6].

Worldwide, a great variety of pain assessment tools have been developed. Both pain therapists and researchers should be familiar with their weaknesses and strengths and indicators of when to use which tool. For cognitively intact persons, these instruments vary between simple self-rating scales, which focus on pain intensity to extensive pain questionnaires with sophisticated combinations of assessment focusing on pain quality, pain affect, and pain history [39–41].

A proper pain management should monitor the effect of the treatment with a pain assessment instrument, which has been demonstrated to be responsive to change over time [52, 59]. Thus far, few studies have investigated the treatment responsiveness of pain tools for patients with dementia [21, 53]. Following the COSMIN recommendations [52], the MOBID-2 Pain Scale [32, 35–37] proved to be responsive to decrease in pain intensity after pain treatment over time [34]. This psychometric responsiveness is needed to be confident that an improvement in individual patients is not merely measurement error. Importantly, a responsive pain instrument is a prerequisite for investigating the effect of pain management on both the pain intensity score and NPSs.

In patients with advanced dementia and inability to rate and communicate pain, instruments should be based on the observation of behaviors, as recommended by the American Geriatric Society (AGS) [6]. Typical behavior related to pain such as change in facial expression, vocalization, or defense should be assessed and differed from behavior that might be related to NPSs in dementia [6]. A number of promising assessment tools are available, but most of these instruments require further validation and reliability testing in people with dementia.

Following this development, a recent initiative from a group of European researchers has led to the review of pain assessment tools [23], aiming to identify key items with both *theoretic* and *empirical* value to develop a new comprehensive pain assessment tool (The COST Action TD1005 *Pain Assessment in Patients with Impaired Cognition, especially in Dementia*).

Summary: Assessing Symptoms and Clinically Relevant Change in Patients with Dementia

- A key challenge in pain assessment is the differentiation between pain and NPSs.
- Typical behavior may be related to pain or to dementia; some symptoms/behaviors of pain may overlap symptoms of dementia.
- Several pain assessment instruments use symptoms defined as NPSs to identify pain in people with dementia.
- Only very few studies prove the validity of NPSs to identify pain in these individuals.
- The evaluation of the effectiveness of pain treatment intervention is imperative.
- A proper pain assessment tool for people with dementia must be responsive to detect change in pain intensity after pain treatment.

RECOMMENDATIONS

All of these following behaviors, vocalizations, facial expressions, and body movements are frequently the most prominent, or even the only observable feature of pain in patients with dementia. These symptoms are often not recognized as pain, but frequently interpreted as a symptom of dementia. Reversely, the more severe the dementia, the more likely the patient is to display these overlapping symptoms as a result of dementia and not necessarily due to pain [23, 30, 54].

With these facts and clinical recommendations in mind, let us return to our patient Elsa B. What are her chances for receiving proper, skilled pain assessment and pain management? This chapter has highlighted the importance of considering NPSs when assessing and treating possible pain conditions in patients with dementia. Using validated and reliable pain assessment tools together with the awareness of the similarity of pain and dementia symptoms represents an important step toward appropriate care of this population.

As illustrated in Fig. 7-1, the evaluation and treatment of both pain and behavioral symptoms are an ongoing cyclic process. For Elsa B., agitation and anxiety were found to be both a symptom of pain (agitation) and a psychological issue (anxiety). In addition to musculoskeletal pain, the MOBID-2 uncovered lower abdominal pain due to a urinary infection. This illustrates the importance of pain assessment not only to facilitate high quality pain treatment, but also to detect and treat other basic medical conditions. The agitation was reduced with antibiotics together with pain treatment. Meanwhile, her anxiety did not recede until environmental interventions were introduced (shielding her from other NH patients). Although agitation has been shown to correlate with pain and be responsive to

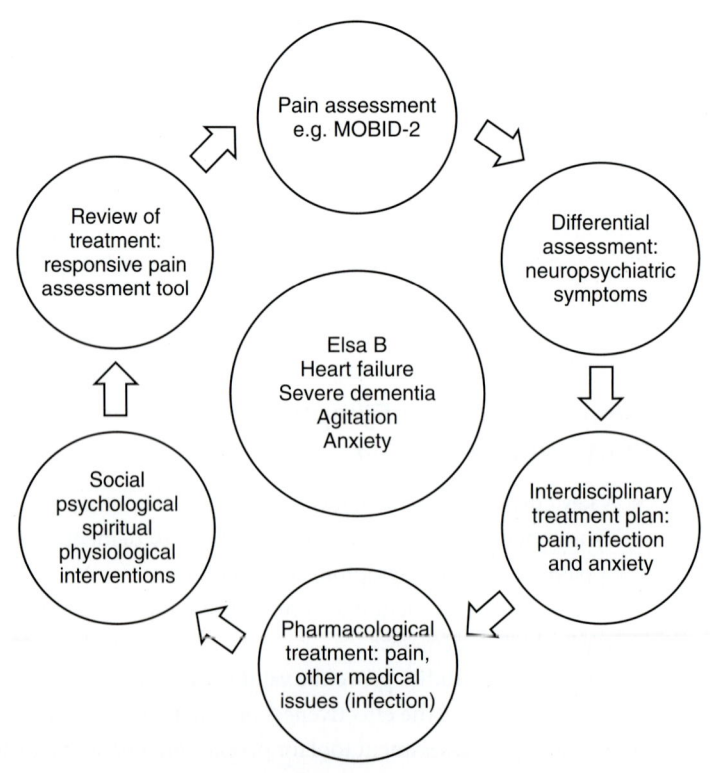

FIGURE 7-1 Example of a comprehensive pain management cycle.

pain treatment, anxiety may not respond. Awareness of the behaviors that are more or less likely to signify pain may facilitate an individualized and monitored treatment plan for patients like Elsa B.

REFERENCES

1. Aarsland D, Bronnick K, Ehrt U, De Deyn PP, Tekin S, Emre M, Cummings JL. Neuropsychiatric symptoms in patients with Parkinson's disease and dementia: frequency, profile and associated care giver stress. J Neurol Neurosurg Psychiatry 2007;78:36–42.
2. Achterberg WP, Pieper MJ, van Dalen-Kok AH, de Waal MW, Husebo BS, Lautenbacher S, Kunz M, Scherder EJ, Corbett A. Pain management in patients with dementia. Clin Interv Aging 2013;8:1471–82.
3. Ahn H, Horgas A. The relationship between pain and disruptive behaviors in nursing home residents with dementia. BMC Geriatr 2013;13:14.
4. Alexopoulos GS, Abrams RC, Young RC, Shamoian CA. Cornell scale for depression in dementia. Biol Psychiatry 1988;23:271–84.
5. Allen GJ, Hartl TL, Duffany S, Smith SF, VanHeest JL, Anderson JM, Hoffman JR, Kraemer WJ, Maresh CM. Cognitive and motor function after administration of hydrocodone bitartrate plus ibuprofen, ibuprofen alone, or placebo in healthy subjects with exercise-induced muscle damage: a randomized, repeated-dose, placebo-controlled study. Psychopharmacology 2003;166:228–33.
6. American Geriatrics Society (AGS). The management of chronic pain in older persons: AGS panel on chronic pain in older persons. J Am Geriatr Soc 1998;46:635–51.
7. American Psychiatric Association (APA). Diagnostic and statistical manual of mental disorders, 5th edition. Washington, DC: APA; 2013.
8. Ballard C, Corbett A, Chitramohan R, Aarsland D. Management of agitation and aggression associated with Alzheimer's disease: controversies and possible solutions. Curr Opin Psychiatry 2009;22:532–40.
9. Ballard C, Day S, Sharp S, Wing G, Sorensen S. Neuropsychiatric symptoms in dementia: importance and treatment considerations. Int Rev Psychiatry 2008;20:396–404.
10. Ballard C, Gray A, Ayre G. Psychotic symptoms, aggression and restlessness in dementia. Rev Neurol 1999;155:S44–52.
11. Ballard C, Hanney ML, Theodoulou M, Douglas S, McShane R, Kossakowski K, Gill R, Juszczak E, Yu LM, Jacoby R. The dementia antipsychotic withdrawal trial (DART-AD): long-term follow-up of a randomised placebo-controlled trial. Lancet Neurol 2009;8:151–7.
12. Ballard C, Smith J, Husebo BS, Aarsland D, Corbett A. The role of pain treatment in managing the behavioural and psychological symptoms of dementia (BPSD). Int J Palliat Nurs 2011;17:420–24.
13. Bartels SJ, Horn SD, Smout RJ, Dums AR, Flaherty E, Jones JK, Monane M, Taler GA, Voss AC. Agitation and depression in frail nursing home elderly patients with dementia: treatment characteristics and service use. Am J Geriatr Psychiatry 2003;11:231–8.
14. Bergh S, Engedal K, Røen I, Selbæk G. The course of neuropsychiatric symptoms in patients with dementia in Norwegian nursing homes. Int Psychogeriatr 2011;23:1231–9.
15. Black BS, Finucane T, Baker A, Loreck D, Blass D, Fogarty L, Phillips H, Hovanec L, Steele C, Rabins PV. Health problems and correlates of pain in nursing home residents with advanced dementia. Alzheimer Dis Assoc Disord 2006;20:283–90.
16. Bozeat S, Gregory CA, Ralph MAL, Hodges JR. Which neuropsychiatric and behavioural features distinguish frontal and temporal variants of frontotemporal dementia from Alzheimer's disease? J Neurol Neurosurg Psychiatry 2000;69:178–86.
17. Brummel-Smith K, London MR, Drew N, Krulewitch H, Singer C, Hanson L. Outcomes of pain in frail older adults with dementia. J Am Geriatr Soc 2002;50:1847–51.
18. Chibnall JT, Tait RC, Harman B, Luebbert RA. Effect of acetaminophen on behavior, well-being, and psychotropic medication use in nursing home residents with moderate-to-severe dementia. J Am Geriatr Soc 2005;53:1921–9.
19. Cohen-Mansfield J. Conceptualization of agitation: results based on the Cohen-Mansfield agitation inventory and the agitation behavior mapping instrument. Int Psychogeriatr 1997;8:309–15.
20. Cohen-Mansfield J, Libin A. Assessment of agitation in elderly patients with dementia: correlations between informant rating and direct observation. Int J Geriatr Psychiatry 2004;19:881–91.
21. Cohen-Mansfield J, Lipson S. The utility of pain assessment for analgesic use in persons with dementia. Pain 2008;134:16–23.

22. Cohen-Mansfield J, Werner P. Predictors of aggressive behaviors: a longitudinal study in senior day care centers. J Gerontol B Psychol Sci Soc Sci 1998;53:P300–10.
23. Corbett A, Husebo BS, Malcangio M, Staniland A, Cohen-Mansfield J, Aarsland D, Ballard C. Assessment and treatment of pain in people with dementia. Nat Rev Neurol 2012;8:264–74.
24. Crowley K. Sleep and sleep disorders in older adults. Neuropsychol Rev 2011;21:41–53.
25. Cummings JL. The neuropsychiatric inventory assessing psychopathology in dementia patients. Neurology 1997;48:S10–6.
26. Cummings JL, Mega M, Gray K, Rosenberg-Thompson S, Carusi DA, Gornbein J. The Neuropsychiatric Inventory: comprehensive assessment of psychopathology in dementia. Neurology 1994;44:2308–14.
27. Douzjian M, Wilson C, Shultz M, Berger J, Tapnio J. A program to use pain control medication to reduce psychotropic drug use in residents with difficult behavior Ann Long-Term Care 1998;6:174–79.
28. Ferrell BA, Ferrell BR, Osterweil D. Pain in the nursing home. J Am Geriatr Soc 1990;38:409–14.
29. Foley D, Ancoli-Israel S, Britz P, Walsh J. Sleep disturbances and chronic disease in older adults: Results of the 2003 National Sleep Foundation Sleep in America Survey. J Psychosom Res 2004;56:497–502.
30. Husebo BS, Ballard C, Aarsland D. Pain treatment of agitation in patients with dementia: a systematic review. Int J Geriatr Psychiatry 2011;26:1012–8.
31. Husebo BS, Ballard C, Cohen-Mansfield J, Seifert R, Aarsland D. The response of agitated behavior to pain management in persons with dementia. Am J Geriatr Psychiatry 2014;22:708–17.
32. Husebo BS, Ballard C, Sandvik R, Nilsen OB, Aarsland D. Efficacy of treating pain to reduce behavioural disturbances in residents of nursing homes with dementia: cluster randomised clinical trial. BMJ 2011;343:d4065.
33. Husebo BS, Corbett A. Dementia: pain management in dementia-the value of proxy measures. Nat Rev Neurol 2014;10:313–4.
34. Husebo BS, Ostelo R, Strand LI. The MOBID-2 Pain Scale: reliability and responsiveness to pain in patients with dementia. Eur J Pain 2014;18:1419–30.
35. Husebo BS, Strand LI, Moe-Nilssen R, Husebo SB, Ljunggren AE. Pain behaviour and pain intensity in older persons with severe dementia: reliability of the MOBID Pain Scale by video uptake. Scand J Caring Sci 2009;23:180–9.
36. Husebo BS, Strand LI, Moe-Nilssen R, Husebo SB, Ljunggren AE. Pain in older persons with severe dementia. Psychometric properties of the Mobilization–Observation–Behaviour–Intensity–Dementia (MOBID-2) Pain Scale in a clinical setting. Scand J Caring Sci 2010;24:380–91.
37. Husebo BS, Strand LI, Moe-Nilssen R, Husebo SB, Snow AL, Ljunggren AE. Mobilization-Observation-Behavior-Intensity-Dementia Pain Scale (MOBID): development and validation of a nurse-administered pain assessment tool for use in dementia. J Pain Symptom Manag 2007;34:67–80.
38. International Psychogeriatric Association (IPA). The IPA complete guides to BPSD—specialists guide. Milwaukee, WI: IPA; 2012.
39. Jensen MP, Karoly P. Self-report scales and procedures for assessing pain in adults. In: Turk DC, Melzack, R, editors. Handbook of pain assessment. New York: The Guilford Press; 2001. p. 15–34.
40. Jensen MP, Karoly P, Braver S. The measurement of clinical pain intensity: a comparison of six methods. Pain 1986;27:117–26.
41. Jensen MP, Turner JA, Romano JM, Fisher LD. Comparative reliability and validity of chronic pain intensity measures. Pain 1999;83:157–62.
42. Kalaria RN, Maestre GE, Arizaga R, Friedland RP, Galasko D, Hall K, Luchsinger JA, Ogunniyi A, Perry EK, Potocnik F, et al. Alzheimer's disease and vascular dementia in developing countries: prevalence, management, and risk factors. Lancet Neurol 2008;7:812–26.
43. Kovach CR, Logan BR, Noonan PE, Schlidt AM, Smerz J, Simpson M, Wells T. Effects of the Serial Trial Intervention on discomfort and behavior of nursing home residents with dementia. Am J Alzheimers Dis Other Demen 2006;21:147–55.
44. Kovach CR, Noonan PE, Griffie J, Muchka S, Weissman DE. Use of the assessment of discomfort in dementia protocol. Appl Nurs Res 2001;14:193–200.
45. Kunik ME, Snow AL, Davila JA, Steele AB, Balasubramanyam V, Doody RS, Schulz PE, Kalavar JS, Morgan RO. Causes of aggressive behavior in patients with dementia. J Clin Psychiatry 2010;71:1145–52.
46. Lautenbacher S, Kundermann B, Krieg JC. Sleep deprivation and pain perception. Sleep Med Rev 2006;10:357–69.
47. Lyketsos CG, Lopez O, Jones B, Fitzpatrick AL, Breitner J, DeKosky S. Prevalence of neuropsychiatric symptoms in dementia and mild cognitive impairment: results from the cardiovascular health study. JAMA 2002;288:1475–83.

48. Lyketsos CG, Olin J. Depression in Alzheimer's disease: overview and treatment. Biol Psychiatry 2002; 52:243–52.
49. Lyketsos CG, Steinberg M, Tschanz JT, Norton MC, Steffens DC, Breitner JC. Mental and behavioral disturbances in dementia: Findings from the Cache County study on memory in aging. Am J Psychiatry 2000;157:708–14.
50. Manfredi PL, Breuer B, Wallenstein S, Stegmann M, Bottomley G, Libow L. Opioid treatment for agitation in patients with advanced dementia. Int J Geriatr Psychiatry 2003;18:700–5.
51. Mayer G, Jennum P, Riemann D, Dauvilliers Y. Insomnia in central neurologic diseases -occurrence and management. Sleep Med Rev 2011;15:369–78.
52. Mokkink LB, Terwee CB, Patrick DL, Alonso J, Stratford PW, Knol DL, Bouter LM, de Vet HC. The COSMIN checklist for assessing the methodological quality of studies on measurement properties of health status measurement instruments: an international Delphi study. QoL Res 2010;19:539–49.
53. Morello R, Jean A, Alix M, Sellin-Peres D, Fermanian J. A scale to measure pain in non-verbally communicating older patients: the EPCA-2 Study of its psychometric properties. Pain 2007;133:87–98.
54. Pieper MJ, van Dalen-Kok AH, Francke AL, van der Steen JT, Scherder EJ, Husebo BS, Achterberg WP. Interventions targeting pain or behaviour in dementia: a systematic review. Ageing Res Rev 2013;12:1042–55.
55. Seignourel PJ, Kunik ME, Snow L, Wilson N, Stanley M. Anxiety in dementia: a critical review. Clin Psychol Rev 2008;28:1071–82.
56. Selbaek G, Kirkevold O, Engedal K. The course of psychiatric and behavioral symptoms and the use of psychotropic medication in patients with dementia in Norwegian nursing homes—a 12-month follow-up study. Am J Geriatr Psychiatry 2008;16:528–36.
57. Srikanth S, Nagaraja AV, Ratnavalli E. Neuropsychiatric symptoms in dementia-frequency, relationship to dementia severity and comparison in Alzheimer's disease, vascular dementia and frontotemporal dementia. J Neurol Sci 2005;236:43–48.
58. Steele C, Rovner B, Chase GA, Folstein M. Psychiatric symptoms and nursing home placement of patients with Alzheimer's disease. Am J Psychiatry 1990;147:1049–51.
59. Terwee CB, Bot SD, de Boer MR, van der Windt DA, Knol DL, Dekker J, Bouter LM, de Vet HC. Quality criteria were proposed for measurement properties of health status questionnaires. J Clin Epidemiol 2007;60:34–42.
60. Tosato M, Lukas A, van der Roest HG, Danese P, Antocicco M, Finne-Soveri H, Nikolaus T, Landi F, Bernabei R, Onder G. Association of pain with behavioral and psychiatric symptoms among nursing home residents with cognitive impairment: results from the SHELTER study. Pain 2012;153:305–10.
61. Volicer L, Frijters DH, Van der Steen JT. Relationship between symptoms of depression and agitation in nursing home residents with dementia. Int J Geriatr Psychiatry 2012;27:749–54.
62. Voyer P, McCusker J, Cole MG, St-Jacques S, Khomenko L. Factors associated with delirium severity among older patients. J Clin Nurs 2007;16:819–31.
63. Wood S, Cummings JL, Ming-Ann H, Barclay T, Wheatley MV, Yarema KT, Schnelle JF. The use of the neuropsychiatric inventory in nursing home residents: characterization and measurement. Am J Geriatr Psychiatry 2000;8:75–83.

CHAPTER 8

Pain in Other Types of Cognitive Impairment with a Focus on Developmental Disability

Ruth Defrin

Cognitive impairment is a broad term that refers to all the conditions in which the cognitive process is limited or altered. Cognitive deficits can be global or specific, congenital or acquired, and may appear at various points during the course of life. Given the vast number of individuals with cognitive impairment, the underdetection and undertreatment of pain among this population is a serious, worldwide concern that requires our attention. Some of the challenges of identifying pain, measuring pain, and adequately treating pain may be common to individuals with Alzheimer's disease, mental retardation (MR), and other types of cognitive impairment, yet specific challenges and features may characterize specific entities of cognitive impairment.

This chapter will concentrate on pain and cognitive impairment among individuals with developmental disability, in which the symptoms begin during the developmental period. In contrast to most other conditions, in which cognitive impairment develops in adulthood (e.g., Alzheimer's disease), individuals with developmental disability encounter the consequences of the aforementioned challenges already in early childhood and throughout their life time. Yet, the literature on this population with regard to pain and the challenges of its management is insufficient. Therefore, raising the awareness for this topic and encourage further research is important.

DEVELOPMENTAL DISABILITY—DEFINITIONS

Developmental disability is the broad term for "a diverse group of severe chronic conditions that are due to mental and/or physical impairments, which include autism, *cerebral palsy and intellectual disability*" [17]. Many individuals in each of these conditions exhibit some sort of cognitive impairment (see Section 2, below).

Autism spectrum disorders (ASD), of which *autism* is the best described and most severe of these developmental disorders, are characterized by impairment in the social interaction and communication domain (such as responding inappropriately in conversations, misreading nonverbal interactions, or having difficulty building friendships), restricted repetitive and stereotyped patterns of behavior, interests, and activities, and/or abnormal functioning. Asperger syndrome, Rett syndrome, childhood disintegrative disorder (CDD), and pervasive developmental disability (PDD) are also included under ASD. Individuals with ASD must show symptoms from early childhood, even if those symptoms are not recognized until later [1].

Cerebral palsy is a group of movement, muscle tone, and posture disorders that are often accompanied by disturbances of sensation, perception, cognition, communication, and behavior. In general, cerebral palsy causes impaired movement associated with exaggerated reflexes, floppiness or rigidity of the limbs and trunk, abnormal posture, involuntary movements, unsteadiness of walking, or some combination of these. Signs and symptoms appear during infancy or preschool years [82].

Intellectual disability (ID), previously termed MR, is a neurodevelopmental disorder characterized by impairments of general mental abilities that impact adaptive functioning in three domains; the conceptual domain includes skills in language, reading, writing, math, reasoning, knowledge, and memory. The social domain refers to empathy, social judgment, interpersonal communication skills, the ability to make and retain friendships, and similar capacities. The practical domain centers on self-management in areas such as personal care, job responsibilities, money management, recreation, and organizing school and work tasks. While ID does not have a specific age requirement, individual's symptoms must begin during the developmental period and are diagnosed based on the severity of deficits in adaptive functioning [1]. Individuals with ID have limited ability to learn, reason, make decisions, and solve problems (usually with an intelligence quotient [IQ] score of 70–75 and less) as well as difficulties in the ability to communicate effectively, interact with others, and take care of themselves. ID is the most common developmental disability, affecting about 1–3% of the population [56].

DEVELOPMENTAL DISABILITY—ETIOLOGY AND PREVALENCE OF COGNITIVE IMPAIRMENT

ASD has a strong genetic basis, although environmental factors have also been suggested to interact with the underlying mechanisms. Most children with autism, which is the most prevalent conditions of all ASD, present impairments in at least one area of cognitive functioning [94]. According to one survey, most children with autism have mild cognitive impairment, while the minority (3–7%) have severe and profound cognitive impairment [102]. Cognitive impairment is also characteristic of Rett syndrome and PDD; the prevalence rate of the different levels of cognitive impairment among these conditions is not clear.

Cerebral palsy is caused by abnormal development of, or damage to, motor control centers of the brain. The prevalence rate of cognitive impairment among individuals with cerebral palsy varies from 23% to 44% depending on the type of cerebral palsy and the presence or absence of epilepsy [71]. The underlying mechanism of ID is identifiable in only 25% of patients. The etiology may be related to infections which are present at birth or occur after birth; chromosomal abnormalities, such as Down syndrome and fragile X; environmental, metabolic or nutritional causes, toxic insults (intrauterine exposure to alcohol, cocaine, amphetamines, etc.), and trauma before and after birth [86].

About 85% of individuals with ID have the mild form as diagnosed by the IQ score and adaptive skills. The proportion of individuals with moderate, severe, and profound ID is 10%, 4% and 1%, respectively [1]. Individuals with severe to profound ID experience a decreased life expectancy due to the underlying etiology and additional complications that may include respiratory infections, immobility, significant oral motor incoordination, dysphagia, aspiration, and internal organ pathologies. Life expectancy of individuals with mild ID does not differ from that of the general population [73].

EXPOSURE TO PAIN AMONG INDIVIDUALS WITH DEVELOPMENTAL DISABILITY

Many individuals with developmental disability and in particular those with profound and multiple disabilities have substantial, sustained, and complex health-care needs which often involve pain [57, 71]. Sources of pain are abundant among individuals with developmental disability: neurological impairments, motor disabilities, and coordination disorders leading to pathological gait and posture patterns, increased/decreased muscle tone, and general difficulties in activity of daily living are known sources of pain, especially in cerebral palsy and in individuals with severe ID. Dislocated joints, pressure sores, and overuse injuries due to the aforementioned pathologies and to the use of assistive devices are additional sources of pain. Assistive technologies used for feeding and breathing may potentially cause painful bruises or injuries and hence pain. Primary and secondary pathologies of internal organs are also a source of pain, discomfort. and general poor health among individuals with ID [15, 69].

A specific syndrome may be associated with specific pathologies. For example, Rett syndrome is characterized by scoliosis, joint deformities, spasticity, and kyphosis [43]. Neuropathy, fibromyalgia, and joint laxity were associated with fragile-X syndrome [22]. The rates of arthritis and osteoporosis are especially high among adults with Down's syndrome as well as other signs of premature aging [14]. Beyond the above mentioned, individuals with developmental disability in general are subject to more injuries, falls, and accidents than their nondisabled peers [38]. As a result, these individuals are exposed, more than usual, to painful medical procedures related to the etiology of the disability or its consequences, in turn leading to greater risk of suffering from acute or chronic pain [15, 67, 82, 99]. Thus, pain of musculoskeletal, visceral, or neuropathic origin is likely to develop in individuals with developmental disabilities.

Estimates on the prevalence rate of pain among individuals with ASD are not abundant. Most of the literature deals with chronic gastrointestinal symptoms which include but are not restricted to abdominal pain. Abdominal pain was identified in 24–50% of children with ASD [46, 66]. The prevalence rates of pain among individuals with cerebral palsy based on large cohort studies vary from 50% to 83% depending on the level of motor impairment and comorbid conditions [33, 84]. However, the rates of pain among those individuals with cerebral palsy who also have cognitive impairment are less known.

The prevalence of pain among individuals with ID varies according to the reporting source. A survey based on caregivers' impressions reported that 15.4% of 7544 community-dwelling adults with mild to moderate ID experienced chronic pain for an average of 6.3 years. A significant proportion of the individuals with chronic pain also experienced limitations in several aspects of daily living, emotional distress, and reduced quality of life suggesting that chronic pain is a significant problem in this population [99]. Interestingly, the level of ID was not found to be associated with the presence of pain. In another survey based on caregivers' reports, 13.4% of 157 adults with moderate to severe ID had chronic pain with an average duration of 6 years. The authors found a higher prevalence of chronic pain in group homes compared with family homes, possibly due to the higher proportion of people with severe and profound ID associated with more complex health problems living in residential homes [63]. A recent survey found that 18% of 255 residents with ID living in a representative special care facility suffered from acute pain either at the present or during the preceding week [4]. On the other hand, interviews with adults with mild to severe ID resulted in higher prevalence rates for acute or chronic pain, varying between 23.5% and 76.2% [20, 80, 101], suggesting perhaps that caregivers are not familiar or aware of acute or chronic pain among the people they care for.

With regard to children, caregivers' reports on the prevalence of pain in 94 children and adolescents with moderate to profound ID was as high as 62% [10]. A recent multi-center cross-sectional European survey on 490 children with cerebral palsy reported prevalence rates of 60–73% [72]. This is not surprising considering that in another study, 72% of ambulatory children with ID at a day care had at least one injury, compared with only 25% of children without impairments [54].

UNDERTREATMENT OF PAIN AMONG INDIVIDUALS WITH DEVELOPMENTAL DISABILITY

Despite the high prevalence of pain, children and adults with ID are prescribed with significantly less analgesic medications [28, 37, 56] compared with cognitively intact individuals. For example, a significantly lower percentage of children with ID received smaller doses of analgesic medications, for less postoperative days after spinal fusion compared to cognitively intact children [56]. In another study, 40% of older adults with ID who underwent hip fracture did not receive analgesic medication in the 3 weeks post operation despite complaints of severe pain [36]. Recently, 85% of residents in special care facilities who suffered from pain had no analgesic prescription, even when the pain was severe [4].

A delay in diagnosis and management of painful medical conditions as well as setbacks in hospitalization is often experienced by individuals with ID. One study found that 92% of 191 individuals with profound and multiple IDs who were physically examined had a previously undetected but treatable condition [64]. In addition, 87% of 53 such individuals attending a health check required one or more health interventions [58]. Individuals with ID may even experience increased, unnecessary death rates that could have been prevented if pain could be adequately monitored [85, 100].

Jancar and Speller [47], for example, retrospectively analyzed hospital records about pain observed in 32 people with ID who died from intestinal obstruction. The study found that pain and distress were recorded in nine patients and five displayed signs of tenderness and guarding. The authors suggested that pain was not communicated clearly by individuals with more severe IDs, or that medical staff did not perceive the episodes as serious because signs of illness were less apparent than expected. In 2007, following the deaths of six people with ID in nursing home care, Mencap (a leading UK charity for people with learning disability) published *Death by Indifference*, which exposed the unequal health-care and institutional discrimination that people with ID often experience in nursing homes. In 2013, the Confidential Inquiry published the findings of its 2-year investigation on the subject. The investigation showed that people with a learning disability receive fewer screening tests and fewer health investigations. It showed that people with a learning disability are less likely to get the health care they need. The Inquiry concluded that 37% of deaths of people with ID were avoidable and probably resulted from health-care professionals' lack of understanding and mistaken beliefs about patients with a learning disability that they have a high pain threshold [65].

This horrendous state of affairs may result from the tendency of individuals with ID not to report pain in potentially harmful situations, and from the difficulty in assessing pain in these individuals due to their poor communication capabilities. LaChapelle et al. [49] showed that as the level of ID increases in children, verbal reports of pain decrease. In adults as well, the more serious the ID, the less pain is self-reported [23]. It is noteworthy, however, that, although self-report is the preferred assessment technique by clinicians [7], verbal skills do not guarantee adequate pain reports. Turk et al. [96] interviewed 19 adults with ID about experiences of general practitioner consultations. Four of them said they did not tell anyone when they experienced pain, and had not consulted their general practitioner over the previous year [96]. In addition, Donovan [32] cited a nurse who described a very bright and verbal patient with ID who told the nurse he had had a pain in his foot for the past few days. A large piece of glass was found embedded in his foot upon examination [32]. These characteristics of individuals with ID and the difficulty of caregivers to identify painful conditions have led to the premise that individuals with ID are less sensitive to pain in comparison with their cognitively intact peers [2, 45]. Observation of self-injurious behavior among some individuals with ID has also contributed to this premise.

ARE INDIVIDUALS WITH DEVELOPMENTAL DISABILITY LESS SENSITIVE TO PAIN?

Sensitivity to pain can be directly evaluated by measuring pain threshold. The psychophysical concept of the sensory threshold reflects the idea that sensory events have to be stronger than a critical level in order to be perceived. According to this view, a sensory threshold is defined as the smallest amount of stimulus energy necessary to produce a sensation [39] and pain threshold is defined as the smallest stimulus energy necessary to produce pain. This energy amount can be quantified with several methods that are either stimulus-dependent or response-dependent. In the former methods, represented by the method of limits, the dependent variable is the amount of stimulus intensity (or time) corresponding to a fixed response which is detection of pain. In the latter methods, represented by the method of levels, the dependent variable is the subjects' response corresponding to various fixed stimulus intensities (for more details, please see also Chapter 11).

Obviously, the success of these methods depends on the collaboration of the subjects, their understanding, and their communication ability. They cannot therefore be applied to individuals with severe levels of ID. Indeed, the number of studies in which pain threshold was actually measured in individuals with ID is small. Table 8-1 summarizes these studies which are presented in chronological order.

In the first study of its kind, Hennequin et al. [45] measured cold-pain threshold in 26 individuals with Down's syndrome (9 children and 17 adults) by measuring the time elapsed from the application of an ice cube on the wrist or temple to the first verbal expression of pain. The onset of pain response following the ice cube application was longer in individuals with Down's syndrome compared with controls. This led the authors to conclude that, although the former individuals are not insensitive to pain, they have a higher pain threshold than normal. Noteworthy is that this stimulus-dependent method includes

TABLE 8-1 Summary of Psychophysical Studies Measuring Pain Threshold among Individuals with Developmental Disability

Authors	Type of Developmental Disability	Participants	Stimulation	Testing Method	Pain Threshold Compared to Controls
Hennequin et al. [45]	Down's syndrome	26 (children and adults)	Ice cube	Modified limits	Higher
Defrin et al. [30]	Down's syndrome and nonspecified intellectual disability	25 (adults)	Computerized heat and cold	Limits Levels	Normal Lower
Cascio et al. [16]	Autism spectrum disorders	8 (adults)	Computerized heat and cold	Limits	Lower
Priano et al. [76]	Prader–Willi syndrome	11 (adolescents)	Computerized heat and cold	Limits	Higher
Riquelme and Montoya [81]	Cerebral palsy	15 (children)	Pressure algometer	Modified limits	Lower

a reaction time artifact which is the time it takes the individual to respond verbally to the sensation evoked by the ice cube rendering the threshold confounded by this artifact.

In 2004, Defrin and coworkers [30] measured heat-pain threshold in 25 individuals with ID, 11 of which had Down's syndrome and 14 with nonspecified ID. Pain threshold in the forearms was measured using a computerized thermal stimulator with two different methods; the method of limits, which includes a reaction-time artifact (as subjects are required to press a switch upon pain detection, thereby ceasing the stimulus), and the reaction-time-free method of levels (as subjects report postfactum whether a predetermined stimulus intensity was painful or not). The authors found that individuals with ID had a similar pain threshold to that of controls when measured with the method of limits; however, they had a significantly lower pain threshold compared to controls when measured with the method of levels (see Fig. 8-1).

The measurement of heat-pain threshold with reaction time–dependent and –independent methods enabled the calculation of the reaction time and nerve conduction velocity of the participants [30]. Reaction time was found to be significantly slower in individuals with ID compared with controls and nerve conduction velocity (compatible with that of C fibers) tended to be slower, more so in individuals with Down's syndrome compared with controls (see Fig. 8-2). Since reaction time is intrinsic to the method of limits, slow reaction time induces an artificial elevation of the pain threshold. Thus, the lack of elevation in heat-pain threshold in individuals with ID despite slower reaction time using the method of limits and the decreased heat-pain threshold measured with the method of levels implies that individuals with ID indeed have lower pain threshold compared to normal. The results of this study suggested that contrary to previous belief, individuals with MR are even more sensitive to pain than the normal population; however, they may seem less sensitive to pain due to slow reactions. These authors thus proposed that measurements of pain threshold in these individuals should be conducted using methods that do not rely on reaction time.

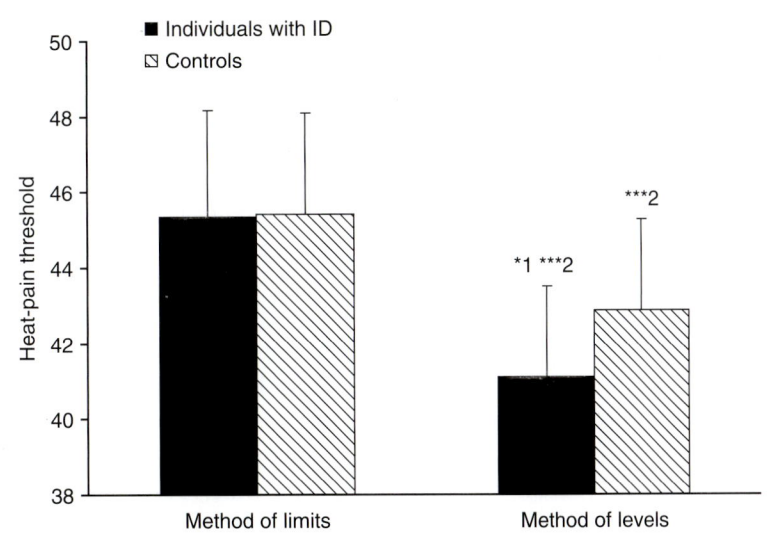

FIGURE 8-1 Individuals with intellectual disability (ID) had similar heat-pain threshold as controls when measured with the reaction-time-dependent method of limits. However, individuals with ID had significantly lower heat-pain threshold compared to controls when measured with the reaction-time-free method of levels (*1, $P < 0.05$). In both groups, heat-pain thresholds measured with the method of levels were significantly lower than those measured with the method of limits (***2, $P < 0.0001$). Bars denote group means ± SD.

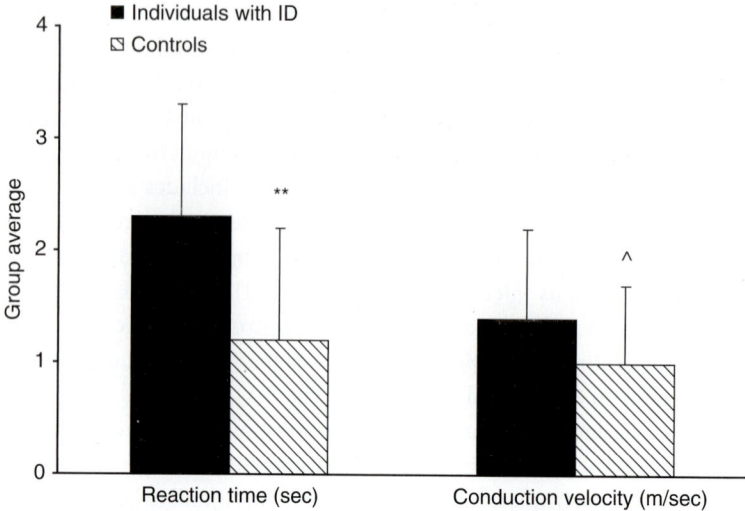

FIGURE 8-2 Individuals with intellectual disability (ID) had significantly slower reaction time than controls (**$P < 0.01$) and tended to have slower nerve conduction velocity than controls (^$P = 0.064$) as calculated from the two pain threshold measurements. Bars denote group mean ± SD.

Cascio et al. [16] measured heat- and cold-pain thresholds with computerized thermal stimulator among eight adults with high functioning autism (either *autistic disorder* or *Asperger disorder*). The authors used the method of limits and found that pain thresholds were significantly lower than in matched control. Priano et al. [76] too measured heat- and cold-pain thresholds using computerized thermal stimulator with the method of limits in 14 adolescents with Prader–Willi syndrome, a neurogenetic developmental disorder with a tendency to self-injury. The authors found that the thresholds of the participants, measured in the hands were increased compared to controls and concluded that these individuals are hyposensitive to pain. The authors also found that the latencies and conduction velocities of the median and ulnar nerves subserving the hand are slower than those of controls; however, their measurements reflected the large myelinated fibers not involved in heat and cold conduction. Therefore, it was not clear whether the increased pain thresholds were due to the slower nerve conduction velocity.

Riquelme and Montoya [81] recently found that children (but not adults) with cerebral palsy had increased sensitivity to pressure pain in the lips than controls when measured with a modified method of limits. Noteworthy, however, is that out of 29 participants, only 15 had ID and their contribution to the results was not examined.

Peripheral and central nerve conduction in ID was evaluated in only a few more studies with inconsistent results. To the best of our knowledge, all the electrophysiological recordings in this population were done with innocuous stimuli, and therefore, the results may not be applied to the pain system. For example, as in the study of Priano et al. [76], slower median nerve conduction velocities and lower nerve action potential amplitudes compared to controls were also found in five children with Down's syndrome [5] but not in five children with Prader–Willi syndrome [6]. The latter exhibited normal somatosensory-evoked potentials measured in the scalp as in Priano et al. [76] but also lower than normal amplitudes, as in the case of children with cerebral palsy with and without ID [81]. Normal median nerve conduction velocity was also seen in two patients of brothers with ID suffering from hereditary [74] and congenital [50] insensitivity to pain associated with self-injury;

however, nerve biopsies from these two patients revealed low numbers of myelinated and unmyelinated nerve fibers. Prolonged latencies of somatosensory-evoked potentials as well as of brain stem auditory-evoked potentials and visual-evoked potentials found in infants with Down's syndrome [18] may suggest that they may suffer from various sensory deficits including the nerve conduction of noxious stimuli. The above-mentioned findings suggest that myelinization of sensory nerve fibers and the number of normal nerve fibers may be affected in some but not all ID syndromes. Further studies are needed to determine whether alterations exist also in nerve conduction of noxious stimuli.

In the absence of additional studies, in which pain threshold was directly measured, and on the basis of the electrophysiological findings, we may conclude that individuals with ID especially those with Down's syndrome or otherwise non-specified ID are certainly not less sensitive to pain than normal and may even be more sensitive to pain than normal. The inconsistent evidence with regard to pain threshold among the different disability types (see Table 8-1) could reflect differences in pain processing between the syndromes. We may also conclude that alterations in peripheral and/or central nerve conduction of sensory signals may be responsible for the delayed responses seen in methods that include reaction time. Due to the possibility that individuals with developmental disability exhibit alterations in nerve conduction, measuring pain threshold with methods that bypass this limitation, that is, reaction-time-free methods are preferable.

PAIN SCALING ABILITIES OF INDIVIDUALS WITH DEVELOPMENTAL DISABILITY

Ability to self-report is the basis not only for threshold measurements but also for freely communicating pain during interviews. Interviewing individuals with developmental disability is important; although depending on their cognitive impairment, they sometimes are still the best source of information regarding their health. The results of studies are inconsistent with regard to the ability of individuals with developmental disability to use pain scales. For example, Dagnan and Ruddick [27] found that 25 out of 29 individuals with mild and moderate ID were able to give reliable responses using visual analog scale consisting of two pictorial anchors (one smiling and one crying) with a 5-inch line between them. Validity of self-report was also obtained using colored analog scale in children and adults with mild ID [41, 60]. Furthermore, adults with mild to moderate ID were found to reliably use the 21-point (0–100) box scale to rate their chronic pain over time [19]. The scale has a row of 21 boxes labeled from 0 to 100, in increments of five. The 0 anchor is labeled "no pain," while the 100 anchor is labeled "pain as bad as it could be." To complete the scale, respondents indicate the box that best represents their pain. It is noteworthy that reliability was inversely correlated with the ID level, with those less affected being more reliable in their ratings.

In contrast, LaChapelle et al. [49] found that 35% of individuals with severe ID were not able to respond to a simple question on their pain intensity in response to an injection, and those who responded provided an unreliable pain rating. Furthermore, their pain reports did not correspond with their facial expression during injection [49]. Similarly, Defrin et al. [29] found that adults with various levels of ID could not reliably use a five-faces scale to report their pain. These individuals choose either the smiling face (which indicates no pain) or the face in the middle of the scale, which has no particular expression regardless of whether they were at rest or subject to needle stick. Here again, their pain reports using the faces scale did not correspond with their facial expression or their bodily movements during injection [29]. In another study, 60% of children with cerebral palsy failed a validity test designed to assess their understanding of a faces pain scale [52]. It is possible that these subjects simply cannot use faces scale because they do not comprehend the meaning of ranks and cannot dispose their pain experience onto faces. Furthermore, it has been postulated that short scales (2–6 points) have an increased risk of scale attenuation effect, resulting in reduced rating variability and discrimination [19]. Other, graphical or three-dimensional, tangible scales might be more suitable. The poker chip tool is a good example. The tool was found suitable for small children as well consists of four chips that represent "pieces of hurt", with one chip indicating a "little hurt" and all four chips indicating "the most hurt a person could have."

In summary, it appears that not all individuals with developmental disability are able to use scales to report pain; nor is every scale suitable for every individual. Further study is needed to explore the best rating scale for different levels of developmental disability. Nevertheless, the inability to use pain rating scales does not necessarily preclude the ability to provide free verbal report on the existence of pain or grossly quantify its intensity, which has considerable clinical significance.

BEHAVIORAL INDICES OF PAIN IN INDIVIDUALS WITH DEVELOPMENTAL DISABILITIES

Although self-report is considered a gold standard of pain assessment, pain threshold and direct scaling cannot be applied to individuals who have a limited verbal ability to report pain. In these instances other methods that do not rely on direct communication should be applied. Facial activity is perhaps the most immediate and intuitive sources of information available, and hence the analysis of facial expressions of pain is the most common way to study pain among noncommunicative individuals with and without ID. A specific method termed facial action coding system (FACS) was developed by Ekman and Friesen [35], on the premise that the face displays considerable plasticity and expresses stereotypical reactions to different situations including pain. The movements of a single or a group of muscles in the face called "action units" (AUs) are coded, and the frequency or intensity of these AUs are quantified. A substantial body of work has been published, mostly by Craig and colleagues on the validity and reliability of the FACS as a measurement tool for pain in newborns and children and later in elderly people with dementia [26, 42, 48, 51, 88].

In addition to facial expressions, body gestures, vocalization, and other behavioral expressions have been coded among individuals with developmental disability, using various tools. One example is the noncommunicating children's pain checklist (NCCPC) developed by McGrath and coworkers [12, 62]. The NCCPC allows the observer to score the frequency of occurrence of behaviors comprising the following categories: vocal, eating, sleeping, social, facial, activity, body and limb, and physiological signs. Additional tools include, but are not restricted to, the pain and discomfort scale (PADS) [3] and the face legs activity cry and consolability (FLACC) behavioral pain assessment tool [55].

Facial expressions among individuals with ID were analyzed during acute and chronic pain conditions. Facial expressions during acute pain are usually analyzed before and during a medical procedure deemed painful such as needle stick associated with vaccination or blood draw and dental cleaning. In several studies, the overall facial activity of individuals with ID was increased compared to their baseline level [12, 29, 34, 42, 49, 75, 98]. Most of these studies lacked a control group of cognitively intact individuals, and therefore, it is not clear whether the increase in facial expression was different than normal. The two studies that had such a control group revealed that children [34] or adults [29] with mild–moderate ID displayed changes in pain behavior similar to those of controls, whereas children who were unable to verbalize their pain [34] or adults with severe-profound ID [29] exhibited elevated or atypical facial expressions at baseline compared with controls that affected the magnitude of the change in pain behavior. Expressions such as closing and squinting of eyes, grimacing, brow furrowing, and mouth opening are common in these individuals during pain. However, other facial expressions that are not intuitively associated with pain also appear during acute painful conditions. These may include moving the eyes from side to side, tongue protrusion, and a smile [29].

Facial reactions to pain were also examined in children with ASD. Here again, facial expressions were increased during acute pain compared to baseline and to a greater extent and longer duration after the end of the venipuncture compared with controls [68, 79, 95]. Furthermore, individuals with ASD displayed a significantly increased heart rate in response to venipuncture that was significantly greater than in controls [95]. These findings contradict the commonly held view on insensitivity to pain among individuals with ASD. One study did not find an increase in facial expression of adolescents with cerebral palsy during vaccination compared to sham control; however, the subjects were reported to suffer from chronic pain which might have affected their response [70]. It may thus be concluded that prior reports of reduced pain sensitivity in ID and ASD are related to a different mode of pain expression rather than to insensitivity to pain.

In the minority of facial expression studies on individuals with ID, experimental rather than clinical stimuli were used [87, 90]. These authors administered four innocuous (warm, cold, pressure, and light touch) and one presumably noxious (pin prick) stimulation modalities to 44 adults with severe and profound of ID. The authors found increased facial activity during the application of all the stimuli compared to baseline but did not find differences in facial activity between the different stimulation modalities.

As with facial expression, general bodily movements were also increased in individuals with ID and ASD during acute painful medical procedures compared to baseline [29, 34, 75, 79, 91]. Here again, individuals with more severe ID had more pronounced or atypical body gestures than those with milder ID. In one study, the increase in bodily movements was more pronounced among individuals with self-injurious behavior as compared to those without self-injurious behavior [91]. It should be pointed out that as with facial expression, behaviors that are not intuitively associated with pain might appear. For example, Defrin et al. [29] reported that many individuals ID presented "freezing behavior" during vaccination, that is, lowering the level of their reactions, significantly more so in individuals with severe–profound ID than those with mild–moderate ID or controls. Weiner et al. [100] have also identified behavioral patterns similar to freezing in individuals with ID and named them "stillness". During freezing, the individuals might appear detached and as if not bothered by the pain. Therefore, freezing jeopardizes the detection of pain perceived by individuals especially with severe–profound ID and has probably led care takers to the impression that these individuals are actually insensitive to pain.

Conditions of chronic pain also induce an increase in facial expressions [8, 99] and in general pain behavior, including vocalization, agitation, guarded movements, or stereotypical movements such as teeth clenching and hand waving; these conditions also cause problems in eating and sleeping [24, 34, 42, 62, 97, 99]. Biersdorff [2] studied the impressions of third parties (service providers and family members) while freely observing 123 individuals with ID or with other types of developmental disabilities. Although about half (52%) showed typical pain responsiveness and 11% seemed hyperresponsive, 37% were deemed hyporesponsive due to slow reactions and unusual pain behavior. Biersdorff warned that staff members "may miss signs of illness or injury because they are looking for the more obvious pain signals" [2]. Breau and colleagues [10] also found that if pain expression was lacking or atypical among individuals with ID, a child's pain could remain unrelieved, and this in turn could adversely affect functioning.

A small number of studies explored the effect of the level of ID or the ability to communicate pain on pain behavior. For example, LaChapelle et al. [49] found no differences in the frequency or intensity of facial expression (analyzed with FACS) between individuals capable and not capable to verbally report the perceived pain. Defrin et al. [29] studied pain behavior of 132 individuals with four levels of ID (mild, moderate, severe, and profound) and 38 cognitively intact controls. The facial expressions (analyzed with FACS) of individuals with severe–profound ID were significantly increased compared to those with mild–moderate ID and cognitively intact controls at baseline (see Fig. 8-3). Perhaps as a result of this baseline difference, facial expressions increased significantly during vaccination relative to baseline only in individuals with mild and moderate ID and in controls but not in individuals with severe–profound ID (see Fig. 8-3). Similarly, baseline level of body and facial pain behavior (analyzed with NCCPC-revised [NCCPC-R] form) was significantly higher in individuals with severe–profound ID than that of individuals with mild–moderate ID and those of controls. Nevertheless, significant elevation in NCCPC-R scores was observed in all the groups during vaccination relative to baseline values (see Fig. 8-4). These results suggest that not all behavioral tools are suitable to all levels of ID and that the NCCPC-R can detect changes in all levels of ID whereas the FACS seems more suitable to those with mild–moderate ID [29].

In summary, studies assessing pain behavior among individuals with ID and other types of developmental disabilities show how these individuals respond with a noticeable

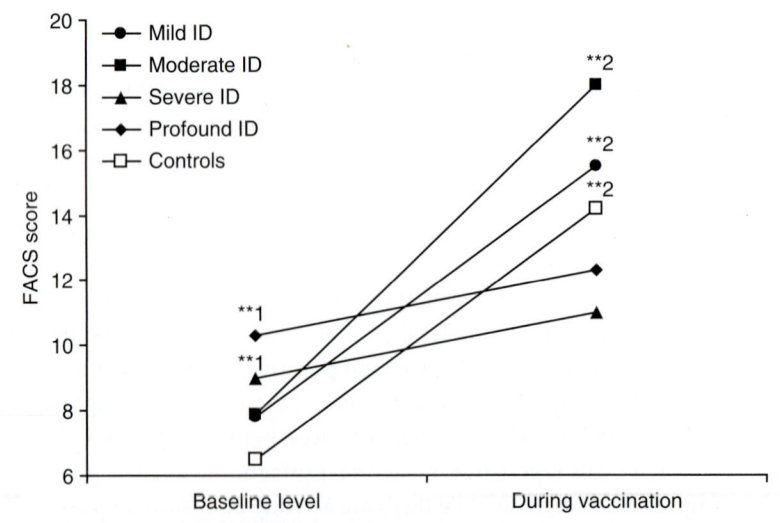

FIGURE 8-3 Baseline facial action coding system (FACS) scores of individuals with severe–profound intellectual disability (ID) were significantly higher than those of mild–moderate ID and of cognitively intact controls (**1, $P < 0.001$). During vaccination, FACS scores significantly increased relative to baseline values only in individuals with mild–moderate ID and in controls (**2, $P < 0.001$). Values denote group means.

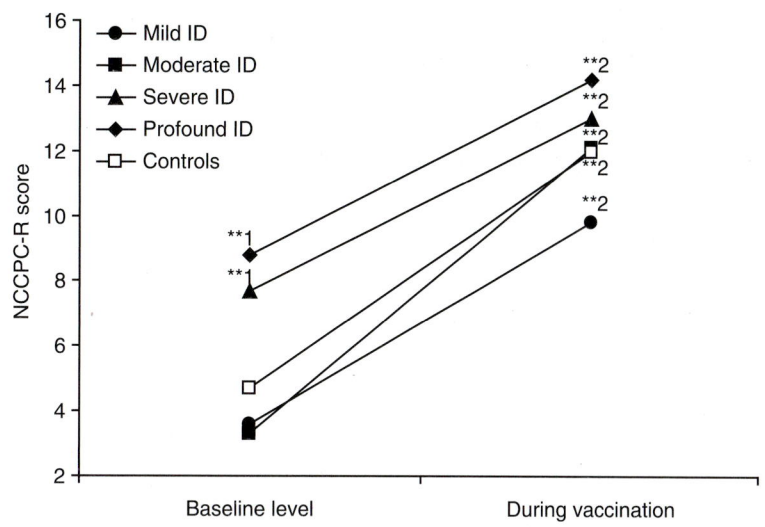

FIGURE 8-4 Baseline NCCPC-R scores of individuals with severe and profound intellectual disability (ID) were significantly higher than those of individuals with mild–moderate ID and of cognitively intact controls (**1, $P < 0.001$). All groups exhibited a significant elevation in NCCPC-R score during vaccination relative to baseline values (**2, $P < 0.001$) with no significant differences in delta scores between the groups. Values denote group means.

and sometimes robust increase in facial and bodily reactions during painful insults similar to their nonimpaired peers. Facial expressions may include frowning, grimacing, distorted expression, rapid blinking but also smiling. Body reactions may include guarding movements, rigidity, restlessness, increased pacing/rocking, but also freezing. Vocalizations such as moaning, shouting, crying, and verbal abuse can also be present, as well as general changes in behavior and habits such as increased aggression and irritability, reduced appetite, sleep disturbances, and distress. The findings contradict the previously held view that noncommunicative individuals are insensitive to pain. It is noteworthy that some behaviors are atypical and seem inappropriate to a painful condition (smile, freeze); however, they should not be considered as reflecting indifference or insensitivity to pain.

CHALLENGES AND BIASES IN PAIN MEASUREMENT AMONG INDIVIDUALS WITH DEVELOPMENTAL DISABILITIES

Facial and bodily responses to pain are perhaps the most intuitive way that caregivers and parents used to identify a state of pain in individuals with ID. Parents of children with ID reported that vocalization, social behavior and facial expressions were the indices by which they identified pain conditions in their children [25, 89]. Yet, observing behavior is confounded by many biases that should be taken into consideration. Even observing a person who is familiar to the observer might turn out to be a difficult task. Hennequin et al. [44] found that parents of children with Down's syndrome have difficulties in discerning if their child was in pain with a prevalence of 28–32%. Clarke and Thompson [21] asked parents of adults with ID about their experience of caring for their son/daughter who had a diagnosed health condition. They found that a majority did not perceive their son/daughter in much pain, which was generally attributed to their being healthy or receiving suitable treatment.

It has been suggested that parents may be underestimating the presence of pain in their children with ID, which serves as an unconscious defense mechanism against feelings of guilt or distress [13].

Facial and behavioral expressions of pain are shaped by the immediate surrounding and by culture among other factors. In individuals with ID an additional diversity in pain behavior exists due to the nature of the condition. McGrath and colleagues [61] observed that behaviors typically associated with pain in nonimpaired people might be hard to interpret in those with ID and that their behavioral limitations may actually mask the expression of pain. Biases in interpreting pain behavior exists also due to the fact that in many studies on individuals with ID, behavioral analyses of pain responses are done while the observers are not blind to the application of the painful insult (e.g., needle injection). Observers may thus be aware of the timing of the event and perhaps of the intensity of pain it evokes, producing a bias in their judgment.

Prkachin et al. [77] found that, although observers can distinct between patients' pain states, they are not especially sensitive and are likely to systematically downgrade patients' suffering. Underestimation bias was found more pronounced in more experiences caregivers than in inexperienced ones [24, 51, 78]. Observers are also subject to biases related to the age, sex, and physical attractiveness of the observed [25, 40, 49] and to stereotyped beliefs about individuals with ID [13, 49]. Thus, different observers/caregivers may interpret pain behaviors differently.

Pain assessment is foundational to the understanding of the pain experience and to planning and conducting proper management. Biases and mistaken beliefs about pain behavior and pain sensitivity among individuals with developmental disability may lead to inadequate treatment of pain. The combined use of self-report, behavioral observations as well as physiological and psychophysical measurements may provide sufficient data for proper evaluation of the individual's condition. Educating and training caregivers in evidence-based pain assessment tools and in possible biases and pitfalls of these tools might improve pain assessment and hence pain management of individuals with developmental disabilities. Considering that behavior among these individuals may be routinely irregular, continuous monitoring of behavior in seemingly nonpainful conditions may better serve to identify changes in behavior associated with painful conditions.

SELF-INJURIOUS BEHAVIOR

Self-injurious behavior is a behavior that causes physical injury to the individual's own body. The prevalence rates of self-injurious behavior among individuals with developmental disability vary from 1.7% to 93% depending on the methodology, the definition of self-injurious behavior, and the cohort evaluated [31]. As many as 70% of ASD patients may show self-injurious behavior at some point in their lives, but this is typically found in more severely affected individuals and takes on many forms including head banging, scratching, bruising, and biting [83]. Self-injurious behavior impedes physical and social development, interferes with community participation, and affects a person's quality of life. In addition, self-injurious behavior may provoke negative emotions and stress upon caregivers and can thus influence their quality of life.

The underlying mechanism of self-injurious behavior is unknown. Often individuals occupied with self-injurious behavior are deemed insensitive to pain. However, two recent studies in which pain behavior of noncommunicating individuals with ID was recorded with the FACS [90] and the NCCPC [91] showed that in contrast to this view individuals who self-injured expressed more facial and bodily reaction than those who did not. In fact, self-injurious behavior might indicate the presence of painful conditions. For example, Carr and Owen-DeSchryver [15] studied 11 individuals with ID and found that problematic behaviors (e.g., aggression toward others, stereotypic movement disorders, and tantrums) as well as self-injurious behavior, were more evident on days when the patients were ill than on days when they were well and when higher levels of pain and discomfort were identified. Caregivers too reported that their impression is that self-injurious behavior occurs in individuals who seem to suffer from acute or chronic pain [89, 99].

If self-injurious behavior is related to acute or chronic pain it may be regarded as a coping mechanism of pain perhaps via the release of opioids resulting from the painful nature of this behavior. However, administrating the μ-opioid receptor antagonist naltrexone was found to attenuate self-injurious behavior in 50–80% of individuals with ID [92]. Alternatively, self-injurious behavior may induce pain relief via the diffuse noxious inhibitory control (DNIC) loop. It has been suggested that noxious stimulus applied to one body region exerts an inhibitory effect onto pain in another, remote body region via the activation of the subnucleus reticularis dorsalis in the brain stem [53]. Self-injurious behavior may thus function as the conditioning stimulus exerting inhibition over acute or chronic pain. A recent finding of Symons et al. [93] showing elevated levels of cortisol and α-amylase among individuals with self-injurious behavior compared with matched individuals may support the role of this behavior in inducing stress analgesia or alternatively suggest that self-injurious behavior may be related to altered stress regulation. On the other hand, Breau et al. [11] found that nonverbal children with ID who suffered from chronic pain tended to engage in self-injurious behavior less frequently, injure a smaller body area, and target the site where pain originated, while those without identifiable pain who engaged in self-injurious behavior tended to self-injure more frequently and in a diffuse pattern. The authors concluded that there may be qualitatively different forms of self-injurious behavior initiated and propagated for different reasons.

Further study is needed to elucidate the nature and purpose of self-injurious behavior among individuals with ID. Challenging behaviors including self-injurious behavior can exist alongside chronic or undetected pain. A thorough health assessment is important whenever challenging or self-injurious behavior are significant causes for concern.

CLINICAL IMPLICATIONS

Individuals with developmental disability are at an increased risk of acute and/or chronic pain, yet these individuals receive inadequate pain management. Steps are to be taken in order to prevent this situation. First and foremost, care takers should be aware of the potential high risk of individuals with ID to experience pain alongside their altered ability to adequately express the pain at the time they experience it. A constant monitoring of any potential sign/symptom should be undertaken and individuals should be encouraged to communicate about any sensation they perceive either freely or with aids such as body maps and simple, preferably symbolic pain scales which can be used to help ascertain the location, intensity, and duration of the pain experienced.

When individuals with ID arrive to health service facilities, a thorough assessment for possible pain and underlying medical problems should take place including the evaluation of intensity, location in the body, duration of pain, and functional limitations due to the pain. Due to communication problems, additional diagnostic tests should be done in addition to the physical examination. The use of proxy reports by people who know the person best (family members, caregivers, or professionals) is also advised.

When noncommunicating individuals are assessed, caregivers and health-care professionals should be aware of their own beliefs and perceptions regarding pain in individuals with ID, including views about sensitivity to pain and the behaviors that represent pain. It is important to be aware of the fact that pain may be reflected by odd and possibly paradoxical behaviors which may confuse the evaluator (e.g., smiling and freezing).

Finally, multidisciplinary studies are needed to better understand the pain experience of this population, explore the behavioral aspects of pain, examine the functions of self-injurious behavior and other challenging behaviors, and develop valid pain assessment tools.

REFERENCES

1. American Psychiatric Association (APA). Diagnostic and statistical manual of mental disorders, 5th edition. Arlington, VA: American Psychiatric Publishing; 2013.
2. Biersdorff KK. Incidence of significantly altered pain experience among individuals with developmental disabilities. Am J Mental Retard 1994;98:619–31.
3. Bodfish JW, Harper VN, Deacon JR, Symons FJ. Identifying and measuring pain in persons with developmental disabilities: a manual for the Pain and Discomfort Scale (PADS). Western Carolina Center Research Reports, Morganton; 2001.
4. Boerlage AA, Valkenburg AJ, Scherder EJ, Steenhof G, Effing P, Tibboel D, van Dijk M. Prevalence of pain in institutionalized adults with intellectual disabilities: a cross-sectional approach. Res Dev Disabil 2013; 34:2399–406.
5. Brandt BR, Rosén I. Impaired peripheral somatosensory function in children with Down syndrome. Neuropediatrics 1995;26:310–2.
6. Brandt BR, Rosén I. Impaired peripheral somatosensory function in children with Prader–Willi syndrome. Neuropediatrics 1998;29:124–6.
7. Breau LM, Burkitt C. Assessing pain in children with intellectual disabilities. Pain Res Manag 2009;14:116–20.
8. Breau LM, Camfield C. The relation between children's pain behaviour and developmental characteristics: a cross-sectional study. Dev Med Child Neurol 2011;53:1–7.
9. Breau LM, Camfield CS, McGrath PJ, Finley GA. The incidence of pain in children with severe cognitive impairments. Arch Pediatr Adolesc Med 2003;157:1219–26.
10. Breau LM, Camfield CS, McGrath PJ, Finley GA. Pain's impact on adaptive functioning. J Intellect Disabil Res 2007;51:125–34.
11. Breau LM, Camfield CS, Symons FJ, Bodfish JW, Mackay A, Finley GA. Relation between pain and self-injurious behavior in nonverbal children with severe cognitive impairments. J Pediatr 2003;142:498–503.
12. Breau LM, Finley GA, McGrath PJ, Camfield CS. Validation of the Non-Communicating Children's Pain Checklist—postoperative version. Anesthesiology 2002;96:528–35.
13. Breau LM, MacLaren J, McGrath PJ, Camfield CS, Finley GA. Caregivers' beliefs regarding pain in children with cognitive impairment: relation between pain sensation and reaction increases with severity of impairment. Clin J Pain 2003;19:335–44.
14. Carmeli E, Coleman R. The clinical characteristics of aging adults with mental retardation. Phys Ther Rev 2002;6:267–71.
15. Carr EG, Owen-DeSchryver JS. Physical illness, pain, and problem behavior in minimally verbal people with developmental disabilities. J Autism Dev Disord 2007;37:413–24.
16. Cascio C, McGlone F, Folger S, Tannan V, Baranek G, Pelphrey KA, Essick G. Tactile perception in adults with autism: a multidimensional psychophysical study. J Autism Dev Disord 2008;38:127–37.
17. Centers for Disease Control and Prevention. Developmental disabilities 2004. Accessed at http://www.cdc.gov/ncbddd/dd/default.htm
18. Chen YJ, Fang PC. Sensory evoked potentials in infants with Down syndrome. Acta Paediatr 2005;94:1615–8.

19. Chibnall JT, Tait RC. Pain assessment in cognitively impaired and unimpaired older adults: a comparison of four scales. Pain 2001;92:173–86.
20. Chou YC, Lu ZXJ, Wang FTY, Lan CF, Lin LC. Meanings and experiences of menstruation: perceptions of institutionalized women with an intellectual disability. J Appl Res Intellect Disabil 2008;21:575–84.
21. Clarke ZJ, Thompson AR. Parents' experiences of pain and discomfort in people with learning disabilities. Br J Learn Disabil 2007;36:84–90.
22. Coffey SM, Cook K, Tartaglia N, Tassone F, Nguyen DV, Pan R, Bronsky HE, Yuhas J, Borodyanskaya M, Grigsby J, et al. Expanded clinical phenotype of women with the FMR1 premutation. Am J Med Genet A 2008;146:1009–16.
23. Cohen-Mansfield J, Marx MS. Pain and depression in the nursing home: corroborating results. J Gerontol 1993;48:96–7.
24. Collignon P, Giusiano B. Validation of a pain evaluation scale for patients with severe cerebral palsy. Eur J Pain 2001;5:433–42.
25. Craig KD, Korol CT, Pillai RR. Challenges of judging pain in vulnerable infants. Clinics Perinatol 2002;29:445–57.
26. Craig KD, Prkachin KM, Grunau R. The facial expression of pain. In: Turk D, Melzack R, editors. Handbook of pain assessment. New York: Guilford Press; 1992. p. 257–76.
27. Dagnan D, Ruddick L. The use of analogue scales and personal questionnaires for interviewing people with learning disabilities. Clin Psychol Forum 1995;79:21–4.
28. Dawson P. Cognitively impaired residents receive less pain medication than non-cognitively impaired residents. Perspectives 1998;22:16–7.
29. Defrin R, Lotan M, Pick CG. The evaluation of acute pain in individuals with cognitive impairment: a differential effect of the level of impairment. Pain 2006;124:312–20.
30. Defrin R, Pick CG, Peretz C, Carmeli E. A quantitative somatosensory testing of pain threshold in individuals with mental retardation. Pain 2004;108:58–6.
31. Denis J, Van den Noortgate W, Maes B. Self-injurious behavior in people with profound intellectual disabilities: a meta-analysis of single-case studies. Res Dev Disabil 2011:32;911–23.
32. Donovan, J. Learning disability nurses' experiences of being with clients who may be in pain. J Adv Nurs 2002;38:458–66.
33. Doralp S, Bartlett DJ. The prevalence, distribution, and effect of pain among adolescents with cerebral palsy. Pediatr Phys Ther 2010;22:26–33.
34. Dubois A, Capdevila X, Bringuier S, Pry R. Pain expression in children with an intellectual disability. Eur J Pain 2010;14:654–60.
35. Ekman P, Friesen W. Investigators guide to the facial action coding system. Palo Alto, CA: Consulting Psychologist Press, 1978.
36. Feldt KS, Finch M. Older adults with hip fractures. J Gerontol Nurs 2002;8:27–3.
37. Feldt KS, Ryden MB, Miles S. Treatment of pain in cognitively impaired compared with cognitively intact older patients with hip-fracture. J Am Geriatr Soc 1998;46:1079–85.
38. Finlayson J, Morrison J, Jackson A, Mantry D, Cooper SA. Injuries, falls and accidents among adults with intellectual disabilities: prospective cohort study. J Intellect Disabil Res 2010;54:966–80.
39. Gescheider GA. Psychophysics, method, theory and application. New-Jersey: Lawrence Erlbaum, 1985.
40. Hadjistavropoulos HD, Ross M, Von Baeyer C. Are physicians' ratings of pain affected by patients' physical attractiveness? Soc Sci Med 1990;31:69–72.
41. Hadjistavropoulos T, LaChapelle DL, MacLeod FK, Hale C, O'Rourke N, Craig KD. Cognitive functioning and pain reactions in hospitalized elders. Pain Res Manag 1998;3:145–51.
42. Hadjistavropoulos T, LaChapelle DL, MacLeod FK, Snider B, Craig KD. Measuring movement-exacerbated pain in cognitively impaired frail elders. Clin J Pain 2000;16:54–63.
43. Halbach NSJ, Smeets EEJ, Schrander-Stumpel CTRM, Van Schrojenstein Lantman, de Valk HHJ, Maaskant MA, Curfs LMG. Aging in people with specific genetic syndromes: Rett syndrome. Am J Med Genet A 2008;146:1925–32.
44. Hennequin M, Faulks D, Allison PJ. Parents' ability to perceive pain experienced by their child with Down syndrome. J Orofac Pain 2003;17:347–53.
45. Hennequin M., Morin C, Feine JS. Pain expression and stimulus localization in individuals with Down's syndrome. Lancet 2000;356:1882–7.
46. Horvath K, Perman JA. Autistic disorder and gastrointestinal disease. Curr Opin Pediatr 2002;14:583–7.

47. Jancar J, Speller CJ. Fatal intestinal obstruction in the mentally handicapped. J Intellect Disabil Res 1994;38:413–22.
48. Kunz M, Scharmann S, Hemmeter U, Schepelmann K, Lautenbacher S. The facial expression of pain in patients with dementia. Pain 2007;133:221–8.
49. LaChapelle, DL, Hadijistavropoulos R, Craig KD. Pain Measurement in persons with intellectual disability. Clin J Pain 1999;15:13–23.
50. Larner AJ, Moss J, Rossi ML, Anderson M. Congenital insensitivity to pain: a 20 year follow up. J Neurol Neurosurg Psychiatr 1994;57:973–4.
51. Lautenbacher S, Niewelt BG, Kunz M. Decoding pain from the facial display of patients with dementia: a comparison of professional and nonprofessional observers. Pain Med 2013;14:469–77.
52. LeBaron S, Zeltzer L. Assessment of acute pain and anxiety in children and adolescents by self-reports, observer reports, and a behavior checklist. J Consult Clin Psychol 1984;52:729–38.
53. Le Bars D. The whole body receptive field of dorsal horn multireceptive neurons. Brain Res Rev 2002;40:29–44.
54. Leland NL, Garrard J, Smith DK. Comparison of injuries to children with and without disabilities in a day-care center. J Dev Behav Pediatr 1994;15;402–8.
55. Malviya S, Voepel-Lewis T, Burk C, Merkel S, Tait A. The revised FLACC observational pain tool: improved reliability and validity for pain assessment in children with cognitive impairment. Paediatr Anaesth 2006;16:258–65.
56. Malviya S, Voepel-Lewis T, Tait AR, Merkel S, Lauer A, Munro H, Farley F. Pain management in children with and without cognitive impairment following spine fusion surgery. Paediatr Anaesth 2001;11:453–8.
57. Mansell J. Raising our sights: services for adults with profound intellectual and multiple disabilities. London: Department of Health; 2010.
58. Martin G, Philip L, Bates L, Warwick J. Evaluation of a nurse-led annual review of patients with severe intellectual disabilities, needs identified and needs met, in a large group practice. J Learn Disabil 2004;8:235–46.
59. Maulik PK, Mascarenhas MN, Mathers CD, Dua T, Saxena S. Prevalence of intellectual disability: a meta-analysis of population-based studies. Res Dev Disabil 2011;32:419–36.
60. McGrath PA, Seifert SE, Speechley KN, Booth JC, Stitt L, Gibson MC. A new analoge scale for assessing children's pain. Pain 1996;64:435–43.
61. McGrath PJ. Behaviour measures of pain. In: Finley GA, McGrath PJ, editors. Measurement of pain in infants and children, Seattle, WA: IASP Press; 1998. p. 93–102.
62. McGrath PJ, Rosmus C, Canfield C, Campbell MA, Hennigar A. Behaviours caregivers use to determine pain in non-verbal, cognitively impaired individuals. Dev Med Child Neurol 1998;40:340–3.
63. McGuire BE, Daly P, Smyth F. Chronic pain in people with intellectual disability under-recognised and under-treated. J Intellect Disabil Res 2010;54:240–5.
64. Meehan S, Moore G, Barr O. Specialist services for people with learning disabilities. Nurs Times 1995;91:33–5.
65. Mencap. Death by indifference. London: Mencap; 2013.
66. Molloy CA, Manning-Courtney P. Prevalence of chronic gastrointestinal symptoms in children with autism and autistic spectrum disorders. Autism 2003;7:165–71.
67. Morgan CL, Baxter H, Kerr MP. Prevalence of epilepsy and associated health service utilization and mortality among patients with intellectual disability. Am J Ment Retard 2003;108:293–300.
68. Nader R, Oberlander TF, Chambers CT, Craig KD. Expression of pain in children with autism. Clin J Pain 2004;20:88–97.
69. Nocon A. Equal treatment: closing the gap—background evidence for the DRC's formal investigation into health inequalities experiences by people with learning disabilities or mental health problems. Manchester: Disability Rights Commission; 2006.
70. Oberlander TF, Gilbert CA, Chambers CT, O'Donnell ME, Craig KD. Biobehavioral responses to acute pain in adolescents with a significant neurological impairment. Clin J Pain 1999;15:201–9.
71. Odding E, Roebroeck ME, Stam HJ. The epidemiology of cerebral palsy: incidence, impairments and risk factors. Disabil Rehabil 2006;28:183–91.
72. Parkinson KN, Gibson L, Dickinson HO, Colver AF. Pain in children with cerebral palsy: a cross-sectional multicentre European study. Acta Paediatr 2010;99:446–51.
73. Patja K, Mölsä P, Iivanainen M. Cause-specific mortality of people with intellectual disability in a population-based, 35-year follow-up study. J Intellect Disabil Res 2001;45:30–40.

74. Pavone L, Huttallocher L, Siciliano L, Micoli G, Rizzo R, Anastosi M, Woolmann R. Two brothers with a variant of hereditary sensory neuropathy. Neuropediatrics 1992;23:92–5.
75. Phan A, Edwards CL, Robinson EL. The assessment of pain and discomfort in individuals with mental retardation. Res Dev Disabil 2005;26:433–9.
76. Priano L, Miscio G, Grugni G, Milano E, Baudo S, Sellitti L, Picconi R, Mauro A. On the origin of sensory impairment and altered pain perception in Prader–Willi syndrome: a neurophysiological study. Eur J Pain 2009;13:829–35.
77. Prkachin KM, Berzins S, Mercer SR. Encoding and decoding of pain expressions: a judgement study. Pain 1994;58:253–9.
78. Prkachin KM, Craig KD. Expressing pain: the communication and interpretation of facial pain signals. J Nonverbal Behav 1995;19:191–205.
79. Rattaz C, Dubois A, Michelon C, Viellard M, Poinso F, Baghdadli A. How do children with autism spectrum disorders express pain? A comparison with developmentally delayed and typically developing children. Pain 2013;154:2007–13.
80. Reid BC, Chenette R, Macek MD. Prevalence and predictors of untreated caries and oral pain among Special Olympic athletes. Spec Care Dent 2003;23:139–42.
81. Riquelme I, Montoya P. Developmental changes in somatosensory processing in cerebral palsy and healthy individuals. Clin Neurophysiol 2010;121:1314–20.
82. Rosenbaum P, Paneth N, Leviton A, Goldstein M, Bax M. A report. The definition and classification of cerebral palsy, April 2006. Dev Med Child Neurol J 2007;49:8–14.
83. Ross-Russell M, Sloan P. Autoextraction in a child with autistic spectrum disorder. Br Dent J 2005;198:473–4.
84. Roth-Isigkeit A, Thyen U, Stöven H, Schwarzenberger J, Schmucker P. Pain among children and adolescents: restrictions in daily living and triggering factors. Pediatrics 2005;115:152–62.
85. Roy A, Simon GB. Intestinal obstruction as a cause of death in the mentally handicapped. J Ment Defic Res 1987;31:193–7.
86. Shapiro BK, Batshaw ML. Intellectual disability (Chap. 33). In: Kliegman RM, Behrman RE, Jenson HB, Stanton BF, editors. Nelson textbook of pediatrics. 19th edition. Philadelphia, PA: Elsevier Saunders; 2011.
87. Shinde SK, Danov S, Chen CC, Clary J, Harper V, Bodfish JW, Symons FJ. Convergent validity evidence for the Pain and Discomfort Scale (Pads) for pain assessment among adults with intellectual disability. Clin J Pain 2014;30:536–43.
88. Simons W, Malabar R. Assessing pain in elderly patients who cannot respond verbally. J Adv Nurs 1995;22:663–9.
89. Solodiuk JC, Scott-Sutherland J, Meyers M, Myette B, Shusterman C, Karian VE, Harris SK, Curley MA. Validation of the Individualized Numeric Rating Scale (INRS): a pain assessment tool for nonverbal children with Intellectual disability. Pain 2010;150:231–6.
90. Symons FJ, Harper V, Shinde SK, Clary J, Bodfish JW. Evaluating a sham-controlled sensory-testing protocol for nonverbal adults with neurodevelopmental disorders: self-injury and gender effects. J Pain 2010;11:773–81.
91. Symons FJ, Harper VN, McGrath PJ, Breau LM, Bodfish JW. Evidence of increased non-verbal behavioral signs of pain in adults with neurodevelopmental disorders and chronic self-injury. Res Dev Disabil 2009;30:521–8.
92. Symons FJ, Thompson A, Rodriguez MC. Self-injurious behavior and the efficacy of naltrexone treatment: a quantitative synthesis. Mental Retard Dev Disabil Res Rev 2004;10:193–200.
93. Symons FJ, Wolff JJ, Stone LS, Lim TK, Bodfish JW. Salivary biomarkers of HPA axis and autonomic activity in adults with intellectual disability with and without stereotyped and self-injurious behavior disorders. J Neurodev Disord 2011;3:144–51.
94. Szelag E, Kowalska J, Galkowski T, Poppel E. Temporal processing deficits in high functioning children with autism. Br J Psychol 2004;95:269–82.
95. Tordjman S, Anderson GM, Botbol M, Brailly-Tabard S, Perez-Diaz F, Graignic R, Carlier M, Schmit G, Rolland AC, Bonnot O, et al. Pain reactivity and plasma beta-endorphin in children and adolescents with autistic disorder. PLoS One 2009;4:e5289.
96. Turk V, Kerry S, Corney R, Rowlands G, Khattran S. Why some adults with intellectual disabilities consult their general practitioners more than others. J Intellect Disabil Res 2010;54:833–42.
97. Valkenburg AJ, Boerlage AA, Ista E, Duivenvoorden HJ, Tibboel D, van Dijk M. The COMFORT—behavior scale is useful to assess pain and distress in 0- to 3-year-old children with Down syndrome. Pain 2011;152:2059–64.

98. Van der Putten A, Vlaskamp C. Pain assessment in people with profound intellectual and multiple disabilities; a pilot study into the use of the Pain Behaviour Checklist in everyday practice. Res Dev Disabil 2011; 32:1677–84.
99. Walsh M, Morrisson TG, McGuire BE. Chronic pain in adults with an intellectual disability: prevalence, impact, and health service use based on caregiver report. Pain 2011;152:1951–57.
100. Weiner D, Peterson B, Keefe F. Chronic pain-associated behaviors in the nursing home: resident versus caregiver perceptions. Pain 1999;80:577–88.
101. Willis DS, Wishart JG, Muir WJ. Menopausal experiences of women with intellectual disabilities. J Appl Res Intellect Dis 2011;24:74–85.
102. Yeargin-Allsopp M, Rice C, Karapurkar T, Doernberg N, Boyle C, Murphy C. Prevalence of autism in a US metropolitan area. JAMA 2003;289:49.

CHAPTER 9

Methods of Assessing Pain and Associated Conditions in Dementia: Self-report Pain Scales

Sophie Pautex and Stefan Lautenbacher

The application of self-report scales is limited due to the cognitive and linguistic impairments in patients with dementia. Dementia of mild to moderate degrees may still allow the necessary functional prerequisites for successful completion of self-report scales. The chapter will alert how it can be verified that these prerequisites are met. Furthermore, it will inform the readers about the cognitive challenges that are associated with the valid self-report of pain. Finally, the available scales will be reviewed and solutions for best practice will be recommended.

INTRODUCTION ABOUT THE IMPORTANCE OF SELF-ASSESSMENT

Pain is a subjective, complex, and multidimensional experience, for which there are no objective biological markers. Despite decades of effort, there is no neurophysiologic or chemical test that can measure pain in individual patients. Various studies have demonstrated that health-care professionals tend to underestimate a patient's pain intensity, while family caregivers tend to the opposite and overestimate the intensity of pain [10, 42, 46, 47, 53, 62, 65, 72, 76]. To compensate for such evaluation biases, self-report tools should always be used in patients with dementia who can still communicate. Besides these considerations, self-report opens the realm of internal and private states and gains access to information never accessible by observers, making it always a first-choice approach [15, 37, 63].

Furthermore, we cannot assume that older patients automatically report pain, even to health professionals. Many older adults do not report pain for various reasons, including the belief that pain is regular and must be endured, not wanting be a bother, expecting that the health-care provider will anyhow know when pain is present, and fearing of the meaning of pain [30]. Indeed, attitudes of stoicism and cautiousness may contribute to the underreporting of pain symptoms in older people as demonstrated by Yong [77]. Given the higher prevalence of chronic pain with increasing age, older adults may also show more acceptance of chronic pain and may perceive mild aches and pain as normal part of aging. Kamel and colleagues [37] demonstrated in a study conducted in two nursing homes that the systematic use of three pain assessment scales (the visual analog scale [VAS], faces scale, and pain descriptive scale) increased the detection of pain (from 15% to 30%) among nursing home residents.

In conclusion, when an elder patient with dementia presents for an initial evaluation, then a quantitative and qualitative assessment for persistent pain including self-report measures should be performed; thereafter, the patient should be screened for persistent pain at a regular basis [14].

BARRIERS AGAINST AND PREREQUISITES FOR THE SUCCESSFUL COMPLETION OF SELF-REPORT

Cognitive Impairment

Dementia is not a single disease but a complex of different signs and symptoms that often overlap. For example, Alzheimer-type dementia is often characterized predominantly by memory loss, accompanied by impairment in other cognitive functions or "domains," such as language function (aphasia), fine motor functions (apraxia), or recognition (agnosia). Especially cognitive impairments in memory may hinder a person's ability to consider what pain has been during the course of a day, when it started, whether it was related to something, and what its cause might have been. The inability to concentrate and maintain attention can also affect participation in pain assessment. Loss of language (aphasia) and disturbances in visual-spatial skills can further limit the ability to provide detailed information. Visual agnosia, when people with dementia can no longer recognize everyday items, can also affect assessment when visual means become relevant.

Before assessing the pain of the patients, cognitive impairment but also cognitive resources of the patients should be identified. The mini-mental state examination (MMSE), although far from being a perfect tool, is still the most commonly administered psychometric screening assessment of cognitive functioning [22]. The MMSE can be used to screen patients for cognitive impairment, to track changes in cognitive functioning over time, and oftentimes to assess the effects of therapeutic agents on cognitive function. If available, further neuropsychological examination should be used to identify the resources of the patient and to adapt the pain assessment to the patient's capacities. Pain assessment can be a challenging procedure in patients with moderate to strong degrees of cognitive impairment. Accurate self-reporting of pain requires the ability to understand the question posed by a pain rating, to accurately interpret the experience of noxious stimuli as sources of pain, to correctly recall the pain, and to adequately express pain by verbal means.

Sensory Impairment: Assistive Devices

Given that sensory deficits are common in older persons, it is important to determine the presence of any deficit and to evaluate the patient's sensory ability to use available pain scales. Sensory-assistive devices, for example glasses, should be checked to make sure they are working properly. Adjustments to the self-report tool should be made to accommodate patients with poor vision, such as using enlarged type and bold figures or using verbal communication with numerical or verbal scales [18, 30]. Written information should be provided for patients with auditory deficits.

Guidelines for Caregivers on How to Use and Explain the Scales to the Patients

It is important to take the time to find the most appropriate scale for each patient and ensure that they assimilate and respond adequately. Using the same scale over time in one patient is the best approach to track changes reliably. Furthermore, patients with dementia have often limited attention spans and are easily distracted [18]. Therefore, it may be helpful to prepare these patients by limiting distractions in the room. If possible, pain assessment should be performed in a quiet room. It is also important to allow sufficient time for older adults to process and respond to the assessment task [18]. A pain assessment scale should be explained to the patient using a standard text and the patient should demonstrate comprehension of the scales.

SELF-ASSESSMENT OF PAIN

A careful patient history that allows the patient to describe her or his pain is also essential for discriminating the types of pain, identifying the underlying cause and evaluating the impact of pain as well as the efficacy of our treatments. It is also crucial to acknowledge the pain of the patient and to reassure that the health-care professionals will take care of it.

A structured pain interview that includes simple questions related to the presence or absence of pain or discomfort, pain intensity, frequency, location, and impact on daily activities is a feasible approach to pain assessment even in the cognitively impaired patients [17, 50, 73]. This complete pain assessment must, of course, be followed by a complete physical examination focusing on the site of pain and referred pain and with some complementary examinations, if appropriate (for example, X-ray, computed-tomography [CT] scan, magnetic resonance imaging [MRI]).

Onset, Duration, Variations, Rhythms

Patients need to be asked when and how pain occurred. Duration and variations of pain should be assessed with some question such as "Is your pain always there, or does it come and go?" Transitory exacerbation of pain (breakthrough pain) should be assessed.

Exacerbating and Alleviating Factors

Asking the patient to describe the factors that exacerbate or alleviate the pain helps to plan interventions. A typical question might be "What makes the pain better or worse?" Analgesics, nonpharmacologic approaches (massage, relaxation, music or visualization therapy, heat or cold) are some interventions that may relieve the pain. Other factors (movement, physical therapy, activity) may intensify the pain.

Qualitative Description of Pain

Patients should also be encouraged to describe their pain with qualitative terms. For example, patients can describe nociceptive pain with terms that include "burning," "searing," "raw," "numb," "stabbing," and "tingling." Neuropathic pain is described as "electric shock," or "pins and needles" [58]. Some patients with dementia and aphasia do not understand anymore the term of pain but admit some discomfort or other unpleasant sensations such as aching.

Location of Pain

Most (74.9%) of older adults with pain endorsed multiple sites of pain [52]. In this context, establishing the location and spatial extent of pain on a chart consisting of drawings of the human body or body parts, on which the patient maps the pain, can be a very useful approach. Pointing to the body part that hurts has also been shown to be an effective approach with cognitively impaired older adults [75].

Consequences of Pain

The extent to which pain interferes with daily activities increases exponentially with age. The consequences (for example, depression, anxiety, loss of appetite, sleep disturbance, functional disability, behavior trouble, and compromised quality of life) must regularly be assessed [4, 6, 11, 21, 27, 51, 60, 61, 64, 74].

Pain Intensity Scales

First, we have to determine which self-report pain scale is the most adequate for the particular patient. The ability to comprehend and use a self-report scale is closely related to the severity of dementia and, in particular, to the communication ability of the patient [40]. However, scale comprehension is not related to the type of dementia. Patient's failure to complete one type of self-report pain scale does not preclude success with other types of scale. There are several self-report scales, among which the VAS, the Numerical Rating Scale (NRS), the Verbal Rating or Descriptor Scale (VRS, VDS), the Pain Thermometer (PT), and the Faces Pain Scale (FPS) are the most frequently used [69].

Most of these scales have demonstrated an acceptable reliability and validity in older patients and in patients with cognitive impairment in different settings (acute care, pain clinic, nursing home, community dwelling) [30].

The **VAS** consists typically of a 10-cm line anchored by the two extremes of pain, for example, no pain, extreme pain. Patients are asked to position a sliding vertical marker or mark the position by a pen to indicate the level of pain they were experiencing, for example, currently; pain severity is then measured as the distance in millimeter between the zero position and the marked spot [35, 44, 59, 69]. The VAS is one of the most commonly used tools in the clinical setting due to its practicability and availability. However, elderly people can have problems of understanding the VAS; two studies demonstrated a significant correlation between age and incorrect responding to the VAS [35, 38]. The VAS has also been thought to become better intelligible by adding graded colors, usually red, symbolizing more pain, with a higher completion rate in patients with dementia [57].

The **VRS** originated by Melzack is a simple, commonly used pain rating scale [45]. To complete it, subjects select one of six descriptors that represent pain of progressive intensity: none, mild, discomforting, distressing, horrible, or excruciating [48]. It has demonstrated good reliability and validity with older adults and when compared with other pain intensity scales, is often the preferred tool for many older adults [31, 33]. Limitations include the possibility that the words may not have the same meaning for each individual, and the categories between words do not represent equal intervals on the scale [48]. The PT, originally developed by Roland and Morris, is a variation of the VRS and has demonstrated some preferences in elderly patients with moderate to severe cognitive impairment [68].

The **NRS** with a 0–10, 0–20, or 0–100 point scale has wording such as "no pain" at one extreme and "worst pain possible" at the other [49]. Often the value of "4" on a 0–10 point scale is used to confirm the need for further intervention or to document that the patient's goals for analgesia have been achieved [28]. Although validated for use with the elderly, a substantial portion of older adults have difficulty responding to this scale, particularly if administered verbally without showing the number [73, 75]. A similar scale is the modified 21-point box scale. It is a row of 21 boxes labeled from 0 to 100 in increments of five. The 0 anchor was labeled "no pain," while the 100 anchor was labeled "pain as bad as it could be." To complete the scale, respondents indicate the box that best represent their pain [36].

The **FPS** consists of a line drawing of seven faces which express increasing pain (no pain = 0, maximum pain = 6) [2]. It has been adapted for older adults populations from similar pain scales used in pediatric settings [32]. Herr et al. [32] found preliminary support for the construct validity, strong ordinal properties, and strong test–retest reliability of the FPS in a sample of white, elderly individuals in the community. Later, Stuppy evaluated the reliability and validity of the FPS using a sample of 60 patients older than 55. Findings revealed that the FPS was reliable, valid, and sensitive to change and was preferred to the NRS, VAS, and VDS by 53% of the subjects [66].

Different studies have attempted to determine the most appropriate scale for cognitively impaired elderly but report conflicting results. Ferrell and others found completion rates in 287 nursing homes residents that vary from 44% for the VAS to 65% for the present pain intensity subscale of the McGill questionnaire, a combined word and number scale [16]. This is consistent with the findings of Krulewitch et al. [39], who reported the worst completion rate for a VAS (53%) and the faces scale (53%) compared to the pain intensity scale (62%), a combined visual and verbal scale. Scherder and others [57] described a very high completion rate for the CAS, a colored vertical VAS (100% in early AD and 80% in midstage AD). In comparison to NRS, VRS remained more stable as the degree of cognitive impairment increases. Pautex et al. [54, 55] was able to demonstrate that four pain self-assessment scales (verbal, horizontal visual, vertical visual, and FPS) possess high test–retest reliability in a population with dementia. Correlation between the four self-assessment scales was very strong. Correlations were slightly lower in patients with moderate than with mild dementia. The 5-point VRS appeared to perform slightly better in a more recent study among patients with severe cognitive deficits (respectively 57.5% and 95% for the NRS and 5-point VRS) [40].

Whatever the scale chosen, sufficient time must be spent to explain the scale to the patient. For example, for the VAS the scale should be presented horizontally to the patient: "this is a scale that evaluates pain." Then, the sliding vertical marker should be moved on the left side of the scale: "the sliding vertical marker on this side corresponds to no pain at all." Then the sliding vertical marker should be moved on the right part of the scale: "the sliding vertical marker on this side corresponds to an extreme pain." Then, the patient's ability to correctly indicate which position correspond to no pain and which position to the most severe pain should be tested: "move the sliding vertical marker to the place on the scale that corresponds to no pain and then move the sliding vertical marker to the place on the scale that corresponds to an extreme pain." If the patient demonstrates comprehension of the scale, patient should indicate the level of pain, he currently experiences: "to evaluate your current pain, move the sliding vertical marker to indicate where your current pain is."

When the right scale has been found for a patient, it is important to use consistently the same scale with each assessment.

Pain Disability Scale

The Pain Disability Index (PDI) [8] can be used as self-report instrument and appears both suitable and informative for the application in individuals with beginning cognitive impairment. It requires again not more than the proper use of numerical scales ranging from 0 to 10 as also required for pain intensity assessment; therefore, the PDI cannot easily result in cognitive overload. By means of such numerical scales, the functional disruptions by chronic pain can be self-rated for seven domains, family/home responsibilities, recreation, social activities, occupation, sexual behavior, self-care, and life-support activities. It is obvious that these domains are not equally relevant for individuals being already retired for many years and mainly living in nursing homes. However, the focus on functional limitations experienced, which constitute a major impact on the quality of life in the elderly, makes the PDI certainly face-valid. Modified versions excluding irrelevant domains are conceivable. The PDI could already be used to disclose stoic attitudes toward chronic pain in the elderly [8, 12].

Multidimensional Tools

Short-Form McGill Questionnaire

The Short-Form McGill Pain Questionnaire (SF-MPQ) is a valid and reliable tool for the brief assessment of the multidimensional qualities of pain (sensory and affective) as well as pain intensity (VAS, Present Pain Index [PPI; based on a 1–5 intensity scale]) in people with chronic pain, but its applicability in older people requires further investigation. Gagliese and Melzack [24] found similar factor structure, internal consistency, and pattern of subscale correlations in young and elderly individuals. There were also no significant differences between the two age groups when periods with the highest, usual, and lowest pain intensity were considered. However, the elderly group had significantly lower MPQ total and sensory scores and chose fewer words than the young group, suggesting differences in pain quality but not intensity. Gauthier et al. [25] confirmed a similar internal consistency and convergent validity as well as a comparable four-factor solution in older (≥60 years) and younger (<60 years) cancer patients. Older and younger patients selected in this study the same words with the same intensity to describe their pains. Gagliese and Katz [23] investigated male patients after prostatectomy. The correlation between VAS and MPQ scores was significantly lower in the older than younger group. Manias et al. [43] used the SF-MPQ—among other scales—to evaluate a nursing intervention in older hospitalized people with success. In sum, the SF-MPQ has shown its applicability in geriatric pain research, identifying age differences in pain processing. However, most of the studies have not referred to the suitability of the SF-MPQ for use in patients with dementia.

Brief Pain Inventory

The Brief Pain Inventory (BPI-SF), the short form (nine items) of which is considered here, might be validly applied as long as numerical scales from 0 to 10 can be competently used to self-rate internal states. However, patients have to refer repeatedly to periods of 24 hours, a task which might be too difficult for patients with dementia, suffering, by definition, often from memory problems. The advantage of the BPI-SF compared to one-dimensional pain scales is that it assesses pain intensity and its diurnal variations along with the pain-related interference, which are also two basic dimensions for the understanding of pain in dementia. Chen et al. [7] investigated individuals with MMSE scores down to 18, suggesting at least slight degrees of dementia, with a modified version of BPI, which contains only pain severity items and found a completion rate of almost 100%. MMSE scores were correlated with BPI scores, showing more pain in those elderly with cognitive impairments. However, this shortened version got rid of the interference items, which just make the BPI-SF two-dimensional and thus conceptually attractive. Auret et al. [1] tried to preserve the two-dimensionality of the BPI and, nevertheless, reduced its length to increase the usability in residential care facilities. For that purpose, they reduced the BPI further to six items (three for pain intensity and three for pain interference) and substituted the numerical category ratings by verbal descriptors ratings. The authors were aware that this shortened BPI requires further testing but believed that it had already shown adequate internal consistency. Accordingly, the use of the BPI as self-report tool in residents who have some cognitive impairment might have become conceivable by this modification.

Geriatric Pain Measure

A promising instrument for multidimensional pain self-assessment is the Geriatric Pain Measure (GPM), a 24-item questionnaire with versions in various languages, specifically developed and validated for interviewer- and self-administered assessment of pain in older adults. The GPM has been used in community-dwelling and nursing home populations and is easy to administer and to score, although the GPM may still be considered too long [9]. Therefore, a short version with only 12 items has been made available [3]. Ferrell et al. [19] reported good psychometric properties and convergent validity with the MPQ. Pain intensity, disengagement, pain with ambulation, pain with strenuous activities, and pain with other activities were the five factors, which Ferrel et al. [18] extracted. It became obvious in a study by Fisher et al. [20] that this tool depends on the context of application (cognitive status, difficulty of instruction, and time for answers) as many other tools. Results suggest that nursing home residents can provide consistent and reliable self-report of pain with this instrument, given that appropriate time and assistance are provided. A clear correlation between cognitive status and failed responses was obtained for the Likert-scaled questions, but not for the yes/no questions. This means that self-rating may turn into a structured pain interview when the patients can no longer rate pain dimensionally, but only categorically in its simplest form.

DOES THE USE OF SELF-ASSESSMENT SCALES IMPROVE PAIN MANAGEMENT?

Pain assessment of any kind in nursing homes increases the likelihood of better pain management [13], although pain assessment by observers does not guarantee subsequent intervention [78]. This suggest that pain assessment—although being one of the very critical factors for pain management—is embedded in a multifactorial network of determinants of whether adequate pain management is provided to elderly in nursing homes with and without cognitive impairment [67]. There are no data available, suggesting evidence that self-report of pain has a more beneficial influence on subsequent pain management than observer rating. By theory, one might assume that repeated requirements of self-assessing pain might keep elderly individuals aware of this specific source of discomfort and its potential remedies. Thus, it might be an activity of caregivers and nurses worth pursuing to support the self-assessment of the patient, that is, the "validation of pain," instead of switching too early to exclusive observer ratings. However, no empirical corroboration exists so far for this idea.

DIVERGENCE BETWEEN SELF-REPORT AND OBSERVER RATING

There is a clear difference in accessibility of pain by self-report measures and observer ratings. Private events as the subjective experience of pain can only be indicated by self-report following introspection. For most of the common self-report measures, introspection has to take on metric form to become a quantitative parameter. Qualitative assessment of self-report has rarely been used. The observer rating may use the self-report of patients and becomes at this point also dependent on the self-awareness and intellectual as well as linguistic skills of the patients. However, observers can add and integrate further behavioral indicators of pain into their pain evaluation, which are hardly accessible by self-perception. Good examples are involuntary protective or avoidance behaviors, pain-indicative voice formations during vocalization, and spontaneous facial reactions while in pain. Therefore, a complete convergence between self-report and observer rating of pain would be very puzzling, and a moderate correlation would be preferential to suggest that one and the same latent construct, namely pain, is indeed assessed, using however different sources of information. How does this situation present when elderly individuals with and without cognitive impairment are under investigation?

Horgas et al. [34] compared an observational scale (Noncommunicative Patient's Pain Assessment Instrument [NOPPAIN]) when used by nurses with two self-report measures of pain (VDS and NRS) in 20 cognitively intact and 20 impaired individuals. The overall intensity rating by observers was significantly correlated with self-reported pain intensity but only in cognitively intact elderly participants. This suggests that cognitively impaired elderly individuals are less adequately able to verbally report pain. The change was quite drastically: While the MMSE score dropped from 27 in the cognitively intact to 17 in the impaired individuals, the correlations between self-report and observer ratings lost size from around $r = 0.65$ to around $r = 0.10$. The higher correlations may demarcate the convergence which self-reports, and observer rating may at best achieve, and the lower correlations may reflect the progressive loss of validity of self-report in case of dementia. This reasonable conclusion seemed to be completely contradicted by a recent study by Lukas et al. [40]. The authors found surprisingly that the self-report assessed by means of Pain Today (yes/no), Pain Now (yes/no) and PPI-MPQ correlated less with three observer scales (Abbey Pain Scale, Pain Assessment In Advanced Dementia [PAINAD], NOPPAIN) in subjects without cognitive impairment (MMSE: ca. 27 on average) (coefficients between 0.2 and 0.3) than in patients with dementia (MMSE: ca. 14 on average) (coefficients between 0.5 and 0.7). A glimpse of an explanation offers the completion rates for the two groups, which were 100% for the unimpaired and 73% for the impaired participants. Assuming that in the 27% patients with incomplete self-reports the data would not support a relationship with the observer ratings, the correlations for the dementia group as a whole might have been substantially lower. The authors gave another reasonable account by stressing that the observer rating instruments were developed to match the behavioral indicators of pain in patients with dementia and not in cognitively unimpaired individuals.

Not surprisingly, the divergence between self-report and observer rating depends not only on the tools applied for self-report and observer rating but also on the type of observer. van Herk et al. [70] obtained data with low to moderate correlations between the self-report of nursing home residents and the observer ratings of either caregivers or relatives. The exact size of the correlations varied depending on the group of observers.

In sum, the divergence between self-report and observer rating of pain in elderly individuals without and with slight cognitive impairment seems to be comprehensible, considering that the two measures use information from different sources. The divergence likely increases with the progression of dementia until it is complete when the patients are no longer able to self-report the pain.

RECOMMENDATIONS FOR BEST PRACTICE

The attempt to obtain self-report of pain from elderly individuals suspect of being cognitively impaired should be the rule as first step. It can be attained in most patients even with mild to moderate dementia when certain precautions are taken. Older adults with cognitive impairment should be only questioned about present pain and be given repeated instructions as well as adequate time to respond. The self-report of pain may be a simple "yes" or "no," unequivocal vocalizations, or gestures such as hand grasp or eye blink. When self-report is absent or limited, the investigator should indicate why self-report cannot be used and whether further investigations and observations are needed in this matter [29].

As a further recommendation may serve the idea that every pain assessment should be planned at best as single case investigation, considering the individual handicaps and resources of the patient. Of course, there are patients with dementia, presenting with visual spatial dysfunctions [26] and poor fine motor coordination [71], which result into handicaps preventing good use of the VAS. It is known that the decoding of emotional faces is impaired in Alzheimer's disease [56]; nevertheless, many researchers and clinicians trust without hesitation that the FPS is always a valid measure. Patients with dementia may be bad with numbers [5] and words [41]; these are deficits, which make the use of numerical and VRSs for exact pain assessment risky. Furthermore, all scales make it necessary to relate an internal state in a proportional or at least monotonic fashion to at least ordinally stringed numbers, words, faces, line lengths, etc. It is almost common knowledge among experts that all these skills may be hampered in dementia, sometimes in a pathognomonic manner for specific forms of dementia. This means that the ability of self-reporting pain is necessarily variably existent and recommendations of "on average" useful scales are not the best practice but the lesser evil. Of course, it is of help for the caregivers to learn which pain scales have been tested for their usefulness and may be used without major risk of missing pain in their patients. However, the evidence for the appropriateness of such scales has mainly been supplied by group statistics, which are based on the neglect of the individual profiles of sensory, motor, and cognitive dysfunctions. It is agreed that considering individual profiles is time and effort consuming, but it is nevertheless the most adequate approach. For note, the diagnostic category of dementia consists of heterogeneous subcategories, which in turn include heterogeneous clusters of symptoms and dysfunctions. In such a situation, it is hardly possible to have a suitable tool of self-report assessment of pain at hand for all patients without considering the individual case.

Determining the time point when older adults with cognitive impairment can no longer reliably report pain using a standard tool can be challenging for clinicians. When there are first indications that cognition has been worsened, it is recommended to reevaluate the patient to guarantee understanding and ability to use a standard pain scale. This can be done by asking the patients to indicate where on the scale a "severe" pain and where a "mild" pain might be. The reliability of responses can be evaluated by having the patients rate their pain on the selected pain scale, distract them for a few minutes with other activities, and then ask them to rate this pain again. The scores reported should be the same or very similar if patients are still reliably reporting current pain. When questioning about pain, phrasing has been found to have an important impact on the information obtained from older adults. Open-ended questions such as "tell me about your pain, aches, soreness, or discomfort" typically supplies substantially more pain information than the closed-ended question such as "what would you rate your pain, aches, soreness, or discomfort on a 0–10 scale, with 0 being no pain, and 10 equal to the worst pain possible?" Vague questions such as "how are you feeling?" can lead to answers biased by social desirability, stoicism, and misconceptions of the patients. Older adults often deny the presence of "pain" but assert experiencing "discomfort" or express pain by use of other but similar descriptors. Alternative methods of feedback, such as head nods, hand squeezes, eye movements, or finger raising can be used. When investigating patients from a different cultural background, tools translated and validated for that population and the presence of a translator may be required. Individuals with sensory deficits should be accommodated—as needed—with enlarged types, adequate lighting, hearing enhancement, corrective lenses, and clear and simple instruction in both verbal and written forms.

SUMMARY

Self-report assessment of pain should always be attempted in individuals with weak to moderate forms of dementia by using simple scales (NRS, VDS) for assessing pain intensity. More sophisticated tools with multidimensional pain concepts are still awaiting development and evaluation in robust and reliable short forms. Self-report scales cannot be applied in a perfectly standardized fashion because the individual patient with varying sensory, motor, and cognitive deficits has to be considered. The clinicians and caregivers are challenged to determine the time point when alternatives to self-report have to be taken into account. Although even the use of simple self-report approaches is time and effort consuming, the consequence may be very favorable because better pain management is likely and patients with dementia can be actively involved in the "validation" of their pain.

REFERENCES

1. Auret KA, Toye C, Goucke R, Kristjanson LJ, Bruce D, Schug S. Development and testing of a modified version of the brief pain inventory for use in residential aged care facilities. J Am Geriatr Soc 2008;56:301–6.
2. Bieri D, Reeve RA, Champion GD, Addicoat L, Ziegler JB. The Faces Pain Scale for the self-assessment of the severity of pain experienced by children: development, initial validation, and preliminary investigation for ratio scale properties. Pain 1990;41:139–50.

3. Blozik E, Stuck AE, Niemann S, Ferrell BA, Harari D, von Renteln-Kruse W, Gillmann G, Beck JC, Clough-Gorr KM. Geriatric Pain Measure short form: development and initial evaluation. J Am Geriatr Soc 2007; 55:2045–50.
4. Bosley BN, Weiner DK, Rudy TE, Granieri E. Is chronic nonmalignant pain associated with decreased appetite in older adults? Preliminary evidence. J Am Geriatr Soc 2004;52:247–51.
5. Cappelletti M, Butterworth B, Kopelman M. Numeracy skills in patients with degenerative disorders and focal brain lesions: a neuropsychological investigation. Neuropsychology 2012;26:1–19.
6. Casten RJ, Parmelee PA, Kleban MH, Lawton MP, Katz IR. The relationships among anxiety, depression, and pain in a geriatric institutionalized sample. Pain 1995;61:271–6.
7. Chen Q, Hayman LL, Shmerling RH, Bean JF, Leveille SG. Characteristics of chronic pain associated with sleep difficulty in older adults: the Maintenance of Balance, Independent Living, Intellect, and Zest in the Elderly (MOBILIZE) Boston study. J Am Geriatr Soc 2011;59:1385–92.
8. Chibnall JT, Tait RC. The Pain Disability Index: factor structure and normative data. Arch Phys Med Rehabil 1994;75:1082–86.
9. Clough-Gorr KM, Blozik E, Gillmann G, Beck JC, Ferrell BA, Anders J, Harari D, Stuck AE. The self-administered 24-item geriatric pain measure (GPM-24-SA): psychometric properties in three European populations of community-dwelling older adults. Pain Med 2008;9:695–709.
10. Cohen-Mansfield J, Lipson S. Pain in cognitively impaired nursing home residents: how well are physicians diagnosing it? J Am Geriatr Soc 2002;50:1039–44.
11. Cohen-Mansfield J, Marx MS. Pain and depression in the nursing home: corroborating results. J Gerontol 1993;48:P96–7.
12. Cook AJ, Chastain DC. The classification of patients with chronic pain: age and sex differences. Pain Res Manag 2001;6:142–51.
13. de Souto Barreto P, Lapeyre-Mestre M, Vellas B, Rolland Y. Potential underuse of analgesics for recognized pain in nursing home residents with dementia: a cross-sectional study. Pain 2013;154:2427–31.
14. Etzioni S, Chodosh J, Ferrell BA, MacLean CH. Quality indicators for pain management in vulnerable elders. J Am Geriatr Soc 2007;55:S403–8.
15. Faries JE, Mills DS, Goldsmith KW, Phillips KD, Orr J. Systematic pain records and their impact on pain control. A pilot study. Cancer Nurs 1991;14:306–13.
16. Ferrell BA. Pain evaluation and management in the nursing home. Ann Intern Med 1995;123:681–7.
17. Ferrell BA, Ferrell BR, Osterweil D. Pain in the nursing home. J Am Geriatr Soc 1990;38:409–14.
18. Ferrell BA, Ferrell BR, Rivera L. Pain in cognitively impaired nursing home patients. J Pain Symptom Manag 1995;10:591–8.
19. Ferrell BA, Stein WM, Beck JC. The Geriatric Pain Measure: validity, reliability and factor analysis. J Am Geriatr Soc 2000;48:1669–73.
20. Fisher SE, Burgio LD, Thorn BE, Hardin JM. Obtaining self-report data from cognitively impaired elders: methodological issues and clinical implications for nursing home pain assessment. Gerontologist 2006; 46:81–8.
21. Flaherty JH. 'Who's taking your 5th vital sign?'. J Gerontol A Biol Sci Med Sci 2001;56:M397–9.
22. Folstein MF, Folstein SE, McHugh PR. 'Mini-mental state'. A practical method for grading the cognitive state of patients for the clinician. J Psychiatr Res 1975;12:189–98.
23. Gagliese L, Katz J. Age differences in postoperative pain are scale dependent: a comparison of measures of pain intensity and quality in younger and older surgical patients. Pain 2003;103:11–20.
24. Gagliese L, Melzack R. Age-related differences in the qualities but not the intensity of chronic pain. Pain 2003;104:597–608.
25. Gauthier LR, Young A, Dworkin RH, Rodin G, Zimmermann C, Warr D, Librach SL, Moore M, Shepherd FA, Pillai Riddell R, et al. Validation of the short-form McGill pain questionnaire-2 in younger and older people with cancer pain. J Pain 2014;15:756–70.
26. Geldmacher DS. Visuospatial dysfunction in the neurodegenerative diseases. Front Biosci 2003;8:e428–36.
27. Giron MS, Forsell Y, Bernsten C, Thorslund M, Winblad B, Fastbom J. Sleep problems in a very old population: drug use and clinical correlates. J Gerontol A Biol Sci Med Sci 2002;57:M236–40.
28. Hartrick CT, Kovan JP, Shapiro S. The numeric rating scale for clinical pain measurement: a ratio measure? Pain Pract 2003;3:310–6.
29. Herr K, Coyne PJ, McCaffery M, Manworren R, Merkel S. Pain assessment in the patient unable to self-report: position statement with clinical practice recommendations. Pain Manag Nurs 2011;12:230–50.
30. Herr KA, Garand L. Assessment and measurement of pain in older adults. Clin Geriatr Med 2001;17:457–78.

31. Herr KA, Mobily PR. Comparison of selected pain assessment tools for use with the elderly. Appl Nurs Res 1993;6:39–46.
32. Herr KA, Mobily PR, Kohout FJ, Wagenaar D. Evaluation of the Faces Pain Scale for use with the elderly. Clin J Pain 1998;14:29–38.
33. Herr KA, Spratt K, Mobily PR, Richardson G. Pain intensity assessment in older adults: use of experimental pain to compare psychometric properties and usability of selected pain scales with younger adults. Clin J Pain 2004;20:207–19.
34. Horgas AL, Nichols AL, Schapson CA, Vietes K. Assessing pain in persons with dementia: relationships among the non-communicative patient's pain assessment instrument, self-report, and behavioral observations. Pain Manag Nurs 2007;8:77–85.
35. Jensen MP, Karoly P, Braver S. The measurement of clinical pain intensity: a comparison of six methods. Pain 1986;27:117–26.
36. Jensen MP, Miller L, Fisher LD. Assessment of pain during medical procedures: a comparison of three scales. Clin J Pain 1998;14:343–9.
37. Kamel HK, Phlavan M, Malekgoudarzi B, Gogel P, Morley JE. Utilizing pain assessment scales increases the frequency of diagnosing pain among elderly nursing home residents. J Pain Symptom Manag 2001;21:450–5.
38. Kremer E, Atkinson JH, Ignelzi RJ. Measurement of pain: patient preference does not confound pain measurement. Pain 1981;10:241–8.
39. Krulewitch H. Assessment of pain in cognitively impaired older adults: a comparison of pain assessment tools and their use by nonprofessional caregivers [comment]. Issues Law Med 2000;16:143–65.
40. Lukas A, Niederecker T, Gunther I, Mayer B, Nikolaus T. Self- and proxy report for the assessment of pain in patients with and without cognitive impairment: experiences gained in a geriatric hospital. Z Gerontol Geriatr 2013;46:214–21.
41. Macoir J, Laforce R Jr, Monetta L, Wilson M. Language deficits in major forms of dementia and primary progressive aphasias: an update according to new diagnostic criteria. Geriatr Psychol Neuropsychiatr Vieil 2014;12:199–208.
42. Madison JL, Wilkie DJ. Family members' perceptions of cancer pain. Comparisons with patient sensory report and by patient psychologic status. Nurs Clin North Am 1995;30:625–45.
43. Manias E, Gibson SJ, Finch S. Testing an educational nursing intervention for pain assessment and management in older people. Pain Med 2011;12:1199–215.
44. McGrath PA, Seifert CE, Speechley KN, Booth JC, Stitt L, Gibson MC. A new analogue scale for assessing children's pain: an initial validation study. Pain 1996;64:435–43.
45. Melzack R. The McGill Pain Questionnaire: major properties and scoring methods. Pain 1975;1:277–99.
46. Monroe TB, Misra SK, Habermann RC, Dietrich MS, Cowan RL, Simmons SF. Pain reports and pain medication treatment in nursing home residents with and without dementia. Geriatr Gerontol Int 2013.
47. Nekolaichuk CL, Bruera E, Spachynski K, MacEachern T, Hanson J, Maguire TO. A comparison of patient and proxy symptom assessments in advanced cancer patients. Palliat Med 1999;13:311–23.
48. Ohnhaus EE, Adler R. Methodological problems in the measurement of pain: a comparison between the verbal rating scale and the visual analogue scale. Pain 1975;1:379–84.
49. Paice JA, Cohen FL. Validity of a verbally administered numeric rating scale to measure cancer pain intensity. Cancer Nurs 1997;20:88–93.
50. Parmelee PA. Pain in cognitively impaired older persons. Clin Geriatr Med 1996;12:473–87.
51. Parmelee PA, Smith B, Katz IR. Pain complaints and cognitive status among elderly institution residents. J Am Geriatr Soc 1993;41:517–22.
52. Patel KV, Guralnik JM, Dansie EJ, Turk D. C. Prevalence and impact of pain among older adults in the United States: findings from the 2011 National Health and Aging Trends Study. Pain 2013;154:2649–57.
53. Pautex S, Berger A, Chatelain C, Herrmann F, Zulian GB. Symptom assessment in elderly cancer patients receiving palliative care. Crit Rev Oncol Hematol 2003;47:281–6.
54. Pautex S, Herrmann F, Le Lous P, Fabjan M, Michel JP, Gold G. Feasibility and reliability of four pain self-assessment scales and correlation with an observational rating scale in hospitalized elderly demented patients. J Gerontol A Biol Sci Med Sci 2005;60:524–9.
55. Pautex S, Michon A, Guedira M, Emond H, Le Lous P, Samaras D, Michel JP, Herrmann F, Giannakopoulos P, Gold G. Pain in severe dementia: self-assessment or observational scales? J Am Geriatr Soc 2006;54:1040–5.

56. Phillips LH, Scott C, Henry JD, Mowat D, Bell JS. Emotion perception in Alzheimer's disease and mood disorder in old age. Psychol Aging 2010;25:38–47.
57. Scherder EJ, Bouma A. Visual analogue scales for pain assessment in Alzheimer's disease. Gerontology 2000;46:47–53.
58. Scherder EJ; Plooij B. Assessment and management of pain, with particular emphasis on central neuropathic pain, in moderate to severe dementia. Drugs Aging 2012;29:701–6.
59. Scott J, Huskisson EC. Graphic representation of pain. Pain 1976;2:175–84.
60. Scudds RJ, Robertson, J. Empirical evidence of the association between the presence of musculoskeletal pain and physical disability in community-dwelling senior citizens. Pain 1998;75:229–35.
61. Sengstaken EA, King SA. The problems of pain and its detection among geriatric nursing home residents. J Am Geriatr Soc 1993;41:541–4.
62. Shega JW, Hougham GW, Stocking CB, Cox-Hayley D, Sachs GA. Factors associated with self- and caregiver report of pain among community-dwelling persons with dementia. J Palliat Med 2005;8:567–75.
63. Simons W, Malabar R. Assessing pain in elderly patients who cannot respond verbally. J Adv Nurs 1995; 22:663–9.
64. Skevington SM. Investigating the relationship between pain and discomfort and quality of life, using the WHOQOL. Pain 1998;76:395–406.
65. Solomon PE, Prkachin KM, Farewell V. Enhancing sensitivity to facial expression of pain. Pain 1997; 71:279–84.
66. Stuppy DJ. The Faces Pain Scale: reliability and validity with mature adults. Appl Nurs Res 1998;11:84–9.
67. Swafford KL, Miller LL, Tsai PF, Herr KA, Ersek M. Improving the process of pain care in nursing homes: a literature synthesis. J Am Geriatr Soc 2009;57:1080–7.
68. Taylor LJ; Herr KA. Pain intensity assessment: a comparison of selected pain intensity scales for use in cognitively intact and cognitively impaired African American older adults. Pain Manag Nurs 2003; 4:87–95.
69. Tiplady B, Jackson SH, Maskrey VM, Swift CG. Validity and sensitivity of visual analogue scales in young and older healthy subjects. Age Ageing 1998;27:63–6.
70. van Herk R, van Dijk M, Biemold N, Tibboel D, Baar FP, de Wit R. Assessment of pain: can caregivers or relatives rate pain in nursing home residents? J Clin Nurs 2009;18:2478–85.
71. Villardita C. Alzheimer's disease compared with cerebrovascular dementia: neuropsychological similarities and differences. Acta Neurol Scand 1993;87:299–308.
72. Weiner D, Peterson B, Keefe F. Chronic pain-associated behaviors in the nursing home: resident versus caregiver perceptions. Pain 1999;80:577–88.
73. Weiner D, Peterson B, Ladd K, McConnell E, Keefe F. Pain in nursing home residents: an exploration of prevalence, staff perspectives, and practical aspects of measurement. Clin J Pain 1999;15:92–101.
74. Wilson KG, Watson ST, CurrieSR. Daily diary and ambulatory activity monitoring of sleep in patients with insomnia associated with chronic musculoskeletal pain. Pain 1998;75:75–84.
75. Wynne CF, Ling SM, Remsburg R. Comparison of pain assessment instruments in cognitively intact and cognitively impaired nursing home residents. Geriatr Nurs 2000;21:20–3.
76. Yeager KA, Miaskowski C, Dibble SL, Wallhagen M. Differences in pain knowledge and perception of the pain experience between outpatients with cancer and their family caregivers. Oncol Nurs Forum 1995; 22:1235–41.
77. Yong HH, Bell R, Workman B, Gibson SJ. Psychometric properties of the Pain Attitudes Questionnaire (revised) in adult patients with chronic pain. Pain 2003;104:673–81.
78. Zwakhalen SM, van't Hof CE, Hamers JP. Systematic pain assessment using an observational scale in nursing home residents with dementia: exploring feasibility and applied interventions. J Clin Nurs 2012; 21:3009–17.

CHAPTER 10

Observational Pain Tools

Sandra Zwakhalen, Keela A. Herr, and Kristen Swafford

The self-assessment tools discussed in the previous chapter (see Chapter 9) can be valuable for assessing pain in older persons with dementia, and their use should always be considered. Research suggests that for most persons with mild-to-moderate dementia, self-reports can be used in a valid and reliable way [15, 50, 86]. However, evidence shows that older persons with a score below 18 on the Mini-Mental Status Examination (MMSE) [27] tend to be unreliable and invalid in their responses on self-reports [15]. When dementia progresses and the person becomes less verbally responsive, observational pain tools become more important. Research on pain in persons with dementia is largely dominated by studies on the development of pain assessment tools to detect the presence of pain, with a tremendous increase in the development of behavioral pain assessment tools for nonverbal persons with dementia during the last two decades. Observational pain tools typically focus on direct observation of pain-related behaviors, and also may include changes in behavior and functioning. In this chapter, the necessity of using observational tools for the assessment of pain in persons with moderate to severe dementia is explained. Based on reviews of the state-of-the-art use of observational tools, the scope and quality of the available tools regarding validity, reliability, and usability will be addressed. Furthermore, benefits of tools for persons and for care workers will be discussed. Finally, directions for future developments to improve the recognition and quantification of pain in persons with dementia will be given.

BACKGROUND

Statistics indicate that 45–80% of institutionalized older persons experience the presence of daily pain [96], although prevalence rates vary. Methods used to assess the prevalence of pain in institutionalized older adults differ enormously, and often lack reliability and validity. Underassessment is frequently highlighted as one of the most important reasons for undertreatment of pain in dementia [19].

The underassessment of pain is, in large part, directly related to the complexity of assessment in nonverbal persons, many of whom have dementia. Dementia complicates the assessment of pain because of memory, judgment, and verbal impairment [37]. These issues and the impact on the ability to communicate are probably the most challenging factors in the process of pain assessment. As a result, pain is often extremely difficult to assess. Unrecognized, untreated persistent pain in people with dementia causes unnecessary suffering and can result in additional loss of functioning such as cognitive problems or behavioral problems [2].

REVIEWS ON THE ASSESSMENT OF PAIN IN DEMENTIA BY OBSERVATIONAL TOOLS

During the last decade, several systematic reviews addressed the current state-of-the-art observational tools. They all aimed to identify pain assessment tools for older persons with limited verbal capacity and evaluate their psychometric quality and usefulness.

An overview of the reviews and their conclusions is presented in Table 10-1.

The reviews show that currently many tools are available. These tools use different formats in terms of items and scoring methods. Some tools are more extensive than others because they specify behaviors that are sometimes clustered into categories or cluster items in slightly different categories, although they refer to similar behavior. This means that some tools use similar cues to measure pain, but they split up the cues into smaller items to be observed (e.g., the cue facial expression is split into opening mouth or squeezing eyes).

The American Geriatric Society (AGS) Panel on Persistent Pain in Older Persons identified six categories of behavior changes that are typically found in cognitively impaired older adults who are in pain (Table 10-2) [2]. Some of these categories include very common pain expressions (e.g., facial expressions), while others are more subtle or require specific knowledge about the person being observed (e.g., irritability, changes in sleep patterns).

Measures of these AGS indicators of pain are often used in reviews to indicate the comprehensiveness of the tools available.

Based on current insights, two of the main questions regarding behavioral observation are (1) which of the AGS categories is most sensitive to detecting pain in older persons suffering from dementia and (2) whether all the subcategories and behaviors included in each category are required for assessing pain. Recent research suggests that the category making up facial expressions of pain is one of the strongest indicators of pain in older persons with dementia. These facial expressions seem particularly useful and sensitive to assess pain in dementia [53, 57, 89].

All reviews presented above conclude that no single scale could be recommended across all populations and settings and further testing of tools is needed. Currently, no tool is accepted as the best silver standard when self-report as the gold standard is lacking. However, development is still ongoing and psychometric evaluation of tools has resulted in the establishment of some sound behavioral pain assessment tools.

The most frequently recommended tools include PACSLAC, PAINAD, Abbey, Dololus-2, MOBID, and DS-DAT. Furthermore, lately there seems to be a trend to tailor pain tools toward more specific subpopulations/groups of dementia (e.g., orofacial pain, paramedic care). This trend underlines that one size does not fit all. An examination of observational pain tools and their psychometric properties follows.

OBSERVATIONAL PAIN TOOLS, CLOSELY EXAMINED

Because of the large volume of tools in various stages of development and testing, a synthesis of the existing work on each tool is provided in Table 10-3. We have attempted to be

TABLE 10-1 Overview of Systematic Reviews on Pain in Older Nonverbal Adults

Author	Target Population	Tools Reviewed	Overall Conclusion
Stolee et al. [92]	Cognitive impairment	Behavior checklist and facial grimace scale; CNPI; DS-DAT, Doloplus2; EPCA; FACS; MDS; PAINAD; PADE; PBM; Proxy pain questionnaire	There is a need for further development and testing. Instruments demonstrated weak validity and reliability data. No specific recommendations were made for one tool (DS-DAT and PAINAD scored adequate).
Zwakhalen et al. [107]	Severe dementia	Doloplus2; EPCA; ECS; Observational pain behavior tool; CNPI; PACSLAC; PAINAD; PADE; RaPID; Abbey; NOPPAIN; Pain assessment scale for use with cognitively impaired adults	All tools demonstrated moderate psychometric qualities; Doloplus-2 and PACSLAC appeared to be most promising.
Herr et al. [33]	Dementia	Abbey; ADD; CNPI; DS-DAT; Doloplus 2; FLACC; NOPPAIN; PACSLAC; PADE; PAINAD	No standardized tool in English is recommended for broad adoption in clinical practice. Results indicate that, although further testing and development is required, DS-DAT and NOPPAIN are promising, followed by CNPI, PACSLAC, and Doloplus-2.
Van Herk et al. [101]	Cognitive impairments or communication difficulties	FACS; PBM; DS-DAT; Doloplus2; Behavior checklist cognitively impaired older adults ; CNPI; ADD; PAINAD; PATCOA; PADE; PACSLAC; NOPPAIN; Abbey	Based on the validation studies, PAINAD, FACS, PACSLAC, and DS-DAT show most promising findings. However, PAINAD seems to be most feasible in clinical practice.
Lord [61]	Paramedic assessment in cognitive impaired	Used tools detected by two previous performed reviews	No tools are designed for paramedic use and only one tool was designed to assess pain in acute care. The Abbey pain scale may have implications in paramedic assessment of pain.
Park et al. [74]	Nonverbal cognitive impaired	Abbey; ADD; Behavioral checklist; CNPI; DS-DAT; NOPPAIN; PACSLAC; PADE; PAINAD; PATCOA; MOBID	Various tools are available; psychometric evaluation is required. Although more psychometric testing of the 24-item version of the PACSLAC is recommended, its use was supported.
Lobbezoo et al. [60]	Orofacial pain in dementia	ADD, DS-DAT, Doloplus-2, PACSLAC, PAINAD	No tools available for dental pain, so no scale could be recommended.
Husebo et al. [41]	Patients with dementia	PADE; PAINE; Abbey; DS-DAT; CNPI; PAINAD; Doloplus-2; PACSLAC; ADD; NOPPAIN; EPCA-2; MOBID-2	An impressive number of scales have been developed. Implementation is lacking and high-quality studies (RCTs) are lacking.

Source: Used with permission from S. Zwakhalen, Maastricht University, The Netherlands.

TABLE 10-2 AGS Categories of Behavior Changes in Cognitively Impaired Older Adults

Facial expressions (such as grimacing)
Verbalizations and vocalizations (such as moaning)
Body movements (such as guarding)
Changes in interpersonal interactions (such as withdrawn socially)
Changes in activity patterns or routines (such as a change in appetite or sleep pattern)
Mental status changes (such as irritability)

comprehensive and include information on each tool available in English, as well as current references describing original development and subsequent further evaluation. Tools were not included if they were developed and had primary testing for a population other than persons with dementia (e.g., the Multidimensional Objective Pain Assessment Tool [MOPAT] [65], the Disability Distress Assessment Tool [Dis DAT]) [84], their translatability to another setting/culture was not possible because of the data capture required (e.g., Discomfort Behavior Scale [DBS]) [91], or they were developed for a single pain etiology (e.g., Pain Behaviors for Osteoarthritis Instrument for Cognitively Impaired Elders [PBOI-CIE]) [98]. Table 10-3 provides our judgment regarding reliability and validity based on the cumulative evidence available on each tool. Key summary points are provided to assist readers in considering the utility of a given tool for their setting and population. For a more in-depth discussion of each tool, we refer readers to the City of Hope Pain and Palliative Care Resource Center (http://prc.coh.org/PAIN-NOA.htm).

THE EFFECTIVENESS OF OBSERVATIONAL PAIN ASSESSMENT IN OLDER PERSONS WITH DEMENTIA

Assessing pain is challenging, especially for staff caring for older persons with dementia. A pressing question is whether improved recognition and assessment of pain in dementia actually leads to treatment and improvement in quality of life. Several studies suggest that pain assessment by using an observational tool increases awareness of pain and may facilitate an improvement in the assessment and management of pain in dementia [53, 59, 62, 64, 83, 89]. Lukas et al. [62] showed that the use of instruments such as pain tools improved recognition of the presence or absence of pain by over 25% above chance. Furthermore, it seems that tools with items capturing facial action units common in pain demonstrated higher levels of sensitivity, reliability, and validity [89].

All observational tools rely on a proxy report that is most often performed by nursing staff. The regular assessment and attention to pain shows not only positive effects on residents' outcomes, but also improves staff outcomes such as work stress [30].

DIRECTIONS OF FUTURE DEVELOPMENTS TO IMPROVE THE RECOGNITION AND QUANTIFICATION OF PAIN IN PERSONS WITH DEMENTIA

Although pain research in persons with dementia has expanded greatly in the past decade, several key aspects of pain assessment remain poorly understood. Although progress has

TABLE 10-3 Tool-Specific Information

Nonverbal Pain Behavior Scale	Description	Validity	Reliability	Feasibility and Clinical Utility	Languages and Settings	Summary
The Abbey Pain Scale (The APS) [1, 58, 62, 70]	• 6 items including vocalization, facial expression, change in body language, behavioral change, physiological change, and physical change. • Items scored on a 4-point scale for intensity of the behavior with a total score of intensity of pain (0–18)	• Good concurrent and construct validity • Differentiates between pre- and postintervention	• Moderate internal consistency • Strong interrater reliability • Sufficient test–retest reliability	• Reported completion 1 min • Scoring interpretation provided, but relationship with self-report of pain severity questionable • Cutoff of 3.5 for pain/no pain determined using ROC analysis	**Languages:** • English • Japanese [94] • Italian [93] **Settings:** • Australian residential aged care facilities (RACF) • Hong Kong nursing homes • Japanese nursing homes • Italian hospitals	• Clinically usable, brief measure of observable pain behaviors • Evidence of reliability and validity is established • Issues related to scoring level of pain severity • "Physical change" item may need revision based on consistent problems across studies
Algoplus [8, 81, 83]	• Five items/categories (facial expressions, look, complaints, body position, atypical behaviors) with 3–6 basic pain behaviors in each category. • Items scored yes if one basic behavior observed • Total score 0–5	• Discriminant validity differentiating acute pain and non-acute pain patients • Convergent validity in correlation between Algoplus and pain ratings of cognitively intact patients • Sensitivity to change between rest and movement and before and after analgesia	• Sufficient overall internal consistency, although some items may underestimate pain intensity particularly in Cambodian patients • Strong interrater reliability overall, but individual item ratings fair to strong	• Training time unclear • Time to administer/score 1 min • Cutoff of 2 for acute pain recommended based on ROC analysis	**Languages:** • French only—although translated into English **Settings:** • French hospital, emergency departments, rehabilitation units and long-term care facilities • Cambodian emergency department	• Only tool focused on identification of acute pain • Short, reliable tool for rapid evaluation of acute pain • Good preliminary psychometrics, but needs further evaluation in persons with advanced dementia • Testing in other cultures warranted

(continued)

TABLE 10-3 Tool-Specific Information (continued)

Nonverbal Pain Behavior Scale	Description	Validity	Reliability	Feasibility and Clinical Utility	Languages and Settings	Summary
Checklist of Nonverbal Pain Indicators (CNPI) [24, 25, 46, 57, 70, 71]	• 6 items including nonverbal vocalizations, facial grimacing or wincing, bracing, rubbing, restlessness, vocal complaints • Items scored present or absent at rest and on movement • Total score range from 0 to 12	• Convergent validity with other tools • Discriminates between baseline and pain conditions and between pain at rest and on movement.	• Moderate internal consistency reliability, although low for observations at rest • Good interrater reliability • Good to very good intrarater reliability • Moderate to good test-retest	• Easy to use • Time to complete not specified, but likely 5 min or less • Scoring instructions provided • No evidence that any number of pain behaviors from the CNPI corresponds with levels of pain intensity	**Languages:** • English • Norwegian **Settings:** • US nursing homes and hospitals • Canadian nursing homes • Australian RACF • Norwegian nursing homes	• Clinically usable, brief measure of observable pain behaviors • One of few tools with testing in hospital setting • Further evaluation of total score use (versus comparison of score at rest and movement) warranted
CNA Pain Assessment Tool (CPAT) [9–11]	• 5 items including facial expression, behavior, mood, body language, and activity level • Items scored 0 or 1 with different criteria based on item • Total score range 0–5	• Construct validity established with differences before and after a painful event; before and after intervention • Criterion validity established with concurrent administration of established research discomfort tool	• Strong interrater reliability • Sufficient internal consistency • Fair test-retest	• Training of 45 min required • Observation and scoring requires 1 min • A score of 1 or greater requires further action by the nursing assistant and high scores are to be evaluated by the nursing staff.	**Languages:** • English **Settings:** • US nursing homes	• Clinically usable, brief measure of observable pain behaviors by CNAs • Further evaluation of item scoring criteria and evaluation of tool sensitivity in controlled design recommended • Testing in other cultures and settings warranted

DOLOSHORT [78]	• 5 item, shortened version of Doloplus-2 with items significantly correlated with VAS scores in a multiple regression model • Scoring range not provided	• Construct validity established with differences before and after pain intervention • Convergent and discriminant validity established in French-speaking Swiss sample • Moderately high degree of sensitivity and specificity using suggested cutoff scores	• Sufficient internal consistency • Further reliability testing warranted	• Reported to be quick and easy to use • Cutoff score suggested at 3 via ROC analysis • Administration, scoring unclear	**Languages:** • French **Settings:** • Swiss hospital	• High convergent and discriminant validity and strong responsiveness of tool to treatment in preliminary testing • Testing in other cultures and settings warranted
Doloplus-2 [13, 32, 34, 35, 54, 67, 70, 77, 79, 80, 97, 105, 108]	• 10 items, 3 dimensions of somatic ($n = 5$), psychomotor ($n = 2$), psychosocial ($n = 3$) • Scoring range 0–30, reflects progression of experienced pain severity, not current pain experience	• Construct, concurrent, convergent and discriminant validity established in French and other cultures • Recent construct validity established in English version • Distinguishes between pain/no pain moderately well	• Good or excellent test–retest and interrater reliability in French, English, Italian, Portuguese and Spanish • Moderate test–retest and interrater reliability in Dutch • intrarater reliability • Strong internal consistency	• Appears easy to use • Estimated time to complete 5 min • Suggest score of 5 as threshold for pain • Considerable training resource materials available in several languages • Use by health and social care providers, as well as family; however, question regarding training and administration skills • Electronic tool available	**Languages:** • French primary and follow-up studies [32, 54, 77, 79, 105] • Japanese [3] • Italian [67, 73] • English [80] • Portuguese [80] • Spanish [80] • Dutch [80, 108] • Norwegian [34, 35, 97] • Chinese [13] **Settings:** • Hospitals • Nursing homes • Geriatric clinics • Palliative care	• Clinically useful tool, unclear how score interpreted if some domains not scored • Substantial psychometric support and use in Europe • Limited information on psychometric qualities of English version • Training needs among diverse users not yet clarified • Most translated of nonverbal pain tools • Differences in tool performance (particularly psychosocial domain) may relate to cultural or institutional differences

(*continued*)

TABLE 10-3 Tool-Specific Information (continued)

Nonverbal Pain Behavior Scale	Description	Validity	Reliability	Feasibility and Clinical Utility	Languages and Settings	Summary
DS-DAT [21, 36, 39, 40, 58, 66, 75, 99, 106]	• 9 items including noisy breathing, negative vocalizations, content facial expression, sad facial expression, frightened facial expression, frown, relaxed body language, tense body language, and fidgeting • Items measured for presence/absence, then for frequency, duration, and intensity during 5-min observation period • Each item is scored 0–3 with scoring range 0–27	• Content validity established in English, Italian, and Dutch • Evidence for discriminant validity moderately strong • Moderate convergent validity with pain tools • Construct validity: No consistency of model identified in confirmatory factor analysis in OA pain sample	• Good internal consistency • Moderately strong interrater reliability • Fair test-retest after 1 h with independent raters • Strong intrarater reliability	• Complex administration and scoring • Potentially requires extensive training (30+ h) • Time for completion reported 7–10 min	**Languages:** • English • Italian [21] • Dutch [36] • US hospitals and nursing homes • Italian nursing homes • Dutch nursing homes	• Time for training and for proper administration may be barrier to use • Construct validity issues and complex administration suggests tool refinement may be useful • Preliminary support for use by clinical users
Elderly Pain Caring Assessment (EPCA-2) [68]	• 8 items divided into 2 subscales: • Signs outside caregiving (facial expression, spontaneous posture adopted at rest, movement of	• Tool developers bring strong evidence for good convergent and discriminant validity and responsiveness of the EPCA-2.	• Initial reliability tests are favorable. • Internal consistency established for the global scale and for each subscales. • Good interrater reliability	• Pilot study measured approximate time of 15 min to complete, including 5 min observation before and 5 min after caregiving and 5 min to score.	**Languages:** • French only **Settings:** • French hospitals	• High convergent and discriminant validity and strong responsiveness of tool to treatment in preliminary testing. • Purports to measure pain severity rather than presence of pain only

	the patient out of bed or in bed, interaction with other people) • Signs during caregiving (anxious anticipation of intervention, reactions during caregiver intervention, reactions of the patient when painful part nursed, complaint voices in course of caregiving) • Each item scored on a 5-point scale (0 = no pain to 4 = extremely intense pain) • Total score 0–20	• Factor analysis confirmed the 2 factors of rest and caregiving pain and explained 56% of the variation in EPCA scores.	• A manual explaining the rating of each item and precautions for using the EPCA2 in day-to-day practice is available from the authors.	• Time for proper administration may be barrier to use • Not validated in English speaking populations or in long-term care settings—testing in other cultures and settings warranted
Mahoney Pain Scale (MPS) [63]	• 4 items addressing facial expression, vocalizations, body language, and breathing changes rated on 0–3 scale of minimal pain to severe pain. • 4 items on agitated behavior, change in activities, physiological state, current or history of painful conditions • Identifies location of physical pain problems on proxy pain maps • Total score 0–24	• Construct validity established with changes across activities and across groups in MPS score • Concurrent validity between nursing assistants' global pain ratings and nurses score on MPS, although gold standard questionable • Good interrater reliability during aversive activity for all tool items, except breathing • Sufficient internal consistency for pain severity items and fair for items differentiating pain and agitation	• Observation of 5 min required • Scoring overall is unclear with limited validation of item weighting • Initial study proposes general pain score cutoff of 4.5 for severity of pain, and cutoff score on pain vs. agitation of 2.75 **Languages:** • English **Settings:** • Australian nursing homes	• Addresses common pain behaviors and also incorporates aspects of pain assessment beyond direct observation of behaviors • Requires knowledge of normal behavior to rate changes in behavior • Rating schema and assumptions about pain severity ratings need further validation • Testing in other languages and settings needed

(continued)

TABLE 10-3 Tool-Specific Information (continued)

Nonverbal Pain Behavior Scale	Description	Validity	Reliability	Feasibility and Clinical Utility	Languages and Settings	Summary
Mobilization-Observation-Behavior-Intensity-Dementia (MOBID and MOBID-2) [42–45]	• 11-point NRS for 3 AGS behaviors: • MOBID includes 3 items (pain noises, facial expression, and defense), rating each on pain intensity from 0 to 10 during guided movement • Includes overall pain intensity rating on an 11-point NRS. • MOBID-2 adds section on pain intensity rating of pain behavior related to head, internal organs, and skin; and body diagram	• Concurrent validity established with MOBID detecting increased pain with movement, but did not connect number of pain behaviors with pain intensity among familiar caregivers. • MOBID-2 demonstrates construct validity with correlations with overall pain score and concurrent validity associating score with other pain-related variables	• Good internal consistency among external raters • Wide range in interrater reliability for the presence of pain behaviors but better interrater reliability for pain intensity • Variable test-retest reliability • MOBID-2 • Sufficient internal consistency • Moderate to strong interrater reliability for pain intensity scores • Moderate to strong test-retest	• One to 2 h training in reports, however no information on time to administer/score • No information on scoring cutoff or interpretation • MOBID testing with clinical caregivers with 2 h training, reported less than 5 min average to complete	Languages: • Norwegian Settings: • Norwegian nursing homes	• Evidence for use in research established and preliminary support for use by clinical users • Further evidence of validity of inferred pain intensity from behavior observation warranted • Testing in other cultures and settings warranted
Noncommunicating Patient's Pain Assessment Instrument (NOPPAIN) [26, 38, 57, 90]	• Nursing assistant administered instrument for observing and rating pain in patients with dementia. 4 parts: • Self-report • Observed behavior response to	• Construct: • Specificity: moderate to low • Sensitivity: moderate to strong • Convergent: strong when compared to self-report of presence/absence	• Internal consistency Low • Interrater reliability: Good to very good across all studies • Test-retest moderate at 1 wk on a video sample	• Provides pictures and text for ease of understanding, • Scoring and interpretation unclear, though cutoff of 4.5 for pain-no pain determined using ROC analysis in follow-up study	Languages: • English • Italian [26] • Brazilian Portuguese [5] translation only; no psychometrics to date	• Internal consistency and discriminant validity findings suggest need for further refinement of tool • Clinical utility would be enhanced with scoring and interpretation guidelines

	daily activities (i.e., words, noises, pain faces, bracing, rubbing, restlessness) on 6-point Likert scale • Pain location • VDS pain thermometer for proxy report of global pain intensity	of pain; moderate when compared to self-report of pain intensity • Discriminant: positive correlations with anger, depression, and anxiety constructs	Effect size very large in discriminating pain states vs. baseline	• Scoring and Reported rating time range: <30"–85.2" by direct care providers • Minimal training required	**Settings:** • US nursing home • Australian nursing home • Italian hospital
Pain Assessment in the Cognitively Impaired (PACI) [49, 51, 52]	• Direct care provider-administered screening tool, 7 items in three dimensions: facial expression ($n = 3$), verbalizations ($n = 2$), and body movements ($n = 2$) • Rate present or absent • Scoring range 0–7	• Construct, concurrent and convergent validity supported • Able to differentiate between painful states during activity and at rest	• Internal consistency psychometrics are not available • Moderate interrater reliability during both periods of activity and rest	• Scoring is clear (0–7) with 0 = no pain and 7 = high pain, but debate exists about use of scales to infer pain intensity • Minimal training required • Definitions of behavioral terms provided	• Further testing to assess sensitivity and specificity as well as responsiveness to treatment effects needed • Internal consistency data needed • Testing in other cultures and settings warranted **Languages:** • English only **Settings:** • Canadian nursing homes
The Pain Assessment Scale for Seniors with Severe Dementia (PACSLAC) [4, 14, 23, 28–30, 32, 49, 57, 58, 72, 82]	• 60 items in four dimensions: facial expression ($n = 13$), activity/body movements ($n = 20$), social/personality/mood ($n = 12$), physiological/eating/sleeping/vocal ($n = 15$) • Rate present or absent • Scoring range 0–60	• Construct, concurrent and discriminant validity demonstrated • Ability to detect differences in levels of pain • Sensitive to treatment effects	• Good to very good internal consistency • Almost perfect agreement in interrater reliability testing • Interrater reliability strong for both caregivers and qualified nurses • Strong intrarater reliability	• Long list of items • Simple instructions • 5-min estimated completion time • Preliminary cutoffs for pain presence suggested • Nurses and direct care providers report clinical usefulness	• Substantial psychometric support • Comprehensive in behavioral indicators • Factor analysis in English speaking samples with older adults in diverse settings is warranted • Cultural background and perceptions may affect interpretation of behavioral indicators **Languages:** • English primary • French [6] • Portuguese [85] • Japanese [95] • Dutch [108] **Settings:** • Nursing homes

(*continued*)

TABLE 10-3 Tool-Specific Information (continued)

Nonverbal Pain Behavior Scale	Description	Validity	Reliability	Feasibility and Clinical Utility	Languages and Settings	Summary
PACSLAC-D [109, 110, 112]	• Modified Dutch version of PACSLAC, direct observation scale with 24 items covering 3 subscales: facial and vocal expression ($n = 10$); resistance/defense ($n = 6$); and social-emotional aspects/mood ($n = 8$) • Rate present or absent • Scoring range 0–24	• Tool developed with factor analysis–guided refinement of original PACSLAC • Highly correlated with original PACSLAC • High degree of sensitivity and specificity using suggested cutoff scores	• Very good internal consistency for overall tool and subscales • Strong intrarater reliability for whole scale, moderate to strong for subscales	• Minimal training required (30 min) • Easy to use • Scoring instructions available to enhance interpretation	**Languages:** • Dutch only (translated to English, but no psychometrics to date) **Settings:** • Dutch nursing homes	• Larger, more diverse samples and settings needed to establish normative values • Further testing in larger English-speaking samples with increased diversity needed
PACSLAC 2 [12]	• Screening tool for both direct care providers and nurses. • 31 dichotomously scored items in 6 pain behavior categories: facial expressions ($n = 11$), verbalizations ($n = 5$), body	• Construct, convergent and discriminant established • Strong effect size • Accounts for unique variance even with contributions of all other tools, including PACSLAC	• Sufficient internal consistency sufficient • Moderate interrater reliability	• Clinical usefulness tested in Canadian nursing homes • Used by both direct care providers and nurses who report feasibility • Authors advise individualized scoring rather than population-based scoring	**Languages:** • English **Settings:** • Canadian nursing homes	• Promising preliminary testing • Easy-to-use, brief tool • Further testing to establish sensitivity to detect treatment effects needed

	movements (n = 11), changes in interpersonal interactions (n = 2), changes in activity patterns (n = 1), mental status changes (n = 1) • Scoring range 0–31			
Pain Assessment in Dementing Elders (PADE) [18, 57, 103]	24 items, 3 parts: • Part I—13 distinct observed behaviors (rating intensity on a semi-VDS scale); • Part II—proxy assessment of global pain intensity; and • Part III—chart review of 10 activities of daily living including dressing, feeding, transfers from wheelchair to bed (using 4 point Likert scale rating)	Construct validity: • As a whole, weakly differentiates between pain and no pain groups; improved differentiation with Part I only • Concurrent validity not yet established • Moderate correlation with agitation scale (all parts) and moderate correlation with other pain scales (Part I only) • Discriminant validity supported (Part I only)	• Variable internal consistency range through several studies • Fair/moderate (Part II) to moderate/strong (Parts I,III) interrater reliability • Low/moderate (Part II) to moderate/high (Parts I/III) test–retest reliability	• Long list of items with complex format and different scaling approaches within tool • Authors report 5–10 min to complete with practice • Administration instructions not clear • No score interpretation provided • Unknown training requirements	**Languages:** • English only **Settings:** • US nursing homes	• Addresses common pain behaviors and also incorporates aspects of pain assessment beyond direct observation • Further validation needed if entire tool is to be used, or refinement of those parts with low reliability • Feasibility and clinical utility issues remain uncertain
The Pain Assessment in Advanced Dementia Scale (PAINAD) [4, 18, 22, 24, 47, 48, 55–58, 62, 69, 76, 104]	• 5 categorical items: breathing, negative vocalizations, facial expression, body language, consolability • Scoring range 0–10 • 0–2 scale	• Convergent, concurrent validity established with other pain scales and self-report • Construct validity established with differences before and after pain interventions	• Sufficient internal consistency • Good to very good interrater reliability • Strong test–retest reliability	• Simple to use • Easy-to-follow definitions of terms provided • Scoring instructions provided • Cutoff of 3.5 for pain/no pain determined using ROC analysis	**Languages:** • English • German [88] • Chinese [56] • Spanish [31] • Dutch [108] • Italian [20] • Portuguese [7]	• "Breathing" item may need revision based on consistent problems across studies • Reliability and validity established

(continued)

TABLE 10-3 Tool-Specific Information (continued)

Nonverbal Pain Behavior Scale	Description	Validity	Reliability	Feasibility and Clinical Utility	Languages and Settings	Summary
		• Confirmatory factor analysis model with a good fit identified only when item "breathing" was removed • Factor analysis explained the variance of 61.09% of PAINAD scores in Portuguese version		• Time to complete 1–3 min • Limited training required • Tested in long-term care and acute care	**Settings:** • Acute care • Nursing home	• Further study of tool sensitivity needed to address identification of false positives
Pain Assessment in noncommunicative elderly persons (PAINE) [16–18]	• 22 items rated for the past week in 3 dimensions: repetitive physical movements, repetitive vocalizations, physical signs of pain, and changes in behaviors • Items are scored for frequency of occurrence on a scale of 1–7 • Summary score includes mean of moaning and rigidity ratings and count based on all other variables	• Concurrent validity with moderate to good correlations with other informant ratings • Low correlations with self-report and observational measures • Sensitive to treatment effects	• Sufficient internal consistency • Moderate interrater reliability • Test-retest sufficient after 1 wk	• Time to complete unknown • Scoring somewhat complex	**Languages:** • English only **Settings:** • Nursing homes	• Preliminary data support need for further evaluation with larger samples • Clinical usefulness undetermined • Testing with direct care providers is needed

Rotterdam Elderly Pain Observation Scale (REPOS) [100, 102]	• 10-item tool with dichotomously scored after a 2-min observation period • Items cover facial expression, emotional status, physical behavior, and vocalizations • Scoring range 0–10 • Total score of 3 or higher indicative of chronic pain	• Construct validity established with a good fit in one-dimensional multiple linear regression model • Convergent validity supported with one other pain scale • Observations made during movement • Sensitive to presence of pain in those with advanced dementia	• Moderate internal consistency • Strong interrater reliability • Moderate intrarater agreement	• Easy to use and score • Decision tree provided to assist with interpretation of score • Optimal cutoff score determined maintaining sufficient sensitivity and specificity • Encourages use of self-report in tandem with REPOS score	**Languages:** • Dutch, translated to English **Settings:** • Nursing homes in Netherlands	• Promising preliminary findings suggest validity, reliability, and clinical utility • Larger samples in diverse settings and cultures warranted for confirming normative values • Further testing to establish sensitivity to detect treatment effects needed

Source: Used with permission from K. Herr, PhD, RN, AGSF, FAAN, College of Nursing, The University of Iowa.

been made, many areas require further research. However, the state of the science on available tools must consider the developmental stage of tool evolution. Clinical utility is a key factor that drives acceptability and use of these tools. Less useful scales slowly disappear while better tools remain. Yet no available tool meets all required standards of psychometric soundness and generalizability across setting/populations. The goal of a common tool used across all countries and settings is not likely to be met, although it is clear from the summary in Table 10-2 that many tools are being translated and tested in different countries. The benefit of examining differences in pain experience and response across settings and countries would be advanced with valid tool translations and psychometric testing.

The proliferation of nonverbal pain tools reinforces the lack of a single acceptable standard tool, but also suggests there may be more benefit focusing on refinement of existing tools, rather than continued development of new tools unless they really open up new possibilities. This problem can be addressed by additional refinement that focuses on usability and establishing reliability and validity across populations and by future collaboration between experts in this multidisciplinary field of science. Within Europe, there is an action entitled, "Pain assessment in patients with impaired cognition, especially dementia." This European Cooperation in Science and Technology (COST) Action, enabled by the EU Research and Technological Development of the seventh Framework Program, brings together experts from a wide range of scientific disciplines to develop a comprehensive and internationally accepted assessment toolkit for older adults targeting various subtypes of dementia (http://www.cost-td1005.net.).

Further efforts are needed, and we will address some of the future challenges. To improve the value and clinical usefulness of behavioral tools, one of the first challenges will be to clarify what observational behavioral pain cues are most sensitive to pain for which persons. Challenging behavior displayed by persons with dementia, such as agitation, resistance, and screaming, are signals for possible existence of pain. However, these behaviors can also be caused by the dementia or by dementia-related anxiety or depression. There is an urgent need to better understand the complex relationship between pain and challenging behavior.

Currently, all tools are quite generic in terms of items used, and, in general, tools are developed to assess pain in the broad category of nonverbal older persons with dementia. However, persons with dementia are very heterogeneous in terms of neuropathology, type of dementia, cognitive and physical impairments, and severity of the dementia. At this point, though, our knowledge in differentiating pain indicators among these groups is in its infancy. Growth in this area will be crucial given findings regarding the impact of neuropathology on pain behaviors. For example, persons with Alzheimer dementia (AD) may report less pain while vascular dementia (VaD) persons may show enhanced pain responses [87]. In addition, pain behaviors may be dependent on dementia stages, as a very recent study by Kaasalainen and colleagues [50] showed that persons with intact verbal capacity displayed different behaviors compared to nonverbal dementia persons. However, the interrelatedness of neuropathology and dementia stages on pain behaviors is not fully known.

Nursing homes are the most common setting for conducting research on pain in dementia. The context always needs to be taken into consideration, but little research is available to guide assessment practices and decisions in settings other than nursing homes. There are differences between the assessment of pain in acute hospital care and in institutionalized long-term care facilities, not only in the type of pain experiences but also in terms of interpersonal professional relations between the staff and the person with dementia.

In-depth knowledge of the older adult and their needs is definitely an advantage when it comes to the assessment of pain in this nonverbal population. These contextual aspects are rarely addressed.

Another key area for the near future of pain research in dementia relates to the scoring methods and cutoffs of observational pain tools available to improve the interpretation of scores and enhance their value in evaluating pain. Most of the tools use a total score by summing up the individual items. Usually there is no weighting of items, and recent evidence regarding the sensitivity of facial items suggests attention to the importance of selected indicators is needed. On the other hand, certain specific behaviors are strongly related (e.g., grimacing and frowning). Hardly any of the scales have clear proven cutoff scores, something urgently needed in daily clinical practice to guide treatment decisions. Some of the more frequently used and more mature tools do report on (preliminary) cutoffs to enhance scoring interpretation, such as the PAINAD [111]. While studies predominantly focus on the presence of pain, recent literature suggests that behavioral tools may also be used to determine pain intensity in older persons with moderate–severe cognitive impairment [62]. The study of Lukas and colleagues [62] was the first to provide support for the use of observational pain assessment tools to help identify both the presence and also the intensity of pain. While others are more hesitant to link behavioral cues to pain intensity, research by Horgas and colleagues suggested that the total number of pain behaviors was significantly related to self-reported pain intensity in cognitively intact older people [37].

However, a gap remains in determining what level or score on an observational tool represents mild, moderate, or severe pain. Although more evidence is needed to support this possible linearity, having an observational tool that would be helpful in assessing pain intensity would be a step toward usability.

The feasibility of pain assessment in nonverbal older adults with dementia may be enhanced through innovative opportunities and possibilities. Many digital applications are currently being developed to ease the scoring of tools at the bedside. An example is the Abbey scale, now available as an application for Android and IPad. More advanced innovative systems based on behavioral facial expressions to monitor pain automatically are also being developed.

Last but not least, we emphasize that proper assessment and management of pain in older people with dementia using behavioral pain cues does require staff training—not only to help the staff become acquainted with tools available but also to discuss the potential barriers and their beliefs about pain in dementia. Because universal pain-specific cues do not exist, nurses and caregivers should know the person with dementia and their relatives in order to consult all possible resources that could reveal unique and individualized pain information. An approach in which the observational pain tool is only one aspect of an overall pain assessment process is the rule in the assessment and management of pain in dementia.

SUMMARY

The aim of this chapter was to present the current state of behavioral pain tools available to assess pain in people with dementia and to discuss challenges and possible future developments. Ongoing studies and innovative developments in pain research are likely to inform the selection of observational tools available for use in the near future.

REFERENCES

1. Abbey J, Piller N, De Bellis A, Esterman A, Parker D, Giles L, Lowcay B. The Abbey pain scale: a 1-minute numerical indicator for people with end-stage dementia. Int J Palliat Nurs 2004;10:6–13.
2. AGS Panel on Persistent Pain in Older Persons. The management of persistent pain in older persons. J Am Geriatri Soc 2002;50:S205–24.
3. Ando C, Hishinuma M. Development of the Japanese DOLOPLUS-2: a pain assessment scale for the elderly with Alzheimer's disease. Psychogeriatrics 2010;10:131–7.
4. Apinis C, Tousignant M, Arcand M, Tousignant-Laflamme Y. Can adding a standardized observational tool to interdisciplinary evaluation enhance the detection of pain in older adults with cognitive impairments? Pain Med 2013;15:32–41.
5. Araujo RS, Pereira LV. Brazilian version of the Non-communicative Patient's Pain Assessment Instrument (NOPPAIN): conceptual, item, and semantic equivalence [in Portuguese]. Cad Saude Publica 2012; 28:1985–92.
6. Aubin M, Verreault R, Savoie M, LeMay S, Hadjistavropoulos T, Fillion L, Beaulieu M, Viens C, Bergeron R, Vézina L, et al. Validity 'and Utilities' clinic of a grid observation (PACSLAC-F) to evaluate the pain in seniors with dementia's living in the long-term care [in French]. Can J Aging 2008;27:45–55.
7. Batalha LMC, et al. Cultural adaptation and psychometric properties of the Portuguese version of the Pain Assessment in Advanced Dementia Scale [Portuguese]. Revista Cientifica da Unidade de Investigacao em Ciencias da Saude: Dominio de Enfermagem 2012;8:7–10.
8. Bonin-Guillaume S, Rat P, Jouve E. A cut-off score of Algoplus (R) to assess pain in elderly patients visiting Emergency Room. J Am Geriatr Soc 2011;59:S174.
9. Cervo FA, Bruckenthal P, Chen JJ, Bright-Long LE, Fields S, Zhang G, Strongwater I. Pain assessment in nursing home residents with dementia: psychometric properties and clinical utility of the CNA Pain Assessment Tool (CPAT). J Am Med Dir Assoc 2009;10:505–10.
10. Cervo FA, Bruckenthal P, Fields S, Bright-Long LE, Chen JJ, Zhang G, Strongwater I. The role of the CNA Pain Assessment Tool (CPAT) in the pain management of nursing home residents with dementia. Geriatr Nurs 2012;33:430–8.
11. Cervo FA, Raggi RP, Bright-Long LE, Wright WK, Rows G, Torres AE, Levy RB, Komaroff E. Use of the certified nursing assistant pain assessment tool (CPAT) in nursing home residents with dementia. Am J Alzheimer's Dis Other Demen 2007;22:112–9.
12. Chan S, Hadjistavropoulos T, Williams J, Lints-Martindale A. Evidence-based development and initial validation of the pain assessment checklist for seniors with limited ability to communicate-II (PACSLAC-II). Clin J Pain 2014;30:816–24.
13. Chen YH, Lin LC, Watson R. Evaluation of the psychometric properties and the clinical feasibility of a Chinese version of the Doloplus-2 scale among cognitively impaired older people with communication difficulty. Int J Nurs Stud 2010;47:78–88.
14. Cheung G, Choi P. The use of the pain assessment checklist for seniors with limited ability to communicate (PACSLAC) by caregivers in dementia care. N Z Med J 2008;121:21–9.
15. Chibnall JT, Tait RC. Pain assessment in cognitively impaired and unimpaired older adults: a comparison of four scales. Pain 2001;92:173–86.
16. Cohen-Mansfield J. Pain assessment in noncommunicative elderly persons—PAINE. Clin J Pain 2006;22: 569–75.
17. Cohen-Mansfield J. The relationship between different pain assessments in dementia. Alzheimer Dis Assoc Disord 2008;22:86–93.
18. Cohen-Mansfield J, Lipson S. The utility of pain assessment for analgesic use in persons with dementia. Pain 2008;134:16–23.
19. Cohen-Mansfield J, Thein K, Marx MS, Dakheel-Ali M. What are the barriers to performing nonpharmacological interventions for behavioral symptoms in the nursing home? J Am Med Dir Assoc 2012;13:400–5.
20. Costardi D, Rozzini L, Costanzi C, Ghianda D, Franzoni S, Padovani A, Trabucchi M. The Italian version of the Pain Assessment in advanced dementia (PAINAD) scale. Arch Gerontol Geriatr 2007;44:175–80.
21. Dello Russo C, Di Giulio P, Brunelli C, Dimonte V, Villani D, Renga G, Toscani F. Validation of the Italian version of the Discomfort Scale—dementia of Alzheimer type. J Adv Nurs 2008;64:298–304.
22. DeWaters T, Popovich J, Faut-Callahan M. An evaluation of clinical tools to measure pain in older people with cognitive impairment. Br J Community Nurs 2003;8:226–34.
23. Eritz, H, Hadjistavropoulos T. Do informal caregivers consider nonverbal behavior when they assess pain in people with severe dementia? J Pain 2011;12:331–9.

24. Ersek M, Herr K, Neradilek MB, Buck HG, Black B. Comparing the psychometric properties of the Checklist of Nonverbal Pain Behaviors (CNPI) and the Pain Assessment in Advanced Dementia (PAIN-AD) instruments. Pain Med 2010;11:395–404.
25. Feldt KS. The checklist of nonverbal pain indicators (CNPI). Pain Manag Nurs 2000;1:13–21.
26. Ferrari R, Martini M, Mondini S, Novello C, Palomba D, Scacco C, Toffolon M, Valerio G, Vescovo G, Visentin M. Pain assessment in non-communicative patients: the Italian version of the Non-Communicative Patient's Pain Assessment Instrument (NOPPAIN). Aging Clin Exp Res 2009;21:298–306.
27. Folstein MF, Folstein SE, McHugh PR. "Mini-mental state". A practical method for grading the cognitive state of patients for the clinician. J Psychiatr Res 1975;12:189–98.
28. Fuchs-Lacelle S, Hadjistavropoulos T. Development and preliminary validation of the pain assessment checklist for seniors with limited ability to communicate (PACSLAC). Pain Manag Nurs 2004;5:37–49.
29. Fuchs-Lacelle S, Hadjistavropoulos H. Inter-rater reliability and additional psychometric information on the pain assessment checklist for seniors with limited ability to communicate (PACSLAC). Seattle: IASP Press; 2005.
30. Fuchs-Lacelle S, Hadjistavropoulos T, Lix L. Pain assessment as intervention: a study of older adults with severe dementia. Clin J Pain 2008;24:697–707.
31. García-Soler Á, Sánchez-Iglesias I, Buiza C, Alaba J, Navarro AB, Arriola E, Zulaica A, Vaca R, Hernández C. Adaptation and validation of the Spanish version of the Pain Evaluation Scale in patients with advanced dementia: PAINAD-Sp [in Spanish]. Rev Esp Geriatr Gerontol 2014;49:10–4.
32. Hadjistavropoulos T, Voyer P, Sharpe D, Verreault R, Aubin M. Assessing pain in dementia patients with comorbid delirium and/or depression. Pain Manag Nurs 2008;9:48–54.
33. Herr K, Bjoro K, Decker S. Tools for assessment of pain in nonverbal older adults with dementia: a state-of-the-science review. J Pain Symptom Manag 2006;31:170–92.
34. Holen JC, Saltvedt I, Fayers PM, Bjørnnes M, Stenseth G, Hval B, Filbet M, Loge JH, Kaasa S. The Norwegian Doloplus-2, a tool for behavioural pain assessment: translation and pilot-validation in nursing home patients with cognitive impairment. Palliat Med 2005;19:411–7.
35. Holen JC, Saltvedt I, Fayers PM, Hjermstad MJ, Loge JH, Kaasa S. Doloplus-2, a valid tool for behavioural pain assessment? BMC Geriatr 2007;7:29.
36. Hoogendoorn LI, Kamp S, Mahomed CA, Adèr HJ, Ooms ME, van der Steen JT. The role of observer for the reliability of Dutch version of the Discomfort Scale-Dementia of Alzheimer Type (DS-DAT) [in Dutch]. Tijdschr Gerontol Geriatr 2001;32:117–21.
37. Horgas AL, Elliott AF, Marsiske M. Pain assessment in persons with dementia: relationship between self-report and behavioral observation. J Am Geriatr Soc 2009;57:126–32.
38. Horgas AL, Nichols AL, Schapson CA, Vietes K. Assessing pain in persons with dementia: relationships among the non-communicative patient's pain assessment instrument, self-report, and behavioral observations. Pain Manag Nurs 2007;8:77–85.
39. Hurley AC, Volicer L. Evaluation of pain in cognitively impaired individuals. J Am Geriatr Soc 2001;49:1397–8.
40. Hurley AC, Volicer BJ, Hanrahan PA, Houde S, Volicer L. Assessment of discomfort in advanced Alzheimer patients. Res Nurs Health 1992;15:369–77.
41. Husebo B, Achterberg WP, Lobbezoo F, Kunz M, Lautenbacher S, Kappesser J, Tudose C, Strand LI. Pain in patients with dementia: a review of pain assessment and teatment challenges. Nor Epidemiol 2012;22:243–51.
42. Husebo BS, Strand LI, Moe-Nilssen R, Borgehusebo S, Aarsland D, Ljunggren AE. Who suffers most? Dementia and pain in nursing home patients: a cross-sectional study. J Am Med Dir Assoc 2008;9:427–33.
43. Husebo BS, Strand LI, Moe-Nilssen R, Husebo SB, Ljunggren AE. Pain behaviour and pain intensity in older persons with severe dementia: reliability of the MOBID Pain Scale by video uptake. Scand J Caring Sci 2009;23:180–9.
44. Husebo BS, Strand LI, Moe-Nilssen R, Husebo SB, Ljunggren AE. Pain in older persons with severe dementia. Psychometric properties of the Mobilization-Observation-Behaviour-Intensity-Dementia (MOBID-2) Pain Scale in a clinical setting. Scand J Caring Sci 2010;24:380–91.
45. Husebo BS, Strand LI, Moe-Nilssen R, Husebo SB, Snow AL, Ljunggren AE. Mobilization-Observation-Behavior-Intensity-Dementia Pain Scale (MOBID): development and validation of a nurse-administered pain assessment tool for use in dementia. J Pain Symptom Manag 2007;34:67–80.
46. Jones KR, Fink R, Hutt E, Vojir C, Pepper GA, Scott-Cawiezell J, Mellis BK. Measuring pain intensity in nursing home residents. J Pain Symptom Manag 2005;30:519–27.
47. Jordan A, Hughes J, Pakresi M, Hepburn S, O'Brien JT. The utility of PAINAD in assessing pain in a UK population with severe dementia. Int J Geriatr Psychiatry 2011;26:118–26.

48. Jordan A, Regnard C, O'Brien JT, Hughes JC. Pain and distress in advanced dementia: choosing the right tools for the job. Palliat Med 2012;26:873–8.
49. Kaasalainen S, Crook J. An exploration of seniors' ability to report pain. Clin Nurs Res 2004;13:199–215.
50. Kaasalainen S, Akhtar-Danesh N, Hadjistavropoulos T, Zwakhalen S, Verreault R. A comparison between behavioral and verbal report pain assessment tools for use with residents in long term care. Pain Manag Nurs 2013;14:e106–14.
51. Kaasalainen S, Stewart N, Middleton J, Knezacek S, Hartley T, Ife C, Robinson L. Development and evaluation of the Pain Assessment in the Communicatively Impaired (PACI) tool: part I. Int J Palliat Nurs 2011;17:387–91.
52. Kaasalainen S, Stewart N, Middleton J, Knezacek S, Hartley T, Ife C, Robinson L. Development and evaluation of the Pain Assessment in the Communicatively Impaired (PACI) tool: part II. Int J Palliat Nurs 2011;17:431–8.
53. Kunz M, Scharmann S, Hemmeter U, Schepelmann K, Lautenbacher S. The facial expression of pain in patients with dementia. Pain 2007;133:221–8.
54. Lefebre-Chapiro L, Doloplus C. The Doloplus 2 scale—valuating pain in the elderly. Eur J Palliat Care 2001;8:191–4.
55. Leong IY, Chong MS, Gibson SJ. The use of a self-reported pain measure, a nurse-reported pain measure and the PAINAD in nursing home residents with moderate and severe dementia: a validation study. Age Ageing 2006;35:252–6.
56. Lin PC, Lin LC, Shyu YI, Hua MS. Chinese version of the Pain Assessment in Advanced Dementia Scale: initial psychometric evaluation. J Adv Nurs 2010;66:2360–8.
57. Lints-Martindale AC, Hadjistavropoulos T, Lix LM, Thorpe L. A comparative investigation of observational pain assessment tools for older adults with dementia. Clin J Pain 2012;28:226–37.
58. Liu JY, Briggs M, Closs SJ. The psychometric qualities of four observational pain tools (OPTs) for the assessment of pain in elderly people with osteoarthritic pain. J Pain Symptom Manag 2010;40:582–98.
59. Liu JY, Pang PC, Lo SK. Development and implementation of an observational pain assessment protocol in a nursing home. J Clin Nurs 2012;21:1789–93.
60. Lobbezoo F, Weijenberg RA, Scherder EJ. Topical review: orofacial pain in dementia patients. A diagnostic challenge. J Orofac Pain 2011;25:6–14.
61. Lord B. Paramedic assessment of pain in the cognitively impaired adult patient. BMC Emerg Med 2009;9:20.
62. Lukas A, Barber JB, Johnson P, Gibson SJ. Observer-rated pain assessment instruments improve both the detection of pain and the evaluation of pain intensity in people with dementia. Eur J Pain 2013;17:1558–68.
63. Mahoney AE, Peters L. The Mahoney Pain Scale: examining pain and agitation in advanced dementia. Am J Alzheimer's Dis Other Demen 2008;23:250–61.
64. Manias E, Gibson SJ, Finch S. Testing an educational nursing intervention for pain assessment and management in older people. Pain Med 2011;12:1199–215.
65. McGuire DB, Reifsnyder J, Soeken K, Kaiser KS, Yeager KA. Assessing pain in nonresponsive hospice patients: development and preliminary testing of the multidimensional objective pain assessment tool (MOPAT). J Palliat Med 2011;14:287–92.
66. Miller J, Neelon V, Dalton J, Ng'andu N, Bailey D Jr, Layman E, Hosfeld A. The assessment of discomfort in elderly confused patients: a preliminary study. J Neurosci Nurs 1996;28:175–82.
67. Monacelli F, Vasile Nurse A, Odetti P, Traverso N. Doloplus-2 pain assessment: an effective tool in patients over 85 years with advanced dementia and persistent pain. Clin Ter 2013;164:E23–5.
68. Morello R, Jean A, Alix M, Sellin-Peres D, Fermanian J. A scale to measure pain in non-verbally communicating older patients: the EPCA-2 Study of its psychometric properties. Pain 2007;133:87–98.
69. Mosele M, Inelmen EM, Toffanello ED, Girardi A, Coin A, Sergi G, Manzato E. Psychometric properties of the pain assessment in advanced dementia scale compared to self assessment of pain in elderly patients. Demen Geriatr Cogn Disord 2012;34: 38–43.
70. Neville C, Ostini R. A psychometric evaluation of three pain rating scales for people with moderate to severe dementia. Pain Manag Nurs 2014;15:798–806.
71. Nygaard HA, Jarland M. The Checklist of Nonverbal Pain Indicators (CNPI): testing of reliability and validity in Norwegian nursing homes. Age Ageing 2006;35: 79–81.
72. Pannerden SCVT, Candel MJ, Zwakhalen SM, Hamers JP, Curfs LM, Berger MP. An item response theory-based assessment of the Pain Assessment Checklist for Seniors with Limited Ability to Communicate (PACSLAC). J Pain 2009;10:844–53.
73. Paoletti F, Moretto G, Sossi V, Raunikar A, Bello M, Garavelli E, De Vuono C. Valutazione del dolore in soggetti anziani con deterioramento cognitivo: indagine di prevalenza attraverso l'utilizzo della scala Doloplus-2. [Pain

evaluation in nursing home patients with cognitive impairment who don't respond to self-report scales: a cross sectional study using Doloplus-2 scale.] Riv L'Infermiere 2013;3.

74. Park J, Castellanos-Brown K, Belcher J. A review of observational pain scales in nonverbal elderly with cognitive impairments. Res Soc Work Pract 2010;20:651–64.
75. Pasman HR, Onwuteaka-Philipsen BD, Kriegsman DM, Ooms ME, Ribbe MW, van der Wal G. Discomfort in nursing home patients with severe dementia in whom artificial nutrition and hydration is forgone. Arch Intern Med 2005;165:1729–35.
76. Paulson-Conger M, Leske J, Maidl C, Hanson A, Dziadulewicz L. Comparison of two pain assessment tools in nonverbal critical care patients. Pain Manag Nurs 2011;12:218–24.
77. Pautex S, Herrmann F, Le Lous P, Fabjan M, Michel JP, Gold G. Feasibility and reliability of four pain self-assessment scales and correlation with an observational rating scale in hospitalized elderly demented patients. J Gerontol Ser A Biol Sci Med Sci 2005;60:524–9.
78. Pautex S, Herrmann FR, Le Lous P, Gold G. Improving pain management in elderly patients with dementia: validation of the Doloshort observational pain assessment scale. Age Ageing 2009;38:754–7.
79. Pautex S, Herrmann FR, Michon A, Giannakopoulos P, Gold G. Psychometric properties of the Doloplus-2 observational pain assessment scale and comparison to self-assessment in hospitalized elderly. Clin J Pain 2007;23:774–9.
80. Pickering G, Gibson SJ, Serbouti S, Odetti P, Ferraz Gonçalves J, Gambassi G, Guarda H, Hamers JP, Lussier D, Monacelli F, et al. Reliability study in five languages of the translation of the pain behavioural scale Doloplus (R). Eur J Pain 2010;14:545.e1–10.
81. Pickering ME, Bunna P, Rat P, Madeline G, Lebost C, Serrie A, Pereira B. Acute pain evaluation with Algoplus (R) Scale in Cambodian patients. Pain Med 2013;14:1971–6.
82. Pieper MJ, Achterberg WP, Francke AL, van der Steen JT, Scherder EJ, Kovach CR. The implementation of the serial trial intervention for pain and challenging behaviour in advanced dementia patients (STA OP!): a clustered randomized controlled trial. BMC Geriatr 2011;11:12.
83. Rat P, Jouve E, Pickering G, Donnarel L, Nguyen L, Michel M, Capriz-Ribière F, Lefebvre-Chapiro S, Gauquelin F, Bonin-Guillaume S. Validation of an acute pain-behavior scale for older persons with inability to communicate verbally: Algoplus (R). Eur J Pain 2011;15:198.e1–10.
84. Regnard C, Reynolds J, Watson B, Matthews D, Gibson L, Clarke C. Understanding distress in people with severe communication difficulties: developing and assessing the Disability Distress Assessment Tool (DisDAT). J Intellect Disabil Res 2007;51:277–92.
85. Santos R, Castro-Caldas A, Hadjistavropoulos T. Adaptação Cultural e Validação Da Pain Assessment Checklist for Seniors with Limited Ability to Communicate (PACSLAC). Para a População Portuguesa 2012;20:5–10.
86. Scherder EJ, Bouma A. Visual analogue scales for pain assessment in Alzheimer's disease. Gerontology 2000;46:47–53.
87. Scherder EJ, Sergeant JA, Swaab DF. Pain processing in dementia and its relation to neuropathology. Lancet Neurol 2003;2:677–86.
88. Schuler MS, Becker S, Kaspar R, Nikolaus T, Kruse A, Basler HD. Psychometric properties of the German "Pain Assessment in Advanced Dementia Scale" (PAINAD-G) in nursing home residents. J Am Med Dir Assoc 2007;8:388–95.
89. Sheu E, Versloot J, Nader R, Kerr D, Craig KD. Pain in the elderly: validity of facial expression components of observational measures. Clin J Pain 2011;27:593–601.
90. Snow AL, Weber JB, O'Malley KJ, Cody M, Beck C, Bruera E, Ashton C, Kunik ME. NOPPAIN: a nursing assistant-administered pain assessment instrument for use in dementia. Demen Geriatr Cogn Disord 2004;17:240–6.
91. Stevenson KM, Brown RL, Dahl JL, Ward SE, Brown MS. The Discomfort Behavior Scale: a measure of discomfort in the cognitively impaired based on the Minimum Data Set 2.0. Res Nurs Health 2006;29:576–87.
92. Stolee P, Hillier LM, Esbaugh J, Bol N, McKellar L, Gauthier N. Instruments for the assessment of pain in older persons with cognitive impairment. J Am Geriatr Soc 2005;53:319–26.
93. Storti M. The validation of a pain assessment scale for patients with cognitive impairment: the Italian version of Abbey's scale [in Italian]. Recenti Prog Med 2009;100:405–9.
94. Takai Y, Yamamoto-Mitani N, Chiba Y, Nishikawa Y, Hayashi K, Sugai Y. Abbey Pain Scale: development and validation of the Japanese version. Geriatr Gerontol Int 2010;10:145–53.
95. Takai Y, Yamamoto-Mitani N, Chiba Y, Nishikawa Y, Sugai Y, Hayashi K. Prevalence of pain among residents in Japanese nursing homes: a descriptive study. Pain Manag Nurs 2013;14:e1–9.

96. Takai Y, Yamamoto-Mitani N, Okamoto Y, Koyama K, Honda A. Literature review of pain prevalence among older residents of nursing homes. Pain Manag Nurs 2010;11:209–23.
97. Torvik, K., Kaasa S, Kirkevold Ø, Saltvedt I, Hølen JC, Fayers P, Rustøen T. Validation of Doloplus-2 among nonverbal nursing home patients—an evaluation of Doloplus-2 in a clinical setting. BMC Geriatr 2010;10:9.
98. Tsai PF, Beck C, Richards KC, Phillips L, Roberson PK, Evans J. The Pain Behaviors for Osteoarthritis Instrument for Cognitively Impaired Elders (PBOICIE). Res Gerontol Nurs 2008;1:116–22.
99. Van Der Steen JT, Pasman HR, Ribbe MW, Van Der Wal G, Onwuteaka-Philipsen BD. Discomfort in dementia patients dying from pneumonia and its relief by antibiotics. Scand J Infect Dis 2009;41:143–51.
100. van Herk R, Boerlage AA, Baar FP, Tibboel D, de Wit R, van Dijk M. Evaluation of a pilot project for implementation of REPOS in daily practice. J Pain Symptom Manag 2009;1:357–65.
101. van Herk R, van Dijk M, Baar FP, Tibboel D, de Wit R. Observation scales for pain assessment in older adults with cognitive impairments or communication difficulties. Nurs Res 2007;56:34–43.
102. van Herk R, van Dijk M, Tibboel D, Baar F, de Wit R. The Rotterdam Elderly Pain Observation Scale (REPOS): a new behavioral pain scale for non-communicative adults and cognitively impaired elderly persons. J Pain Manag 2009;1:367–78.
103. Villanueva MR, Smith TL, Erickson JS, Lee AC, Singer CM. Pain Assessment for the Dementing Elderly (PADE): reliability and validity of a new measure. J Am Med Dir Assoc 2003;4:1–8.
104. Warden V, Hurley AC, Volicer L. Development and psychometric evaluation of the Pain Assessment in Advanced Dementia (PAINAD) scale. J Am Med Dir Assoc 2003;4:9–15.
105. Wary B, Doloplus C. Doloplus-2, a scale for pain measurement [in French]. Soins Gerontol 1999;19:25–7.
106. Young DM, Pain in institutionalized elders with chronic dementia. Iowa City: University of Iowa; 2001.
107. Zwakhalen SM, van't Hof CE, Hamers JP. Systematic pain assessment using an observational scale in nursing home residents with dementia: exploring feasibility and applied interventions. J Clin Nurs 2012;21:3009–17.
108. Zwakhalen SM, Hamers JP, Abu-Saad HH, Berger MP. Pain in elderly people with severe dementia: a systematic review of behavioural pain assessment tools. BMC Geriatr 2006;6:3.
109. Zwakhalen SM, Hamers JP, Berger MP. Improving the clinical usefulness of a behavioural pain scale for older people with dementia. J Adv Nurs 2007;58:493–502.
110. Zwakhalen SM, Hamers JP, Berger MP. The psychometric quality and clinical usefulness of three pain assessment tools for elderly people with dementia. Pain 2006;126:210–20.
111. Zwakhalen SM, van der Steen JT, Najim MD. Which score most likely represents pain on the observational PAINAD pain scale for patients with dementia? J Am Med Dir Assoc 2012;13:384–9.
112. Zwakhalen SM, Koopmans RT, Geels PJ, Berger MP, Hamers JP. The prevalence of pain in nursing home residents with dementia measured using an observational pain scale. European journal of pain 2009;13:89–93.

CHAPTER 11

Behavioral Approaches and Psychophysics

Miriam Kunz and Stefan Lautenbacher

The chapter will give an overview of the behavioral assessment of pain in dementia with a specific focus on facial activity beyond the use of observational scales. Especially for research purposes, it is important to study possible dementia-related alterations in the pain system by psychophysical procedures. Appropriate procedures and their results will also be reviewed.

BEHAVIORAL RESPONSES TO PAIN

For practical reasons, pain is often considered to be what the individual says it is, at least in cognitively unimpaired individuals. However, in patients with dementia—whose ability to provide self-report is often critically diminished—the presence of pain becomes dependent on the decision of observers/health-care professionals/caregivers. Such a decision is most often based on the patients' nonverbal behavior, like body postures, facial expressions, and paralinguistic vocalizations. However, then the question arises of whether these behavioral responses are specific and distinct enough to always correctly inform about the internal state of the patient. In the last decades, several studies have been conducted that aimed at answering this question by trying to objectively assess, analyze, and describe behavioral responses to pain using specialized tools (e.g., the Facial Action Coding System; FACS [8]). Although most of these specialized tools may not be suitable for pain assessment in routine clinical settings, they do allow for an objective and valid characterization of behavioral pain responses. The crucial need for such objective and valid characterizations of behavioral pain responses becomes evident when looking at the variability of items that are used as pain-indicative behaviors in the various observational scales for assessing pain in patients with dementia. For example, items for pain-indicative facial responses range from "looking blank" (DOLOPLUS 2 [36]) to "grimacing" (Mobilization-Observation-Behavior-Intensity-Dementia; MOBID-2 [19]) to "anxious look on the face" (Elderly Pain Caring Assessment 2; ECPA-2 [41]), three descriptions which are quite different. Accordingly, no agreement on the specific contents of the facial expression of pain has been reached. So, how do nonverbal responses to pain really look like? The aim of this chapter is to answer this question. To do this, this chapter will review empirical findings on behavioral responses to pain (of healthy individuals as well as of patients with dementia) that were assessed using objective and reliable tools for behavioral assessment, in order to get a clearer picture of how nonverbal responses to pain can best be described and whether they are changed in the course of dementia.

Facial Responses to Pain

Among the three categories of nonverbal behavioral responses to pain, namely facial expressions, vocalizations, and body movements, the *facial expression* of pain has been studied most extensively. Especially in the last two decades a considerable number of studies have been conducted that tried to analyze how the face of pain looks like and which bio–psycho–social factors modulate the way we facially express pain. The main reason why research on pain behavior has mostly focused on facial expressions of pain is that they are readily accessible, highly sensitive and are believed to be the most specific pain behavior in humans [53]. Therefore, it is not surprising that facial expressions are typically included in behavioral pain assessment tools developed for patients with dementia—although the items used to describe the supposed pain-indicative facial responses vary substantially between tools [17, 55] (see also Chapter 10).

Which Methods Can be Used to Analyze Facial Responses?

One of the first instruments developed for the assessment of nonverbal behavior is the FACS, which focuses exclusively on facial expressions [8]. Nearly all studies so far that have investigated facial responses to pain in healthy individuals as well as in patients with dementia used the FACS. The FACS is based on the anatomical analysis of visible facial movements which are categorized as Action Units (AUs). The FACS lists 44 different AUs; each AU being based on discrete movements of specific muscles or, in a few patients, on groups of muscles of the face. FACS analyses of facial expressions are not carried out in real time but instead the videotaped facial expressions are coded in slow-motion and stop-frame feedback. Certificated FACS coders, who undergo an approximately 100- to 200-hour training [8], identify which AUs are displayed, their on- and offset, and their intensity during specified time intervals. Not only is the sufficient FACS training rather long but also the FACS coding itself is very time consuming, thus making FACS analyses difficult to use in clinical settings. For research purposes, however, the FACS has enabled us to better describe and understand facial responses occurring during the experience of pain.

Although the FACS is considered the gold standard when analyzing facial expressions of pain (as well as of other affective states), FACS analyses have one methodological shortcoming, namely that they only measure clearly visible movements of the face and consequently, very subtle facial expressions might be missed. In order to definitely assess such very subtle facial activity, the use of a sufficiently amplified electromyogram (*EMG*) is necessary. However, so far, very few studies have used facial EMG to assess facial responses to pain [39, 54] because only a limited number of facial muscles can be assessed simultaneously, which makes it difficult to monitor all facial key activities for pain in parallel. Since EMG electrodes have to be attached to the skin of the face for that purpose, a placement of not more than three or four electrodes is advisable because otherwise electrodes would become too obtrusive and would interfere with the facial expression [18]. Moreover, the ability to isolate the activity of a single facial muscle is much poorer when using surface EMG (due to EMG crosstalk among neighboring muscles) compared to FACS analyses [18]. Altogether, when investigating how the facial expression of pain looks like and which muscle groups are involved in the expression, facial EMG is less useful compared to FACS analyses.

Besides FACS and EMG analyses, new developments in visual computer techniques have rendered the possibility of developing *automated recognition systems* for facial expressions of pain. Several attempts in this direction have been made [2, 16]. However, the development is still at its beginning and not ready to be used in clinical or most research contexts. The most important shortcoming so far has been that most attempts to validate automatic recognition systems for facial pain displays have used video material with posed facial expressions that depict "caricatures" of pain expressions that lack naturally occurring variations; in other words, only intensified pain-prototypical facial expressions have been used to feed the machine learning algorithms. However, it is crucial that such a system is capable to detect pain despite the occurrence of the wide variations in natural facial expressions.

In summary: Which methods can be used to analyze facial responses? The Facial Action Coding system (FACS) is still the gold standard to objectively and reliably assess facial responses to pain, although FACS coding is very time consuming, and thus not practical for clinical settings. Although still in the developmental phase, new progresses in computer vision systems and machine learning seem very promising and might render an automatic analyzes of facial responses to pain possible in the next decades. Such systems would be of special interest for pain detection in patients with dementia given that they would allow a constant monitoring of potential pain-indicative facial expressions.

How do Facial Expressions of Pain Look Like?

Using the FACS to analyze facial responses occurring in the context of pain, facial activity during pain is not unspecific grimacing but seems to convey pain specific information [11, 53]. Evidence for this can be mainly taken from two sources. First, despite some variability, there seems to be a subset of facial movements that repeatedly occur across different types of pain (ranging from different types of experimental pain-induction procedures to clinical pain [44, 45]) as well as across individuals (male/female [25]; young/old [28]). This subset includes as the most prominent facial movements tightening of the muscles surrounding the eyes (AU6_7), furrowed brows (AU4), raising the upper lip/nose wrinkling (AU9_10), and eye closure (AU43) [44, 45]. Images of these facial movements are displayed in Fig. 11-1 (upper four rows). The combination of these facial movements is often referred to as the "prototypical facial expression of pain." Evidence for the existence of pain-specific facial expressions is also provided by the observation that—when actors are taught to display this subset of "pain-prototypical" facial movements—observers can recognize pain among other emotions above chance level [49].

It is, however, important to keep in mind that—although these key facial movements reliably occur during pain—this does not imply only one uniform facial expression of pain that can be observed at all time and in each individual [7]. Instead, the frequencies of occurrence of the single key movements during pain usually range only from 10% to 60% [23, 26]. Therefore, the likelihood that all four key facial movements occur simultaneously or in other words the likelihood that an individual experiencing pain displays the complete "prototypical expression of pain" is very low. Rather, individuals often display only parts of this subset, sometimes even blending it with a limited range of other facial movements (e.g., smiling [15, 30, 31]). We could recently show that it might be more helpful to

A		**Furrowed brows (AU4)**
		- part of the prototypical expression of pain -
B		**Tightening of the muscles surrounding the eyes (AU6 7)** (most prominent facial response to pain)
		- part of the prototypical expression of pain -
C		**Raising the upper lip/nose wrinkling (AU9 10)**
		- part of the prototypical expression of pain -
D		**Eye closure (AU43)**
		- part of the prototypical expression of pain -
E		**Opening the mouth (AU25 26 27)** (very frequent facial response to pain in patients with dementia)

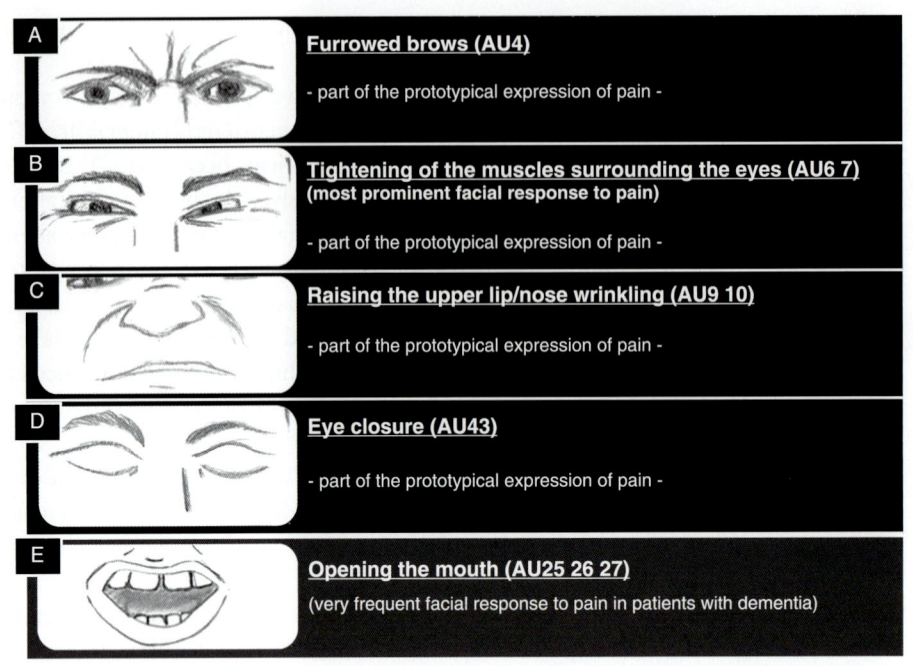

FIGURE 11-1 Pain-indicative facial movements: Shown are those facial movements that are frequently displayed in the context of experimental as well as clinical pain conditions. Facial responses to pain have mostly been analyzed using the facial action coding system (FACS) which categorizes facial responses in different Action Units (AUs). Each picture illustrates a single AU. **A–D:** Depicts those AUs that have been shown to be the key facial activities reliably occurring during pain ("prototypical facial expressions of pain"). In addition, **(E)** depicts an AU that is often found to be pain indicate for patients with dementia.

differentiate between at least three *different facial activity patterns of pain* that are displayed in the context of pain and which are composed of different combinations of facial movements [26]. These were tightening of the muscles surrounding the eyes with furrowed brows and wrinkled nose (pattern I; combination of A + B + C of Fig. 11-1); furrowed brows with tightening of the muscles surrounding the eyes (pattern II; combination of A + B of Fig 11-1), and opened mouth with tightening of the muscles surrounding the eyes (pattern III; combination of B + D of Fig. 11-1). These different facial activity patterns all have one facial movement in common, namely the tightening of the muscles surrounding the eyes (AU 6_7). This facial movement is indeed the most frequent, and thus possibly the most important movement occurring during pain [7]. Moreover, the tightening of the muscles surrounding the eyes is also the one facial movement that helps to differentiate the very similar facial expressions of pain and disgust, which is crucial for clinical practice since facial expressions of pain and of disgust are very frequently mistaken for each other [29]. Last but not least, when describing how facial responses to pain look like, it is also important to mention that a considerable percentage of individuals (approximately 15–25%) do not show any visible facial responses during the experience of pain at all in the laboratory, although they do report moderate to even strong pain intensities [26]. This is important to keep in mind when judging pain based on facial expressions, because this indicates that individuals might be experiencing pain, although they do not show any pain-related facial activity and that a "stoic face" is thus not necessarily incompatible with the experience of pain [7, 26]!

In summary: How do facial expressions of pain look like? There is a subset of facial actions that are frequently displayed in the context of pain and these pain-indicative facial actions are shown in Fig. 11-1. These single facial movements are rather seldom displayed simultaneously when individuals are experiencing pain, but instead individuals most often show different combinations of these single facial movements. Most frequently, tightening of the muscles surrounding the eyes is paired with one or two of these other pain-indicative facial movements. However, it is also possible that no visible facial expression is displayed, even though an individual is experiencing pain.

Are Facial Expressions of Pain "Hardwired" or a Learned Behavior?

Given that dementia is associated with a decline in cognitive capacities, it is important to understand to which degree facial expressions of pain are "hardwired" or a learned behavior. If they are mostly a learned behavior, the possibility that facial expressions of pain are affected by the dementia-related cognitive decline seems more likely. Based on empirical findings, it is acknowledged that facial responses to pain are a mixture of biological dispositions as well as of social learning [11]. As for their biological dispositions, infants (including neonates) [7] and congenitally blind individuals [24] display similar patterns of facial movements in response to pain as sighted adults do (see also Fig. 11-1 for a list of the most frequent pain-indicative facial movements). These findings clearly suggest that the basis of the facial expressions of pain is indeed "hardwired." This is an important conclusion especially when considering facial expressions of pain in patients with dementia. Given that the capacity to facially express pain appears mainly inborn, it seems unlikely that patients with dementia unlearn how to facially express pain across the course of cognitive decline, at least in its early phases. Therefore, facial responses to pain might remain unaltered in patients with dementia and can be used as a valid diagnostic indicator of pain. We will further discuss this topic later on (see section on dementia-related changes in facial responses).

Despite facial expressions of pain having been shown to be strongly "hardwired," it is also acknowledged that facial responses become modifiable across early and late childhood through social learning experiences [11]. One very important modification regards the degree to which we express pain via our face. Whereas young children tend to show vigorous facial expressions of pain, older children and adults seem to have learned to effectively downregulate their facial expressions of pain [35]. In line with this finding, a recent functional imaging study could show that a low degree of facial expressiveness to pain was associated with higher activation in frontostriatal structures [23]. Given that these frontostriatal structures are known to be involved in motor inhibition, this finding suggests that low-expressive individuals actively suppress their facial expression of pain [23]. When trying to interpret these findings, it has been argued that individuals learn to suppress the facial display of negative affect (including pain) following culturally/socially learned "display rules." These display rules represent social norms about when, where, and how one should express affective states [9] and are learned already at a young age. Based on this theory, facially responding to pain would be the "default" that individuals learn to suppress due to social/cultural demands (e.g., "big boys don't cry," "one mustn't be oversensitive to pain"). In accordance with this theory, it has been demonstrated in previous studies that social learning and the social context do indeed influence the degree of facial expressiveness to pain. The presence of others can reduce (e.g., when being together with a stranger) as well as increase (when being together with a loved one) the amount of pain-indicative facial responses depending on the nature of the relationship between interactants [21, 50]. Furthermore, it has also been shown that the degree of facial expressions due to pain can be effectively modulated by operant learning, with facial responses increasing or decreasing dependent on the contingency of reinforcement [32].

In summary: Are facial expressions of pain "hardwired" or a learned behavior? The basic algorithms of facial expressions of pain (determining which facial movements are displayed in the context of pain) seem to be "hardwired". This is a crucial prerequisite in order to reliably communicate one's affective state across developmental stages, ranging from neonatal stages up to older age, as well as largely independent of one's cognitive status. The degree to which we communicate pain via our face, however, seems to be also affected by social learning, with individuals mainly learning to downregulate their facial expressions of pain when inappropriate.

Are Facial Expressions of Pain Changed in Patients with Dementia?

So far, only a few studies have investigated facial responses to pain in patients with dementia [12–14, 27, 33, 37, 42]. Facial responses during experimental pain induction (pressure and electrical stimulation [27, 33, 37], flu injections [12], venipuncture [13, 42], and exacerbation of chronic musculoskeletal pain during physical exercise [14]) were videotaped and later analyzed using the FACS [7]. Although these studies differed immensely with regard to the way of pain induction, the findings are surprisingly homogeneous. First of all, it was consistently found that facial responses to increasing pain intensified in patients with dementia [27, 33, 37]. This means that facial expressions still encode the intensity of pain in patients with dementia. Moreover, even patients who were verbally compromised still facially displayed pain properly [27, 33, 42]. Furthermore, these facial expressions were composed of the same types of facial movements as can be found in elderly individuals without dementia in response to pain [33]. There is only one facial action that was displayed much more frequently in patients with dementia, namely the opening of the mouth (AU25_26_27) [33]. Given its high frequency of occurrence in patients with dementia we also included this facial movement in Fig. 11-1 (last row). Although opening of the mouth is not listed among the prototypical facial movements occurring during pain, this facial movement has nevertheless been frequently reported in the context of pain even in cognitively unimpaired individuals [7]. Thus, opening of the mouth is not an atypical facial response to pain, but this facial response seems to be especially pain-indicative in patients with dementia.

The similarity in types of facial movements being displayed by patients with dementia and healthy controls is illustrated in Fig. 11-2. Here, examples of facial expressions are shown that were displayed in response to painful pressure stimulation. When comparing these expressions to the pain-indicative facial responses shown in Fig. 11-1, it should become evident that the "pain typicality" of facial expressions of pain is not reduced in patients with dementia.

These findings are very promising, given that they clearly suggest that the face seems to specifically encode the experience of pain and that this specific encoding does not change in the course of dementia. Considering the degree of specific facial expressiveness during pain, facial responses in patients with dementia seem to be augmented compared to responses in cognitively unimpaired controls [14, 27, 33, 42]. So far, one can only speculate why patients with dementia show an increased facial expressiveness in response to pain. One reason might be that the increase in facial responses indicates an intensified processing

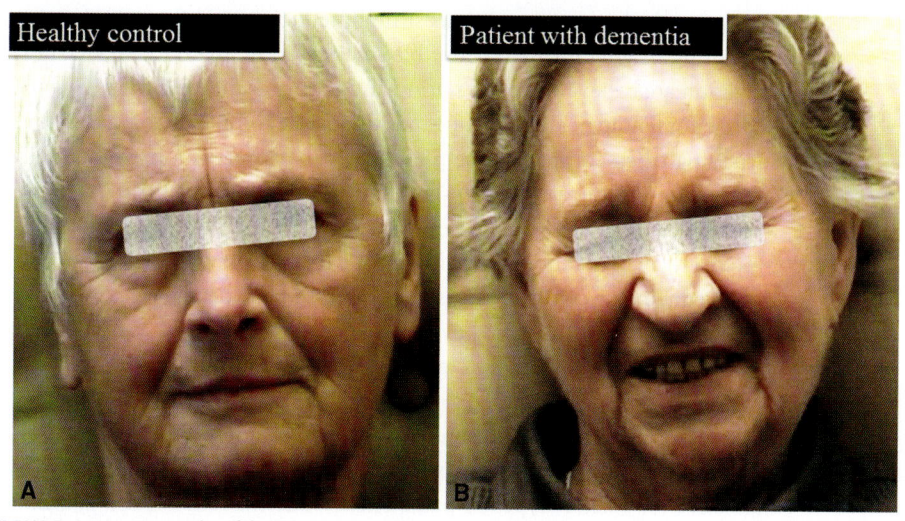

FIGURE 11-2 Example of facial responses to a 5-kg pressure stimulus in healthy individuals and in patients with dementia.

of noxious stimulation in demented patients. This perspective was also supported by recent imaging studies on cerebral responses to noxious stimulation in patients with dementia (see Chapter 5 on brain imaging and pain in patients with dementia). The intensified pain responses might in turn be due to the decline in capacity to anticipate pain and cope with pain. These changes may have physiological and psychological components.

Moreover, it may also be that the increase in facial expressiveness has nothing to do with pain itself but instead facial responses to noxious stimulation are increased simply because the cognitive ability in demented patients to control the impulse to facially display their inner state is impaired. As discussed above, we mainly learn in the course of childhood to inhibit the facial display of negative affective states, such as pain, owing to certain display rules, and this ability to suppress facial responses to pain might be impaired in patients with dementia.

In summary: Are facial expressions of pain changed in patients with dementia? Patients with dementia display the same types of facial movements in response to pain. Thus, the pain typicality of their facial expression is not reduced. This implicates that facial expressions of pain have the potential to serve as an alternative pain indicator in patients with dementia, even in patients with compromised self-report. Over a series of studies, the facial expression of pain in patients with dementia has appeared to be rather enhanced than reduced, suggesting no dampening of nociception and pain processing.

Body Movements

Although it is unquestionable that the experience of pain is typically accompanied by body movements, little research has been conducted so far that aimed at classifying or describing body movements accompanying pain. Reasons for the lack of research might stem from the complexity and variability of bodily movements and the lack of instruments to objectively assess them. Interestingly, within the group of nonverbal behavioral responses to pain, body movements are believed to have as primary function the control of pain [43, 53]. For example, rubbing or holding the affected body part seem to mainly serve the purpose of protecting the body from noxious stimuli, reducing pain through counterstimulation, and promoting healing through better blood circulation. In contrast, facial expression and vocalization are believed to have a primary communicative function. Given these differences, the phenomenological variability and functional complexity of body movements seem less surprising when comparing them to those behavioral responses that mainly serve as facial codes for communicative purpose. Because body movements do not mainly serve communicative purposes, they do not need to be as recognizable and distinct as facial expressions. Moreover, given that body areas being affected can vary immensely, body movements aiming at reducing or controlling the pain can also be expected to vary immensely. Because of this diversity, several authors have tried to characterize body movements that are indicative only for a specific type of pain (e.g., lung cancer pain [52], back pain [22], rheumatoid arthritis [40]) instead of looking for universal body movements of pain.

Nevertheless, despite this enormous diversity, there seem to be some body movements that have repeatedly been observed across different types of pain and that might be pain indicative for various types of pain. These body movements are guarding (protecting affected area, holding body part, avoiding touch, moving away), bracing (a stiff and static position), and rubbing the painful area [34]. The question is whether these three descriptors of body movements are also pain indicative for patients with dementia. Many researchers believe so, given that "guarding," "bracing," and "rubbing" are included in most of the observational scales for pain assessment in patients with dementia [17, 55]. Nevertheless, some authors have issued the concern that these body movements might be less indicative in frail elderly patients with dementia [51]. Indeed, elderly patients with dementia may have difficulties in moving or may show stiffness for other reasons, for example, due to arthritis or due to Parkinson's disease. Therefore, such changes in body movements might under certain circumstances be completely unrelated to pain per se. This might mean that pain is wrongly diagnosed, even though the patient is pain-free (and is "only" functionally impaired) or—as the opposite problem—that pain is overlooked because health-care professionals interpret these changes in body movement simply as further age-related impairments [51].

In summary: How do pain-indicative bodily movements look like in patients with dementia? Body movements occurring during the experience of pain can be extremely variable and are thus more difficult to be recognized as indications of pain compared to the pain-related facial expressions. Given this variability, it seems advisable to not look for body movements that seem to be pain indicative for every type of pain but instead to focus on body movements that are indicative for pain in specific body areas and due to specific sources. It seems especially important to keep this in mind in patients with dementia because the bodily movements associated with pain might be less specific and distinct in this group of patients. First attempts have recently been made in this direction, for example by trying to assess which body movements might be indicative for orofacial pain in patients with dementia [38].

Vocalization

So far, very little is known about changes in paralinguistic vocalization occurring during pain. Although it is acknowledged that pain experiences are accompanied by nonverbal vocalizations and although vocalization items—such as crying, shouting, groaning—are included in nearly all observational scales for pain assessment in patients with dementia

[17, 55], studies are lacking that have tried to investigate these pain-indicative vocalizations using specialized tools. Using voice analysis tools, the following parameters should be assessed in order to better characterize pain-indicative vocalizations: frequency, voice intensity, formants, and voice quality as well as temporal characteristics [48].

Conclusions about Bahavioral Responses to Pain

Although most pain assessment tools for patients with dementia include items describing pain-indicative facial expressions, body movements, and vocalizations [17, 55] (see also Chapter 10), surprisingly little is known about how these pain-indicative nonverbal responses really look like and whether they are changed in patients with dementia. So far, research has mainly focused on facial expressions of pain. Here, some key facial movements have been described that occur frequently in the context of pain and that can also be found in patients with dementia. Thus, patients with dementia seem to communicate pain via their facial expressions as validly and distinctively as cognitively unimpaired individuals do. Interestingly, patients with dementia tend to display more pain via their face compared to healthy controls, either due to an intensification of nociceptive processing or due to a lack of inhibitory mechanisms that control the degree of facial displays. With regard to body movements and vocalizations occurring during the experience of pain, objective and reliable descriptors—especially for patients with dementia—are lacking so far and are urgently needed.

PSYCHOPHYSICS

Besides better understanding of how dementia affects the behavioral indicators of pain, it is also important to investigate how the transmission in the pain system might be altered during the course of dementia. In order to do this, the transmission properties of the pain system should be assessed—among others—by use of psychophysical procedures. So far, several studies have tried to do this by assessing changes in pain thresholds, pain tolerance, pain reflexes, and supra-threshold responses to experimental pain in patients with dementia (mostly with patients with Alzheimer's disease). Psychophysical protocols have the advantage to give fairly complete control of the relationship between noxious stimulus and subjective response, which allows separating the noxious stimulus from the assessed pain response. An overview of the available psychophysical methods for pain assessment is given by Arendt-Nielsen and Lautenbacher [1].

When assessing pain thresholds—here, the individual has to indicate at which physical intensity level a stimulus feels to be barely painful—in patients with dementia and in healthy controls, most studies found no differences in threshold levels between the two groups [3, 4, 10, 20, 37]. Likewise, patients with dementia were also found to rate supra-threshold pain intensities (with stimuli lying above the pain threshold) as equally painful compared to controls [5, 20, 27, 30]. When investigating pain tolerance—here, the individual has to indicate at which physical intensity level further increases feel unbearably painful and would not be tolerated—the findings were more contradictory, with evidence for increased [3], decreased, and unchanged tolerance levels in patients with dementia [20]. An interesting approach has been chosen by Jensen-Dahm et al. [20], who not only reported on the changes in pain psychophysics in patients with dementia but also in parallel on the psychometric quality of their data. Their findings clearly suggest that the pain threshold, pain tolerance, and supra-threshold pain ratings were as reliable in patients with mild degrees of dementia as they were in healthy controls. Thus, we can conclude that the sensitivity to low and moderate noxious stimuli seems unchanged in patients with dementia, whereas it remains unclear how pain tolerance is affected.

Some authors have argued that it might be more appropriate to assess pain responses which are independent of the patients' ability to give a self-report of pain, given the deterioration of cognitive abilities in dementia [32]. Such a response is the nociceptive flexion reflex (NFR; also name RIII-reflex), a polysynaptic reflex allowing for noxious electrical stimuli eliciting an intensity-related withdrawal response. The NFR threshold has been shown to be strongly correlated with the subjective pain threshold (at least in cognitively unimpaired individuals) (for a review see [47]); thus, it is believed to have the potential to serve as a psychophysical-like assessment tool based on nociceptive behavior. Typical parameters are the reflex threshold and the reflex amplitude as well as latency evoked by supra-threshold stimulus intensities. The NFR reflex has been assessed in one study, and it was found that its threshold was significantly decreased in dementia which might point to an increase in nociceptive processing, at least at the spinal level [27]. Another type of evoked responses that is independent of the patients' ability to give a self-report of pain are autonomic responses (e.g., heart rate, skin conductance). Studies showed a decline in autonomic responsiveness in patients with dementia [27, 46]. However, given that it is known that dementia is accompanied by dysfunctions of the autonomic system—even at the earliest stages of dementia [6]—the autonomic response might not be a valid pain indicator in this patient group. With regard to stimulus-related brain responses to pain in patients with dementia, the Chapters 3 and 5 might be of special interest for the reader. Just in short, brain responses to painful stimulation seem either unchanged (when assessing evoked potentials) or even increased (when using functional imaging) in patients with Alzheimer's disease.

Conclusions about Pain Psychophysics

In conclusion, although the psychophysical findings on pain processing in patients with dementia are partially contradictory, most findings seem to suggest that the processing of pain is not diminished in patients with mild to moderate forms of dementia (mostly patients with Alzheimer's disease). When interpreting these findings, one has to keep in mind, however, that these findings are based on patients with only mild to moderate degrees of cognitive impairments, which allow for adhering to verbal instructions and providing self-report of pain. This ability declines strongly in moderate to severe stages of dementia. We therefore do not know whether or how psychophysical pain parameters might be altered in later stages of the disease. Due to methodological and ethical considerations, however, it is difficult to apply psychophysical protocols including the necessary induction of experimental pain in these severe stages of dementia.

As regards recommendations for future studies, research on pain processing in patients with dementia should not solely rely on self-report ratings, especially when investigating patients in later stages of the disease, but use instead multimethod approaches, trying to assess pain in parallel via subjective, behavioral, neural, and autonomic responses.

REFERENCES

1. Arendt-Nielsen L, Lautenbacher S. Assessment of pain perception. In: Lautenbacher S, Fillingim RB, editors. Pathophysiology of pain perception. New York: Kluwer Academic/Plenum Publishers; 2004. p. 25–42.
2. Bartlett MS, Littlewort GC, Frank MG, Lee K. Automatic decoding of facial movements reveals deceptive pain expressions. Curr Biol 2014;24:738–43.
3. Benedetti F, Arduino C, Vighetti S, Asteggiano G, Tarenzi L, Rainero I. Pain reactivity in Alzheimer patients with different degrees of cognitive impairment and brain electrical activity deterioration. Pain 2004;111:22–9.
4. Benedetti F, Vighetti S, Ricco C, Lagna E, Bergamasco B, Pinessi L, Rainero I. Pain threshold and tolerance in Alzheimer's disease. Pain 1999;80:377–82.
5. Cole LJ, Farrell MJ, Duff EP, Barber JB, Egan GF, Gibson SJ. Pain sensitivity and fMRI pain-related brain activity in Alzheimer's disease. Brain 2006;129:2957–65.
6. Collins O, Dillon S, Finucane C, Lawlor B, Kenny RA. Parasympathetic autonomic dysfunction is common in mild cognitive impairment. Neurobiol Aging 2012;33:2324–33.
7. Craig KD, Prkachin KM, Grunau RVE. The facial expression of pain. In Turk DC, Melzack R, editors. Handbook of pain assessment, 3rd edition. New York: Guilford; 2011. p. 117–33.
8. Ekman PE, Friesen WV. Facial action coding system. Palo Alto, CA: Consulting Psychologists Press; 1978.
9. Ekman PE, Sorenson ER, Friesen WV. Pan-cultural elements in facial displays of emotions. Science 1969;164:86–8.
10. Gibson SJ, Voukelatos X, Ames D, Flicker L, Helme RD. An examination of pain perception and cerebral event-related potentials following carbon dioxide laser stimulation in patients with Alzheimer's disease and age-matched control volunteers. Pain Res Manag 2001;6:126–32.
11. Hadjistavropoulos T, Craig KD, Duck S, Cano A, Goubert L, Jackson PL, Mogil JS, Rainville P, Sullivan MJ, de C Williams AC, et al. A biopsychosocial formulation of pain communication. Psychol Bull 2011;137:910–939.
12. Hadjistavropoulos T, Craig KD, Martin N, Hadjistavropoulos H, McMurtry B. Toward a research outcome measure of pain in frail elderly in chronic care. Pain Clin 1997;10:71–9.
13. Hadjistavropoulos T, LaChapelle D, MacLeod F, Hale C, O'Rourke N, Craig KD. Cognitive functioning and pain reactions in hospitalized elders. Pain Res Manag 1998;3:145–51.
14. Hadjistavropoulos T, LaChapelle DL, MacLeod FK, Snider B, Craig KD. Measuring movement-exacerbated pain in cognitively impaired frail elders. Clin J Pain 2000;16:54–63.
15. Hale C, Hadjistavropoulos T. Emotional components of pain. Pain Res Manag 1997;2:217–25.
16. Hammal Z, Kunz M, Arguin M, Gosselin F. Spontaneous pain expression recognition in video sequences. Proceedings of BCS International Academic Conference—Visions Comp Science; 2008. p. 191–210.
17. Herr K, Bjoro K, Decker S. Tools for assessment of pain in nonverbal older adults with dementia: a state-of-the-science review. J Pain Symptom Manag 2006;31:170–92.
18. Hess U. Facial EMG. In Harmon-Jones E, Beer JS, editors. Methods in social neuroscience. New York, NY: Guilford Press; 2009. p. 70–91.
19. Husebo BS, Strand LI, Moe-Nilssen R, Husebo SB, Ljunggren AE. Pain in older persons with severe dementia. Psychometric properties of the Mobilization-Observation-Behaviour-Intensity-Dementia (MOBID-2) Pain Scale in a clinical setting. Scand J Caring Sci 2010;24:380–91.
20. Jensen-Dahm C, Werner MU, Dahl JB, Jensen TS, Ballegaard M, Hejl AM, Waldemar G. Quantitative sensory testing and pain tolerance in patients with mild to moderate Alzheimer's disease compared to healthy control. Pain 2014;155:1439–45.
21. Karmann AJ, Lautenbacher S, Bauer F, Kunz M. The influence of communicative relations on facial responses to pain: does it matter who is watching? Pain Res Manag 2014;19:15–22.
22. Keefe FJ, Block AR. Development of an observation method for assessing pain behavior in low back pain patients. Behav Ther 1982;13:363–76.
23. Kunz M, Chen JI, Lautenbacher S, Vachon-Presseau E, Rainville P. Cerebral regulation of facial expressions of pain. J Neurosci 2011;31:8730–38.
24. Kunz M, Faltermeir N, Lautenbacher S. Impact of visual learning on facial expressions of physical distress: a study on voluntary and evoked expressions of pain in congenitally blind and sighted individuals. Biol Psychol 2012;89:467–76.
25. Kunz M, Gruber A, Lautenbacher S. Sex differences in facial encoding of pain. J Pain 2006;7:915–28.
26. Kunz M, Lautenbacher S. The faces of pain: a cluster analysis of individual differences in facial activity patterns of pain. Eur J Pain 2014;18:813–23.
27. Kunz M, Mylius V, Scharmann S, Schepelman K, Lautenbacher S. Influence of dementia on multiple components of pain. Eur J Pain 2008;13:317–25.

28. Kunz M, Mylius V, Schepelmann K, Lautenbacher S. Impact of age on the facial expression of pain. J Psychos Res 2008;64:311–8.
29. Kunz M, Peter J, Huster S, Lautenbacher S. Pain and disgust: the facial signaling of two aversive bodily experiences. PLoS One 2013;8:e83277
30. Kunz M, Prkachin K, Lautenbacher S. The smile of pain. Pain 2009;145:273–5.
31. Kunz M, Prkachin K, Lautenbacher S. Smiling in pain: explorations of its social motives. Pain Res Treatment 2013;2013:128093.
32. Kunz M, Rainville P, Lautenbacher S. Operant conditioning of facial displays of pain. Psychosom Med 2011;73:422–431.
33. Kunz M, Scharmann S, Hemmeter U, Schepelmann K, Lautenbacher S. The facial expression of pain in patients with dementia. Pain 2007;133:221–18.
34. Labus JS, Keefe FJ, Jensen MP. Self-reports of pain intensity and direct observations of pain behavior: when are they correlated? Pain 2003;102:109–124.
35. Larochette AC, Chambers CT, Craig KD. Genuine, suppressed and faked facial expressions of pain in children. Pain 2006;126:64–71.
36. Lefebvre-Chapiro S. The Doloplus 2 scale—evaluating pain in the elderly. Eur J Palliat Care 2001;8:191–194.
37. Lints-Martindale A, Hadjistavropoulos T, Barber B, Gibson S. A psychophysical investigation of the facial action coding system as an index of pain variability among older adults with and without Alzheimer's disease. Pain Med 2007;8:678–89.
38. Lobbezoo F, Weijenberg RAF, Scherder EJA. Topical review: orofacial pain in dementia patients. A diagnostic challenge. J Orofac Pain 2011;25:6–14.
39. Mailhot J-P, Vachon-Presseau E, Jackson PL, Rainville P. Dispositional empathy modulates vicarious effects of dynamic pain expressions on spinal nociception, facial responses and acute pain. Eur J Neurosci 2012;35:271–8.
40. McDaniel LK, Anderson KO, Bradley LA, Young LD, Turner RA, Agudelo CA, Keefe FJ. Development of an observation method for assessing pain behavior in rheumatoid arthritis patients. Pain 1986;24:165–84.
41. Morello R, Jean A, Alix M, Sellin-Peres D, Fermanian J. A scale to measure pain in non-verbally communicating older patients: the EPCA-2 study of its psychometric properties. Pain 2007;133:87–98.
42. Porter FL, Malhotra KM, Wolf CM, Morris JC, Miller JP, Smith MC. Dementia and response to pain in the elderly. Pain 1996;68:413–21.
43. Prkachin KM. Pain behavior is not unitary. Behav Brain Sci 1986;9:754–755.
44. Prkachin KM. The consistency of facial expressions of pain: a comparison across modalities. Pain 1992;51:297–306.
45. Prkachin KM, Solomon PE. The structure, reliability and validity of pain expression: evidence from patients with shoulder pain. Pain 2008;139:267–74.
46. Rainero I, Vighetti S, Bergamasco B, Pinessi L, Benedetti F. Autonomic responses and pain perception in Alzheimers's disease. Eur J Pain 2000;4:267–74.
47. Sandrini G, Serrao M, Rossi P, Romaniello A, Cruccu G, Willer JC. The lower limb flexion reflex in humans. Prog Neurobiol 2005;77:353–95.
48. Scherer KR, Johnstone T, Klasmeyer G. Vocal expression of emotion. In Davidson R, Scherer KR, GoldsmithH, editors. Handbook of the affective sciences. New York: Oxford University Press. 2003. p 433–56.
49. Simon D, Craig KD, Gosselin F, Belin P, Rainville P. Recognition and discrimination of prototypical dynamic expressions of pain and emotions. Pain 2008;135:55–64.
50. Vervoort T, Goubert L, Eccleston C, Verhoeven K, De Clerq A, Buysse A, Crombez G. The effects of parental presence upon the facial expression of pain: The moderating role of child catastrophizing. Pain 2008;138:277–285.
51. Weiner D, Peterson B, Keefe F. Chronic pain-associated behaviors in the nursing home: resident versus caregiver perceptions. Pain 1999;80:577–88.
52. Wilkie DJ, Keefe FJ, Dodd MJ, Copp LA. Behavior of patients with lung cancer: description and associations with oncologic and pain variables. Pain 1992;51:231–240.
53. Williams AC. Facial expression of pain: an evolutionary account. Behav Brain Sci 2002;25:439–55.
54. Wolf K, Mass R, Kiefer F, Naber D, Wiedemann K. The face of pain—a pilot study to validate the measurement of facial pain expression with an improved electromyogram method. Pain Res Manag 2005;10:15–19.
55. Zwakhalen SM, Hamers JP, Abu-Saad HH, Berger MP. Pain in elderly people with severe dementia: a systematic review of behavioural pain assessment tools. BMC Geriatr 2006;6:3.

CHAPTER 12

Assessment of Specific Forms of Pain in Dementia: Orofacial Pain

Frank Lobbezoo, Suzanne Delwel, and Roxane A. F. Weijenberg

P ain is not a uniform phenomenon, but can take many clinical forms. For example, the assessment of neuropathic pain differs considerably from that of cancer pain or orofacial pain. This is even more challenging when dealing with pain in dementia. Using orofacial pain as an example, this chapter will stress the need to assess specific forms of pain, and not only pain in general. In addition, orofacial pain will be used to exemplify the requirements, which have to be met when specific forms of pain are to be assessed.

OROFACIAL PAIN

According to the *Guidelines for assessment, diagnosis, and management of orofacial pain* of the American Academy of Orofacial Pain (AAOP), orofacial pain refers to pain that is associated with the hard and soft tissues of the mouth and face [7]. The guidelines describe orofacial pain as a debilitating and prevalent condition. A large-scale study in the United States showed that about 22% of the general population suffered from one or more types of orofacial pain in the previous 6 months [26]. The most commonly reported orofacial pain in that survey was dentoalveolar pain (tooth ache; 12.2%), followed by pain in the temporomandibular joint (5.3%) and face/cheek pain (1.4%). Orofacial pain can be a symptom of many conditions, like headaches; neurogenic, musculoskeletal, and psychophysiological pathologies; cancer, infection, and autoimmune phenomena; and tissue trauma [7]. The International Association for the Study of Pain (IASP) has proclaimed 2014 as the Global Year against Orofacial Pain. Within that framework, concise but informative fact sheets have been produced describing the characteristics of eight common orofacial pain conditions, viz, neurovascular orofacial pain, persistent dentoalveolar pain disorder, odontogenic/dental pain, burning mouth syndrome, temporomandibular disorders (TMDs), persistent idiopathic facial pain, glossopharyngeal neuralgia, and trigeminal neuralgia [19]. Clearly, with such a wide range of orofacial pain conditions, the etiology must be multifaceted and multifactorial as well. In addition, orofacial pain may have multiple consequences for the patient, most notably socioeconomic ones with a large impact on (oral health-related) quality of life. Finally, the prevention, diagnosis, and treatment of orofacial pain conditions are in the hands of many specialists, among which oral hygienists, general dentists, and physicians as well as several dental specialists (e.g., orofacial pain specialists, oral surgeons), nurses, medical specialists (e.g., neurologists, anesthesiologists), and physiotherapists. It is outside the scope of this chapter to describe these issues in detail. Please refer to De Leeuw and Klasser [7] for more information.

Orofacial Pain in Healthy Older Persons

While a lot is known about the prevalence of orofacial pain in the general population, there is a striking lack of data describing the epidemiological characteristics of orofacial pain in older persons. The few studies that do report on this issue suggest a high prevalence. Lester et al. [25] studied several aspects of dental status in a group of frail and functionally dependent persons of 60 years of age and older, almost half of whom were living in long-stay residential facilities while the others resided in sheltered or private housing. The authors reported that 22% of the examined individuals suffered from oral pain over the four previous weeks—a figure that is similar to the general adult population prevalence of orofacial pain reported by Lipton et al. [26]. An even higher percentage of 37.2% of oral or facial pain in the previous 4 weeks was reported by Locker [28], who studied oral disorders in independent, community-dwelling persons of 50 years and over. A recent large-scale longitudinal population study by Ekbäck et al. [9] focused on pain related to the musculoskeletal structures of the masticatory system (TMD pain) in elderly people, over a 20-year period. About 8% of the examined older individuals reported some TMD pain, and about 2% of the 50- to 70-year-old individuals even reported rather great or severe TMD-related pain, which suggests that a not-negligible part of this age group might need proper treatment for their TMD pain. The total percentage of self-reported TMD-related pain in this group of older persons is similar to the approximately 10% that is reported for TMD pain in the general adult population [24]. Taking all evidence together, orofacial pain in older persons, either community-dwelling or institutionalized, seems a rather prevalent condition, a considerable part of which may be TMD-related.

Orofacial Pain in Older Persons with Dementia

Worldwide, about 35.6 million people suffer from dementia, and this percentage is on the rise [1]. Aging is the largest risk factor for dementia (10–35% of persons 85 years and older suffer from dementia, while only 1% of those between 60 and 65 years of age are afflicted [21]). Other risk factors are illiteracy, low educational level, low socialeconomic status, inactive lifestyle, head trauma, genetic predisposition (e.g., the presence of the apolipoprotein-E4 allele), cardiovascular factors (e.g., hypertension), overweight, diabetes mellitus, smoking, and even loss of teeth (for a review on the latter, see [48]). Pain is a common finding in older persons with dementia. For example, Maxwell et al. [29] reported that up to about 80% of older home care clients suffer from current daily pain. However, others reported lower percentages, but this may very well be due to an underreporting or an underdetection of pain in this largely nonverbal population, which in turn can lead to an undertreatment of the painful conditions [6, 13, 35]. Indeed, even when older persons with dementia suffer from the same painful conditions as do older persons without dementia (e.g., postoperative pain after hip fracture surgery), they are being prescribed less analgesics [30, 33, 37]. Whether or not pain pathways are actually altered due to the pathology associated with several types of dementia, is still under debate, although there is some evidence suggesting that pain centers in the medial pain system (involved in the emotional rather than sensory evaluation of pain) are degenerated in Alzheimer's disease [4, 41]. On the other hand, central neuropathic pain, due to white matter lesions which are commonly seen in vascular dementia and mixed type dementia, is very likely both present and untreated in older persons with dementia [39]. In other words, pain is a common condition in older persons with dementia, while the pain modulation capacities in dementia may be affected due to the condition's pathology [40].

It is tempting to extrapolate the current knowledge on pain in older persons with dementia, as outlined above, to the various aspects of orofacial pain in this population. However, there is a striking lack of studies on issues like the epidemiological characteristics of orofacial pain in older persons with dementia. Although the case-control design that was used in the study by de Souza Rolim et al. [8] does not allow strong conclusions to be drawn on the prevalence of orofacial pain in older persons with Alzheimer's Disease (AD), orofacial pain was observed in 20.7% of the 29 examined AD individuals—a percentage that resembles the ones reported by Lipton et al. [26] and Lester et al. [25]. This finding suggests that orofacial pain needs to be considered when caring for older persons with dementia. Importantly, professional caregivers as well as family members of these persons consider being free from orofacial pain the number one outcome for the long-term oral care [20]. It is therefore an unfortunate fact that as yet, there is no specific instrument available for the assessment of orofacial pain in nonverbal individuals [27]. However, since there have been some recent studies in this area, *the first aim* of this chapter is to describe the efforts undertaken so far to develop such specific tool for orofacial pain assessment in older persons with dementia.

Many orofacial pain conditions, notably TMD pain, affect the masticatory process. Especially in frail older persons with dementia, impaired chewing may lead to malnutrition, which in turn may yield poorer physical health and decreased activity. Such decrease in bodily functionality hampers the consumption of energy, thus reducing appetite, and thereby setting up a vicious cycle (for a review, see [27]). This cycle needs to be interrupted, the more so because impaired mastication seems to be detrimental for many cognitive functions as well [48]. Hence, *the second aim* of this chapter is to provide an overview of the relationship between mastication and cognition in older persons without and with a dementia.

ASSESSMENT OF OROFACIAL PAIN IN DEMENTIA

Assessment of Pain in Older Persons with Dementia

In otherwise healthy individuals, self-report scales like verbal descriptor scales, 0–10 numerical rating scales, and 100-mm visual analog scales are considered a first step in the assessment of pain, while in persons with mild to moderate cognitive impairments, pain thermometers and faces pain scales are commonly recommended, depending on the abilities of the individual [35, 38, 50]. In individuals with a more advanced stage of dementia, however, the ability to communicate is frequently lost. Further, these individuals often lack insight into their condition. Consequently, most persons with a dementia are not able to provide the clinician with relevant information about their pain. Hence, other approaches are needed to increase caregivers' awareness and to assess pain in this group.

A commonly used approach to the assessment of pain in nonverbal individuals is the observation of specific behaviors that could be associated with the presence of pain. Apart from a painful condition being present or absent, the clinician would also be interested in determining the intensity of the observed pain, as well as its location. The ideal observational pain assessment tool would enable the determination of all pain characteristics. However, not only is pain a subjective and highly complex condition, in dementia there is also a substantial overlap between pain-related behavior and dementia-related behavior, which prevents the development of the ideal tool [15, 16]. Nevertheless, many observational pain tools have been developed over the years for use in nonverbal individuals, of which the strengths and limitations as well as the psychometric properties have been reviewed extensively by Smith [42] and Herr et al. [11] (for an updated review, see http://prc.coh.org/pain-noa.htm). From those reviews, it can be concluded that despite all efforts, no tool is currently available that can be recommended for widespread application. It is therefore an important development that an international multidisciplinary consortium, supported by the European Cooperation in Science and Technology (COST Action TD-1005 Pain Assessment in Patients with Impaired Cognition, especially Dementia; www.cost-td1005.net), has set off in 2011 to develop an observational tool that would meet the characteristics of the ideal tool as closely as possible. The roadmap toward the development of the Pain Assessment in Impaired Cognition (PAIC) tool is described extensively in Corbett et al. [5].

Assessment of Orofacial Pain in Older Persons with Dementia

The PAIC tool [5] will be the core of a comprehensive toolkit that will include additional instruments for the assessment of, among others, specific pain conditions like back pain and orofacial pain. The challenge of assessing orofacial pain in older persons with dementia was already recognized in the comprehensive review on this topic by Lobbezoo et al. [27]. The authors performed a literature search in PubMed (viz, [orofacial pain OR dental pain OR TMD] AND dementia) as to identify all scientific articles that were published on orofacial pain and dementia. Their search yielded 44 applicable papers, which were supplemented with another 30 papers from the authors' personal collections and the reference lists of the selected papers. Surprisingly, even though orofacial pain is highly prevalent in older persons with dementia, no specific tool for its assessment could be identified. Therefore, the authors decided to scrutinize all eight observational pain assessment tools that had appeared in their search for their possible qualities to assess orofacial pain [2, 3, 10, 12, 14, 17, 18, 22, 23, 44].

The orofacial aspects in the eight identified tools are shown in Table 12-1. In half of the identified tools, viz, the Assessment of Discomfort in Dementia (ADD) [22, 23], the Certified Nursing Assistant (CNA) Pain Assessment Tool (CPAT) [2], the Doloplus 2 [12], and the Mobilization-Observation-Behavior-Intensity-Dementia (MOBID) [17, 18], no orofacial aspects were included, apart from an item regarding decreased appetite in the ADD [22, 23], which could be indicative of, but is not specific for, orofacial pain. The MOBID did contain an orofacial pain item in the initial testing phase of the tool, viz, the observation of teeth/mouth care. Unfortunately, since this item seemed to assess dementia-related behaviors, such as surprise and confusion, rather than pain-related behaviors, the item was removed from the instrument. Three of the eight identified instruments included observations of orofacial behavior, namely "a slack or unclenched jaw" (Discomfort Scale—Dementia of Alzheimer Type (DS-DAT; [14]), tooth clenching and opening the mouth (Pain Assessment Checklist for Seniors with Limited Ability to Communicate (PACSLAC); [10]), and "the jaw may be clenched" (Pain Assessment in Advanced Dementia (PAINAD); [44]). Although these observations do relate to the orofacial area, they cannot be considered specific behaviors characterizing orofacial pain. Only with one of the eight identified tools,

TABLE 12-1 Orofacial Aspects of the Observational Pain Assessment Tools Which Were Identified in the Literature Search by Lobbezoo et al. [27]

Pain Aassessment Tool	Orofacial Aspects	Remarks
ADD: Assessment of Discomfort in Dementia [22, 23]	None	None
C-PAT: Certified Nursing Assistant—Pain Assessment Tool [2]	None	None
DS-DAT: Discomfort Scale for Dementia of the Alzheimer Type [14]	Observation of "a slack unclenched jaw"	Observation not specific for orofacial pain being absent
Doloplus 2 [12]	None	None
MOBID: Mobilization-Observation-Intensity-Dementia Pain Scale [17, 18]	None	In the process of the development of the MOBID, observation of teeth/mouth care was removed from the instrument [18]
OHAT: Oral Health Assessment Tool [3]	Dental pain identified as follows: Score 1: verbal or behavioral signs of pain such as pulling a face, chewing lips, not eating, aggression. Score 2: same as score 1, *plus* physical pain signs (swelling of cheek or gum, broken teeth, ulcers)	While the reliability was found to be substantial, the validity of this tool is reason for concern
PACSLAC: Pain Assessment Checklist for Seniors with Limited Ability to Communicate [10]	Observations of tooth clenching and opening the mouth	Observations not specific for orofacial pain being present
PAINAD: Pain Assessment in Advanced Dementia Scale [44]	Observation of "the jaw may be clenched"	Observation not specific for orofacial pain being present

the Oral Health Assessment Tool (OHAT) [3], the presence of dental pain was established on the basis of both orofacial behavioral observations and specific intraoral findings. Unfortunately, even though the OHAT had a substantial reliability, the validity was insufficient. Hence, this tool cannot be recommended for the assessment of dental pain in older persons with dementia.

Lobbezoo et al. [27] conclude that there is a striking lack of literature on the assessment of orofacial pain in older persons with dementia, let alone that specific tools are available that can be recommended as reliable and valid instruments for such assessments. From their review, the authors did gather some suggestions as to how to compose an observational tool for the assessment of orofacial pain. The suggested orofacial pain indicators are summarized in Table 12-2. As an additional requirement, the authors indicated that the instrument should be easy to use in the elderly care clinic.

TABLE 12-2 Suggested Orofacial Pain Indicators to Be Included in a Specific Observational Tool for the Assessment of Orofacial Pain [27]

Orofacial Pain Indicator
The patient holds or rubs his or her orofacial area.
The patient limits his or her mandibular movements.
The patient modifies his or her oral behavior (e.g., eating).
The patient is uncooperative or resistant to oral care.

New Developments in Orofacial Pain Assessment

Although there are no papers so far that report on the development of a reliable, valid, and easy-to-use instrument for the assessment of orofacial pain in patients with dementia, some developments are worth reporting at this stage. Toxopeus et al. [43] report on the secondary analysis of the video uptakes that were used during the initial testing phase of the MOBID [17, 18], during which the teeth/mouth care item was removed for the reason stated above. Since the observers of the video uptakes during the initial testing phase of the MOBID consisted of nondental professionals only, Toxopeus et al. [43] presented the recordings to a group of experienced elderly care dentists. These observers were asked to score the video fragments for the presence of orofacial pain-/discomfort-related behaviors (viz, pain noises, facial expressions, or defense) and for the presence of dementia-related behaviors (viz, anxiety, aggression, or confusion), using the thus-composed orofacial MOBID pain scale. The scoring was done at two occasions, as to establish the reliability of the observations. Despite the vast experience of the observers in dealing with older persons with dementia, they were not able to reliably score the teeth/mouth care item in terms of pain/discomfort-related behavior or dementia-related behavior. Hence, the orofacial MOBID pain scale cannot be recommended for the assessment of orofacial pain in older persons with dementia. In conclusion, the findings of Toxopeus et al. [43] support the decision of Husebo et al. [18] to remove the teeth/mouth care item from the initial version of the MOBID.

As indicated above, the PAIC tool [5] for the assessment of pain in cognitively impaired individuals, notably those with dementia, will be the core of a comprehensive toolkit that will include additional instruments for the assessment of, among others, orofacial pain. Following the structure of the PAIC tool, a specific observational tool has been developed for the assessment of orofacial pain at rest, during oral functions like eating and drinking, and during mouth care. During these activities, observations will be made of facial activities, body movements, and vocalizations. In addition, the observer will note specific orofacial behaviors like limiting jaw movements, refusing dentures, and drooling. This tool, the Orofacial Pain Scale for Nonverbal Individuals (OPS-NVI) is currently being tested for its user-friendliness and psychometric properties by one of us (SD). Until the outcomes of that study are known, clinicians are suggested to follow the approach described by Herr et al. [11]; see Table 12-3. Importantly, since a person suffering from dementia who is being admitted to institutionalized care might already be suffering from a painful condition, establishing baseline behavior (Table 12-3) might best be done in a "guaranteed pain-free condition," that is, while being prescribed analgesics.

TABLE 12-3 Stepwise Assessment of Orofacial Pain in Nonverbal Individuals in the Absence of a User-Friendly, Reliable, and Valid Observational Tool [11]

Steps in Orofacial Pain Assessment

Anticipate the presence of pain with—or following—disease, injury, or surgery.
Establish baseline behavior as to enable the observation of pain-related behavioral changes.
Identify less obvious pain indicators, for example, agitation and aggression.
In case of doubt, administer analgesics and look for behavioral changes.

OROFACIAL PAIN AND IMPAIRED CHEWING IN OLDER PERSONS WITH DEMENTIA

As indicated in the introductory paragraph, many orofacial pain conditions negatively affect the masticatory process. In turn, impaired mastication has been associated with cognitive decline. The comprehensive review of Weijenberg et al. [48] describes the evidence for this association, based on both animal studies and human work. For example, when senescence-accelerated (i.e., genetically prone to pathological aging) mice have undergone a reduced chewing intervention, like consuming a soft diet [51] or having their teeth cut [32, 45], they show impaired cognitive abilities, like reduced spatial memory function as tested in a Morris water maze (i.e., a behavioral procedure during which the mouse is placed in a large circular pool and is supposed to find a submerged platform that allows it to escape the water using visual clues). The association of this finding with older age is further underlined by the observation that the effects of reduced chewing interventions are larger in middle-aged and old mice than in young specimens [46]. Interestingly, the cognitive decline is in part reversible by fitting crowns to the cut teeth [45]. This evidence, along with the many other studies reviewed by Weijenberg et al. [48], suggests that a causal association exists between impaired chewing and cognitive decline.

Besides animal evidence for a causal relation between mastication and cognition, also human experimental studies suggest the existence of such association. In Table 2 of Weijenberg et al. [48], studies are summarized that have demonstrated, by means of brain scanning techniques like positron emission tomography and functional magnetic resonance imaging, that various brain areas (viz, prefrontal cortex, supplementary motor area, sensory–motor cortex, parietal cortex, insula, cerebellum, and thalamus) are being activated during mastication, both in young/middle-aged adults and in older persons of 60 years of age and older [31, 34].

Apart from such experimental works, Scherder et al. [36] reported the outcomes of a clinical study to the association between the functional status of the masticatory system in older (i.e., 60 years of age and older) persons without dementia and their episodic memory (i.e., memory of experiences and specific events in time in a serial form, from which actual events can be reconstructed that took place at any given point in one's life) and executive functions (e.g., divided attention, set-shifting, and inhibition). The authors found significant negative associations between edentulousness and wearing a complete denture on both episodic memory and executive functioning [36]. This suggests the existence of a relationship between diminished dental function and decreased cognitive abilities.

Whereas the study by Scherder et al. [36] dealt with older persons without dementia, Weijenberg et al. [47] set out to study the association between oral mixing ability and cognition in older persons with dementia. Oral mixing ability was assessed by means of a two-color chewing gum. The better the chewing ability of an individual, the better both colors were mixed. This technique, which included a fully automated computerized analysis of the samples, was found to be feasible and reliable [49], and could thus be applied in the clinical study to the association between oral mixing ability and cognition. Weijenberg et al. [47] examined a group of older persons with dementia. Apart from the mixing ability test, cognition was assessed with a multidomain neuropsychological test battery. Significant correlations were found between reduced masticatory ability and declines in global cognition and verbal fluency (i.e., the ability to quickly produce words of a certain category or type), which is in line with the above-summarized results of animal studies and experimental human works.

The implications of the above-mentioned results are compelling: they stress the urgent need for the development of prevention strategies to be applied by caretakers in nursing homes. Good oral care that yields better, pain-free masticatory function may stabilize or even improve cognition in older persons, especially in those with dementia.

CONCLUSION

Orofacial pain is most likely a common condition in older persons with dementia. So far, however, strong data that demonstrate the prevalence of orofacial pain in dementia are lacking, in part because the assessment of orofacial pain in nonverbal individuals is complicated by the absence of a reliable, valid, and user-friendly observational tool. A promising prospect is the recent development of the Pain Assessment in Impaired Cognition (PAIC) toolkit that will also include a specific orofacial pain tool, the Orofacial Pain Scale for Nonverbal Individuals (OPS-NVI). When, after thorough psychometric testing, this tool will become available, important issues like the effects of orofacial pain on mastication in older persons with dementia can be further studied. The outcomes of such studies will undoubtedly be pivotal to clarifying to opinion leaders and policy makers the urgent need to improve oral health care in older persons with dementia. Pain-free oral functioning will lead to a higher quality of life and might even help stabilizing or even improving cognition in this frail and vulnerable patient population. Importantly, this orofacial pain project will serve as an example for the development of other tools that aim at the assessment of specific forms of pain in dementia, like back pain and neuropathic pain.

REFERENCES

1. Alzheimer's Disease International. World Alzheimer Report, 2009. Accessed at http://www.alz.co.uk/research/files/WorldAlzheimerReport.pdf
2. Cervo FA, Raggi RP, Bright-Long LE, Wright WK, Rows G, Torres AE, Levy RB, Komaroff E. Use of the certified nursing assistant pain assessment tool (CPAT) in nursing home residents with dementia. Am J Alzheimers Dis Other Demen 2007;22:112–9.
3. Chalmers JM, King PL, Spencer AJ, Wright FA, Carter KD. The oral health assessment tool—validity and reliability. Aust Dent J 2005;50:191–9.
4. Cole LJ, Gavrilescu M, Johnston LA, Gibson SJ, Farrell MJ, Egan GF. The impact of Alzheimer's disease on the functional connectivity between brain regions underlying pain perception. Eur J Pain 2011;15:568.e1–11.
5. Corbett A, Achterberg W, Husebo B, Lobbezoo F, de Vet H, Kunz M, Strand LI, Constantinou M, Tudose C, Kappesser J, et al. An international road map to improve pain assessment in people with impaired cognition: the development of the Pain Assessment in Impaired Cognition (PAIC) tool. BMC Neurol 2014;14:229.
6. Cornali C, Franzoni S, Gatti S, Trabucchi M. Diagnosis of chronic pain caused by osteoarthritis and prescription of analgesics in patients with cognitive impairment. J Am Med Dir Assoc 2006;7:1–5.
7. De Leeuw R, Klasser GD, editors. Orofacial pain: guidelines for assessment, diagnosis, and management. Chicago, IL: Quintessence Publishing; 2013. 301pp.
8. de Souza Rolim T, Fabri GM, Nitrini R, Anghinah R, Teixeira MJ, de Siqueira JT, Cestari JA, de Siqueira SR. Oral infections and orofacial pain in Alzheimer's disease: a case-control study. J Alzheimers Dis 2014;38:823–9.
9. Ekbäck G, Unell L, Johansson A, Ordell S, Carlsson GE. Changes in dental status and prevalence of symptoms related to temporomandibular disorders in 50- to 70-year-old subjects. Longitudinal and cross-sectional results. J Craniomandib Funct 2013;5:317–31.

10. Fuchs-Lacelle S, Hadjistavropoulos T. Development and preliminary validation of the pain assessment checklist for seniors with limited ability to communicate (PACSLAC). Pain Manag Nurs 2004;5:37–49.
11. Herr K, Bjoro K, Decker S. Tools for the assessment of pain in nonverbal older adults with dementia: a state-of-the-science review. J Pain Symptom Manag 2006;31:170–92.
12. Hølen JC, Saltvedt I, Fayers PM, Bjørnnes M, Stenseth G, Hval B, Filbet M, Loge JH, Kaasa S. The Norwegian Doloplus-2, a tool for behavioural pain assessment: translation and pilot-validation in nursing home patients with cognitive impairment. Palliat Med 2005;19:411–7.
13. Huffman JC, Kunik ME. Assessment and understanding of pain in patients with dementia. Gerontologist 2000;40:574–81.
14. Hurley AC, Volicer BJ, Hanrahan PA, Houde S, Volicer L. Assessment of discomfort in advanced Alzheimer patients. Res Nurs Health 1992;15:369–77.
15. Husebo BS, Achterberg WP, Lobbezoo F, Kunz M, Lautenbacher S, Kappesser J, Tudose C, Strand LI. Pain in patients with dementia: an overview of pain assessment and treatment challenges. Nor Epidemiol 2012; 22:243–51.
16. Husebo BS, Kunz M, Achterberg WP, Lobbezoo F, Kappesser J, Tudose C, Strand LI, Lautenbacher S. Pain assessment and treatment challenges in patients with dementia. [Scherzmessung und –behandlung bei Patienten mit Demez.] Zeitschr Neuropsychol 2012;23:237–46.
17. Husebo BS, Strand LI, Moe-Nilssen R, Husebo SB, Ljunggren AE. Pain behaviour and pain intensity in older persons with severe dementia: reliability of the MOBID Pain Scale by video uptake. Scand J Caring Sci 2009;23:180–9.
18. Husebo BS, Strand LI, Moe-Nilssen R, Husebo SB, Snow AL, Ljunggren AE. Mobilization-Observation-Behavior-Intensity-Dementia Pain Scale (MOBID): development and validation of a nurse-administered pain assessment tool for use in dementia. J Pain Symptom Manag 2007;34:67–80.
19. International Association for the Study of Pain, 2013. Accessed at http://www.iasp-pain.org/Content/NavigationMenu/GlobalYearAgainstPain/GlobalYearAgainstOrofacialPain/FactSheets/default.htm
20. Jones JA, Brown EJ, Volicer L. Target outcomes for long-term oral health care in dementia: a Delphi approach. J Public Health Dent 2000;60:330–4.
21. Kester M, Scheltens P. Dementia. Neurol Pract 2009;9:241–51.
22. Kovach CR, Griffie J, Muchka S, Noonan PE, Weissman DE. Nurses' perceptions of pain assessment and treatment in the cognitively impaired elderly. It's not a guessing game. Clin Nurse Spec 2000;14: 215–20.
23. Kovach CR, Weissman DE, Griffie J, Matson S, Muchka S. Assessment and treatment of discomfort for people with late-stage dementia. J Pain Symptom Manag 1999;18:412–9.
24. LeResche L. Epidemiology of temporomandibular disorders: implications for the investigation of etiologic factors. Crit Rev Oral Biol Med 1997;8:291–305.
25. Lester V, Ashley FP, Gibbons DE. The relationship between socio-dental indices of handicap, felt need for dental treatment and dental state in a group of frail and functionally dependent older adults. Community Dent Oral Epidemiol 1998;26:155–9.
26. Lipton JA, Ship JA, Larach-Robinson D. Estimated prevalence and distribution of reported orofacial pain in the United States. J Am Dent Assoc 1993;124:115–21.
27. Lobbezoo F, Weijenberg RA, Scherder EJ. Topical review: orofacial pain in dementia patients. A diagnostic challenge. J Orofac Pain 2011;25:6–14.
28. Locker D. The burden of oral disorders in a population of older adults. Community Dent Health 1992; 9:109–24.
29. Maxwell CJ, Dalby DM, Slater M, Patten SB, Hogan DB, Eliasziw M, Hirdes JP. The prevalence and management of current daily pain among older home care clients. Pain 2008;138:208–16.
30. Nègre-Pagès L, Regragui W, Bouhassira D, Grandjean H, Rascol O, DoPaMiP Study Group. Chronic pain in Parkinson's disease: the cross-sectional French DoPaMiP survey. Mov Disord 2008;23:1361–9.
31. Onozuka M, Fujita M, Watanabe K, Hirano Y, Niwa M, Nishiyama K, Saito S. Age-related changes in brain regional activity during chewing: a functional magnetic resonance imaging study. J Dent Res 2003; 82:657–60.
32. Onozuka M, Watanabe K, Mirbod SM, Ozono S, Nishiyama K, Karasawa N, Nagatsu I. Reduced masticatory function stimulates impairment of spatial memory and degeneration of hippocampal neurons in aged SAMP8 mice. Brain Res 1999;826:148–53.
33. Plooij B, van der Spek K, Scherder EJ. Pain medication and global cognitive functioning in dementia patients with painful conditions. Drugs Aging 2012;29:377–84.

34. Sasaguri KI, Sato S, Hirano Y, Aoki S, Ishikawa T, Fujita M, Watanabe K, Tomida M, Ido Y, Onozuka M. Involvement of chewing in memory processes in humans: an approach using fMRI. Int Congr Ser 2004;1270:111–6.
35. Scherder E, Herr K, Pickering G, Gibson S, Benedetti F, Lautenbacher S. Pain in dementia. Pain 2009;145:276–8.
36. Scherder E, Posthuma W, Bakker T, Vuijk PJ, Lobbezoo F. Functional status of the masticatory system, executive function, and episodic memory in older persons. J Oral Rehabil 2008;35:324–36.
37. Scherder EJ, Bouma A. Is decreased use of analgesics in Alzheimer disease due to a change in the affective component of pain? Alzheimer Dis Assoc Disord 1997;11:171–4.
38. Scherder EJ, Bouma A. Visual analogue scales for pain assessment in Alzheimer's disease. Gerontology 2000;46:47–53.
39. Scherder EJ, Plooij B. Assessment and management of pain, with particular emphasis on central neuropathic pain, in moderate to severe dementia. Drugs Aging 2012;29:701–6.
40. Scherder EJ, Sergeant JA, Swaab DF. Pain processing in dementia and its relation to neuropathology. Lancet Neurol 2003;2:677–86.
41. Schmidt ML, Zhukareva V, Perl DP, Sheridan SK, Schuck T, Lee VM, Trojanowski JQ. Spinal cord neurofibrillary pathology in Alzheimer disease and Guam Parkinsonism–Dementia complex. J Neuropathol Exp Neurol 2001;60:1075–86.
42. Smith M. Pain assessment in nonverbal older adults with advanced dementia. Perspect Psychiatr Care 2005;41:99–113.
43. Toxopeus AH, Husebo BS, Strand LI, Delwel S, van Wijk AJ, Scherder EJA, Lobbezoo F. The mouth care item of the MOBID Pain Scale: secondary analyses of video uptakes by dental professionals. Gerodontology 2014. doi:10.1111/ger.12115
44. Warden V, Hurley AC, Volicer L. Development and psychometric evaluation of the pain assessment in advanced dementia (PAINAD) scale. J Am Med Dir Assoc 2003;4:9–15.
45. Watanabe K, Ozono S, Nishiyama K, Saito S, Tonosaki K, Fujita M, Onozuka M. The molarless condition in aged SAMP8 mice attenuates hippocampal Fos induction linked to water maze performance. Behav Brain Res 2002;128:19–25.
46. Watanabe K, Tonosaki K, Kawase T, Karasawa N, Nagatsu I, Fujita M, Onozuka M. Evidence for involvement of dysfunctional teeth in the senile process in the hippocampus of SAMP8 mice. Exp Gerontol 2001;36:283–95.
47. Weijenberg RA, Lobbezoo F, Visscher CM, Scherder EJ. Oral mixing ability and cognition in elderly persons with dementia. J Oral Rehabil 2015;42:481–6.
48. Weijenberg RA, Scherder EJ, Lobbezoo F. Mastication for the mind—the relationship between mastication and cognition in ageing and dementia. Neurosci Biobehav Rev 2011;35:483–97.
49. Weijenberg RA, Scherder EJ, Visscher CM, Gorissen T, Yoshida E, Lobbezoo F. Two-colour chewing gum mixing ability: digitalization and spatial heterogeneity analysis. J Oral Rehabil 2013;40:737–43
50. Wheeler MS. Pain assessment and management in the patient with mild to moderate cognitive impairment. Home Healthc Nurse 2006;24:354–9.
51. Yamamoto T, Hirayama A. Effects of soft-diet feeding on synaptic density in the hippocampus and parietal cortex of senescence-accelerated mice. Brain Res 2001;902:255–63.

CHAPTER 13

Guidelines and Practical Approaches for the Effective Pain Assessment of the Patient with Dementia

Thomas Hadjistavropoulos

Pain is a complex experience that involves the interplay of physical, emotional, behavioral, and cognitive components and is influenced by social, cultural, and situational factors [22, 42]. Given its subjectivity, verbal and nonverbal pain communication becomes important in pain assessment. For many patients with dementia, however, severe cognitive dysfunction impairs ability to provide meaningful verbal report of pain. This creates special challenges with respect to health professionals' ability to understand the subjective pain state, that these patients are experiencing, and underscores the importance of nonverbal responses in pain assessment.

A FRAMEWORK FOR CONSTRUING PAIN ASSESSMENT

The challenges of pain assessment in dementia can be conceptualized through a communications framework of pain [22]. This framework construes the process of pain communication as consisting of three stages: (1) the subjective internal experience of pain and all of the factors that influence it (e.g., biological, psychological, situational), (2) the manner in which this experience is encoded in expressive behavior (i.e., self-report of pain and nonverbal pain behaviors such as grimaces or altered gait), and (3) the decoding of expressive behavior by observers who could potentially respond to palliate the pain experience.

The internal experience of pain is complex. Emotions such as fear, anger, and disgust are often elements of that experience [30]. Moreover, the functional, emotional, cognitive, and social consequences, that a given pain problem may lead to, vary from person to person. Although, sometimes, the term "pain assessment" is equated with "assessment of pain intensity," a complete understanding of a patient's pain condition would require thorough examination of all of the elements comprising the pain experience and its influences regardless of whether these elements are physical or psychosocial.

The Communications Framework of Pain [21, 22] describes the two main pathways of encoding pain into expressive behavior. These pathways are verbal expression and nonverbal communication. The framework professes that the two pathways differ along the dimensions of cognitive executive mediation and reflexive automaticity. That is, self-report of pain is dependent upon higher cognitive processes and is typically characterized by greater clarity than nonverbal reactions which can be more ambiguous. In contrast, nonverbal pain responses such as grimacing tend to be more automatic and less subject to voluntary control than is self-report. Compared to self-report, nonverbal responses may often be more difficult to decode and correctly interpret by observers. That is, a behavioral reaction may be indicative of pain, but it could also be indicative of other types of non–pain-related distress (e.g., fear).

While both verbal and nonverbal pain responses are important for all pain assessments, nonverbal expressions become increasingly critical as patient cognitive functions (and, thus, ability to provide reliable and valid verbal report) deteriorate. Systematic research on nonverbal pain expressions of patients with dementia has been conducted [27, 36, 38] and has included a focus on the development and validation of a variety of observational tools designed to assess pain behavior (i.e., Pain Assessment in Advanced Dementia [PAINAD] [49]; DOLOPLUS-2 [50]; Abbey Pain Scale [1]; Pain Assessment Checklist for Seniors with Limited Ability to Communicate [PACSLAC] [16]; Noncommunicative Patient's Pain Assessment Instrument [NOPPAIN] [48]).

Given advances in pain assessment, including tool development, expert groups and organizations have produced guidelines and recommendations for the assessment of the dementia patient. Key guidelines and recommendations are reviewed in this chapter, which concludes with discussion of a practical approach to the pain assessment of the dementia patient. This practical approach borrows heavily from the preexisting literature.

PAIN ASSESSMENT GUIDELINES

The focus of the physical examination of the patient with dementia does not differ much from that of the patient without dementia other than that the dementia patient may require additional guidance and support. As such, the focus of this chapter is on assessment of pain intensity, psychological functioning, and environmental aspects that may impact pain. Given overlap among various guidelines, Table 13-1 shows key recommendations that have been made along with the various guidelines that articulate each recommendation. In considering the information on the table, it is important to note that, most often, a guideline may have omitted a specific recommendation not because of disagreement with that recommendation but because it might have fallen outside its aims or scope. To summarize, some of the key recommendations, derived from the various guidelines, include the following:

1. Integrate the results of physical examinations, clinical history, test results, etc.
2. Use self-report approaches where possible/always attempt self-report.
3. Use observational approaches to pain assessment.
4. Solicit relevant information from caregivers/collaborative informants.
5. It is often useful to assess pain during movement because movement is more likely to elicit pain behavior.
6. Adopt an individualized assessment comparing results over time.
7. Make adaptations for the capabilities of the individual (e.g., simplify language, use larger fonts as needed).
8. Consider pain assessment before and after the administration of a pain management intervention (e.g., an analgesic trial).
9. Recognize the limitations of screening tools (i.e., these tools are not definitive indicators of pain, and they may sometimes fail to identify pain, whereas, other times, they may incorrectly signal the presence of pain).

TABLE 13-1 Recommendations of Major Guidelines for the Pain Assessment of the Older Adult with Dementia

Recommendations	American Geriatrics Society [3, 4]	American Medical Directors Association Pain Management Guideline [5]	Australian and New Zealand Society for Geriatric Medicine [52]	The British National Guideline for Assessment of Pain in Older People [46]	International Interdisciplinary Consensus Statement on Pain Assessment in Older Persons [24]	National Nursing Home Pain Collaborative [31]	Pain in Residential Aged Care Facilities [7]	Task Force of the American Society for Pain Management Nursing [32]	Transforming Long-Term Care Pain Management in North America Guidelines [28]
Integrate results of physical examinations, history, etc.	✓	✓	✓		✓	✓	✓	✓	
Use self-report approaches where possible	✓	✓	✓	✓	✓	✓	✓	✓	✓
Use observational approaches	✓	✓	✓	✓	✓	✓	✓	✓	✓
Solicit caregiver report	✓	✓		✓	✓	✓	✓		
Assess during movement (when it is more likely to elicit pain behavior)	✓			✓	✓	✓	✓		
Adopt an individualized approach comparing scores over time		✓			✓	✓		✓	✓
Recommends specific self-report tools					✓		✓		
Recommends specific observational tools						✓	✓		
Make adaptations for the capabilities of the individual (e.g., use of simplified language)	✓	✓		✓	✓		✓	✓	

(continued)

TABLE 13-1 Recommendations of Major Guidelines for the Pain Assessment of the Older Adult with Dementia (continued)

Recommendations	American Geriatrics Society [3, 4]	American Medical Directors Association Pain Management Guideline [5]	Australian and New Zealand Society for Geriatric Medicine [52]	The British National Guideline for Assessment of Pain in Older People [46]	International Interdisciplinary Consensus Statement on Pain Assessment in Older Persons [24]	National Nursing Home Pain Collaborative [31]	Pain in Residential Aged Care Facilities [7]	Task Force of the American Society for Pain Management Nursing [32]	Transforming Long-Term Care Pain Management in North America Guidelines [28]
Recognize limitations of screening tools (i.e., false positives, false negatives)	✓	✓	✓			✓		✓	
Outlines specific domains of pain behavior that should be attended to	✓	✓	✓	✓	✓	✓	✓	✓	
Recommendations about assessment frequency/need to assess over time	✓	✓		✓	✓	✓	✓		✓
Assess pain before and after pain management intervention	✓	✓			✓	✓	✓	✓	✓

Note: It is recognized that there was subjectivity in creating this table. Sometimes recommendations were implicit or a subjective judgment was made on whether or not to include some of the check marks on this table.

Some guidelines recommend specific standardized assessment tools while others do not. In addition, guidelines generally recognize that pain assessment is a complex process and should not be restricted to the evaluation of pain intensity. As such, emphasis should be placed on functional limitations, emotional functioning, social environment, and other related domains. The following is a summary of key points from various guideline documents.

American Geriatrics Society

The American Geriatrics Society (AGS) [4] has adopted a guideline for the pharmacological management of persistent pain in older persons but did not elaborate much on assessment. Instead, the AGS 2009 [4] document refers the reader to previous literature [24] including previous guidelines [3]. In fact, the AGS 2002 [3] guideline included more detailed information on pain assessment but much of the focus was on older adults who can self-report pain. Nonetheless, the AGS 2002 [3] task force identified the following domains as being important in the pain assessment of older adult with cognitive impairments: facial expressions, verbalizations and vocalizations, body movements, changes interpersonal interactions, changes in activity patterns or routines, and mental status changes. These domains can form the basis for the evaluation of the comprehensiveness of any pain assessment that involves the dementia patient.

Pain in Residential Aged Care Facilities (Australian Pain Society) [7]

The guideline recognizes the challenges of pain assessment in patients with dementia and provides recommendations for both assessment and management. Only the pain assessment recommendations are considered here. The guideline emphasizes a comprehensive approach to pain assessment and stresses the importance of obtaining self-report where possible, use of adaptations to simplify procedures as necessary (e.g., use of simplified language), and informant reports. Staff members are encouraged to look for the behavioral pain expressions falling under the AGS expressive domains mentioned above and to evaluate the impact of pain (e.g., on mood, ambulation). The importance of multidisciplinary collaboration is also emphasized. The Abbey Pain Scale [1] was recommended as a useful standard for pain assessment and the Resident's Verbal Brief Pain Inventory [7] (a modified version of the Brief Pain Inventory) [14] was recommended as the standard for the assessment of residents with sufficient cognitive ability (in addition to use of numeric and verbal descriptors scales). The Australian guideline, however, was produced prior to a proliferation of psychometric research, development, and refinement of long term care (LTC) assessment tools focusing on patients with dementia. As such, the specific tool recommendations did not take into account the more recent literature.

Australian and New Zealand Society for Geriatric Medicine [52]

This document focuses on pain in older persons and contains a brief section of pain assessment that discusses pain in dementia. The section is quite general but recognizes that persons with mild to moderate dementia are often able to self-report pain as well as the importance of behavioral observation and use of observational tools. No specific tools are recommended.

American Medical Directors' Association (AMDA) Pain Management Guideline [5]

Despite a primary focus on pain management, the AMDA guideline discusses assessment in some detail. It is directed to members of interdisciplinary teams working in long-term care (LTC) facilities. There is emphasis on physical examination and test results, along with history information, including collateral informant reports, as well as on an effort to identify the cause of pain. Staff are encouraged to look for signs and symptoms that may suggest pain. Use of a specialized assessment tool is suggested (and tool examples are given with appended copies of a few self-report and observational tools), although no tool is specifically recommended. Assessors are encouraged to make determinations of the impact of pain on mood, activity, and quality of life.

International Interdisciplinary Consensus Statement on Pain Assessment in Older Persons [24]

This consensus document represents, perhaps, the most significant international and interdisciplinary effort to develop guidelines for effective pain assessment in older persons and to cover all key aspects of assessment (e.g., physical, psychological, pharmacological, pain intensity, review of specific tools) [24]. While the document was intended to provide guidelines for seniors with and without dementia, only the sections focusing on dementia are discussed here. The large international group of authors adopted a broad focus and did not only consider guidelines for the assessment of pain (based on both observation and self-report, where available) but also outlined approaches to history taking physical examination (including mobility and balance, neurological examination, medication history, cognitive status evaluation, and assessment of psychological functioning). Most aspects of the physical examination were focused on older adults in general and were not unique to the patients with dementia. As such, they are not reviewed here.

Specific recommendations for older adults with dementia stress the importance of history, physical examination and interview information (including interview with collaborative informants), use of both self-report and observational procedures where possible [19], recommendations for specific unidimensional scales that have been shown to be useful in the assessment of older persons with mild to moderate dementia (e.g., Colored Analog Scale [CAS] [41, 47], numeric rating scales (e.g., 0 = no pain; 10 = pain as severe as it can be), or verbal rating scale, involving verbal descriptors of pain such as mild, moderate, and severe), recognition that pain assessment during movement is most likely to elicit pain behaviors, examination of whether use of analgesics results in reduced pain behaviors, use of an individualized approach to assessment involving the collection of baseline scores for each patient, consistent use of assessment tools over time (i.e., tools must be used under consistent circumstances such as during a specific transfer or program of physiotherapy), and recognition of the limitations of screening tools in pain assessment. Specific promising assessment tools such as the PACSLAC [16] and the DOLOPLUS-2 [50] are mentioned with the caution that more research was needed (i.e., no one tool was specifically recommended for the assessment of patients with dementia).

National Nursing Home Pain Collaborative [31]

Although many consensus guidelines had not recommended specific observational pain assessment tools for older adults with dementia, the National Nursing Home Pain

Collaborative did so based on systematic examination of the literature, psychometric properties, and expert consensus. Specifically, the collaborative recommended use of two tools by LTC facilities: the PAINAD [49] and the PACSLAC [16]. They argued that the PAINAD is useful for daily assessment including follow-up evaluations of pain interventions, whereas the PACSLAC, being more comprehensive, was recommended as a baseline and monthly or quarterly maintenance assessment tool to reflect broader changes in behavior and activity. The PACSLAC was also recommended to facilitate integration of ongoing pain monitoring with Minimum Data Set (MDS) [10] documentation because of good correspondence to MDS indicators. It is noted that, since the National Nursing Home Pain Collaborative made these recommendations, the PACSLAC has been refined and shortened without compromising comprehensive coverage of the pain assessment domains deemed important by the AGS [11].

In addition to recommending specific tools, the Collaborative emphasized the importance of eliciting verbal report where possible, the need for comprehensive pain assessments, the need for repeated pain assessment, integration with MDS [10] and federal United States requirements, the advantages of pain assessment during movement, development of policies to ensure facility-wide pain screenings with accountable staff, and the need for continuing pain education of all front-line staff.

The British National Guideline for Assessment of Pain in Older People [46]

Together with the British Geriatrics Society and the Royal College of Physicians, the British Pain Society developed a national guideline for the pain assessment of older persons. The guideline recognizes the need for comprehensive pain assessments for all older adults as well as the limitations that people with dementia may face in the communication of pain. As such, it stresses the need for observational assessment. Domains to be assessed by observation, similar to those recommended by the AGS [3], are also outlined. The guideline emphasizes the need to attempt self-report with all patients and to adapt self-report scales, as necessary, for older adults with communication impairments. The specific tool that was recommended for observational pain assessment was the Abbey Scale [1]. Especially useful in the guideline is the presentation of an algorithm for the assessment of pain in older persons (see Fig. 13-1).

Task Force of the American Society for Pain Management Nursing [32]

This document addresses a variety of populations with limited ability to communicate (e.g., persons with intellectual disabilities, infants and persons with advanced dementia). In other words, the document is less specialized than other recommendation and guideline documents presented here. This American Society for Pain Management Nursing (ASPMN) task force recommended that a pain assessment hierarchy be established that should involve attempted self-report, search for potential causes of the pain, observation of pain behaviors, use of proxy reporting, and attempt of an analgesic trial (and evaluation of the extent to which this reduces pain indicators). The task force also recommended use of a psychometrically valid pain assessment tool and minimization of emphasis on physiological indicators (such as heart rate changes) because the correlation of such indicators with self-reported pain tends to be weak or absent. Postintervention assessment and documentation

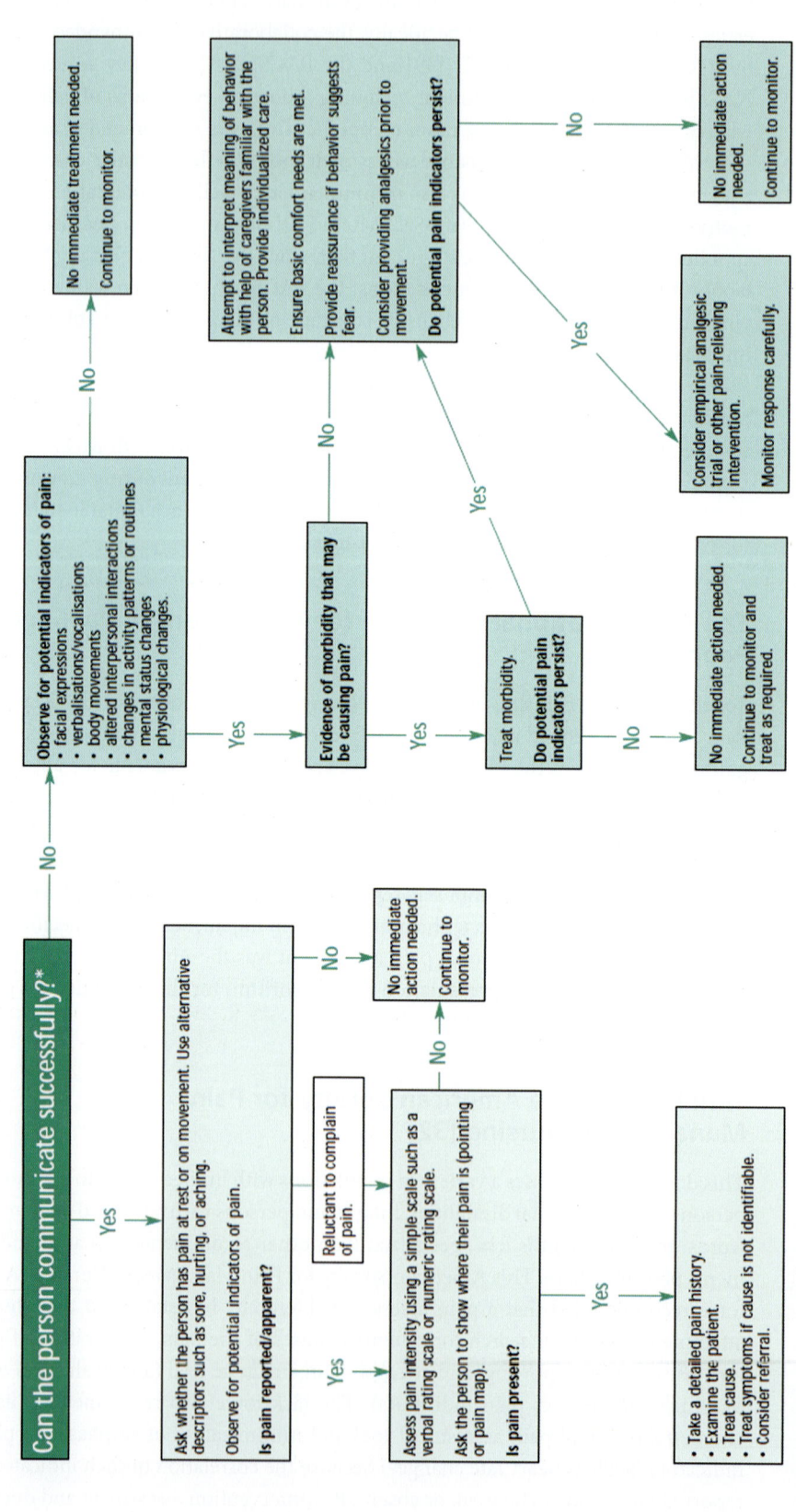

FIGURE 13-1 Copyright © 2007 Royal College of Physicians. Reproduced from Royal College of Physicians et al. [46], with permission. Algorithm for the assessment of pain in older people.

were also recommended. Specific assessment tools designed for seniors with dementia are mentioned, but the reader is referred to the work of the National Nursing Home Pain Collaborative document [31] reviewed above.

Transforming Long-Term Care Pain Management in North America Guidelines [28]

Despite advances in the area of pain assessment in dementia as well as guideline development by credible and influential groups, best practices in pain assessment have not been implemented on a large scale basis. As a result, pain problems continue to go undetected [15, 24, 33, 39, 44]; behavioral disturbance due to pain is managed by psychotropic medication [13], which has been shown to hasten death and lead to unnecessary polypharmacy [8, 9, 26]. Given the absence of wide scale implementation, a group of pain and public policy experts addressed the question of wide-scale implementation failure [28]. The group concluded that most pain assessment guidelines do not take into account regulatory and resource realities. With this in mind, they proposed a model of a pain assessment/management approach that was felt to be feasible and realistic for application within facilities that care for those with dementia. The group proposed specifically as follows:

a. That pain be assessed for all residents on admission and at least once a week thereafter. More frequent pain assessment was recommended in situations that involve suspicion of pain. The group clarified that, in most cases, the pain assessments could be a screening for pain taking only a few minutes to complete.
b. Implementation of a treatment plan within 24 hours of pain assessment suggesting pain (with the clarification that many treatment plans could be as simple as administration of acetaminophen or more frequent repositioning of patient with limited mobility)
c. Reassessment of pain and any side effects of treatment within 24 hours of treatment plan implementation
d. Pain assessment processes and treatment outcomes should be a component of any ongoing quality improvement program to improve care and outcomes for residents.

The group suggested that successful implementation of this plan may be dependent on the assignment of a pain champion within each facility (e.g., a senior nurse responsible for ensuring best practices in pain assessment and management, including communication with physicians as necessary). The group also recognized that additional changes at the policy level may be necessary for effective pain assessment to be implemented.

In a survey of front-line LTC staff, this approach to pain assessment was rated as highly desirable and feasible [25]. Despite its simplicity, this plan would require some, albeit relatively limited, resources (e.g., time release for a nurse so that she can specifically focus on pain assessment/management). In the era of constrained budgets, even small changes to resource allocations may remain challenging. Nursing staff report that they would like to engage in pain assessment as recommended by Hadjistavropoulos et al. [24] but note that they often lack central management support and associated resources [18]. For their part, administrators recognize the importance of pain management but find the reallocation of their very limited resources to be a challenge despite the demonstrated benefits of regular pain assessment on patient outcomes. It is noted, however, that despite existing resource constraints, facilities place considerable resources in approaches to patient care that have yet to show demonstrable benefits on patient outcomes [53] and do not allocate as many resources to regular, facility-wide, evidence-based pain assessments.

A PRACTICAL APPROACH TO PAIN ASSESSMENT

The practical approach to pain assessment, suggested by several of the above guidelines, is summarized here. Effective pain assessment begins with recognition of the complexities of the pain experience and will take into consideration not only indicators of present pain intensity but also results of physical examinations, functional evaluations, patient psychological functioning, environmental context, self-report (if available), and observations of pain behavior. Physical examinations and functional evaluations are beyond the scope of this chapter.

History

Effective pain assessment takes into account patient history [24]. Although the emphasis should be on problem history (and related medical issues), including antecedents and consequences of the pain problem, a thorough and effective history will take into account the full biopsychosocial context of the patient (e.g., psychosocial contributors to pain experience or expression) [22].

Attempting Self-Report

It is highly recommended that self-report of pain be attempted in all cases [24, 32]. Patients with mild to moderate dementia are often able to provide valid self-report of pain [19]. As a rule of thumb, based on the literature [12, 51], it has been suggested [19] that persons with MMSE scores of 18 and higher are typically capable of responding to simple self-report procedures about pain (e.g., 0–10 numeric rating scales which are explained clearly and verbal rating scales that involve use of descriptors such as "mild pain" and "severe pain" with each descriptor corresponding to a number that can be recorded). While no test can determine with certainty whether a patient is capable of providing self-report of pain, procedures to assist with the evaluation of such capacity exist. Most notably, Scherder and Bouma [47] described an effective protocol to assess dementia patient capacity to provide valid responses to the CAS [41, 47]. Specifically, prior to CAS administration, these authors asked patients to point to the scale, point to the marker that slides up and down, point to the points that indicate the highest and lowest levels of pain, and demonstrate how they would move the marker. Several authors and guidelines [24, 31, 32] have emphasized the importance of adaptations for the sensory capabilities of the individual (e.g., use of larger fonts to accommodate vision limitations).

Use of an Observational Pain Assessment Tool

Nonverbal expressions of pain are important to consider in any pain assessment but are essential in cases where reliable and valid verbal report is unavailable due to severe dementia. Use of a specialized and well-validated pain assessment tool [11, 17, 49] is imperative. It is also important to consider that most of the available tools have limited validation information for acute care settings and have been primarily validated with LTC populations.

In using an observational pain assessment tool, several factors have to be taken into consideration. These are the following:

a. It has been recommended that *cutoff scores not be* used in observational pain assessments involving older adults with dementia [11]. This recommendation was made because assessment tool scores can be affected by a variety of factors. For example, duration of observation could influence scores with longer observation periods likely resulting in higher scores. The nature of the activity being observed would also affect such scores as would patient individual differences. Patients with dementias primarily affecting the frontal lobes of the brain, for instance, may be more disinhibited and more expressive of pain than those whose dementia primarily affects other regions of the brain. In addition, patients with limited mobility would have a lower repertoire of behavioral pain expression than patients with full mobility.

b. Instead of using cutoff scores, *an individualized approach to assessment is recommended*. Under ideal circumstances, observational pain assessment should occur regularly and the clinician would observe fluctuations in patient scores over time [20]. An unexpected rise in scores would be indicative of a pain problem. Obtaining scores before and after the administration of analgesics or other intervention [32] would help determine the extent to which the intervention was effective in alleviating pain.

c. Given that, as stated above, the duration of observation and situational variables could affect pain scores, it is important to *conduct assessments under consistent circumstances* (e.g., during a specific necessary but discomforting transfer or during a structured physical examination or program of physical therapy), keeping duration, activity as well as other relevant variables constant. Successful pain assessment has also been conducted by observing the patients (as practicable) over the course of a nursing shift and recording behaviors as they occur [6, 17].

d. It is important to recognize that pain would be more likely to be expressed during movement than during rest [32]. Husebo et al. [34] recommended a standard protocol which can be used to observe the patient. It is noted, however, that use of this protocol would require supervision/clearance from a qualified health professional given the frailty of many patients with dementia. Husebo et al.'s [34] protocol, which can be conducted while the patient is lying down, is as follows: (1) guide to open both hands (one hand at a time), (2) guide to stretch both arms toward the head (one arm at a time), (3) guide to stretch both hips and knees (one leg at a time), (4) guide to turn in bed to both sides, and (5) guide to sit at the bedside. The Husebo et al. [34] protocol has the advantage that it mobilizes the patient in standardized ways that would likely result in the detection pain related to a wide variety of musculoskeletal pain problems.

e. It is important to be aware that certain manifestations of conditions that may be unrelated to pain (e.g., delirium and depression) could mimic and be confused as signs of pain [29]. Selecting a pain assessment tool that has been designed to minimize overlap of its items with those of delirium and associated psychological scales [11] would be important. Moreover, given that delirium is transient, reassessment of pain after the delirious state has ended would also be recommended.

Information from Collateral Informants

The use of collaborative informants is vital, especially in the case of seniors with moderate to severe dementia, both for the purposes of obtaining complete history information but also for gaining a better understanding of the patient's pain (e.g., functional limitations, expressions of pain, possible behavioral disturbance due to pain) outside the context of the clinical examination.

Recognize the Limitations of Pain Assessment Tools

It is important to stress that clinicians should not consider the self-report and observational assessment of pain as being equivalent but as providing complementary information. In fact, the two types of assessment results are not always correlated [37] as they each tap on different aspects of the pain experience (e.g., the observational assessment captures immediate and reflexive aspects of the pain experience, whereas self-report can be subject to situational demand characteristics). Similarly, it should be recognized that the types of pain assessment tools discussed in this chapter should be considered to be screening instruments rather than definitive indicators of pain. As such, they may sometimes incorrectly suggest the presence of pain and other times may miss pain that is present. As such these tools cannot be construed as substitutes for a thorough assessment by a qualified health professional.

Frequency of Pain Assessment

Consistent with literature recommendations [3, 28] pain should be assessed for all patients on admission, at least weekly thereafter and more frequently if a pain problem is presented or suspected.

Evaluate Psychological States that may Result from or Contribute to the Pain Experience

Pain can contribute to the development of a variety of conditions including delirium and depression. It is important that these states be systematically assessed. Delirium may be assessed psychometrically using the Confusion Assessment Method (CAM) [35] and the Delirium Index (DI) [40]. Preexisting guidelines [24] emphasized the importance of assessment of functional and emotional status (at minimum an assessment for symptoms of depression should be conducted). Depression in the nonverbal patient with dementia can be assessed using the Cornell Scale for Depression in Dementia [2] which relies on information from collaborative informants. A variety of psychological domains could also be assessed using the Alzheimer Disease Related Quality of Life (ADRQL) scale [45], based on collaborative informant input. These domains are social interaction, awareness of self, feelings and mood, enjoyment of activities, and response to surroundings.

CONCLUSIONS

It is encouraging to observe that existing pain assessment guidelines, developed by a variety of different groups, share key common elements that include, among others, the importance of observational assessment for seniors with dementia, the need for adaptations of self-report approaches, recognition of the comprehensiveness of the pain assessment process, and others. The focus of this chapter was on professional associations and major consensus groups. Similar guidelines, however, based on the literature [24, 32] have also been elaborated upon by specific authors [23, 43].

While guidelines often fall short from recommending specific pain assessment tool, expert consensus recommendations for use of specific tools is likely to become increasingly common given the advances in tool validation and refinement that we have seen in recent years. Many such advances in the tool development, validation, and refinement followed the creation of most of the aforementioned guidelines. As such, there is a need to update the guidelines presented herein, particularly when it comes to recommendations for specific tools.

A key challenge that remains is that, although useful guidelines exist, these are not usually implemented on a wide-scale basis, often due to resource constraints and lack of familiarity of front line staff with assessment approaches and relevant recommendations [28, 39]. Much remains to be done in the public policy arena to ensure guideline implementation and appropriate resource allocation that would facilitate such implementation.

REFERENCES

1. Abbey J, Piller N, De Bellis A, Esterman A, Parker D, Giles L, Lowcay B. The Abbey pain scale: a 1-minute numerical indicator for people with end-stage dementia. Int J Palliat Nurs 2004;10:6–13.
2. Alexopoulos GS, Abrams RC, Young RC, Shamoian CA. Cornell scale for depression in dementia. Biol Psychiatry 1988;23:271–84.
3. American Geriatrics Society (AGS). The management of persistent pain in older persons. J Am Geriatr Soc 2002;50:S205–24.
4. American Geriatrics Society (AGS). Pharmacological management of persistent pain in older persons. J Am Geriatr Soc 2009;57:1331–46.
5. American Medical Directors Association (AMDA). Pain management in the long term care setting. Columbia, MD: American Medical Directors Association (AMDA); 2012.
6. Aubin M, Verreault R, Savoie M, Lemay S, Hadjistavropoulos T, Fillion L, Beaulieu M, Viens C, Bergeron R, Vezina L, Misson L, Fuchs-Lacelle S. Validite et utilite clinique d'une grille d'observation (PACSLAC-F) pour evaluer la douleur chez des aines atteints de demence vivant en milieu de soins de longue duree. Can J Aging 2008;27:45–55.
7. Australian Pain Society. Pain in residential aged care facilities: management strategies. Sydney, NSW: Australian Pain Society; 2005.
8. Balfour JE, O'Rourke N. Older adults with Alzheimer disease, comorbid arthritis and prescription of psychotropic medications. Pain Res Manag 2003;8:198–204.
9. Ballard C, Hanney ML, Theodoulou M, Douglas S, McShane R, Kossakowski K, Gill R, Juszczak E, Yu L. The dementia antipsychotic withdrawal trial (DART-AD): long-term follow-up of a randomised placebo-controlled trial. Lancet Neurol 2009;8:151–7.
10. Centers for Medicare & Medicaid Services. MDS 3.0 for nursing home. Baltimore, MD: Centers for Medicare & Medicaid Services; 2009.
11. Chan S, Hadjistavropoulos T, Williams J, Lints-Martindale A. Evidence-based development and initial validation of the Pain Assessment Checklist for Seniors with Limited Ability to Communicate-II (PACSLAC-II). Clin J Pain 2014;30:816–24.
12. Chibnall JT, Tait RC. Pain assessment in cognitively impaired and unimpaired older adults: a comparison of four scales. Pain 2001;92:173–86.
13. Cipher DJ, Clifford PA, Roper KD. Behavioral manifestations of pain in the demented elderly. J Am Med Dir Assoc 2006;7:355–65.
14. Cleeland CS, Ryan KM. Pain assessment: global use of the Brief Pain Inventory. Ann Acad Med Singapore 1994;23:129–38.
15. Ferrell BR, Novy D, Sullivan MD, Banja J, Dubois MY, Gitlin MC, Hamaty D, Lebovits A, Lipman AG, Lippe PM, Livovich J. Ethical dilemmas in pain management. J Pain 2001;2:171–80.
16. Fuchs-Lacelle S, Hadjistavropoulos T. Development and preliminary validation of the pain assessment checklist for seniors with limited ability to communicate (PACSLAC). Pain Manag Nurs 2004;5:37–49.

17. Fuchs-Lacelle S, Hadjistavropoulos T, Lix L. Pain assessment as intervention: a study of older adults with severe dementia. Clin J Pain 2008;24:697–707.
18. Gagnon M, Hadjistavropoulos T, Williams J. Development and mixed methods evaluation of a pain assessment training program for long-term care staff. Pain Res Manag 2013;18:307–12.
19. Hadjistavropoulos T. Pain assessment in dementia patients. In: Gibson SJ, Weiner DK. Pain in older persons. Seattle: IASP Press, 2005. p. 135–51.
20. Hadjistavropoulos T, Breau L, Craig KD. Pain assessment in adults and children with limited ability to communicate. In: Turk DC, Melzack R, editors. Handbook of pain assessment. New York: Guilford Press, 2011. p. 260–80.
21. Hadjistavropoulos T, Craig KD. A theoretical framework for understanding self-report and observational measures of pain: a communications model. Behav Res Ther 2002;40:551–70.
22. Hadjistavropoulos T, Craig KD, Duck S, Cano A, Goubert L, Jackson PL, Mogil JS, Rainville P, Sullivan MJL, de C Williams AC, et al. A biopsychosocial formulation of pain communication. Psychol Bull 2011;137:910–39.
23. Hadjistavropoulos T, Fitzgerald TD, Marchildon G. Practice guidelines for assessing pain in older persons who reside in long-term care facilities. Physiother Can 2010;62:104–13.
24. Hadjistavropoulos T, Herr K, Turk DC, Fine PG, Dworkin RH, Helme R, Jackson K, Parmelee PA, Rudy TE, Beattie BL, et al. An interdisciplinary expert consensus statement on assessment of pain in older persons. Clin J Pain 2007;23:S1–43.
25. Hadjistavropoulos T, Janzen Claude JA, Hadjistavropoulos HD, Marchildon GP, Kaasalainen S, Gallagher R, Beattie BL. Stakeholder opinions on a transformational model of pain management in long-term care. J Gerontol Nurs 2011;37:40–51.
26. Hadjistavropoulos T, Kaasalainen S, Williams J, Zacharias R. Improving pain assessment practices and outcomes in long-term care facilities: a mixed methods investigation. Pain Manag Nurs 2014;15:748–59.
27. Hadjistavropoulos T, LaChapelle D, Hadjistavropoulos HD, Green S, Asmundson GJG. Using facial expressions to assess musculoskeletal pain in older persons. European Journal of Pain 2002;6:179–87.
28. Hadjistavropoulos T, Marchildon G, Fine P, Herr K, Palley H, Kaasalainen S, Beland F. Transforming long-term care pain management in North America: the policy clinical interface. Pain Med 2009;10:506–20.
29. Hadjistavropoulos T, Voyer P, Sharpe D, Verreault R, Aubin M. Assessing pain in dementia patients with comorbid delirium and depression. Pain Manag Nurs 2008;9:48–54.
30. Hale C, Hadjistavropoulos T. Emotional components of pain. Pain Res Manag 1997;2:217–25.
31. Herr K, Bursch H, Ersek M, Miller LL, Swafford K. Use of pain-behavioral assessment tools in the nursing home: expert consensus recommendations for practice. J Gerontol Nurs 2010;36:18–31.
32. Herr K, Coyne PJ, McCaffery M, Manworren R, Merkel S. Pain assessment in the patient unable to self-report: position statement with clinical practice recommendations. Pain Manag Nurs 2011;12:230–50.
33. Horgas AL, Nichols AL, Schapson CA, Vietes K. Assessing pain in persons with dementia: relationships among the non-communicative patient's pain assessment instrument, self-report, and behavioral observations. Pain Manag Nurs 2007;8:77–85.
34. Husebo BS, Strand LI, Moe-Nilssen R, Husebo SB, Snow AL, Ljunggren AE. Mobilization-observation-behavior-intensity-dementia pain scale (MOBID): development and validation of a nurse-administered pain assessment tool for use in dementia. J Pain Symptom Manag 2007;34:67–80.
35. Inouye SK. Delirium in older persons. N Engl J Med 2006;354:1157–65.
36. Kunz M, Scharmann S, Hemmeter U, Schepelmann K, Lautenbacher S. The facial expression of pain in patients with dementia. Pain 2007;133:221–8.
37. Labus JS, Keefe FJ, Jensen MP. Self-reports of pain intensity and direct observations of pain behavior: when are they correlated? Pain 2003;102:109–24.
38. Lints-Martindale AC, Hadjistavropoulos T, Barber B, Gibson SJ. A psychophysical investigation of the Facial Action Coding System as an index of pain variability among older adults with and without Alzheimer's disease. Pain Med 2007;8:678–89.
39. Martin R, Williams J, Hadjistavropoulos T, Hadjistavropoulos HD, MacLean M. A qualitative investigation of seniors' and caregivers' views on pain assessment and management. Can J Nurs Res 2005;37:142–64.
40. McCusker J, Cole M, Bellavance F, Primeau F. Reliability and validity of a new measure of severity of delirium. Int Psychogeriatr 1998;10:421–33.
41. McGrath PA, Seifert CE, Speechley KN, Booth JC, Stitt L, Gibson MC. A new analogue scale for assessing children's pain: an initial validation study. Pain 1996;64:435–43.
42. Melzack R, Wall PD. Pain mechanisms: a new theory. Science 1965;150:971–9.

43. Misson L, Savoie M, Aubin M, Hadjistavropoulos T, Verreault R. Les défis de l'évaluation de la douleur chez la personne âgée avec des capacités réduites à communiquer en raison d'une démence avancée. Douleurs 2011;12:55–64.
44. Morrison RS, Siu AL. A comparison of pain and its treatment in advanced dementia and cognitively intact patients with hip fracture. J Pain Symptom Manag 2000;19:240–8.
45. Rabins PV, Kasper JD, Kleinman L, Black BS, Patrick D. Concepts and methods in the development of the ADRQL: an instrument for assessing health-related quality of life in persons with Alzheimer's disease. J Mental Health Aging 1999;5:33–48.
46. Royal College of Physicians, British Geriatrics Society and British Pain Society. The assessment of pain in older people: national guidelines. Concise guidance to good practice series, No 8. London: RCP; 2007. p. 8.
47. Scherder EJ, Bouma A. Visual analogue scales for pain assessment in Alzheimer's disease. Gerontology 2000;46:47–53.
48. Snow AL, Weber JB, O'Malley KJ, Cody M, Beck C, Bruera E, Ashton C, Kunik ME. NOPPAIN: a nursing assistant-administered pain assessment instrument for use in dementia. Demen Geriatr Cogn Disord 2004;17:240–6.
49. Warden V, Hurley AC, Volicer L. Development and psychometric evaluation of the Pain Assessment in Advanced Dementia (PAINAD) scale. J Am Med Dir Assoc 2003;4:9–15.
50. Wary B, Serbouti SD, Doloplus CD. Validation d'une échelle d'évaluation comportementale de la douleur chez la personne âgée. Douleurs 2001;2:35–38.
51. Weiner D, Peterson B, Ladd K, McConnell E, Keefe F. Pain in nursing home residents: an exploration of prevalence, staff perspectives, and practical aspects of measurement. Clin J Pain 1999;15:92–101.
52. White C, Katz B. Position statement no. 21: Pain in older people. Sydney, NSW: ANZSGM; 2012.
53. Williams J, Hadjistavropoulos T, Ghandehari OO, Yao X, Lix L. An evaluation of a person-centred care program for long-term care facilities. Ageing Soc 2015;35:457–88.

CHAPTER 14

Assessment of Behavioral and Mood Symptoms in Dementia Patients Suffering from Pain

Michael A. Rapp

Modern conceptualizations of pain emphasize a biopsychosocial perspective, and hence, it becomes important to be able to monitor all of these multidimensional attributes when attempting to assess the pain experience in persons with dementia. Recent studies suggest a strong relationship between pain and the occurrence of behavioral and affective symptoms of dementia (agitation, aggression, restlessness, repetitive vocalization, wandering, depression, and apathy). In moderate and severe stages of dementia, the ability to verbalize pain experiences is likely to decrease, and distress caused by pain may emerge at different levels of behavior as well as affective and emotional responses. This chapter will systematically review the available assessment tools for monitoring behavioral and mood disturbances in persons with dementia. Particular emphasis will be given to potential pain-related impacts. Available evidence of the types of behavior and mood disturbances most strongly associated with pain in persons with dementia will be reviewed.

Behavioral and mood symptoms belong to the most common symptoms in patients suffering from moderate to severe dementia [33, 42, 48, 86, 88]. High prevalence rates of between 75% [76] and more than 90% [18] have been reported for behavioral symptoms related to dementia. The most prevalent classes of symptoms are agitation and depressed mood, and both have been related to the experience of pain [29], in that specific types of agitation may be enhanced in dementia patients suffering from pain, while mood symptoms may both be exacerbated by pain and exacerbate pain symptoms in dementia [11, 41, 43, 65]. These observations are accompanied by the clinical assumption that patients in moderate to severe stages of dementia are less likely to report pain in a verbal manner, and that pain may thus be expressed through other behaviors [4].

The term *agitation* refers to a heterogeneous group of behavioral disorders, including, for example, verbally and physically aggressive behavior [16, 17, 18]. Agitated behaviors are associated with decreased quality of life for patients and caregivers [68], early institutionalization [83], and frequent hospitalizations [82]. Furthermore, agitation leads to increased prescription of antipsychotics [64, 66], which are known to be associated with severe side effects in the elderly [36] and enhanced mortality, especially in demented patients suffering from Alzheimer disease [3]. With respect to caregivers, agitated behaviors are known to lead to less job satisfaction [31] and increased professional burden [25] and risk for a burn-out [75]. Overall, agitation as one of the most frequent challenging behaviors results in enhanced costs for national health systems [8].

Mood symptoms are common in all stages of dementia [12, 62], showing prevalence rates between 30% and 50% [40]. Depressive episodes in a patient's history have been shown to be a risk factor for dementia [58] and vice versa; that is, persistent symptoms of depression might accelerate cognitive and functional decline in cognitively impaired subjects [69]. In contrast to agitation, mood symptoms in nursing home residents with dementia are often underdiagnosed [5, 63] by caregivers and physicians, as (1) they overlap with other symptoms such as apathy [42, 51], (2) they might present differently compared to depression in cognitively unimpaired subjects [28, 37], and (3) patients with severe dementia might be unable to express emotional distress adequately [40].

In the following, available tools for the assessment of (i) behavioral and (ii) mood symptoms in moderate and severe dementia will be reviewed first. A selected number of tools that have been commonly used in the last two decades will be presented. In the second part, studies on the association between pain and behavioral as well as mood symptoms in moderate to severe dementia will be reviewed using the available evidence. One focus of this overview is on the utility of continuous scales of behavioral symptoms that capture degrees of severity in contrast to categorical assessments of the presence versus absence of symptoms. A review of the treatment of behavioral and mood symptoms in moderate to severe dementia is beyond the scope of this chapter. However, it is to be noted that beyond the treatment of pain alone, both nonpharmacological and pharmacological interventions should be considered in patients with dementia suffering from both pain and behavioral disorders [3, 24, 44, 47, 70]; for an excellent review, see [4]. It is concluded with an assessment of future research needs and possibilities.

ASSESSMENT OF BEHAVIORAL SYMPTOMS IN DEMENTIA

The assessment of behavioral symptoms in dementia has been significantly facilitated by the development of standardized observant-based rating scales in the late 80s and the 90s in the last century. A seminal set of papers can be found in a supplement of the *Journal International Psychogeriatrics* in 1996 (Vol. 8, Suppl. 3).

The available assessments can be broadly classified based on the targeted symptoms and the observant for which the assessment was constructed (e.g., nursing staff, caregivers, and physicians). Based on the scope, there are a number of assessments that measure a broad range of behavioral symptoms (which may be referred to as comprehensive assessments), such as the Neuropsychiatric Inventory (NPI [20, 21]), the Nurses' Observation Scale for Geriatric Patients (NOSGER [72]), and the Behavioral Pathology in Alzheimer Disease Rating Scale (BEHAVE-AD [59]). In the United States, a Minimum Data Set (MDS) is mandatory in all nursing homes that participate in Medicare and Medicaid. The MDS measures a broad range of symptoms based on frequency and severity and can be accessed online (http://www.resdac.org/cms-data/files/mds-3.0). A more specific scale is the Cohen-Mansfield Agitation Inventory for the assessment of agitation and aggression (CMAI [18, 19], for which a brief version has been developed (Brief Agitation Rating Scale [19]), and a four-item agitation assessment is available with the Pittsburgh Agitation Scale (PAS [61]).

The Neuropsychiatric Inventory

The NPI was originally developed for clinicians, specifically, neuropsychiatrists, and is based on an extended mental state examination geared toward the assessment of psychopathological alterations in dementia [20, 21]. In 2000, a nursing home version was presented, which was elaborated toward use by nursing home staff and included an item for assessing professional caregiver burden. The original version of the NPI included 10 items, and was extended to 12 items including sleep and eating-related symptoms [20, 21]. In 1998, a caregiver distress rating was added [35]. The original 10 items cover symptoms including hallucinations, delusions, agitation/aggression, dysphoria/depression, anxiety, irritability, disinhibition, euphoria, apathy, and aberrant motor behavior. Symptoms are in a first step rated for their presence or absence, and, if present, rated on a four-point scale for frequency and a three-point scale for severity. Time to complete varies accordingly from 5 to up to 30 minutes. The assessment process requires a clinician to obtain information in a standardized manner from the professional or family caregiver.

Several studies assessed the reliability and validity of the NPI, and most have shown satisfactory reliability and validity [20, 21, 38, 65, 66]. Furthermore, the NPI has been considered to be sensitive to interventions [53]. However, a more recent study reported moderate test–retest reliability and interrater reliability in a nursing home setting [88], which has raised the question whether the initial dichotomous structure of the rating (i.e., absent versus present), together with a focus on mental state examination items, may hamper the reliability and sensitivity to change, especially in cases where behavioral symptoms are of modest severity and/or occur rarely or in a fluctuating manner.

The Behavioral Pathology in Alzheimer Disease Rating Scale

The BEHAVE-AD was originally developed as a broad measure of behavioral and psychological symptoms in dementia [59] and has been extended in 2001 to include a frequency-weighted severity measure (BEHAVE-AD-FW [60]). The BEHAVE-AD is an informant-based interview that takes 10–20 minutes to complete. The scale comprises seven domains, each consisting of several items assessing delusions, hallucinations, activity disturbances, aggressiveness, diurnal rhythm disturbances, affective disturbances, and anxiety; and a global rating assessing the degree of caregiver distress. Each domain is captured with a combined frequency/severity rating on a four-point scale. The scale has shown excellent interrater reliability [54] and has shown to be sensitive to change in a number of pharmacological trials aimed at alleviating behavioral symptoms [9, 22]. It has recently been argued that the scale's sensitivity to change in intervention trials may be due to its comprehensive assessment of symptoms within each domain; for example, not only is delusional ideation rated as present or absent, but specific delusional symptoms common to dementia such as delusions of theft and other misinterpretations of environment and persons related to dementia are also specifically included in the scale [60].

The Nurses' Observation Scale for Geriatric Patients

The NOSGER was originally developed in Switzerland and has been translated into and validated in the English language [72]. Based on 30 items, it assesses a broad range of domains, including cognition, activities of daily living, mood, and social and disruptive behavior. The

30 items are scored for their presence versus absence over the past 2 weeks. It takes about 15 minutes to complete. The scale has shown moderate to good interrater reliability (ranging from 0.53 for disruptive behavior to 0.80 for extended activities of daily living), but high (>0.75) test–retest reliability. The scale has been validated externally and has shown moderate indices of validity for disruptive behavior [72]. Despite these constraints, there is some emerging evidence that the scale may indeed be sensitive to change [77].

The Cohen-Mansfield Agitation Inventory

The CMAI [18, 19] specifically focuses on agitation as well as aggression and can be used by trained nursing staff. It is considered one of the most widely used scales for this type of behavior. The CMAI takes about 20 minutes to complete. Agitation symptoms are assessed with a standardized 29-item version of the CMAI [18, 19], where each item is rated on a seven-point scale of frequency (1 = never; 7 = several times an hour) over the past week. Since the original publication in 1997, several factor analyses have been published [14, 18, 23, 52, 56, 81, 87, 88], showing sufficient construct validity as well as psychometric properties of the scale in general and validating several non-English versions. In most of the studies, similar factor structures were found based on a verbal-physical and an aggressive-nonaggressive dichotomy of agitation symptoms [81]. In an initial factor analysis on 408 nursing home residents [18], four subsyndromes of agitation were found: (1) aggressive behavior, (2) physically nonaggressive behavior, (3) verbally agitated behavior, and (4) hiding and hoarding, which was observed in day shift only. The first three factors have been consistently confirmed by most factor analyses that followed, and only few additional factors have been proposed [56, 81, 88], suggesting that the CMAI is a valid measure of these subtypes of aggression and agitation. In addition, there are recent studies to suggest that the CMAI is sensitive to change in complex interventions [46, 57, 79].

The Pittsburgh Agitation Scale

The PAS [61] was developed as a brief assessment tool for nursing staff familiar with the dementia patient. It takes about 5 minutes to complete and consists of four items measuring aberrant vocalization, motor agitation, aggressive behavior, and resistance to care. Each item is scored on a five-point scale. The scale has shown high interrater reliability (0.80 [61]), but studies on its external validity are lacking [27].

SUMMARY

While the above presentation of assessments for behavioral symptoms in dementia is necessarily selective, it reveals subtle yet important differences, especially when practical questions for researchers of the relationship between pain and behavior in dementia are concerned. As outlined in Table 14-1, the described scales differ by the need for clinicians involved in the assessment and the amount of training required. Furthermore, the scales differ in their reliability, external validity, and the degree to which they have been shown to be sensitive to change. While it is acknowledged that clinically pain (or its treatment) may be related to delusional and hallucinatory symptoms to some degree, we will later see that most of the evidence concerning the pain–behavior association in dementia is based

TABLE 14-1 Summary Characteristics of the Behavioral Assessments under Review

Scale	Time needed to complete	Scope	Specificity	Measurement scale	Reliability	Validity	Sensitivity to change
NPI(-NH)	5–30 min	Broad measure of psychopathological items	12 items, including delusions, hallucinations, agitation/aggression, disinhibition, anxiety, dysphoria/depression, irritability, euphoria, apathy, sleep, appetite, motor alterations	Dichotomous items, severity and frequency rating if present	++	++	+(?)
BEHAVE-AD	20 min	Broad measure of behavioral and psychological symptoms	7 domains, including delusions, hallucinations, activity disturbances, aggression, sleep, affective disturbance and anxiety, caregiver distress	Each domain with several items on a 4-point scale	++	++	++
NOSGER	15 min	Broad range of functions	Domains include cognition, activities of daily living, mood, and social and disruptive behavior	Each domain with several items (presence vs. absence)	+	+	+
CMAI	20 min	Specific assessment of agitation and aggression	Established factorial structure with three factors reflecting aggressive behavior, physically nonaggressive behavior, verbally agitated behavior, and hoarding and hiding	Each factor with several items on a 7-point scale	++	++	++
PAS	5 min	Specific assessment of agitation and aggression	4 items including aberrant vocalization, motor agitation, aggressive behavior, and resistance to care	Each item on a 5-point scale	++	(+)	

Note: See text for details and abbreviations.

Abbreviations: ++, indicates high; +, indicates presence of; (+), indicates first evidence for; (?), indicates conflicting evidence.

on varying degrees and types of agitation and aggressive behavior, and hence, researchers interested in this association may prefer more specific scales rather than general ones. An overview of the behavioral assessment tools is given in Table 14-1.

ASSESSMENT OF MOOD SYMPTOMS IN DEMENTIA

With advancing dementia, the risk for mood symptoms increases especially in nursing home settings [7]. While there are valid self-report scales for depression in older adults, such as the Geriatric Depression Scale (GDS [84]), most studies in moderate and severe dementia will preclude the use of such instruments given restricted reliability of self-report due to cognitive impairments. Hence, most assessments used for moderate to severe dementia rely on observant ratings, which may hamper overall reliability in this population. Furthermore, mood symptoms in dementia patients vary and may present as depressed mood, apathy, or even irritability in many patients [45]. However, there are scales available that have shown satisfactory reliability in dementia for depressed mood (Cornell Scale for Depression in Dementia [CSDD] [2], National Institute of Mental Health [NIMH], Dementia Mood Assessment Scale [DMAS] [73, 74]) and apathy (Apathy Evaluation Scale [AES] [50, 51]), which, in combination with specific scales for irritability and agitation, may enable to capture mood symptoms (and associated behavioral symptoms) in dementia patients suffering from pain.

The Cornell Scale for Depression in Dementia

The CSDD was specifically developed for depression in cognitively impaired individuals [2]. It relies on interviews with caregivers and informants, and an interview and observation of the patient. Assessments are based on the past week. It consists of 19 items, which are scored on a combined three-point frequency/severity measure. Items not only include anxiety, sadness, and anhedonia, but also include irritability and agitation, in addition to lack of interest, retardation, and depressive ideation. Physical symptoms, sleep disturbance, and appetite are included. It takes approximately 20 minutes to administer. A cut-off score of 8 or more has been proposed for the presence of depression in dementia [2]. The CSDD has been shown to be sensitive and specific for the presence of depression in Alzheimer disease (90% sensitivity and 75% specificity [80]). External validity has been shown to be moderate to high [55]. The CSDD has been shown to be sensitive to change in both pharmacological [6] and nonpharmacological interventions [10].

The Dementia Mood Assessment Scale

The DMAS [32, 73, 74] is an instrument developed for the assessment of depressive symptoms in demented patients at the National Institutes of Mental Health. The DMAS is an observer-based rating that takes approximately 10 minutes to complete. It assesses 24 depressive symptoms, and the frequency of each symptom is rated on a seven-point scale (0 = normal; 6 = severely impaired). Items include motor activity, sleep, appetite, energy, irritability, agitation, depressed mood, depressed ideation, and diurnal variation. Factorial analysis suggests two core factors comprising mood-related and cognition-related symptoms [73]. The presence of a depressive syndrome has been associated with a threshold sum score of >17 points [29, 55]. Comparison with the NPI-NH has shown satisfactory validity of the DMAS ($r = 0.71$ [46]). One study suggests the DMAS to be sensitive to change in intervention trails [39].

The Apathy Evaluation Scale

The AES is a specific instrument to assess apathy in patients with dementia, including severe forms of dementia [50, 51]. Different versions of the scale rely on observation by a clinician (AES-C) and a caregiver (AES-I) or on the patient's subjective replies (AES-S). The AES is an 18-point scale that takes 10–20 minutes to administer. Items focus on alterations in overt behavior, cognition, and emotional responsivity. Ratings are based on a four-point scale frequency measure. Scores for the AES range from 18 to 72, and a cut-off of 42 has been suggested for the AES-C. Interrater reliability was found to be excellent (0.94), and internal consistency was high with alpha values ranging from 0.86 to 0.94 [49, 50, 51]. Comparison with the NPI rating scale apathy item [26] showed high external validity of the AES ($r = 0.76$ [46]). The AES has recently been shown to be sensitive to change in nonpharmacological interventions [79].

SUMMARY

The described scales for the assessment of mood symptoms in moderate to severe dementia are a select few; they reflect continuous scales rather than categorical ratings of the presence or absence of symptoms and are thus valid indicators of symptom severity. Given the likely bidirectional nature of the influence between the severity of pain and the severity of behavioral symptoms (compare Fig. 14-1), these tools seem a prerequisite for a better understanding of the pain–mood interaction in dementia. While both the CSDD and the DMAS show stable and comparable psychometric properties, it seems fair to add that the CSDD has been used more frequently and may be seen by some as the gold standard for the assessment of depression in dementia. At the same time, the assessment of apathy in dementia is not free of controversy; however, given that apathy may be a correlate of chronic pain conditions in patients with dementia, further exploration and use of valid scales with continuous severity measures seem to be called for. An overview of the mood assessments is given in Table 14-2.

ASSESSING THE INTERACTION BETWEEN PAIN AND BEHAVIORAL AS WELL AS MOOD SYMPTOMS IN DEMENTIA: WHAT CAN BE LEARNED FROM THE AVAILABLE EVIDENCE?

To evaluate the utility of different assessment tools as well as potential pitfalls in the assessment of behavior and mood symptoms in patients with dementia suffering from pain, key examples from recent intervention and association studies will be presented. These examples are not meant to reflect a systematic review; rather, they were chosen to illustrate potentials and pitfalls in the assessment of mood and behavioral symptoms in dementia patients suffering from pain in order to reach hypotheses and future research needs.

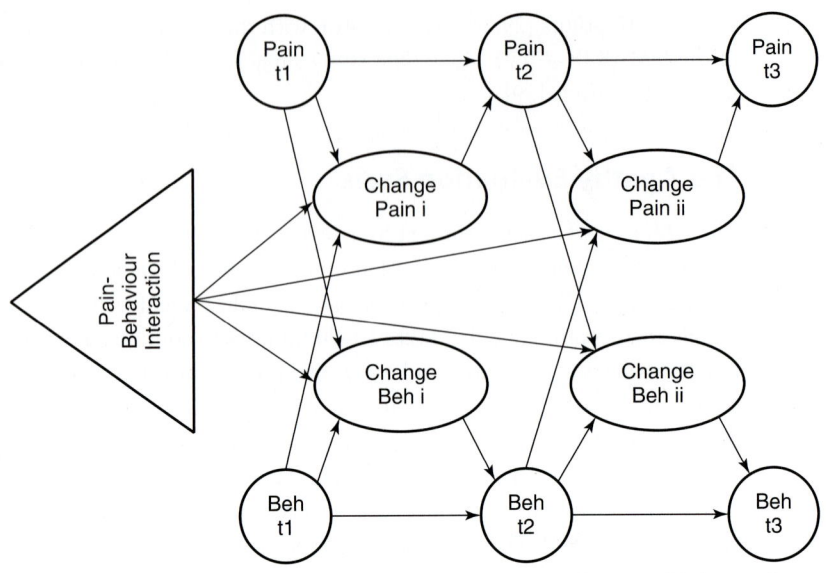

FIGURE 14-1 Schematic representation of the interdependence of pain and behavioral symptoms over time in patients suffering from dementia. Beh indicates behavioral symptoms, t1–t3 indicates measurement points over time, and change i and change ii the respective changes.

For example, Ersek and colleagues [26] used the Iowa Pain Thermometer (IPT) and the Checklist of Nonverbal Pain Indicators (CNPI), together with the CSDD and the PAS, in a multivariate model to predict pain intensity in a sample of 326 nursing home residents (mean age: 83.2 years) suffering from dementia. They found a negative association of pain intensity and PAS agitation in the multivariate model, a finding which they considered unexpected, given that agitation has been shown to be a stable associate of pain in dementia patients. They interpret their finding as either a chance finding or due to the fact that less cognitively impaired residents may have responded to pain with decreased motor behavior since they may be aware that movement increases pain [26] and that more severely cognitively impaired patients may respond to pain with stronger resistance to care. Of note, however, the psychometric properties of the PAS may have precluded the authors from testing differential effects of pain on different types of locomotor behavior. Given that both motor agitation and aggression are both measured with a single item, the PAS did not allow for specifically differentiating between, for example, restless wandering and other types of motor agitation, which have been shown to be differentially associated with pain intensity in another study using the more comprehensive MDS scales for wandering, aggression, and agitation [1]. In a similar vein, Zieber and colleagues [85] found an association between pain and the resistance to care item from the PAS but not to other items assessing aggression and agitation.

Given the potential bidirectional association between negative mood states and pain intensity, that is, the hypothesis that depressed mood may increase pain perception, while increased pain may cause negative mood states (see Fig. 14-1), it seems prudent to consider, both in longitudinal and cross-sectional designs, continuous scales for the assessment of depressed mood in dementia as outlined above, rather than screening tools that are geared toward the dichotomous differentiation between the presence versus the absence of depression. To that end, from a methodological perspective, advanced structural equation modeling techniques as outlined in Fig. 14-1 may be of use. The specific example depicts possible

TABLE 14-2 Summary Characteristics of the Mood Assessments under Review

Scale	Time needed to complete	Scope	Specificity	Measurement scale	Reliability	Validity	Sensitivity to change
CSDD	20 min	Assessment of depression severity in dementia	19 items assessing anxiety, sadness, anhedonia, anergia, apathy, depressive ideation, irritability, and agitation	Items on a 3-point combined frequency/severity scale	++	++	++
DMAS	10 min	Assessment of depression severity in dementia	24 items assessing anxiety, sadness, anhedonia, anergia, apathy, depressive ideation, irritability, and agitation	Items on a 7-point severity scale	++	++	+(+)
AES	10–20 min	Assessment of apathy in dementia	18 items assessing behavior, cognition, and emotional responsivity	Items on a 4-point frequency scale	++	++	+

Note: See text for details and abbreviations.
Abbreviations: ++, indicates high; +(+), indicates moderate; +, indicates presence of.

interactions between longitudinal change over time in pain, and longitudinal change over time in behavior, which can be jointly accounted for in such dual-change score models. Alternatively or additionally, study designs may consider assessing external correlates of pain perception and mood. As an example, Shega and colleagues used a depression screening tool in a sample of 115 community dwelling patients with dementia and their caregivers [67]. They found no association between patient self-report of pain and the mood variables, but an association between caregiver depression and the amount of pain reported. While this finding points to the importance of the reliability and validity of informant-based rating scales using family caregivers who may experience a significant level of stress and depression themselves, it also suggests that levels of depression are difficult to disentangle using depression screening tools, and may thus lead to an underestimation on the influence of depressed mood on pain in dementia patients.

Another concern that is raised here regards the use of dichotomous (presence versus absence) ratings of individual items of behavior and mood disturbance. As an example, despite their relatively large sample, Tosato and colleagues [78] found comparatively small effects of pain on behavioral disturbances in an analytic design that uses the presence versus absence of single items such as delusions, hallucinations, wandering, inappropriate social behavior, and resistance to care. Specifically, in 2822 nursing home residents suffering from dementia, they report odds ratios ranging from 1.37 to 1.48 for resisting care, socially inappropriate behavior, and delusional and hallucinatory symptoms. The respective odds ratios correspond [13] to an effect size in the terminology of Cohen of $d = 0.18–0.22$, which is considered a small effect size [15]. Correlation results with continuous scales report correlations of roughly 0.5, which, assuming an n of 50, corresponds to an effect size of $d = 1.13$, which corresponds to a large effect [15]. Thus, the use of dichotomous rather than continuous rating scales may have precluded this study from finding a clinically relevant effect size.

At the same time, two more recent studies using a comprehensive assessment of agitation and aggression in dementia patients suffering from pain show a differential picture. Husebo et al. [34], in a cluster randomized trial, investigated agitation/aggression using the CMAI in a sample of 352 nursing home residents with moderate to severe dementia and clinically significant behavioral disturbances. The control group homes received treatment as usual, while a stepped pain management approach was implemented in intervention homes. Husebo and colleagues [34] show a decrease across three domains of agitation and aggression, in that verbally agitated behaviors showed the largest significant difference, followed by physically nonaggressive behaviors and aggressive behaviors. Similarly, they found effects of a stepwise protocol for treating pain on the NPI-NH mood cluster and depression, together with improvements in apathy, appetite, and diurnal rhythm disturbances [34]. These two findings from intervention trials clearly highlight the utility of a comprehensive and sufficiently diverse, continuous assessment of both behavioral and mood symptoms, which should also inform natural cross-sectional and longitudinal designs (see also Chapter 7).

The Husebo et al. [34] trials and another recent longitudinal study [71] also point to the need to add state-of-the-art statistical analyses to study designs investigating the pain–behavior interaction in moderate to severe dementia patients. Using mixed longitudinal generalized linear models, Snow et al. [71] were able to control for baseline effects of pain, as well as change over time in pain measures, on the amount of mood and behavioral symptoms reported in a sample of 171 patients over age 60 years diagnosed with dementia in the previous year and with no previous aggression. They found that pain scores at each time period were predictive of increased agitation and depression and decreased pleasant event frequency 4 months later. While such studies cannot clearly disentangle causality in the development of pain and behavioral symptoms, advanced modeling techniques, including the use of multilevel models [58] and dual change score models [30] (Fig. 14-1), should enable a better understanding on the interrelatedness between these important and distressing symptoms in moderate to severe dementia patients.

OVERALL CONCLUSION AND OUTLOOK

Both behavioral and mood symptoms can be reliably assessed in patients with dementia suffering from pain. Available continuous assessments are relatively easy to administer, have proven external validity, and have been shown sensitive to change in intervention trials. Careful choice of outcome and index measures, together with both state-of-the-art and advanced data analysis, should further enhance our understanding of the pain–behavior and pain–mood interaction. Especially longitudinal studies are needed with larger sample to disentangle antecedents, correlates and consequences of pain with respect to behavioral and mood symptoms, and may inform future intervention trials as to the possible utility of pharmacological and nonpharmacological interventions. Such longitudinal studies may also allow for the identification of clusters or profiles of pain and behavioral and mood symptoms, which could allow for the generation of hypotheses for targeted interventions.

REFERENCES

1. Ahn H, Horgas A. The relationship between pain and disruptive behaviors in nursing home residents with dementia. BMC Geriatr 2013;13:14.
2. Alexopoulos GS, Abrams RC, Young RC, Shamoian CA. Cornell scale for depression in dementia. Biol Psychiatry 1988;23:271–84.
3. Ballard C, Hanney ML, Theodoulou M, Douglas S, McShane R, Kossakowski K, Gill R, Juszczak E, Yu LM, Jacoby R, et al. The dementia antipsychotic withdrawal trial (DART-AD): long-term follow-up of a randomised placebo-controlled trial. Lancet Neurol 2009;8:151–7.
4. Ballard CG, Gauthier S, Cummings JL, Brodaty H, Grossberg GT, Robert P, Lyketsos CG. Management of agitation and aggression associated with Alzheimer disease. Nat Rev Neurol 2009;5:245–55.
5. Baller M, Boorsma M, Frijters DH, van Marwijk HW, Nijpels G, van Hout HP. Depression in Dutch homes for the elderly: under-diagnosis in demented residents? Int J Geriatr Psychiatry 2010;25:712–8.
6. Banerjee S, Hellier J, Dewey M, Romeo R, Ballard C, Baldwin R, Bentham P, Fox C, Holmes C, Katona C, et al. Sertraline or mirtazapine for depression in dementia (HTA-SADD): a randomised, multicentre, double-blind, placebo-controlled trial. Lancet 2011;378:403–11.
7. Barca ML, Engedal K, Laks J, Selbaek G. A 12 months follow-up study of depression among nursing-home patients in Norway. J Affect Disord 2010;120:141–8.
8. Beeri MS, Werner P, Davidson M, Noy S. The cost of behavioral and psychological symptoms of dementia (BPSD) in community dwelling Alzheimer's disease patients. Int J Geriatr Psychiatry 2002;17:403–8.
9. Brodaty H, Ames D, Snowdon J, Woodward M, Kirwan J, Clarnette R, Lee E, Lyons B, Grossman F. A randomized placebo-controlled trial of risperidone for the treatment of aggression, agitation, and psychosis of dementia. J Clin Psychiatry 2003;64:134–43.
10. Bruvik FK, Allore HG, Ranhoff AH, Engedal K. The effect of psychosocial support intervention on depression in patients with dementia and their family caregivers: an assessor-blinded randomized controlled trial. Dement Geriatr Cogn Dis Extra 2013;3:386–97.
11. Buffum MD, Miaskowski C, Sands L, Brod M. A pilot study of the relationship between discomfort and agitation in patients with dementia. Geriatr Nurs 2001;22:80–5.
12. Chan SS, Lam LC, Tam CW, Lui VW, Chan WC, Wong S, Wong A, Tham MK, Ho KS, Chan WM, Chiu HF. Prevalence of clinically significant depressive symptoms in an epidemiologic sample of community-dwelling elders with milder forms of cognitive impairment in Hong Kong SAR. Int J Geriatr Psychiatry 2008;23:611–7.

13. Chinn S. A simple method for converting an odds ratio to effect size for use in meta-analysis. Stat Med 2000;19:3127–31.
14. Choy CN, Lam LC, Chan WC, Li SW, Chiu HF. Agitation in Chinese elderly: validation of the Chinese version of the Cohen-Mansfield Agitation Inventory. Int Psychogeriatr 2001;13:325–35.
15. Cohen, J. A power primer. Psychol Bull 1992;112:155–9.
16. Cohen-Mansfield J, Billig N, Lipson S, Rosenthal AS, Pawlson LG. Medical correlates of agitation in nursing home residents. Gerontology 1990;36:150–8.
17. Cohen-Mansfield J, Libin A. Verbal and physical non-aggressive agitated behaviors in elderly persons with dementia: robustness of syndromes. J Psychiatr Res 2005;39:325–32.
18. Cohen-Mansfield J, Marx MS, Rosenthal AS. A description of agitation in a nursing home. J Gerontol 1989;44:M77–84.
19. Cohen-Mansfield J, Dakheel-Ali M, Jensen B, Marx MS, Thein K. An analysis of the relationships among engagement, agitated behavior, and affect in nursing home residents with dementia. Int Psychogeriatr 2012;24:742–52.
20. Cummings JL. The Neuropsychiatric Inventory: assessing psychopathology in dementia patients. Neurology 1997;48:S10–6.
21. Cummings JL, Mega M, Gray K, Rosenberg-Thompson S, Carusi DA, Gornbein J. The Neuropsychiatric Inventory: comprehensive assessment of psychopathology in dementia. Neurology. 1994;44:2308–14.
22. De Deyn PP, Rabheru K, Rasmussen A, Bocksberger JP, Dautzenberg PL, Eriksson S, Lawlor BA. A randomized trial of risperidone, placebo, and haloperidol for behavioral symptoms of dementia. Neurology 1999;53:946–55.
23. de Jonghe JF, Kat MG. Factor structure and validity of the Dutch version of the Cohen-Mansfield Agitation Inventory (CMAI-D). J Am Geriatr Soc 1996;44:888–9.
24. Deudon A, Maubourguet N, Gervais X, Leone E, Brocker P, Carcaillon L, Riff S, Lavallart B, Robert PH. Non-pharmacological management of behavioural symptoms in nursing homes. Int J Geriatr Psychiatry 2009;24:1386–95.
25. Dunkin JJ, Anderson-Hanley C. Dementia caregiver burden: a review of the literature and guidelines for assessment and intervention. Neurology 1998;51:S53–60; discussion S65–7.
26. Ersek M, Polissar N, Neradilek MB. Development of a composite pain measure for persons with advanced dementia: exploratory analyses in self-reporting nursing home residents. J Pain Symptom Manag 2011;41:566–79.
27. Forester B., Oxman T. Measures to assess the noncognitive symptoms of dementia in the primary care setting. J Clin Psychiatry 2003;5:158–63.
28. Gallo JJ, Rabins PV. Depression without sadness: alternative presentations of depression in late life. Am Fam Physician 1999;60:820–6.
29. Geda YE, Rummans TA. Pain: cause of agitation in elderly individuals with dementia. Am J Psychiatry 1999;156:1662–3.
30. Gerstorf D, Lövdén M, Röcke C, Smith J, Lindenberger U. Well-being affects changes in perceptual speed in advanced old age: longitudinal evidence for a dynamic link. Dev Psychol 2007;43:705–18.
31. Gruber-Baldini AL, Boustani M, Sloane PD, Zimmerman S. Behavioral symptoms in residential care/assisted living facilities: prevalence, risk factors, and medication management. J Am Geriatr Soc 2004;52:1610–7.
32. Gutzmann H, Schmidt KH, Richert A, Mayer D. The validity of a German version of the Dementia Mood Assessment Scale (DMAS) by Sunderland. Z Gerontopsychol Psychiatr 2008;21:273–280.
33. Haupt M, Kurz A, Jänner M. A 2-year follow-up of behavioural and psychological symptoms in Alzheimer's disease. Dement Geriatr Cogn Disord 2000;11:147–52.
34. Husebo BS, Ballard C, Cohen-Mansfield J, Seifert R, Aarsland D. The response of agitated behavior to pain management in persons with dementia. Am J Geriatr Psychiatry 2013;S1064:7481.
35. Kaufer DI, Cummings JL, Christine D, Bray T, Castellon S, Masterman D, MacMillan A, Ketchel P, DeKosky ST. Assessing the impact of neuropsychiatric symptoms in Alzheimer's disease: the Neuropsychiatric Inventory Caregiver Distress Scale. J Am Geriatr Soc 1998;46:210–5.
36. Kuehn BM. FDA: antipsychotics risky for elderly. JAMA 2008;300:379–80.
37. Kunik ME, Snow AL, Davila JA, Steele AB, Balasubramanyam V, Doody RS, Schulz PE, Kalavar JS, Morgan RO. Causes of aggressive behavior in patients with dementia. J Clin Psychiatry. 2010;71:1145–52.
38. Lange RT, Hopp GA, Kang N. Psychometric properties and factor structure of the Neuropsychiatric Inventory Nursing Home version in an elderly neuropsychiatric population. Int J Geriatr Psychiatry 2004;19:440–8.

39. Lawlor BA, Aisen PS, Green C, Fine E, Schmeidler J. Selegiline in the treatment of behavioural disturbance in Alzheimer's disease. Int J Geriatr Psychiatry 1997;12:319–22.
40. Lee HB, Lyketsos CG: Depression in Alzheimer's disease: heterogeneity and related issues. Biol Psychiatry 2003;54:353–62.
41. Leonard R, Tinetti ME, Allore HG, Drickamer MA. Potentially modifiable resident characteristics that are associated with physical or verbal aggression among nursing home residents with dementia. Arch Intern Med 2006;166:1295–300.
42. Lyketsos CG, Lopez O, Jones B, Fitzpatrick AL, Breitner J, DeKosky S. Prevalence of neuropsychiatric symptoms in dementia and mild cognitive impairment: results from the cardiovascular health study. JAMA 2002;288:1475–83.
43. Lyketsos CG, Steele C, Galik E, Rosenblatt A, Steinberg M, Warren A, Sheppard JM. Physical aggression in dementia patients and its relationship to depression. Am J Psychiatry 1999;156:66–71.
44. Majić T, Gutzmann H, Heinz A, Lang UE, Rapp MA. Animal-assisted therapy and agitation and depression in nursing home residents with dementia: a matched case–control trial. Am J Geriatr Psychiatry 2013;21:1052–9.
45. Majic T, Pluta JP, Mell T, Aichberger MC, Treusch Y, Gutzmann H, Heinz A, Rapp MA. The pharmacotherapy of neuropsychiatric symptoms of dementia: a cross-sectional study in 18 homes for the elderly in Berlin. Dtsch Arztebl Int 2010;107:320–7.
46. Majić T, Pluta JP, Mell T, Treusch Y, Gutzmann H, Rapp MA. Correlates of agitation and depression in nursing home residents with dementia. Int Psychogeriatr 2012;24:1779–89.
47. Manfredi PL, Breuer B, Wallenstein S, Stegmann M, Bottomley G, Libow L. Opioid treatment for agitation in patients with advanced dementia. Int J Geriatr Psychiatry 2003;18:700–5.
48. Margallo-Lana M, Swann A, O'Brien J, Fairbairn A, Reichelt K, Potkins D, Mynt P, Ballard C. Prevalence and pharmacological management of behavioural and psychological symptoms amongst dementia sufferers living in care environments. Int J Geriatr Psychiatry 2001;16:39–44.
49. Marin RS. Differential diagnosis and classification of apathy. Am J Psychiatry 1990;147:22–30.
50. Marin RS, Biedrzycki RC, Firinciogullari S. Reliability and validity of the Apathy Evaluation Scale. Psychiatry Res 1991;38:143–62.
51. Marin RS, Firinciogullari S, Biedrzycki RC. The sources of convergence between measures of apathy and depression. J Affect Disord 1993;28:117–24.
52. Miller RJ, Snowdon J, Vaughan R. The use of the Cohen-Mansfield Agitation Inventory in the assessment of behavioral disorders in nursing homes. J Am Geriatr Soc 1995;43:546–9.
53. Moniz-Cook E, Vernooij-Dassen M, Woods R, Verhey F, Chattat R, De Vugt M, Mountain G, O'Connell M, Harrison J, Vasse E, et al. A European consensus on outcome measures for psychosocial intervention research in dementia care. Aging Ment Health 2008;12:14–29.
54. Monteiro IM, Boksay I, Auer SR, Torossian C, Sinaiko E, Reisberg B. Reliability of routine clinical instruments for the assessment of Alzheimer's disease administered by telephone. J Geriatr Psychiatry Neurol 1998;11:18–24.
55. Müller-Thomsen T, Arlt S, Mann U, Mass R, Ganzer S. Detecting depression in Alzheimer's disease: evaluation of four different scales. Arch Clin Neuropsychol 2005;20:271–6.
56. Rabinowitz J, Davidson M, De Deyn PP, Katz I, Brodaty H, Cohen-Mansfield J. Factor analysis of the Cohen-Mansfield Agitation Inventory in three large samples of nursing home patients with dementia and behavioral disturbance. Am J Geriatr Psychiatry 2005;13:991–8.
57. Rapp MA, Mell T, Majic T, Treusch Y, Nordheim J, Niemann-Mirmehdi M, Gutzmann H, Heinz A. Agitation in nursing home residents with dementia (VIDEANT trial): effects of a cluster-randomized, controlled, guideline implementation trial. J Am Med Dir Assoc 2013;14:690–5.
58. Rapp MA, Schnaider-Beeri M, Wysocki M, Guerrero-Berroa E, Grossman HT, Heinz A, Haroutunian V. Cognitive decline in patients with dementia as a function of depression. Am J Geriatr Psychiatry 2011;19:357–63.
59. Reisberg B, Borenstein J, Salob SP, Ferris SH, Franssen E, Georgotas A. Behavioral symptoms in Alzheimer's disease: phenomenology and treatment. J Clin Psychiatry 1987;48:9–15.
60. Reisberg B, Monteiro I, Torossian C, Auer S, Shulman MB, Ghimire S, Boksay I, Guillo Benarous F, Osorio R, Vengassery A, et al. The BEHAVE-AD assessment system: a perspective, a commentary on new findings, and a historical review. Dement Geriatr Cogn Disord 2014;38:89–146.
61. Rosen J, Burgio L, Kollar M, Cain M, Allison M, Fogleman M, Michael M, Zubenko GS. The Pittsburg Agitation Scale: a user-friendly instrument for rating agitation in dementia patients. Am J Geriatr Psychiatry 1994;2:52–9.

62. Rosness TA, Barca ML, Engedal K. Occurrence of depression and its correlates in early onset dementia patients. Int J Geriatr Psychiatry 2010;25:704–11.
63. Rovner BW, German PS, Brant LJ, Clark R, Burton L, Folstein MF. Depression and mortality in nursing homes. JAMA 1991;265:993–6.
64. Salzman C, Jeste DV, Meyer RE, Cohen-Mansfield J, Cummings J, Grossberg GT, Jarvik L, Kraemer HC, Lebowitz BD, Maslow K, et al. Elderly patients with dementia-related symptoms of severe agitation and aggression: consensus statement on treatment options, clinical trials methodology, and policy. J Clin Psychiatry 2008;69:889–98.
65. Selbaek G, Kirkevold Ø, Engedal K. The prevalence of psychiatric symptoms and behavioural disturbances and the use of psychotropic drugs in Norwegian nursing homes. Int J Geriatr Psychiatry 2007;22:843–9.
66. Selbaek G, Kirkevold Ø, Engedal K. The course of psychiatric and behavioral symptoms and the use of psychotropic medication in patients with dementia in Norwegian nursing homes—a 12-month follow-up study. Am J Geriatr Psychiatry 2008;16:528–36.
67. Shega JW, Hougham GW, Stocking CB, Cox-Hayley D, Sachs GA. Factors associated with self- and caregiver report of pain among community-dwelling persons with dementia. J Palliat Med 2005;8:567–75.
68. Shin IS, Carter M, Masterman D, Fairbanks L, Cummings JL. Neuropsychiatric symptoms and quality of life in Alzheimer disease. Am J Geriatr Psychiatry 2005;13:469–74.
69. Singh-Manoux A, Akbaraly TN, Marmot M, Melchior M, Ankri J, Sabia S, Ferrie JE. Persistent depressive symptoms and cognitive function in late midlife: the Whitehall II study. J Clin Psychiatry 2010;71:1379–85.
70. Sink KM, Holden KF, Yaffe K. Pharmacological treatment of neuropsychiatric symptoms of dementia: a review of the evidence. JAMA 2005;293:596–608.
71. Snow AL, Chandler JF, Kunik ME, Davila JA, Balasubramanyam V, Steele AB, Morgan RO. Self-reported pain in persons with dementia predicts subsequent decreased psychosocial functioning. Am J Geriatr Psychiatry 2009;17:873–80.
72. Spiegel R, Brunner C, Ermini-Fünfschilling D, Monsch A, Notter M, Puxty J, Tremmel L. A new behavioral assessment scale for geriatric out- and in-patients: the NOSGER (Nurses' Observation Scale for Geriatric Patients). J Am Geriatr Soc 1991;39:339–47.
73. Sunderland T, Hill JL, Lawlor BA, Molchan SE. NIMH Dementia Mood Assessment Scale (DMAS). Psychopharmacol Bull 1988;24:747–53.
74. Sunderland T, Minichiello M. Dementia Mood Assessment Scale. Int Psychogeriatr 1996;8:329–31.
75. Takai M, Takahashi M, Iwamitsu Y, Ando N, Okazaki S, Nakajima K, Oishi S, Miyaoka H. The experience of burnout among home caregivers of patients with dementia: relations to depression and quality of life. Arch Gerontol Geriatr 2009;49:e1–5.
76. Testad I, Aasland AM, Aarsland D. Prevalence and correlates of disruptive behavior in patients in Norwegian nursing homes. Int J Geriatr Psychiatry 2007;22:916–21.
77. Teut M, Schnabel K, Baur R, Kerckhoff A, Reese F, Pilgram N, Berger F, Luedtke R, Witt CM. Effects and feasibility of an Integrative Medicine program for geriatric patients-a cluster-randomized pilot study. Clin Interv Aging 2013;8:953–61.
78. Tosato M, Lukas A, van der Roest HG, Danese P, Antocicco M, Finne-Soveri H, Nikolaus T, Landi F, Bernabei R, Onder G. Association of pain with behavioral and psychiatric symptoms among nursing home residents with cognitive impairment: results from the SHELTER study. Pain 2012;153:305–10.
79. Treusch Y, Majic T, Page J, Gutzmann H, Heinz A, Rapp MA. Apathy in nursing home residents with dementia: results from a cluster-randomized controlled trial. Eur Psychiatry 2015;30:251–7.
80. Vida S, Des Rosiers P, Carrier L, Gauthier S. Depression in Alzheimer's disease: receiver operating characteristic analysis of the Cornell Scale for Depression in Dementia and the Hamilton Depression Scale. J Geriatr Psychiatry Neurol 1994;7:159–62.
81. Weiner MF, Tractenberg RE, Jin S, Gamst A, Thomas RG, Koss E, Thal LJ. Assessing Alzheimer's disease patients with the Cohen-Mansfield Agitation Inventory: scoring and clinical implications. J Psychiatr Res 2002;36:19–25.
82. Wetterling T, Gutzmann H, Haupt K. Reasons for referral to a gerontopsychiatric department [in German]. Nervenarzt 2008;79:340–7.
83. Yaffe K, Fox P, Newcomer R, Sands L, Lindquist K, Dane K, Covinsky KE. Patient and caregiver characteristics and nursing home placement in patients with dementia. JAMA 2002;287:2090–7.
84. Yesavage JA. Geriatric depression scale: consistency of depressive symptoms over time. Percept Mot Skills 1991;73:1032.

85. Zieber CG, Hagen B, Armstrong-Esther C, Aho M. Pain and agitation in long-term care residents with dementia: use of the Pittsburgh Agitation Scale. Int J Palliat Nurs 2005;11:71–8.
86. Zimmer JG, Watson N, Treat A. Behavioral problems among patients in skilled nursing facilities. Am J Public Health 1984;74:1118–21.
87. Zuidema SU, de Jonghe JF, Verhey FR, Koopmans RT. Agitation in Dutch institutionalized patients with dementia: factor analysis of the Dutch version of the Cohen-Mansfield Agitation Inventory. Dement Geriatr Cogn Disord 2007;23:35–41.
88. Zuidema SU, Derksen E, Verhey FR. Prevalence of neuropsychiatric symptoms in a large sample of Dutch nursing home patients with dementia. Int J Geriatr Psychiatry 2007;22:632–8.

CHAPTER 15

Cognitive Screening for Dementia

Samantha Loi, Terence Chong, and David Ames

Cognitive screening is an essential part of the assessment of the patient with suspected dementia. It serves a number of important purposes: (1) meeting with the patient and establishing rapport, (2) exclusion of potential reversible causes of dementia, (3) clarification of cognitive impairment, and (4) management options.

There is no definitive diagnostic test for certain specific types of dementia including the commonest cause, Alzheimer's disease (AD) which can only be diagnosed through histopathological examination of brain tissue. A combination of history of cognitive impairment from the patient and collateral history, examination, investigations, including imaging and neuropsychological assessment, will help guide the diagnosis of the presence of cognitive impairment, and what type, as well as management strategies. With regard to pain, it is important to consider whether a patient has dementia, and if so, what type, as this will alter the method of assessing, and managing the pain.

HISTORY TAKING

Any assessment of cognition requires a thorough history of the emergence, evolution, nature, and extent of any cognitive problems that are present and the impact that these are having on the life of the patient being assessed, and those close to them. Cognitive assessment begins from the moment one lays eyes on the patient. It is important to seek this information from patients themselves, but research indicates that a history of progressive cognitive decline obtained from a reliable informant is the single most important element of information utilized by practitioners when making a diagnosis of dementia. Common presenting symptoms include forgetting where items are, difficulty remembering people's names, and problems recalling recent events or retaining new information. Many patients with early dementia are repetitive, but their families and friends are more likely to be aware of this than the patients themselves. Questions that inquire about each cognitive domain may also reveal and confirm other cognitive deficits such as executive dysfunction, aphasia, agnosia, and dyspraxia [6]. Asking about the duration, onset, and pattern of symptoms is essential. An acute onset of cognitive symptoms following an infection, or change in medications, is likely to be indicative of a delirium, which is potentially reversible. Key features of a delirium include fluctuating conscious state, disorientation, and sleep–wake disturbance.

Medical history including a history of diabetes, smoking, hypertension, and cerebrovascular disease may indicate that a vascular component is likely to be present in the causation of any deficits, especially if these came on suddenly or deteriorated abruptly [6]. However, these features are also risk factors for AD. Head injury or other related trauma may also be significant risk factors for dementia [7]. Commonly seen in women, hypothyroidism may be a cause of reversible cognitive impairment [2]. Liver and renal disease may also impair cognitive function, but are less common causes of dementia [6]. Various neurological disorders including Parkinson's disease and multiple sclerosis are associated with cognitive changes. A history of heavy alcohol use or alcohol dependence may also indicate a frontal-type impairment picture, but it is difficult to measure the extent to which cognitive impairment relates to alcohol consumption [13]. Obtaining a complete and current list of medications, including any recent changes which coincided with the onset of cognitive problems, may suggest a medication-related cause of cognitive impairment.

Previous psychiatric history is important to obtain, as a history of depression can be a risk factor for dementia [17], and current depression can cause symptoms, such as impaired attention and concentration, which may mimic cognitive impairment. In its most severe form, apparent cognitive impairment due to depression is known as "pseudodementia," as described by Madden et al. [19], and then Kiloh [16] who described a case series of patients, some of whose cognition improved with the treatment of depression. Symptoms of depression such as low mood, loss of interest in activities, social withdrawal, changes in appetite or weight, feelings of guilt, hopelessness and helplessness, and suicidal ideation would prompt referral to a psychiatrist for further clarification, prior to diagnosis of cognitive impairment. Screening tools such as the Geriatric Depression Scale (GDS) may assist with detecting depression in older people.

Additionally, acute episodes of anxiety, posttraumatic stress disorder (PTSD), and schizophrenia can also cause cognitive problems, such as impaired attention and registration. A long history of fluctuating schizophrenia may well be associated with executive dysfunction [28]. Behaviors which are different from usual such as being more argumentative, more stubborn, hoarding behavior, or unusual eating habits (such as a propensity for sweet foods) may also indicate changes in cognition.

As some dementias are familial in origin, it is important to know about the patient's family history of disease. Familial AD (FAD) has its age of onset usually under 65 years old, with mutations in one of three genes generally thought to be causative of FAD. These are (1) alterations in amyloid precursor protein (APP, on chromosome 21); (2) mutations in presenilin-1 (PS1) gene, on chromosome 14, have caused the majority of FAD cases, with more than 70 mutations described; and (3) mutations on presenilin-2 (PS2) gene are less common. These three genetic variants account for 30–50% of all autosomal dominant early-onset cases, or about 10% familial early-onset case [3]. Other hereditary diseases that cause dementia include Huntington's disease, primary frontal dementias, and Parkinson's disease [18] (about 5% of dementia cases are familial).

A functional assessment is important as this will determine the practical support and strategies which a patient with dementia will require. The more advanced the dementia, the more dependent the patient will be. In early stages, independent activities of daily living (ADLs) such as showering, dressing, and feeding self will remain intact, but patients may have difficulties with more complex tasks such as shopping, budgeting, and meal preparation and will require assistance with these. The alterations in ADLs are often gradual, and family carers will gradually take over these previous tasks. Legal information including whether wills and power of attorney have been organized are also an important part of a thorough assessment, as is enquiry about driving ability.

Patients do not always initiate assessment. Their family doctor or family members may have prompted a review. Regardless of who has initiated the assessment, obtaining collateral history is crucial with regard to clarifying symptoms and functional abilities. Different perspectives on the cognitive impairment are often obtained from someone other than the patient. Sometimes the family member may be reluctant to speak about the issues in front of the patient, so structuring the initial assessment in such as way so that both the patient and family member have individual time with the specialist and /or a member of the assessment team is important.

MENTAL STATE EXAMINATION

The mental state examination would focus on markers of cognitive and functional impairment. Patients may have impairments in their ability to groom or dress themselves in dementia or lack motivation or effort to do so in depression. Disinhibited or changed behavior may indicate frontal impairment. Speech should be assessed as it can be affected by dementia - patients may demonstrate word-finding or naming difficulties, or difficulties with comprehension. Affect can provide information about conditions that masquerade as cognitive impairment such as depression or anxiety or point toward frontal impairment. Delusions and hallucinations may indicate psychosis as a primary condition or part of dementia. Cognition, insight, and judgment are discussed later in the Cognitive Screening section.

PHYSICAL EXAMINATION

All patients presenting with possible cognitive impairment should have a physical examination. The adage of "look, feel, move, measure" [25] can be used. The general appearance of the patient may provide some insight into the etiology of the cognitive impairment. A shuffling gait as the patient enters the room, the mask-like facies, and tremor may indicate Parkinson's disease. Shortness of breath and eye abnormalities may indicate other medical explanation. Posture and abnormal movements should also be noted.

Vital signs including blood pressure, heart rate, and rhythm should be checked. Examination of the basic systems including cardiovascular, respiratory, gastrointestinal, and peripheral nervous system may all yield important clues.

A cranial nerve examination and assessment for extrapyramidal signs will also be helpful to detect signs of neurological diseases such as facial weakness or abnormal eye movements. Reviewing the patient for other neurological signs such as sensation, weakness, and reflexes may clarify the need for further investigations. Assessing for the presence of primitive reflexes, or frontal release signs such as the snout, grasp, and sucking reflexes may be indicative of advanced or frontal dementias, those these signs are more often elicited in older people as they age. These reflexes are naturally occurring in infants, and can occur with other neurological diseases. The grasp reflex, a flexing of the thumb and fingers, can be elicited by stroking the patient's palm, between their thumb and forefinger. The snout reflex is a contraction of the patient's muscles which causes the mouth to resemble a snout. The sucking reflex is brought about by lightly tapping the patient's lips with an object such as a tongue depressor or the finger. Sometimes the reflex occurs just with approaching the lips with an object. Referral to a neurologist may be required for further clarification.

TABLE 15-1 Biomedical Investigations in Cognitive Screening

Test	Purpose
Full blood count	Anemia, infections
Electrolytes	Renal impairment, hyponatremia
Liver function tests	Hepatitis, obstruction
Thyroid function tests	Hypo- or hyperthyroidism
B_{12}, folate, vitamin D	Deficiency
Urine	Infection

BIOMEDICAL INVESTIGATIONS

Investigations form a vital part of cognitive screening. All patients should have at least basic screening investigations in order to exclude potential reversible causes of dementia. At the very least, a full blood count, electrolytes, liver function and thyroid function tests, and urine specimen are indicated (see Table 15-1).

Anemia, hypothyroidism, and infections can cause cognitive changes, but with treatment, this may improve. Results of cardiovascular risk factors such as fasting glucose and lipids, and an HbA1C (Hemoglobin A1C) test will also provide further information, especially with regard to management. An ECG (electrocardiogram), if there is a history of cardiac problems, or chest X-ray, if there is a history of smoking, may also be recommended, but may not yield much further useful information. Other investigations such as calcium and C-reactive protein may be indicated.

Brain imaging is an important component of cognitive assessment and has been covered in detail in an earlier chapter. A structural brain image obtained with CT (computerized tomography) or MRI (magnetic resonance imaging) should exclude the presence of tumors, hemorrhage, significant stroke, or obstruction of CSF (cerebro-spinal fluid) flow. Focal atrophy may point to the likely presence of a specific cause for dementia (e.g., frontal atrophy in fronto–temporal dementias, hippocampal atrophy in AD), but generalized atrophy is less specific and is quite common in older people with intact cognitive function. Functional imaging such as SPECT (single photon emission computerized tomography) or PET (positron emission tomography) may be useful particularly where the diagnosis is unclear, if available as access will vary across the globe.

COGNITIVE SCREENING FOR DEMENTIA

It is important to emphasize that like a physical examination, the cognitive examination begins as soon as one lays eyes on the patient as opposed to a discrete section of the interaction with the patient. Clues about a patient's cognitive function can be gleaned from the way they interact and converse during the interview and the accuracy, plausibility, and internal consistency of the content of their conversation. Simple demographic questions such as name, age, address, family structure, and current/past occupation can provide invaluable information. For example, a patient living in a nursing home may say that they are only visiting there, forget they are married or have grandchildren, or they may state their age as 35 years when in fact they are 75 years old. These questions also give an indirect indication of premorbid functioning through occupational information and a sense of their support structures.

TABLE 15-2 Domains Measured by Cognitive Screening Tools

Test	Personal Information	Orientation	Short-Term Memory	Remote Memory	Attention	Naming	Visuospatial Visuo-construction	Other
MMSE		*	*		*	*	*	*
3MS	*	*	*		*	*	*	*
AMTS	*	*	*	*	*	*		
SPMSQ	*	*		*	*			
GPCOG		*	*				*	
RUDAS			*				*	*
MOCA		*	*	*	*	*	*	
NUCOG		*	*	*	*	*	*	*

MMSE = Mini Mental State Examination; 3MS = Modified MMSE; AMTS = Abbreviated Mental Test Score; SPMSQ = Short Portable Mental Status Questionnaire; GPCOG = General Practitioner Assessment of Cognition; RUDAS = Rowland Universal Dementia Assessment Scale; MOCA = Montreal Cognitive Assessment; NUCOG = Neuropsychiatry Unit Cognitive Assessment Tool.

The history that is gathered from the patient and informants should provide fairly useful guiding information as your level of suspicion of the presence of cognitive impairment or dementia. It is also important to enquire about level of education, visual and hearing impairment, and language background in selecting and interpreting cognitive tests. The purpose of cognitive screening tools is to assist in the clarification of whether your suspicion is supported and therefore indicates the need for further investigation or specialist referral.

There is a plethora of tools available for use in cognitive screening. An ideal tool for screening is one that requires minimal training or equipment, is rapid to administer, is reliable, and has good sensitivity and specificity. Challenges in this area include accounting for different levels of education, different language backgrounds, different levels of baseline intellectual functioning, and sensory impairments. This chapter will focus on seven of the shorter clinician-administered tools that take up to 20 minutes or less to administer and one tool for informant history. They do not require extensive training to administer. Table 15-2 refers to the domains measured by the clinician administered tools adapted from Flicker 2010 [8].

The most widely used screening tool is Folstein's Mini-Mental State Examination (MMSE) [9]. This is a 30-point tool that tests domains of orientation, short-term memory, attention, naming, and visuospatial function. A score below 24 is suggestive of dementia. This test has been shown to be reliable, internally consistent, and to have useful cutoff points, as shown in Table 15-3 [20, 26]. The psychometric properties show that it is useful at case finding (i.e., high positive predictive value) in clinical settings where there is high pretest probability and also is useful at ruling out dementia (high negative predictive value) in nonclinical settings [20]. A Cochrane review found that for the prediction of conversion from MCI to dementia, the accuracy of baseline MMSE scores had sensitivities of 23–76% and specificities from 40–94% [1]. It concluded that it is not predictive as a stand-alone tool but would still be useful in a screening process. One of its relative weaknesses is a lack of executive function testing. In clinical practice, this is often coupled with the clock-drawing test which assesses executive and visuospatial function [23].

Two modifications of the MMSE are also available: the Standardized Mini-Mental State Examination (SMMSE), which includes more detailed scoring instructions to improve objectivity, and the Modified MMSE Examination (3MS), which has modifications in the content and order of some existing items as well as the addition of four items with the aim of increased standardization of testing, sampling a wider range of cognitive function, and extending the floor and ceiling [5].

TABLE 15-3 Psychometric Properties of MMSE

Setting	Sensitivity (%)	Specificity (%)	Positive Predictive Value (%)	Negative Predictive Value (%)
Memory clinic	79.8	81.3	86.3	73.0
Hospital	71.1	95.6	94.2	76.4
Community	85.1	85.5	34.5	98.5
Primary care	78.4	87.7	53.6	95.7

The Abbreviated Mental Test Score (AMTS) was described by Hodgkinson in 1972 [12]. It is a very quick-to-administer 10-point scale that tests domains of personal information, orientation, short-term and remote memory, attention, and naming. Again, a relative weakness is the lack of executive function testing, but this can be supplemented with the clock-drawing test. Its sensitivity for detecting dementia ranges from 73% to 100% and specificity from 71% to 100% [14].

The Short Portable Mental Status Questionnaire (SPMSQ) is a quick-to-administer 10-item tool which has demonstrated validity and reliability [5] and assesses personal information, orientation, remote memory, and attention.

The General Practitioner Assessment of Cognition (GPCOG) is a tool that combines nine cognitive and six informant items. It tests domains of orientation, short-term memory, and visuospatial function. It is more reliable and superior to the AMTS in detecting dementia as well as being time efficient to administer with cognitive items taking less than 4 minutes and informant items less than 2 minutes [4]. The tool includes a clock-drawing item. General Practitioners responded favorably to this tool [4]. Its sensitivity for detecting dementia from one study is 85% and specificity is 86% [14].

The Rowland Universal Dementia Assessment Scale (RUDAS) was developed with the aim of being valid across cultural groups. This is in contrast to the above tools which were developed and tested in an English-speaking cultural context. The RUDAS takes around 10 minutes to complete and contains six items resulting in 30 points. It tests short-term memory, visuospatial function, and executive function [24]. When using a cutoff score of 23, its sensitivity for detecting dementia was 89% and specificity was 98% [14].

The Montreal Cognitive Assessment (MoCA) assesses the major cognitive domains within 10 minutes and has been validated in a number of different languages which might recommend it for cross-cultural populations [21]. It is currently available in 46 languages and dialects (including five versions of Chinese). An electronic version is also available.

The NUCOG was developed at the Neuropsychiatry Unit, Royal Melbourne Hospital, and is a multidimensional cognitive assessment screening tool with 21 items that cover the five major cognitive domains (executive, attention, language, memory, and visuospatial function), which takes about 20 minutes to administer. It has high levels of reliability and face validity and is able to differentiate patients with dementia from controls and also to differentiate dementia subgroups, when compared to the MMSE. It has a sensitivity of 84% and specificity of 86% for detecting dementia [27]. An electronic version is also available.

The IQCODE is an example of an informant test which can be useful to complement cognitive tools, particularly in situations where patients are uncooperative, acutely unwell, or have low literacy or education levels. The 16-item short version is commonly used and performs well as a screening tool for dementia as well as being relatively unaffected by culture, language, and education [15]. The Cochrane reviews in Table 15-4 demonstrate the

TABLE 15-4 Psychometric Properties of IQCODE

Setting	Cutoff	Sensitivity (%)	Specificity (%)	Positive Likelihood Ratio	Negative Likelihood Ratio
Community	3.3	80	84	5.2	0.23
Secondary care	3.3	91	66	2.7	0.14
Primary care	3.7	75	98		
Primary care	3.2	100	76		

usefulness of the IQCODE, although the primary care data are limited by only being from one study [10, 11, 22].

Other available tools such as the Alzheimer's Disease Assessment Scale Cognitive and Noncognitive Sections (ADAS-Cog and ADAS-Non-Cog) take significantly longer to administer, and thus, they may not be as practical as screening tools.

NEUROPSYCHOLOGICAL ASSESSMENT

Neuropsychological assessment involves a few hours of detailed testing of the various cognitive domains which are consistent with the patient's education, culture, and previous knowledge. Usually specialist training in this area is required. However, not all regions are able to source this type of assessment, nor may this be necessary. Neuropsychological assessment may be indicated when further clarification of the type of cognitive impairment is required. For example, this may be required in a younger patient, or a previously high-functioning patient with suspected memory problems who may be able to "hide" any deficits, and general cognitive screening may not be sufficiently sensitive to uncover these.

It is generally preferable to perform neuropsychological assessment when the patient is "at their best," that is, with glasses, hearing aids, at their best time of the day, etc. This also means when any physical or psychiatric illness is properly treated, for example, depression or schizophrenia. If they have had electroconvulsive therapy (ECT), it is best to wait at least 6 months before attempting neuropsychological assessment. Interpreters, sufficient time, and even assessment in the patient's home may all assist in maximizing the patient's performance.

Neuropsychologists will generally need to know the background of the patient being referred and the specific questions being asked. This will then determine what kind of tests they will do. They will be able to provide a profile of the patient's cognitive domains—memory (long and short term), learning, attention, language, reading, problem-solving, and other behavioral and thinking abilities. The information gathered from this assessment may help clarifying the type of cognitive impairment, and provide a profile of the patient's strengths and weaknesses, and of relevance, strategies to manage their deficits.

MANAGEMENT

The history, examination, investigations, and cognitive examination combined, will all assist in clarifying the type of cognitive impairment and the subsequent management. Discussion and psychoeducation about the diagnosis, ramifications, and prognosis with the patient and their family is necessary. Ongoing review will be required. Referral to the local carer and consumer body, such as the Alzheimer's Association, may also provide additional support. There are limited drug treatments for certain dementias such as AD, and cholinesterase inhibitors such as donepezil, galantamine, and rivastigmine, as well as the *N*-methyl-D-aspartate (NMDA)-receptor antagonist memantine which have been shown to have some benefits in functioning in some people. Adequate control of vascular risk factors such as cholesterol, blood pressure, glucose, smoking, and regular physical activity are also useful management strategies. Psychotropic medications such as risperidone, olanzapine, or quetiapine, often used to treat difficult behaviors seen in dementia, have been found to have increased risk of stroke and sudden death, and alternative nonpharmacological management strategies are first line.

The presence of cognitive impairment will help guide assessment and management of pain. For example patients who have mild-to-moderate cognitive deficits who have some aphasia and word finding difficulties, may not be able to articulate fully the presence of pain, the type, or its precipitants. Hence, the use of alternative pain measures such as the Abbey Pain Scale may yield more information, rather than simply asking. In patients with more severe dementia, questioning them about pain may be futile, and this may have to be gauged by looking at behavior, for example, if agitation is observed in the context of transfers or dressing, or if a person grimaces at certain times. Treating staff will need to regularly assess for pain appropriately, and assessment types may change as the cognitive impairment progresses. It is important to have a high index of suspicion of pain as a cause of agitation or behaviors of concern.

The presence of pain in a person with dementia may also manifest in difficult behaviors such as aggression or withdrawal. These behaviors may be mistakenly treated with inappropriate medications (such as antipsychotics and benzodiazepines) which may cause adverse effects, if pain has not been adequately assessed to be present. Once the presence of pain has been established, appropriate management strategies need to be implemented. Given that the addition of analgesics can cause side effects, nonpharmacological strategies also need to be considered. Heat or ice packs, massage, or splinting may be simple measures. Discussion with the family or carer may also elicit further strategies which may be effective. Remembering to consider that cognition could potentially influence any clinical encounter is the most important first step in cognitive screening for dementia. This then informs our clinical assessment, including history taking, examination and investigation, which consequently improves our treatment of the patient.

REFERENCES

1. Arevalo-Rodriguez I, Smailagic N, Roqué i Figuls M, Ciapponi A, Sanchez-Perez E, Giannakou A, Pedraza OL, Bonfill Cosp X, Cullum S. Mini-Mental State Examination (MMSE) for the detection of Alzheimer's disease and other dementias in people with mild cognitive impairment (MCI). Cochrane Database of Syst Rev 2015;3:CD010783.
2. Begin ME, Langlois MF, Lorrain D, Cunnane SC. Thyroid function and cognition during aging. Curr Gerontol Geriatr Res 2008;474868:1–11.
3. Bird T. Early-onset familial Alzheimer disease. In: Pagon RA, Adam MP, Bird TD, editors. Gene reviews [Internet]. Seattle: University of Washington; 1993 2014. Accessed at http://www.ncbi.nlm.nih.gov/books/NBK1236/
4. Brodaty H, Pond D, Kemp NM, Luscombe G, Harding L, Berman K, Huppert FA. The GPCOG: a new screening test for dementia designed for general practice. J Am Geriatr Soc 2002;50:530–4.
5. Burns A, Lawlor B, Craig S. Assessment scales in old age psychiatry, 2nd edition. London: Taylor and Francis Group; 2004. p. 40–42, 64.

6. Eastley R, Wilcock G. Assessment of the patient with apparent dementia. In: Ames D, Burns A, O'Brien J. Dementia, 4th edition. Great Britain: Hodder Arnold; 2010. p. 48–54.
7. Felminger S, Oliver DL, Lovestone S, Rabe-Hesketh S, Giora A. Head injury as a risk factor for Alzheimer's disease: the evidence 10 years on; a partial replication. J Neurol Neurosurg Psychiatry 2003;74:857–62.
8. Flicker L. Screening and assessment instruments for the detection and measurement of cognitive impairment. In: Ames D, Burns A, O'Brien J. Dementia, 4th edition. Great Britain: Hodder Arnold; 2010. p. 55–60.
9. Folstein MF, Folstein SE, McHugh PR. "Mini-Mental State." A practical method for grading the cognitive state of patients for the clinician. J Psychiatr Res 1975;12:189–98.
10. Harrison JK, Fearon P, Noel-Storr AH, McShane R, Stott DJ, Quinn TJ. Informant Questionnaire on Cognitive Decline in the Elderly (IQCODE) for the diagnosis of dementia within a general practice (primary care) setting. Cochrane Database of Syst Rev 2014;7:CD010771.
11. Harrison JK, Fearon P, Noel-Storr AH, McShane R, Stott DJ, Quinn TJ. Informant Questionnaire on Cognitive Decline in the Elderly (IQCODE) for the diagnosis of dementia within a secondary care setting. Cochrane Database of Syst Rev 2015;3:CD010772.
12. Hodgkinson HM. Evaluation of a mental test score for assessment of mental impairment in the elderly. Age Ageing 1972;1:223–38.
13. Hulse GK, Lautenschlager NT, Tait RJ, Almeida OP. Dementia associated with alcohol and other drug use. Int Psychogeriatr 2005;17:S109–27.
14. Ismail Z, Rajji TK, Shulman KI. Brief cognitive screening instruments: an update. Int J Geriatr Psychiatry 2010;25:111–20.
15. Jorm AF. The informant questionnaire on cognitive decline in the elderly (IQCODE): a review. Int Psychogeriatr 2004;16:275–93.
16. Kiloh LG. Pseudodementia. Acta Psychiatr Scand 1961;37:336–51.
17. Korczyn AD, Halperin L. Depression and dementia. J Neurol Sci 2009;283:139–42.
18. Lesage S, Brice A. Parkinson's disease: from monogenic forms to genetic susceptibility factors. Hum Mol Genet 2009;18:R48–59.
19. Madden JJ, Luhan JA, Kaplan LA. Non-dementing psychosis in older persons. JAMA 1952;150:1567–70.
20. Mitchell AJ. A meta-analysis of the accuracy of the mini-mental state examination in the detection of dementia and mild cognitive impairment. J Psychiatr Res 2009;43:411–31.
21. Nasreddine ZS, Phillips NA, Bedirian V, Charbonneau S, Whitehead V, Colin I, Cummings JL, Chertkow H. The Montreal Cognitive Assessment, MoCA: a brief screening tool for mild cognitive impairment. J Am Geriatr Soc 2005;53:695–9.
22. Quinn TJ, Fearon P, Noel-Storr AH, Young C, McShane R, Stott DJ. Informant Questionnaire on Cognitive Decline in the Elderly (IQCODE) for the diagnosis of dementia within community dwelling populations. Cochrane Database of Syst Rev 2014;4:CD010079.
23. Shulman KI. Clock-drawing: is it the ideal cognitive screening test? Int J Geriatr Psychiatry 2000;15:548–61.
24. Storey JE, Rowland JTJ, Conforti DA, Dickson HG. The Rowland universal dementia assessment scale (RUDAS): a multicultural cognitive assessment scale. Int Psychogeriatr 2004;16:13–31.
25. Talley NJ, O'Connor S. Clinical examination: a systematic guide to physical diagnosis, 6th edition. Australia: Churchill Livingstone; 2010.
26. Tombaugh TN, McIntyre NJ. The mini-mental state examination: a comprehensive review. J Am Geriatr Soc 1992;40:922–35.
27. Walterfang M, Siu R, Velakoulis D. The NUCOG: validity and reliability of a brief cognitive screening tool in neuropsychiatric patients. Aust NZ J Psychiatry 2006;40:995–1002.
28. Wobrock T, Ecker UK, Scherk H, Schneider-AxMann T, Falkai P, Gruber O. Cognitive impairment of executive function as a core symptom of schizophrenia. World J Biol Psychiatry 2009;10:442–51.

CHAPTER 16

Pain-Related Functional Impairment in Dementia

Wilco P. Achterberg, Bart Plooij, and Margot W. M. de Waal

Functional disability is a common accompaniment of persistent pain. In older adults without cognitive impairment pain often interferes with activities of daily life and particularly impacts on discretionary activities, such as social interaction, home maintenance, and hobbies. It remains unclear whether these functional domains are as relevant in persons with moderate to severe dementia and pain. This chapter will explore those domains of function most impacted by and most relevant for pain in persons with dementia and will provide recommendations for specific tools for monitoring these behaviors and activities in routine clinical practice and research. It is, for a large part, based on three recent systematic reviews [30, 31, 44].

A decrease in the level of physical activity is characteristic of older persons, both with and without dementia. Not surprisingly, individuals that are over 90 years of age are less physically active than people aged 60–74 years and those aged 20–34 years [16].

Next to old age, dementia in itself is highly associated with physical impairment, probably in a reciprocal way. It has been found that with increasing cognitive impairment, gait speed during walking decreases, which cannot be explained by demographic variables, for example, education or age [33]. Inversely, increased levels of physical activity may improve cognitive functioning. In formerly sedentary older people, an increase in cognitive functioning has been shown after a walking intervention during 6 months [19]. More specifically, that study showed a more positive effect of aerobic training contrary to anaerobic training on tasks measuring executive functioning. Also in patients with mild cognitive impairment (MCI), physical activity can improve some cognitive functions [37]. The passive behavior that is often encountered in persons with dementia could be considered to be part of the apathy frequently associated with dementia. The question is, however, to what extend this could also be a sign of and caused by pain [31].

The Canadian study of health and aging found that self-rated pain and cognitive impairment are both independently associated with functional impairment, although the role of cognition seems to have a larger effect size. This holds for both basic and instrumental Activities of Daily Living (ADL), terms that will be explained in the next paragraph. In addition, the highest rates of functional impairment in instrumental ADL were found in people with both pain and cognitive impairment. The authors conclude that "This suggests that pain plays an underappreciated and significant role in the development of functional disability among older adults with cognitive impairment." [42]

Therefore, in this chapter we will examine both the effects of dementia and (additional) pain on daily functioning of persons with dementia.

FUNCTION, ACTIVITIES, AND PARTICIPATION: ADL, IADL, AND THE ICF MODEL

When discussing functional impairment, it is good to give an overview of what these impaired functions are, how they can be measured, and how they should be interpreted in the context of scientific literature and every day consequences.

ADL: Activities of Daily Living

In the International Classification of Functioning Disability and Health (ICF), the WHO defined ADL as a complex coaction of physical abilities, environmental conditions, and personal factors [46].

TABLE 16-1 Barthel Index Scoring Form

Feeding	**Toilet Use**
0 = unable 1 = needs help cutting, spreading butter, etc., or requires modified diet 2 = independent	0 = dependent 1 = needs some help, but can do something alone 2 = independent (on and off, dressing, wiping)
Bathing	**Transfers (Bed to Chair and Back)**
0 = dependent 1 = independent (or in shower)	0 = unable, no sitting balance 1 = major help (one or two people, physical), can sit
Grooming	
0 = needs to help with personal care 1 = independent face/hair/teeth/shaving (implements provided)	2 = minor help (verbal or physical) 3 = independent
Dressing	**Mobility (on level surfaces)**
0 = dependent 1 = needs help but can do about half unaided 2 = independent (including buttons, zips, laces, etc.)	0 = immobile or <50 yards 1 = wheelchair independent, including corners, >50 yards 2 = walks with help of one person (verbal or physical) >50 yards 3 = independent (but may use any aid; for example, stick) >50 yards
Bowels	**Stairs**
0 = incontinent (or needs to be given enemas) 1 = occasional accident 2 = continent	0 = unable 1 = needs help (verbal, physical, carrying aid) 2 = independent
Bladder	
0 = incontinent, or catheterized and unable to manage alone 1 = occasional accident 2 = continent	Total score = _____

Note: Above, the Europe scoring of items is used 0/1/2/3 (with range 0–20 points); the USA scoring of items is 0/5/10/15 (with range 0–100 points).

TABLE 16-2 Katz Index of Independence in Activities of Daily Living

Activities Points (1 or 0)	Independence (1 Point) No Supervision, Direction, or Personal Assistance	Dependence (0 Points) With Supervision, Direction, Personal Assistance, or Total Care
Bathing Points: _____	(1 Point) Bathes self completely or needs help in bathing only a single part of the body such as the back, genital area, or disabled extremity	(0 Points) Need help with bathing more than one part of the body, getting in or out of the tub or shower. Requires total bathing
Dressing Points: _____	(1 Point) Get clothes from closets and drawers and puts on clothes and outer garments completely with fasteners. May have help tying shoes	(0 Points) Needs help with dressing self or needs to be completely dressed
Toileting Points: _____	(1 Point) Goes to toilet, gets on and off, arranges clothes, cleans genital area without help	(0 Points) Needs help transferring to the toilet, cleaning self, or uses bedpan or commode
Transferring Points: _____	(1 Point) Moves in and out of bed or chair unassisted. Mechanical transfer aids are acceptable.	(0 Points) Needs help in moving from bed to chair or requires a complete transfer
Continence Points: _____	(1 Point) Exercises completely by self; self-control over urination and defecation	(0 Points) Is partially or totally incontinent of bowel or bladder
Feeding Points: _____	(1 Point) Gets food from plate into mouth without help. Preparation of food may be done by another person.	(0 Points) Needs partial or total help with feeding or requires parenteral feeding

Total points: _____
Scoring: 6 = High (patient independent) 0 = Low (patient very dependent)

ADL refer to daily self-care activities, such as bathing, personal hygiene and grooming, toilet hygiene, walking, and eating. There are several measurement instruments for measuring ADL function. What particular function is considered an ADL function highly depends on the instrument used (examples: Barthel index [27] and Katz index [17], see Tables 16-1 and 16-2).

IADL: Instrumental Activities of Daily Living

IADL are not strictly necessary for basic day-to-day functioning, but are more or less important to live independently in the community. These functions include shopping, housekeeping, accounting, food preparation, use of communication devices such as telephone and computer, but also transportation and doing the laundry.

There are several evaluation tools, such as the Lawton IADL scale [20]; see Table 16-3.

Functions, Activities, and Participation: The ICF Model

The most widely used model to look at consequences of diseases or afflictions such as arthritis, stroke, or pain is the ICF, which was proposed by the WHO (see Fig. 16-1). In this model, a specific health problem influences functions (e.g., moving a leg), activities

TABLE 16-3 Lawton Instrumental Activities of Daily Living (IADL) Scale

Scoring: for each category, circle the item description that most closely resembles the client's highest functional level (either 0 or 1).

A. Ability to Use Telephone
1. Operates telephone on own initiative—looks up, dials numbers, etc. — 1
2. Dials a few well-known numbers — 1
3. Answers telephone but does not dial — 1
4. Does not use telephone at all. — 0

B. Shopping
1. Takes care of all shopping needs independently — 1
2. Shops independently for small purchases — 0
3. Needs to be accompanied on any shopping trip — 0
4. Completely unable to shop — 0

C. Food Preparation
1. Plans, prepares, and serves adequate meals independently — 1
2. Prepares adequate meals if supplied with ingredients — 0
3. Heats, serves, and prepares meals, or prepares meals, or prepares meals but does not maintain adequate diet — 0
4. Needs to have meals prepared and served — 0

D. Housekeeping
1. Maintains house alone or with occasional assistance (e.g., "heavy work domestic help") — 1
2. Performs light daily tasks such as dish washing, bed making — 1
3. Performs light daily tasks but cannot maintain acceptable level of cleanliness — 1
4. Needs help with all home maintenance tasks — 1
5. Does not participate in any housekeeping tasks — 0

E. Laundry
1. Does personal laundry completely — 1
2. Launders small items—rinses stockings, etc. — 1
3. All laundry must be done by others. — 0

F. Mode of Transportation
1. Travels independently on public transportation or drives own car — 1
2. Arranges own travel via taxi, but does not otherwise use public transportation — 1
3. Travels on public transportation when accompanied by another — 1
4. Travel limited to taxi or automobile with assistance of another — 0
5. Does not travel at all — 0

G. Responsibility for Own Medications
1. Is responsible for taking medication in correct dosages at correct time — 1
2. Takes responsibility if medication is prepared in advance in separate dosage — 0
3. Is not capable of dispensing own medication — 0

H. Ability to Handle Finances
1. Manages financial matters independently (budgets, writes checks, pays rent, bills, goes to bank), collects, and keeps track of income — 1
2. Manages day-to-day purchases, but needs help with banking, major purchases, etc. — 1
3. Incapable of handling money — 0

Score _____   Score _____

Total score: _____

A summary score ranges from 0 (low function, dependent) to 8 (high function, independent) for women and 0 through 5 for men to avoid potential gender bias.

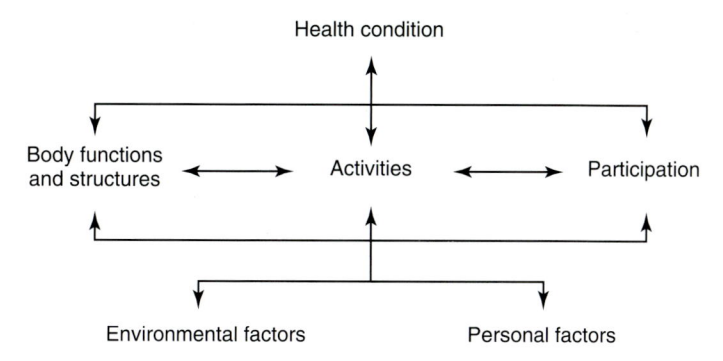

FIGURE 16-1 The International Classification of Functioning, Disability, and Health (ICF), a framework for describing and organizing information on functioning and disability, WHO [46]. It provides a standard language and a conceptual basis for the definition and measurement of health and disability.

(e.g., walking), and participation (e.g., shopping or visiting a relative). It also clarifies, that the strength of the consequences on function, activity, and participation is mediated by other factors, which are related to the individual itself, for instance culture (see Chapter 25) and coping strategies, but also the environment, for instance the presence of a spouse and the presence of formal care [46].

FUNCTIONAL IMPAIRMENT AND DEMENTIA IN THE ICF MODEL

Dementia in itself leads to progressive impairment at each level of the ICF model (function, activities, participation). With disease progression of most subtypes of dementia, participation in general is mostly the first to be impaired because participation functions (such as shopping, visiting friends, work, driving a car) are the most complex activities, requiring complex cognitive tasks skills. In other words, participation tasks heavily rely on higher and more complex cortical functions that are affected early in the disease. Activities and functions are in the course of the disease the next to suffer from the neuropathological changes, affecting the function balance and mobility (leading to falls), and increasing dependence in simple activities, such as bathing and clothing. Apraxia can lead to difficulties in handling even simple tools, such as a knife and fork or a comb. In the end phase of the disease, also simple functions such as moving a limb, urinary and fecal continence, chewing and swallowing are affected.

While the degree of cognitive impairment can be measured with instruments like the Mini-Mental State Examination (MMSE) [12], the severity of the dementia is best measured with instruments that combine cognitive and functional performance. Good examples are the Reisberg Global Deterioration Scale (GDS) [32], the Functional Assessment Staging of Alzheimer's Disease (FAST) [39], or Clinical Dementia Rating (CDR) [29] (see Tables 16-4, to 16-6). On the other hand, it is argued that cognitive decline and functional decline do not always go hand in hand and that functioning is best measured separately, also because cognitive impairment is not the only explanation for functional impairment [11]. (See also paragraph "Measurement Instruments for Function, Activities, and Participation in Dementia" further on.)

TABLE 16-4 Global Deterioration Scale for Assessment of Primary Degenerative Dementia (GDS) (Also Known as the Reisberg Scale)

Diagnosis	Stage	Sign and Symptoms
No dementia	Stage 1: No cognitive decline	In this stage the person functions normally, has no memory loss, and is mentally healthy. People with no dementia would be considered to be in Stage 1.
No dementia	Stage 2: Very mild cognitive decline	This stage is used to describe normal forgetfulness associated with aging, for example, forgetfulness of names and where familiar objects were left. Symptoms are not evident to loved ones or the physician.
No dementia	Stage 3: Mild cognitive decline	This stage includes increased forgetfulness, slight difficulty concentrating, decreased work performance. People may get lost more often or have difficulty finding the right words. At this stage, a person's loved ones will begin to notice a cognitive decline. Average duration: 7 y before onset of dementia.
Early stage	Stage 4: Moderate cognitive decline	This stage includes difficulty concentrating, decreased memory of recent events, and difficulties managing finances or traveling alone to new locations. People have trouble completing complex tasks efficiently or accurately and may be in denial about their symptoms. They may also start withdrawing from family or friends, because socialization becomes difficult. At this stage a physician can detect clear cognitive problems during a patient interview and examination. Average duration: 2 y.
Mid-stage	Stage 5: Moderately severe cognitive decline	People in this stage have major memory deficiencies and need some assistance to complete their daily activities (dressing, bathing, preparing meals). Memory loss is more prominent and may include major relevant aspects of current lives; for example, people may not remember their address or phone number and may not know the time or day or where they are. Average duration: 1.5 y.
Mid-stage	Stage 6: Severe cognitive decline (middle dementia)	People in Stage 6 require extensive assistance to carry out daily activities. They start to forget names of close family members and have little memory of recent events. Many people can remember only some details of earlier life. They also have difficulty counting down from 10 and finishing tasks. Incontinence (loss of bladder or bowel control) is a problem in this stage. Ability to speak declines. Personality changes, such as delusions (believing something to be true that is not), compulsions (repeating a simple behavior, such as cleaning), or anxiety and agitation may occur. Average duration: 2.5 y.
Late Stage	Stage 7: Very severe cognitive decline (late dementia)	People in this stage have essentially no ability to speak or communicate. They require assistance with most activities (e.g., using the toilet, eating). They often lose psychomotor skills, for example, the ability to walk. Average duration: 2.5 y.

TABLE 16-5 Functional Assessment Staging Test (FAST): A Seven-Stage System Based on Level of Functioning

Stage 1: Normal adult
No functional decline

Stage 2: Normal older adult
Personal awareness of some functional decline

Stage 3: Early Alzheimer's disease
Noticeable deficits in demanding job situations

Stage 4: Mild Alzheimer's
Requires assistance in complicated tasks such as handling finances, planning parties, etc.

Stage 5: Moderate Alzheimer's
Requires assistance in choosing proper attire

Stage 6: Moderately severe Alzheimer's
Requires assistance dressing, bathing, and toileting. Experiences urinary and fecal incontinence

Stage 7: Severe Alzheimer's
Speech ability declines to about a half-dozen intelligible words. Progressive loss of abilities to walk, sit up, smile, and hold head up

Note: The FAST focuses more on an individual's level of functioning and activities of daily living versus cognitive decline [39]. A person may be at a different stage cognitively (GDS stage) and functionally (FAST stage).

TABLE 16-6 The Clinical Dementia Rating (CDR) Scale: A Five-Stage System Based on Cognitive (Thinking) Abilities and the Individual's Ability to Function

CDR-0: No dementia

CDR-0.5: Mild
Memory problems are slight but consistent; some difficulties with time and problem-solving; daily life slightly impaired

CDR-1: Mild
Memory loss moderate, especially for recent events, and interferes with daily activities. Moderate difficulty with solving problems; cannot function independently at community affairs; difficulty with daily activities and hobbies, especially complex ones.

CDR-2: Moderate
More profound memory loss, only retaining highly learned material; disoriented with respect to time and place; lacking good judgment and difficulty handling problems; little or no independent function at home; can only do simple chores and has few interests.

CDR-3: Severe
Severe memory loss; not oriented with respect to time or place; no judgment or problem-solving abilities; cannot participate in community affairs outside the home; requires help with all tasks of daily living and with most personal care. Often incontinent.

Note: Commonly used in dementia research. This is the most widely used staging system in dementia research. Here, the person with suspected dementia is evaluated by a health professional in six areas: memory, orientation, judgment and problem-solving, community affairs, home and hobbies, and personal care and one of five possible stages is assigned [29].

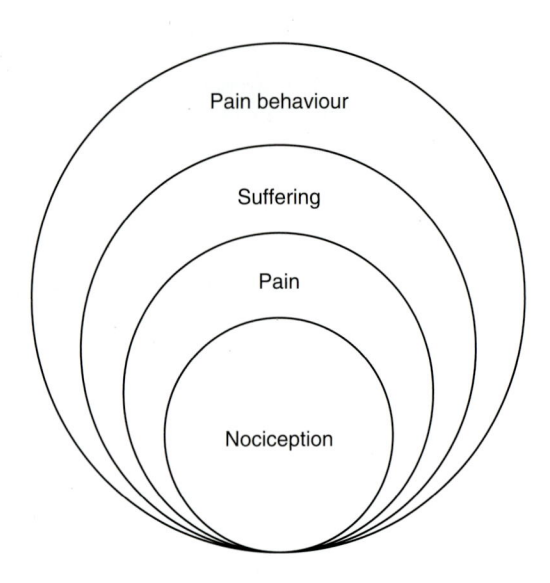

FIGURE 16-2 Loeser's biopsychosocial model of pain.

THE RELATIONSHIP BETWEEN PAIN AND FUNCTIONAL IMPAIRMENT: THE BIOPSYCHOSOCIAL MODEL

The biopsychosocial model of pain by Loeser [22, 23] (see Fig. 16-2) has had a tremendous influence on both pain researchers and pain clinicians. One of the strengths of this model is that it provides an explanatory concept why similar nociceptive stimuli can have different effects on activities and participation in different individuals. In pain research and pain management and rehabilitation practice, especially the pathway to chronic pain and persistent functional impairment (leading to, for instance, the inability to work) is being studied as it has enormous societal, medical, and economic impact. In general, this pathway is as follows: pain may lead to fear of performing certain functions, activities, and participation, and consequently to avoidance of those functions, activities, and participation, which in consequence can lead to persistent disablement. It is however not known if this also applies to persons with dementia.

THE RELATIONSHIP BETWEEN PAIN AND FUNCTIONAL IMPAIRMENT IN PEOPLE *WITHOUT* DEMENTIA

Next to the fact that pain in general can lead to avoidance of activities which trigger the pain, pain in older people without dementia is known to have a negative relationship with the person's physical functioning, including sleeping, eating, and mobility [13, 48]. Moreover, not pain in itself but pain that has consequences on daily functioning will often be the reason to seek help and start treatment.

The relationship of pain with decreased physical functioning is quite strong. The risk of disability and impairment of mobility also is known to increase with the number of painful (musculoskeletal) areas reported [5, 40]. Immobility and avoidance lead to decreased activity and use of muscles, which is a risk factor for (more) pain. This pathway to chronic pain and disability has been described extensively but especially in patients without dementia. It not only provides explanations but also helps to identify targets for treatment. As described above with the model of Loeser, the attitudes and beliefs of older people without dementia influence all aspects of their pain experience, including the effect of pain on functional impairment, and also play an important role in whether and how patients will engage with treatment [1].

THE RELATIONSHIP BETWEEN PAIN AND FUNCTIONAL IMPAIRMENT IN PEOPLE *WITH* DEMENTIA

In people with dementia, it is not expected that attitudes and beliefs have a large influence on the relation between pain and functional impairment. But there are other circumstances that influence the relationship between pain and functional impairment.

First, there is a strong relationship between cognitive impairment (or better: advancing neuropathological changes) and functional impairment. Dementia leads to functional impairment, following the progressive nature of the disease.

Second, persons with dementia experience the effects of both formal and informal caregivers to their health status. When the reaction of the (formal and informal) caregivers is one that tries to be protective and to provide comfort to the persons with dementia, then the avoidance of potential painful activities can be potentiated and independent behavior discouraged. Although this is also the case in patients with other chronic or progressive diseases, this effect in dementia might be larger because the loss of competence that a person with dementia experiences tends to increase the protective behavior of caregivers. This is in line with the operant theory of chronic pain by Fordyce.

Therefore, it is interesting to see what evidence exists on the relationship between pain and functional impairment in people with dementia.

Relationship between Pain and Function in Dementia: Existing Evidence from Cross-Sectional Studies on Pain and Function

Based on a 2014 systematic literature review (van Dalen-Kok et al, 2015), only a small number of studies were identified that describe a relationship between pain and functional limitations in older persons with moderate to severe dementia, like ADL or IADL impairment (six studies), limited mobility or reduced activity/ambulatory status (three studies), and malnourishment (two studies). Interestingly, only few articles report a significant association of pain with functional impairment [21, 41]. The other studies showed no or only weak correlations of pain with functioning. Although one might therefore draw the conclusion that pain is not or only weakly correlated with functional limitations in persons with dementia, we question whether this is appropriate. There is reasonable doubt whether these cross-sectional studies were capable of disentangling the complex relationship between dementia-related and pain-related effects on functional impairment. Interestingly, the study by Lin et al. [21] did find a strong relationship but was different from all the other regular cross-sectional studies. Pain was observed by professionals with the Chinese version of the PAINAD, immediately following instances of routine care. The observed care activities were bathing, assisted transfer from bed to wheelchair, or self-transfer from bed to walking. Pain was observed far more frequently during bathing or assisted transfer than in self-transfer situations: during self-transfer observations, only 1 out of 29 residents (3%) was in pain, whereas during bathing 46% and during assisted transfer 51%. Possibly, pain in dementia is more related to specific functional impairment that is difficult to find using

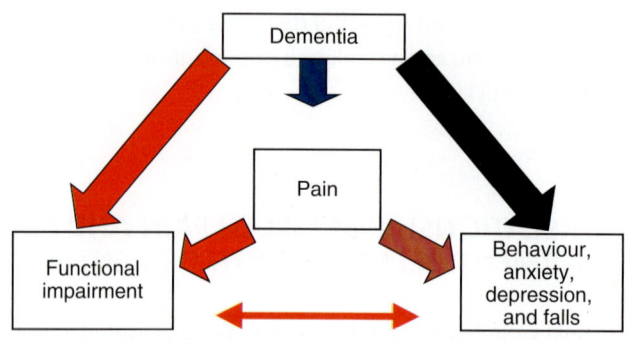

FIGURE 16-3 A schematic model for developing functional impairment in pain and dementia: impairment is directly caused by neuropathological changes in dementia, and by painful conditions or central pain. To a lesser extent, functional impairment is also related to indirect consequences of both pain and dementia: behavioral problems (such as apathy), anxiety, depression and falls, and indirect consequences of these behaviors (physical restraints, psychotropic medication).

more general functional measurement scales. Cipher [7] used path analyses to study the directional influences between cognitive, emotional, and behavioral disturbances and ADLs among residents living in long-term care facilities in the USA. A total of 63% had moderate dementia. The study showed an indirect effect of pain on ADL: pain levels influenced behavioral disturbances and depression, which in turn influenced ADL. One study looked at the activity status [47] and another at the ambulatory status of residents [10]. Again, both found no direct associations between pain and activity or ambulatory status.

To summarize, few cross-sectional studies could show associations between ADL or IADL and presence of pain. One might however have reasonable doubt whether the crude measurement instruments for functional impairment were sensitive enough to pick up the effects of pain, taking into account the complex relationship between dementia-related and pain-related effects on functional impairment. Functional decline can also be the result of other comorbid medical and psychiatric illnesses and sensory impairment [11]. Therefore, we introduce a schematic model to make this complex relationship more comprehensible (see Fig. 16-3). Also, in only one study pain was measured by observations. The study of Lin et al. [21] showed that we might want to observe specific routine care situations more closely.

Relationship between Pain and Function in Dementia: Existing Evidence from Studies of Pain Intervention and Function

Based on a 2012 systematic review on pain interventions in dementia [30] and an additional literature search, two studies were identified that investigated the effect of pain intervention on activities/participation. Treatment with acetaminophen (paracetamol) was studied in a RCT by Chibnall et al. [6]. This crossover study included 25 people with moderate to severe dementia from two nursing homes. Patients were randomly assigned to intervention-placebo or placebo-intervention, consisting of acetaminophen (3000 mg/day) for 4 weeks and placebo for 4 weeks (or vice versa). Between the two phases there was a 1-week washout period. Significant improvement in activities, as measured with the Dementia Care Mapping (DCM) instrument, was reported in patients who received acetaminophen compared to those in the placebo group. More patients participated in media-engagement, work-like activities, and social interaction, and in addition they experienced less unattended distress when they received acetaminophen than when they received placebo. In a large 8-week RCT with follow-up assessment after a 4-week washout period, the effect of pain treatment on ADL was studied among 327 nursing home residents with moderate to severe dementia and significant agitation. Compared to usual care, a stepwise protocol of treating pain (acetaminophen, morphine, buprenorphine transdermal patch, and pregabalin) reduced pain intensity. Although there were no overall improvements in ADL (measured with the Barthel ADL index), in the subgroup receiving acetaminophen ADL improved [35].

MEASUREMENT INSTRUMENTS FOR FUNCTION, ACTIVITIES, AND PARTICIPATION IN DEMENTIA

Objective Measurement of Functions

There are several measurement instruments that give a more-or-less objective evaluation of function (function as defined by the ICF model).

Examples of these instruments are the handheld dynamometer [4], measuring hand grip strength and motricity index [18], measuring movement possibilities of the arm, and mobility and balance tests such as the Berg balance scale [2], POMA [43], and 10-m walking test [34].

These instruments are all tests that rely on the execution of more or less complex instructions. Understanding these instructions requires intact language and other cognitive functions. Performance on these tests is therefore unreliable in advancing dementia.

A recent meta-analysis [28] on performance-based ADL measures in dementia concluded that the DAFS [24] (Direct Assessment of Functional Status) was one of the most commonly used dementia specific performance tests. However, it was not often used in practice, probably because it takes almost 45 minutes to perform. Other ADL performance-based tests take even longer, or are so strongly correlated with cognition (for instance the Test of Everyday Functional Abilities has a correlation of 0.9 with the MMSE), that it seriously raises the question whether they are ADL or cognition tests. Recently, a new performance-based ADL test has been developed for people with moderate to severe dementia, which claims to be more economical: the Erlangen Test for Activities of Daily Living (E-ADL-Test) [26]. Although the first reliability and validity data are promising, the scale has not yet been used in research or in practice. Most dementia performance-based ADL measures were studied in very small samples.

There are some instruments, such as stepmeters and actimeters, that are not dependent on cognitive functions [3]. Although the use for clinical evaluation in everyday practice does not seem very feasible at the moment, they do play an important role in research.

Questionnaires for Measuring Activities and Participation

There are several self-report instruments that can be used to give ratings of one's own functional performance. Some examples are Katz-ADL [17] (measuring basic ADL functions), Lawton IADL [20] (measuring some rather basic instrumental ADL activities), and the Frenchai activity index that measures little more complex functions, which are related to participation in society [38].

Because of deficits in attention, concentration, memory, language, and comprehension of abstract constructs, these instruments are of course difficult to perform reliably by persons with dementia.

Observational Instruments for Measuring Activities and Participation

When the objective measurement of function and self-report is hampered by dementia, the best way to measure function, activities, and participation is by observation. Several instruments are available, such as the Barthel Index [27], Katz and Lawton IADL (see Tables 16-1 to 16-3), all of which can both be filled out by the individual themselves (see Questionnaires for Measuring Activities and Participation), but also by proxy raters (usually care givers), who know the person with dementia well. The instruments mentioned are relatively easy to use and do not require a lot of time to be filled out but are not developed primarily for persons with dementia. Another critical point is that their reliability and validity largely depend on the quality of rating from the proxy. Family members of the person with dementia underestimate the level of impairment [25].

Other more sophisticated instruments exist that do have a specific focus on dementia. DCM is developed to record the activities of a person with dementia [15]. Although this seems to be the most specific, reliable, and valid instrument for measuring performance of persons with dementia living in a long-term care setting and also gives care givers some hints for interventions, the observation time that is needed (several hours!) is certainly a barrier for widespread implementation.

Measures for Assessing Pain Interference

In adults without cognitive impairment it is very common to measure pain-related disability. Persons are asked to self-rate disability as a consequence of pain, for example, in the brief pain inventory [8] or the graded chronic pain scale [45] (see also Chapter 9).

In the systematic review on pain and function [44], only one instrument was identified that was developed to measure actual interference of functioning by pain, which should be rated by observers: the Geriatric Multidimensional Pain and Illness Inventory (GMPI) [9]. It has been designed to assess pain and its functional, social, and emotional consequences and contains 12 items that should be rated by observers. It has three subscales: pain and suffering, interference, and emotional distress. Unfortunately, to our knowledge it did not find its way to regular use in research and clinical practice, and therefore, there is no body of evidence to support the use of this instrument. In addition, attributing disability to pain might be difficult in the presence of much comorbidity.

SO WHAT IS THE ROLE OF PAIN IN FUNCTIONAL IMPAIRMENT IN PERSONS WITH DEMENTIA?

When it comes to defining the exact role of pain in the cascade of impairment of functions, activities, and participation, research literature does not give us a definitive answer. Cross-sectional studies in general do not show significant or clinically important associations, suggesting that there is little effect of pain on functional impairment. We, however, do not agree with this conclusion for several reasons.

1. There is ample evidence that pain is an important causal factor in people without dementia; why should that be different in dementia? One of the reasons could theoretically be that pain in persons with dementia is less hindering actual activities

than in persons without dementia. Although it has been suggested that in some dementia subtypes, for example, Alzheimer's disease, persons with dementia might experience pain less intense [36], others do not agree (see Chapter 3). There is also evidence that persons with dementia react to pain with behavior, among others with withdrawal behavior that is not recognized as pain-related behavior. Further, these behaviors themselves can lead to functional impairment. For instance, withdrawal will almost certainly lead to less activity, and physiologically this has been shown to lead to increased functional impairment ("use it or lose it"). Also, persons with dementia in pain (especially those with agitation) have been found to have a much higher chance of being (chemically and physically) restrained, which certainly has a big effect on physical function [14].

2. Two pain intervention studies that looked at function did find a positive effect of pain management on function [6, 35]. In addition, pain interventions in persons with dementia have shown beneficial effects on behavior and depression, and it is plausible that these effects also will have a positive mediating effect on function as Cipher [7] showed in a pathway analysis.

3. No longitudinal naturalistic studies comparing the course of physical functioning in persons with dementia with and without pain are available. The (few) cross-sectional studies all used rather crude (nonspecific) ADL measures, and the ones that looked more closely at specific functions did find a relationship between pain and function.

Our conclusion therefore is that there probably is an important pathway of pain to functional impairment in dementia, but that studies on pain in persons with dementia in the past have been ignoring this effect, or used inadequate designs and measurement instruments. The effect size of pain on disability may even be larger in persons with dementia because of the stronger behavioral expression of pain in persons with dementia, which is on the one hand, withdrawal, and on the other hand, agitation.

RECOMMENDATIONS FOR RESEARCH

As the effects of pain on the course of physical functioning in persons with dementia have not been studied, there is a great need for this kind of studies: longitudinally and naturalistic. These studies ideally should look at specific functions and activities and not only use a total ADL score. At the moment, because of the scarcity of the literature, no specific instrument can be specifically recommended. DCM and the Barthel ADL index were used in pain intervention studies and proved to be sensitive to change. For evaluation of functioning in intervention studies on a larger scale, the amount of time that DCM takes is however an important drawback.

It is very important that in studies on the effect of pain on the course of physical functioning a (for persons with dementia) a valid pain measurement instrument is used, that is also sensitive to change (see Chapters 9 and 10). In the analysis, several potential confounders or mediating factors, such as sex, age, comorbidity, severity of dementia, behavior, depression, and psychotropic medication, should be accounted for.

Next, we advise that pain intervention studies in persons with dementia should look at functioning as an outcome measure. This is true for future studies, in which functioning should be considered primary outcomes. However, also studies that have been published on pain interventions in persons with dementia with other primary outcome variables but have information on functioning pre- and post-intervention are encouraged to do secondary analyses on the effect of pain management on functioning.

RECOMMENDATIONS FOR CLINICAL PRACTICE: THINK OF PAIN WHEN FUNCTION DETERIORATES!

For clinical practice, it is of the utmost importance to identify functional decline in persons with dementia, in every specific way it presents itself. Whether it is a decline in mobility, eating, bathing, one should always consider pain as a potential causal factor. Therefore, it is very important to try to measure pain during the activity/function that has declined. Although progression of the neuropathology of dementia is a possible cause of functional impairment, one should never assume that this is the only causal factor.

What pain instrument (self-rating or observational instrument) is most adequate, depends on the stage of dementia and the cognitive and communicative functions that are preserved. This is described in the Chapters 9 and 10.

Recognition of decline in function can be achieved with regular, unstructured nursing observations. Regular ADL assessments however are preferred, and we recommend doing them at least once every 3 months. A Barthel or Katz Index takes only a few minutes, and if earlier assessments are stored in a way that change is easily recognizable, it will make the process of recognizing functional impairment easier. In several countries, such as the USA, those regular assessments (with the MDS) are mandatory, and software programs can produce change scores over time.

Although there are now several ADL performance-based assessment instruments available that have been especially developed for dementia, actual implementation and feasibility are still unclear.

Observational instruments, such as the MDS-ADL, Barthel index, or Katz index have proven to be easy to use and feasible in practice, for instance, in long-term care settings, and they have been used in persons with dementia quite often.

Nurses, directors of nursing and medical staff could and should encourage the structured use of these instruments, next to unstructured observations in persons with dementia in order to avoid functional impairment due to pain.

REFERENCES

1. Abdulla A, Adams N, Bone M, Elliott AM, Gaffin J, Jones D, Knaggs R, Martin D, Sampson L, Schofield P. Guidance on the management of pain in older people. Age Ageing 2013;42:i1–57.
2. Berg KO, Wood-Dauphinee SL, Williams JI, Maki B. Measuring balance in the elderly: validation of an instrument. Can J Public Health 1992;83:S7–11.
3. Berlin JE, Storti KL, Brach JS. Using activity monitors to measure physical activity in free-living conditions. Phys Ther 2006;86:1137–45.
4. Bohannon RW. Test-retest reliability of hand-held dynamometry during a single session of strength assessment. Phys Ther 1986;66:206–9.
5. Buchman AS, Shah RC, Leurgans SE, Boyle PA, Wilson RS, Bennett DA. Musculoskeletal pain and incident disability in community-dwelling older adults. Arthritis Care Res (Hoboken) 2010;62:1287–93.
6. Chibnall JT, Tait RC, Harman B, Luebbert RA. Effect of acetaminophen on behavior, well-being, and psychotropic medication use in nursing home residents with moderate-to-severe dementia. J Am Geriatr Soc 2005;53:1921–29.

7. Cipher DJ, Clifford PA. Dementia, pain, depression, behavioral disturbances, and ADLs: toward a comprehensive conceptualization of quality of life in long-term care. Int J Geriatr Psychiatry 2004;19:741–8.
8. Cleeland CS, Ryan KM. Pain assessment: global use of the Brief Pain Inventory. Ann Acad Med Singapore 1994;23:129–38.
9. Clifford PA, Cipher DJ. The Geriatric Multidimensional Pain and Illness Inventory: a new instrument assessing pain and illness in long-term care. Int J Geriatr Psychiatry 2005;19:741–8.
10. D'Astolfo CJ, Humphreys BK. A record review of reported musculoskeletal pain in an Ontario long term care facility. BMC Geriatr 2006;6:5.
11. Desai AK, Grossberg GT, Sheth DN. Activities of daily living in patients with dementia: clinical relevance, methods of assessment and effects of treatment. CNS Drugs 2004;18:853–75.
12. Folstein MF, Folstein SE, McHugh PR. "Mini-mental state". A practical method for grading the cognitive state of patients for the clinician. J Psychiatr Res 1975;12:189–98.
13. Giron MS, Forsell Y, Bernsten C, Thorslund M, Winblad B, Fastbom J. Sleep problems in a very old population: drug use and clinical correlates. J Gerontol A Biol Sci Med Sci 2002;57:M236–40.
14. Hofmann H, Hahn S. Characteristics of nursing home residents and physical restraint: a systematic literature review. J Clin Nurs 2014;23:3012–24.
15. Innes A, Surr C. Measuring the well-being of people with dementia living in formal care settings: the use of Dementia Care Mapping. Aging Ment Health 2001;5:258–68.
16. Johannsen DL, DeLany JP, Frisard MI, Welsch MA, Rowley CK, Fang X, Jazwinski SM, Ravussin E. Physical activity in aging: comparison among young, aged, and nonagenarian individuals. J Appl Physiol (1985) 2008;105:495–501.
17. Katz S, Ford AB, Moskowitz RW, Jackson BA, Jaffe MW. Studies of illness in the aged. The index of ADL: a standardized measure of biological and psychosocial function. JAMA 1963;185:914–9.
18. Kopp B, Kunkel A, Flor H, Platz T, Rose U, Mauritz KH, Gresser K, McCulloch KL, Taub E. The arm motor ability test: reliability, validity, and sensitivity to change of an instrument for assessing disabilities in activities of daily living. Arch Phys Med Rehabil 1997;78:615–20.
19. Kramer AF, Hahn S, Cohen NJ, Banich MT, McAuley E, Harrison CR, Chason J, Vakil E, Bardell L, Boileau RA, Colcombe A. Ageing, fitness and neurocognitive function. Nature 1999;400:418–9.
20. Lawton MP, Brody EM. Lawton instrumental activities of daily living scale (Lawton IADL): handbook of psychiatric measures. Washington, DC: American Psychiatric Press; 2000. p. 131–3.
21. Lin PC, Lin LC, Shyu YI, Hua MS. Predictors of pain in nursing home residents with dementia: a cross-sectional study. J Clin Nurs 2011;20:1849–57.
22. Loeser JD. Pain and suffering. Clin J Pain 2000;16:S2–6.
23. Loeser JD. Perspectives on pain. In: Turner P, editor. Clinical pharmacology and therapeutics. London: MacMillan, 1980. p. 313–6.
24. Loewenstein DA, Amigo E, Duara R, Guterman A, Hurwitz D, Berkowitz N, Wilkie F, Weinberg G, Black B, Gittelman B, Eisdorfer C. A new scale for the assessment of functional status in Alzheimer's disease and related disorders. J Gerontol 1989;44:114–21.
25. Loewenstein DA, Arguelles S, Bravo M, Freeman RQ, Arguelles T, Acevedo A, Eisdorfer C. Caregivers' judgments of the functional abilities of the Alzheimer's disease patient: a comparison of proxy reports and objective measures. J Gerontol B Psychol Sci Soc Sci 2001;56:78–84.
26. Luttenberger K, Schmiedeberg A, Grassel E. Activities of daily living in dementia: revalidation of the E-ADL Test and suggestions for further development. BMC Psychiatry 2012;12:208.
27. Mahoney FI, Barthel DW. Functional evaluation: the Barthel Index. Md State Med J 1965;14:61–5.
28. Martyr A, Clare L. Executive function and activities of daily living in Alzheimer's disease: a correlational meta-analysis. Dement Geriatr Cogn Disord 2012;33:189–203.
29. Morris JC. Clinical dementia rating: a reliable and valid diagnostic and staging measure for dementia of the Alzheimer type. Int Psychogeriatr 1997;9:173–6.
30. Pieper MJ, van Dalen-Kok AH, Francke AL, van der Steen JT, Scherder EJ, Husebo BS, Achterberg WP. Interventions targeting pain or behaviour in dementia: a systematic review. Ageing Res Rev 2013;12:1042–55.
31. Plooij B, Scherder EJ, Eggermont LH. Physical inactivity in aging and dementia: a review of its relationship to pain. J Clin Nurs 2012;21:3002–8.
32. Reisberg B, Ferris SH, de Leon MJ, Crook T. The Global Deterioration Scale for assessment of primary degenerative dementia. Am J Psychiatry 1982;139:1136–39.
33. Rosano C, Simonsick EM, Harris TB, Kritchevsky SB, Brach J, Visser M, Yaffe K, Newman AB. Association between physical and cognitive function in healthy elderly: the health, aging and body composition study. Neuroepidemiology 2005;24:8–14.

34. Salbach NM, Mayo NE, Higgins J, Ahmed S, Finch LE, Richards CL. Responsiveness and predictability of gait speed and other disability measures in acute stroke. Arch Phys Med Rehabil 2001;82:1204–12.
35. Sandvik RK, Selbaek G, Seifert R, Aarsland D, Ballard C, Corbett A, Husebo BS. Impact of a stepwise protocol for treating pain on pain intensity in nursing home patients with dementia: a cluster randomized trial. Eur J Pain 2014;18:1490–500.
36. Scherder EJ, Sergeant JA, Swaab DF. Pain processing in dementia and its relation to neuropathology. Lancet Neurol 2003;2:677–86.
37. Scherder EJ, Van PJ, Deijen JB, Van Der Knokke S, Orlebeke JF, Burgers I, Devriese PP, Swaab DF, Sergeant JA. Physical activity and executive functions in the elderly with mild cognitive impairment. Aging Ment Health 2005;9:272–80.
38. Schuling J, de Haan R, Limburg M, Groenier KH. The Frenchay Activities Index. Assessment of functional status in stroke patients. Stroke 1993;24:1173–77.
39. Sclan SG, Reisberg B. Functional assessment staging (FAST) in Alzheimer's disease: reliability, validity, and ordinality. Int Psychogeriatr 1992;4:55–69.
40. Shah RC, Buchman AS, Boyle PA, Leurgans SE, Wilson RS, Andersson GB, Bennett DA. Musculoskeletal pain is associated with incident mobility disability in community-dwelling elders. J Gerontol A Biol Sci Med Sci 2011;66:82–88.
41. Shega JW, Ersek M, Herr K, Paice JA, Rockwood K, Weiner DK, Dale W. The multidimensional experience of noncancer pain: does cognitive status matter? Pain Med 2010;11:1680–87.
42. Shega JW, Weiner DK, Paice JA, Bilir SP, Rockwood K, Herr K, Ersek M, Emanuel L, Dale W. The association between noncancer pain, cognitive impairment, and functional disability: an analysis of the Canadian study of health and aging. J Gerontol A Biol Sci Med Sci 2010;65:880–6.
43. Tinetti ME, Williams TF, Mayewski R. Fall risk index for elderly patients based on number of chronic disabilities. Am J Med 1986;80:429–34.
44. van Dalen-Kok AH, Pieper MJ, de Waal MW, Lukas A, Husebo BS, Achterberg WP. Association between pain, neuropsychiatric symptoms, and physical function in dementia: a systematic review and meta-analysis. BMC Geriatr. 2015 Apr 19;15:49. d Erratum in: BMC Geriatr. 2015;15:109.
45. Von Korff M, Ormel J, Keefe FJ, Dworkin SF. Grading the severity of chronic pain. Pain 1992;50:133–49.
46. WHO. The International Classification of Functioning, Disability and Health: ICF. Geneva, Switzerland: World Health Organization; 2001.
47. Williams CS, Zimmerman S, Sloane PD, Reed PS. Characteristics associated with pain in long-term care residents with dementia. Gerontologist 2005;45:68–73.
48. Won A, Lapane K, Gambassi G, Bernabei R, Mor V, Lipsitz LA. Correlates and management of nonmalignant pain in the nursing home. SAGE Study Group. Systematic Assessment of Geriatric drug use via Epidemiology. J Am Geriatr Soc 1999;47:936–42.

CHAPTER 17

Nursing Care of Pain in Persons with Dementia

Ann L. Horgas and Toni L. Glover

BACKGROUND AND SIGNIFICANCE

Nurses provide care to older adults with dementia across care settings, including home care, primary care, acute care, and long-term care. Older adults (age 65+) account for half of all hospital inpatient days [48] and approximately 50% of admissions to the intensive care unit (ICU) [37, 46]. It is estimated that five million people currently suffer from Alzheimer's disease (AD) or a related form of dementia in the United States [13]. Globally, this number is estimated as more than 24.3 million people with this disease [16]. Furthermore, with the aging of the population, the number of individuals with dementia is expected to be more than double by 2050 [58]. Thus, nurses should interact with persons with dementia across multiple care settings and need to be knowledgeable about the most effective strategies for managing pain in this population.

Over the past two decades, clinical and empirical efforts have been undertaken to improve the assessment and management of pain in older adults. For instance, in 2001, The Joint Commission (TJC) [31] in the United States mandated pain assessment and management as part of the hospital survey and accreditation process. This accrediting body asserted that patients "have the right to appropriate assessment and management of pain" and declared pain as the "fifth vital sign" [31]. In addition, multiple clinical guidelines have been developed by leading scientific and clinical organizations including the American Geriatrics Society [3, 20], American Pain Society [20], and the American Society for Pain Management Nursing [25]. Despite the TJC mandate and the dissemination of clinical guidelines aimed at improving pain management, there is persistent evidence that pain management for older adults in general, and specifically among persons with dementia, remains suboptimal across care settings [24, 26, 29, 42, 54]. Thus, the purpose of this chapter is to provide the best evidence on the assessment and treatment of pain in older adults with cognitive impairment from a nursing perspective.

NURSING CARE OF PAIN IN PERSONS WITH DEMENTIA

The management of pain is fundamental to the role of the nurse. Pain is defined a complex, multidimensional subjective experience with sensory, cognitive, and emotional dimensions

[3, 39]. In the nursing literature, Margo McCaffery's classic definition of pain remains relevant. She states that "Pain is whatever the experiencing person says it is, existing whenever he says it does" [36]. While focusing on the fact that pain is a subjective experience and that patients' self-report is fundamental to pain assessment, this definition also highlights the difficulty inherent in assessing pain among persons with dementia for whom self-report is often impaired. There is no objective measure of pain; the sensation and experience of pain is subjective. As such, there is a tendency for clinicians to devalue or distrust patients' reports of pain, especially among cognitively impaired adults. Pasero and McCaffery [43] provide a comprehensive chapter on biases, misconceptions, and misunderstandings that hinder clinicians' assessment and treatment of patients who report pain. These issues apply to patients across the life span and across conditions, and led the authors to conclude the following:

> A veritable mountain of literature published during the past three decades attests to the undertreatment of pain. Much of this literature is consistent with the hypothesis that human beings, including health care providers in all societies, have strong tendencies or motivations to deny or discount pain, especially severe pain, and to avoid relieving the pain. Certainly we should struggle to identify and correct personal tendencies that lead to inadequate pain management, but this may not be a battle that can be won. Perhaps it is best to assume that there are far too many biases to overcome and that the best strategy is to establish policies and procedures that protect patients and ourselves from being victims of these influences (p. 48).

Among older adults, there is persistent evidence that pain is underdetected and poorly managed [24, 29, 30, 53]. Unmanaged pain contributes to functional disability, poor sleep, and depression. There are a number of factors that contribute to the undertreatment of pain, including individual- and caregiver-based factors. Individual factors that impair appropriate pain management include the belief that pain is a normal part of aging, concerns about being labeled a hypochondriac or complainer, fear of the meaning of pain in relation to disease progression or prognosis, and fear of opioid addiction and analgesics [2, 19]. Dementia complicates pain assessment and management process because, as the disease progresses, it impairs older adults' ability to recognize, recall, and report pain [29, 53]. In advanced dementia, unmanaged pain exacerbates cognitive impairment and contributes to an increase in disruptive behaviors [4, 34, 40].

Pain assessment and management are also influenced by provider-based factors. Health-care providers often share the mistaken belief that pain is a part of the normal aging process and avoid using opioids due to fear about potential addiction and adverse side effects [43]. Nurses may experience frustration related to difficulties in obtaining an order for pain medications [6]. Dementia also confounds the pain management process.

Evidence indicates that cognitively impaired elders are prescribed and administered significantly less analgesic medication than cognitively intact older adults [30, 41]. This finding may reflect cognitively impaired adults' inability to recall and report the presence of pain to their health-care providers. It may also reflect caregivers' difficulty detecting pain in this population. There are a number of measurement tools currently available to assess pain in this population (see Chapters 9 and 10 for a more thorough discussion of pain measurement). In addition to measurement tools, however, nurses must be vigilant for indicators of pain in older adults with dementia. The most appropriate approach to providing care to this population starts with the acknowledgment that comorbidities (e.g., osteoarthritis, cancer), procedures (e.g., surgery), and activities (e.g., physical manipulation) can cause acute pain or can exacerbate underlying persistent pain. Thus, the assumption should be that pain exists, unless the evidence indicates otherwise. In addition, nurses and other health-care providers should systematically examine their own biases, beliefs, and behaviors about pain management, and should elicit and understand the challenges, beliefs, and preferences their patients bring to the situation as well [43].

The trajectory of dementia is insidious, and there is no cure for this life-limiting disease. Early integration of palliative care is warranted to clarify goals of care, assist with eventual care transitions, and manage symptoms to improve quality of life and maintain optimal function [9, 47, 55] (see Chapter 22 for a more thorough discussion of palliative care). Many caregivers of loved ones with dementia are burdened with health-care decision-making in advanced dementia because they never discussed goals of care and do not know what the patient would have wanted done to preserve life or manage pain and related symptoms with advanced cognitive impairment. Early integration of palliative care can allay patient and caregiver burden. The Dutch End of Life Dementia Study found, on average, only half of residents with dementia in long-term care settings died peacefully, as perceived by their caregivers [10]. Pain was the most common symptom at end of life [22].

Nursing Assessment of Pain in Persons with Dementia

Pain management requires comprehensive assessment, appropriate pain treatment, and regular reassessment. Thus, nurses must utilize a number of resources and skills to assess pain in persons with dementia. Patients' self-report is considered the gold standard for pain assessment [2, 3]. The first principle of pain assessment is to ask about the presence of pain, even among persons with dementia [43]. There is evidence to suggest that persons with moderate to severe dementia are able to provide self-report of pain if asked with a simple question and allowed sufficient time to answer [15, 32, 56].

In patients with dementia who cannot provide self-report, other assessment approaches must be used to identify the presence of pain. A hierarchical pain assessment approach is recommended that includes four steps: (1) attempt to obtain a self-report of pain; (2) search for an underlying cause of pain, such as surgery, procedure, or skin breakdown; (3) observe for pain behaviors; and (4) seek input from family and caregivers [25, 57]. If any of these steps are positive, the nurse should assume that pain is present and initiate a trial of analgesics in addition to nonpharmacological approaches to reduce pain. Reassessment of pain behaviors after an intervention should be observed to evaluate effectiveness.

Observational techniques for pain assessment focus on behavioral or nonverbal indicators of pain [20, 25, 29]. Behaviors such as guarded movement, bracing, rubbing the affected area, grimacing, painful noises or words, and restlessness are often considered pain behaviors [27, 29]. Caregivers should be encouraged to assess for these behavioral indicators of pain. In the acute care setting, vital signs are often considered physiological indicators of pain. It is important to note, however, that elevated vital signs are not considered a reliable indicator of pain, although they can be indicative of the need for pain assessment [25, 43].

Persons with dementia may also express pain in atypical ways [33]. For instance, changes in behavior may signal the presence of pain. Among nursing home residents with dementia, pain contributes to disruptive or challenging behaviors [4]. In a large sample (N = 56,577) of nursing home residents with dementia, residents with more severe pain were less likely to display wandering behaviors, but more likely to display aggressive and agitated behaviors.

Pain was positively correlated with disruptive behaviors such as aggression and agitation, but negatively related to disruptive behaviors that were accompanied by locomotion (e.g., wandering). These findings indicate that effective pain management may help to reduce aggression and agitation, and to promote mobility in persons with dementia.

To summarize, nurses' assessment of pain in persons with dementia requires systematic and thorough assessment, and recognition of the unique expression of pain in this population. Comprehensive pain assessment should include measures of self-reported pain and pain behaviors, as well as observations for changes in individual's behaviors. Family and caregiver input should be elicited, as these observations can provide important supplemental data about specific behaviors, or changes in behavior, that signal pain in the person with dementia [27].

Nursing Management of Pain in Persons with Dementia

Managing pain in older adults with dementia can be challenging. The main goal is to reduce pain and maximize quality of life [24, 57]. Optimal pain treatment uses a multimodal approach, tailored to the patient, that combines pharmacological and nonpharmacological strategies [57]. Pharmacological interventions are an integral component of pain management in older adults [43] (see Chapter 18 for more information on pharmacologic pain treatment). Pharmaceutical pain management is particularly important in elderly persons with dementia, since their ability to participate in some nonpharmacological pain management strategies may be limited by their cognitive capacity [7].

When choosing pain management strategies, consideration should be given to severity of pain; moderate and severe levels of pain require different treatment modalities in order to provide adequate pain relief. Consideration must also be given to the level of cognitive impairment, as this will influence one's ability to report pain and treatment effectiveness and one's ability to adhere to medication self-management and nonpharmacological treatment options [44]. Overall, the goal is to optimize pain relief while minimizing the potential for negative side effects.

Pharmacological Pain Treatment

Pain treatment with medications involves decision-making based on multiple considerations. Ideally, it is a mutual process among health-care providers, patients, and caregivers, with the goal of optimizing quality of life and functioning [57]. An effective pain management strategy for elderly persons includes a careful discussion of risks versus benefits, consideration of patient comorbidities that may influence the choice of pain medication, frequent reviews of medication regimens used by older adults, and the establishment of clear goals of therapy with the patient and family. It is often a process of trial and error that aims to balance medication effectiveness with management of side effects.

Optimal pain management in older adults with dementia is guided by the following principles [7, 18]. First, the treatment of pain should be initiated immediately upon the detection of pain. Secondly, regularly scheduled (rather than as needed) dosing of pain medications should be employed. Additionally, multiple modalities for the evaluation of pain control should be used, including assessment of verbal, behavioral, and functional responses to pain medication. Pain medication should be titrated according to these responses, and a pain medication regimen should be chosen based on what is known about each individual patient. This includes the severity of cognitive impairment and how this affects the patient's ability to express pain, interaction of pain medications with other medications, and knowledge of pain medication side effects, such as constipation.

Analgesic trials have been advocated as a means to reduce pain in persons with dementia, and several systematic studies of this approach have been reported. Horgas and Elliott [12] investigated the effect of the scheduled dosing of extended-release acetaminophen (1.3 g every 8 hours) acetaminophen in reducing observable pain behaviors in persons with moderate to severe dementia. Using a within-subjects ABAB withdrawal design, data on behavioral pain indicators were collected daily for 24 days. The results indicated that, during treatment phases, pain behaviors decreased in both frequency and duration relative to the control and baseline phases and increased when treatment was withdrawn. These finding suggest that acetaminophen alone can reduce pain behaviors associated with musculoskeletal pain in persons with dementia.

Nonpharmacological Pain Treatment

Nondrug strategies are an important component of pain management. Many older adults report using nonpharmacological modalities to manage pain [5, 14, 23]. The most commonly reported nonpharmacological strategies used in the acute care setting were relaxation (e.g., breathing, mediation, imagery, and music), activity restriction, massage, and heat/cold application [57]. Some of these interventions can be used in persons with dementia in place of, or as an adjunct to, analgesics. It would be important to elicit information from the patient and caregiver about prior use, history of effectiveness, and preferences for nonpharmacological pain treatment.

Nonpharmacological pain treatment strategies generally fall into two major categories: physical pain relief modalities and psychological pain relief modalities. Physical pain relief modalities include, but are not limited to, physical therapies, use of heat and cold, massage, and movement. Psychological pain relief modalities focus on changes in the person's perception of the pain and improvement of coping strategies [49]. These include relaxation, distraction, and music therapy, among others. Cognitive behavioral treatment, meditation, and biofeedback are commonly used strategies to treat persistent pain in general populations, but would be difficult to implement in persons with dementia. To date, few of these nonpharmacological strategies have been empirically evaluated for their effectiveness in pain management [57].

For persistent pain, several physical strategies such as exercise and electrical stimulation (e.g., TENS) have been evaluated, but the results are equivocal [17]. The American Geriatrics Society Panel on Exercise and Osteoarthritis provided guidelines on exercise prescriptions for older adults with osteoarthritis pain [1]. Recommendations should be individualized based on person's comorbidities, adherence, personal preference, and feasibility of exercise. Massage therapy may be effective to manage chronic low back pain and can be more beneficial when it is combined with education and exercise [17]. Despite many trials of tai chi, the effectiveness of this intervention for chronic pain in older adults is still inconclusive due to methodological issues in the studies [21]. Furthermore, this intervention would not be feasible in persons with moderate or advanced dementia.

In the acute care setting, relaxation, massage, and music are often used to help manage acute pain [57]. Each of these nondrug approaches have demonstrated mixed results, largely due to individual patient preferences and methodological differences in how the studies were conducted. Thus, there is no conclusive evidence that these modalities relieve pain. Instead, they should be considered on an individualized basis, depending on patient preference and response, and as an adjunct to pharmacologic treatment. Further, the appropriateness of these nonpharmacological pain treatments may depend, in part, on the stage of dementia. Persons with mild dementia may be able to actively engage in some of these treatments, but may be less able to do so as the dementia progresses.

Multisensory stimulation environments to treat pain and dementia have been the focus of recent research in the United States, although this approach has been used for several decades in Europe. Snoezelen (a Dutch word that is roughly equivalent to "sniffing and dozing") is a multisensory intervention designed to promote the optimal level of stimulation for persons with dementia [35]. Snoezelen provides stimulation to the five primary senses of sight, hearing, touch, taste, and smell through soft lighting, meditative music, and essential oil aromatherapy. The rationale for this intervention is that this type of sensory environment reduces demands on cognitive abilities and maximizes residual sensorimotor abilities among persons with dementia. A systematic review of the clinical efficacy of snoezelen for older adults with dementia concluded that there was no significant effect of the intervention on behavior, mood, or interactions [8]. In contrast, Schofield and colleagues [50–52] conducted a series of studies evaluating snoezelen to promote relaxation for nondemented patients with chronic pain. These studies showed significant reductions in pain and improvements in psychosocial and physical pain correlates (e.g., sleep, activity) in patients treated with the multisensory intervention as compared to a comparison group receiving traditional relaxation training [51]. To date, no studies have been conducted in older adults with pain and dementia, although a clinical trial of this combined approach is currently being tested in the Netherlands [45].

Kovach and colleagues conducted a series of investigations using a serial trials intervention protocol [33, 34, 45]. This approach used systematic serial assessments and sequential trials of treatments to identify and treat unmet needs, such as pain, that may contribute to challenging or disruptive behaviors among persons with dementia. Interventions include pharmacological and nonpharmacological treatments, both of which were effective in reducing discomfort among nursing home residents with late-stage dementia. In the Netherlands, a clinical trial is underway to test this intervention for pain, challenging behaviors, depression, and quality of life among nursing home residents with mild or moderate dementia. The systematic intervention protocol (training and intervention of the Dutch STA-OP!) is being compared to a control group receiving general training on pain management and challenging behaviors [45]. The protocol involves a multidimensional approach to reducing discomforts that includes both analgesic medications and nonpharmacological comfort interventions such as snoezelen. The study, when completed, should yield important information about the effectiveness and translation of multidimensional interventions in diverse populations of older adults with dementia.

In summary, nonpharmacological treatments are an important part of pain management. These approaches are challenging to study because it is difficult to find a convincing placebo and to control the dose of the treatment. Further, studies have used different study designs, inconsistent measures, and mixed treatment durations. Thus, studies of these non-drug pain treatments have produced limited evidence to support their use. Nonetheless, patients and families express interest in using nonpharmacological strategies to manage pain [11, 23, 28]. Thus, nurses should consider all possible options for managing pain and discuss these approaches with their patients who are sufficiently cognitively intact to do so.

SUMMARY

Nurses have a critical role in assessing and managing pain. The promotion of comfort and relief of pain is fundamental to nursing practice and, as integral members of interdisciplinary health-care teams, nurses must work collaboratively to effectively assess and treat pain. Given the prevalence of pain in older adults in general and specifically among those with dementia, this nursing role is vitally important. A leading palliative care expert in the United States, Dr. Diane Meier, reminds us that physicians are traditionally trained to diagnose and treat disease and many do not receive adequate education in pain and symptom management [38]. Nurses' education traditionally focuses on a holistic assessment of the individual, comprehensive symptom management, and continuous monitoring and reassessment. Thus, nurses have a key role in monitoring and treating pain. In addition, nurses have the primary responsibility to teach the patient and family about pain and how to manage it both pharmacologically and nonpharmacologically. As such, nurses must be knowledgeable about managing pain in older adults with dementia. Moreover, nurses are responsible for basing their practice on the best evidence available, and thereby helping to bridge the gap between evidence, recommendations, and clinical practice.

REFERENCES

1. AGS. Exercise prescription for older adults with osteoarthritis pain: consensus practice recommendations. A supplement to the AGS Clinical Practice Guidelines on the management of chronic pain in older adults. J Am Geriatr Soc 2001;49:808–23.
2. AGS. The management of persistent pain in older persons. J Am Geriatr Soc 2002;50:1–20.
3. AGS. Pharmacological management of persistent pain in older persons. J Am Geriatr Soc 2009;57:1331–46.
4. Ahn H, Horgas A. The relationship between pain and disruptive behaviors in nursing home residents with dementia. BMC Geriatr 2013;13:1471–2318.
5. Barry LC, Gill TM, Kerns RD, Reid MC. Identification of pain-reduction strategies used by community-dwelling older persons. J Gerontol A Biol Sci Med Sci 2005;60:1569–75.
6. Brorson H, Plymoth H, Ormon K, Bolmsjo I. Pain relief at the end of life: nurses' experiences regarding end-of-life pain relief in patients with dementia. Pain Manag Nurs 2014;15:315–23.
7. Buffum MD, Hutt E, Chang VT, Craine MH, Snow AL. Cognitive impairment and pain management: review of issues and challenges. J Rehabil Res Dev 2007;44:315–30.
8. Chung JC, Lai CK, Chung PM, French HP. Snoezelen for dementia. Cochrane Database Syst Rev 2002;4:CD003152.
9. Crowther J, Wilson KC, Horton S, Lloyd-Williams M. Palliative care for dementia—time to think again? QJM 2013;106:491–4.
10. De Roo ML, van der Steen JT, Galindo Garre F, Van Den Noortgate N, Onwuteaka-Philipsen BD, Deliens L, Francke AL. When do people with dementia die peacefully? An analysis of data collected prospectively in long-term care settings. Palliat Med 2014;28:210–9.
11. Dunn KS, Horgas AL. The prevalence of prayer as a spiritual self-care modality in elders. J Holist Nurs 2000;18:337–51.
12. Elliott AF, Horgas AL. Effects of an analgesic trial in reducing pain behaviors in community-dwelling older adults with dementia. Nurs Res 2009;58:140–5.
13. Fargo K, Bleiler L. Alzheimer's Association report. Alzheimer's Demen 2014;10:e47–92.
14. Ferrell B, Casarett D, Epplin J, Fine P, Gloth FM, Herr K, Katz P, Keefe F, Koo PJS, O'Grady M, et al. The management of persistent pain in older persons. J Am Geriatr Soc 2002;50:S205–24.
15. Ferrell BA, Ferrell BR, Rivera L. Pain in cognitively impaired nursing home patients. J Pain Symptom Manag 1995;10:591–8.
16. Ferri CP, Prince M, Brayne C, Brodaty H, Fratiglioni L, Ganguli M, Hall K, Hasegawa K, Hendrie H, Huang Y, et al. Global prevalence of dementia: a Delphi consensus study. Lancet 2005;366:2112–7.
17. Furlan AD, Imamura M, Dryden T, Irvin E. Massage for low back pain: an updated systematic review within the framework of the Cochrane Back Review Group. Spine (Phila Pa 1976) 2009;34:1669–84.
18. Gordon DB, Dahl JL, Miaskowski C, McCarberg B, Todd KH, Paice JA, Lipman AG, Bookbinder M, Sanders SH, Turk DC, Carr DB. American pain society recommendations for improving the quality of acute and cancer pain management: American Pain Society Quality of Care Task Force. Arch Intern Med 2005;165:1574–80.
19. Gordon DB, Pellino TA, Miaskowski C, McNeill JA, Paice JA, Laferriere D, Bookbinder M. A 10-year review of quality improvement monitoring in pain management: recommendations for standardized outcome measures. Pain Manag Nurs 2002;3:116–30.

20. Hadjistavropoulos T, Herr, K, Turk, D, Fine, P, Dworkin RH, Helme R, Jackson K, Parmelee PA, Rudy TE, Lynn BB, et al. An interdisciplinary expert consensus statement on assessment of pain in older persons. Clin J Pain 2007;23:S1–43.
21. Hall A, Maher C, Latimer J, Ferreira M. The effectiveness of Tai Chi for chronic musculoskeletal pain conditions: a systematic review and meta-analysis. Arthritis Rheum 2009;61:717–24.
22. Hendriks SA, Smalbrugge M, Hertogh CM, van der Steen JT. Dying with dementia: symptoms, treatment, and quality of life in the last week of life. J Pain Symptom Manag 2014;47:710–20.
23. Herr K. Chronic pain in the older patient: management strategies. J Gerontol Nurs 2002;28:28–34.
24. Herr K. Pain in the older adult: an imperative across all health care settings. Pain Manag Nurs 2010;11:S1–10.
25. Herr K, Coyne PJ, Key T, Manworren R, McCaffery M, Merkel S, Pelosi-Kelly J, Wild L. Pain assessment in the nonverbal patient: position statement with clinical practice recommendations. Pain Manag Nurs 2006;7:44–52.
26. Herr K, Titler MG, Schilling ML, Marsh JL, Xie X, Ardery G, Clarke WR, Everett LQ. Evidence-based assessment of acute pain in older adults: current nursing practices and perceived barriers. Clin J Pain 2004;20:331–40.
27. Horgas AL, Dunn K. Pain in nursing home residents: comparison of residents' self-report and nursing assistants' perceptions. J Gerontol Nurs 2001;27:44–53.
28. Horgas AL, Elliott, AF. Pain assessment and management in persons with dementia. Nurs Clin N Am 2004;39:593–606.
29. Horgas AL, Elliott AF, Marsiske M. Pain assessment in persons with dementia: relationship between self-report and behavioral observation. J Am Geriatr Soc 2009;57:126–32.
30. Horgas AL, Tsai PF. Analgesic drug prescription and use in cognitively impaired nursing home residents. Nurs Res 1998;47:235–42.
31. Joint Commission on the Accreditation of Healthcare Organization. Accreditation manual for hospitals. Oakbrook Terrace, IL: JCAHO; 2001.
32. Kaasalainen S, Akhtar-Danesh N, Hadjistavropoulos T, Zwakhalen S, Verreault R. A comparison between behavioral and verbal report pain assessment tools for use with residents in long term care. Pain Manag Nurs 2013;14:e106–14.
33. Kovach CR, Cashin JR, Sauer L. Deconstruction of a complex tailored intervention to assess and treat discomfort of people with advanced dementia. J Adv Nurs 2006;55:678–88.
34. Kovach CR, Noonan PE, Schlidt AM, Reynolds S, Wells T. The Serial Trial Intervention: an innovative approach to meeting needs of individuals with dementia. J Gerontol Nurs 2006;32:18–25; quiz 26–17.
35. Maseda A, Sanchez A, Marante MP, Gonzalez-Abraldes I, Bujan A, Millan-Calenti JC. Effects of multisensory stimulation on a sample of institutionalized elderly people with dementia diagnosis: a controlled longitudinal trial. Am J Alzheimer's Dis Other Demen 2014;29:463–73.
36. McCaffery M. Nursing practice theories related to cognition, bodily pain, and man–environmental interaction. Los Angeles: UCLA Students Store; 1968.
37. McNicoll L, Pisani MA, Zhang Y, Ely EW, Siegel MD, Inouye SK. Delirium in the intensive care unit: occurrence and clinical course in older patients. J Am Geriatr Soc 2003;51:591–8.
38. Meier DE. 'I don't want Jenny to think i'm abandoning her': views on overtreatment. Health Aff (Project Hope) 2014;33:895–8.
39. Melzack R, Casey KL. Sensory, motivational, and central control determinants of pain: a new conceptual model. In: Kenshalo DR, editor. The skin senses. Springfield, IL: Charles C. Thomas Press; 1968. p. 423–43.
40. Monroe TB, Misra SK, Habermann RC, Dietrich MS, Cowan RL, Simmons SF. Pain reports and pain medication treatment in nursing home residents with and without dementia. Geriatr Gerontol Int 2013;11:12130.
41. Morrison RS, Magaziner J, Gilbert M, Koval KJ, McLaughlin MA, Orosz G, Strauss E, Siu AL. Relationship between pain and opioid analgesics on the development of delirium following hip fracture. J Gerontol A Biol Sci Med Sci 2003;58:76–81.
42. Morrison RS, Magaziner J, McLaughlin MA, Orosz G, Silberzweig SB, Koval KJ, Siu AL. The impact of postoperative pain on outcomes following hip fracture. Pain 2003;103:303–11.
43. Pasero C, McCaffery M. Pain assessment and pharmacologic management. St. Louis, MO: Mosby Elsevier; 2011.
44. Pergolizzi J, Boger RH, Budd K, Dahan A, Erdine S, Hans G, Kress HG, Langford R, Likar R, Raffa RB, Sacerdote P. Opioids and the management of chronic severe pain in the elderly: consensus statement of an International Expert Panel with focus on the six clinically most often used World Health Organization Step III opioids (buprenorphine, fentanyl, hydromorphone, methadone, morphine, oxycodone). Pain Pract 2008;8:287–313.
45. Pieper MJ, Achterberg WP, Francke AL, van der Steen JT, Scherder EJ, Kovach CR. The implementation of the serial trial intervention for pain and challenging behaviour in advanced dementia patients (STA OP!): a clustered randomized controlled trial. BMC Geriatr 2011;11:12.

46. Pisani MA, McNicoll L, Inouye SK. Cognitive impairment in the intensive care unit. Clin Chest Med 2003;24:727-37.
47. Raymond M, Warner A, Davies N, Nicholas N, Manthorpe J, Iliffe S. Palliative and end of life care for people with dementia: lessons for clinical commissioners. Prim Health Care Res Dev 2013:1-12.
48. Rosenthal RA, Kavic SM. Assessment and management of the geriatric patient. Crit Care Med 2004;32:S92-105.
49. Rudy TE, Hanlon RB, Markham JR. Psychosocial issues and cognitive-behavioral therapy: from theory to practice. In: Weiner DK, Herr K, Rudy TE, editors. Persistent pain in older adults: an interdisciplinary guide for treatment. New York: Springer, 2002.
50. Schofield P. The effects of snoezelen on chronic pain. Nurs Stand 2000;15:33-4.
51. Schofield P. Evaluating snoezelen for relaxation within chronic pain management. Br J Nurs 2002;11:812-21.
52. Schofield P, Davis B. Sensory stimulation (snoezelen) versus relaxation: a potential strategy for the management of chronic pain. Disabil Rehabil 2000;22:675-82.
53. Smith M. Pain assessment in nonverbal older adults with advanced dementia. Perspect Psychiatr Care 2005;41:99-113.
54. Titler MG, Herr K, Brooks JM, Xie XJ, Ardery G, Schilling ML, Marsh JL, Everett LQ, Clarke WR. Translating research into practice intervention improves management of acute pain in older hip fracture patients. Health Serv Res 2009;44:264-87.
55. Torke AM. Building the evidence base for palliative care and dementia. Palliat Med 2014;28:195-6.
56. Tracy B, Sean Morrison R. Pain management in older adults. Clin Ther 2013;35:1659-68.
57. Wells N, Pasero C, McCaffery M. Improving the Quality of Care Through Pain Assessment and Management. In: Hughes RG, editor. Patient Safety and Quality: An Evidence-Based Handbook for Nurses. Rockville (MD): Agency for Healthcare Research and Quality (US); 2008 Apr. Chapter 17.
58. Wortmann M. Dementia: a global health priority—highlights from an ADI and World Health Organization report: Alzheimers Res Ther 2012;4:40.

CHAPTER 18

Pharmacological Treatment of Pain in Dementia

Gisèle Pickering

Pain is common in older individuals [3]: acute painful conditions are very frequent, as older persons have the highest rates of surgery, procedural pain, and complications [30], and chronic conditions disproportionately affect older adults [42]. Age-related factors influence the pharmacology of drugs and their efficacy/safety ratio, the frequency of comorbidities, the polymedication, drug–drug and drug–disease interactions, the high variability of pharmacological changes, and ensuing analgesic requirements [5]. Over recent years, treatment guidelines for managing pain and prescribing analgesics to older persons have been developed worldwide [2, 4, 6, 9, 37, 57]. They support a more tailored approach based on the patients' individualized risks, an optimization of the treatment strategy, an anticipation of potential medication-related problems (falls, hospitalization) [14], and a multimodal therapeutic regimen. However, pain treatment in older persons with cognitive disorders, communication problems, and especially dementia is a real challenge for a number of reasons: pain assessment is particularly difficult in this population, titration of action and dosage finding are cumbersome, behavioral and psychological symptoms of dementia (BPSD) are easily confused with pain, psychotropic drugs are frequently prescribed and medications, sometimes inappropriate, display their cohort of side effects including delirium. This chapter will review the sequels of dementia on adequate pain management.

PHARMACOLOGICAL CHANGES WITH AGING

Aging is associated with a number of pharmacokinetic and pharmacodynamic changes, and although most published studies were performed in healthy older subjects, a few reports suggest even greater significant pharmacokinetic and pharmacodynamic alterations in frail compared to healthy elderly [49].

Pharmacokinetic Changes

Absorption may be influenced by several factors including comorbidities, medications slowing the gastrointestinal transit, chronic constipation, chronic laxative use, gastroesophageal reflux, and dysphagia [49, 54]. Concerning transdermal absorption, bioavailability of medications in plasters is often unpredictable in older patients, and associated with significant interindividual variability [19].

The consequences of age-related changes in *distribution* are significant. Aging is associated with decreased lean mass, increased fat mass, and decreased total water volume, and consequently changes the distribution of medications in the body [19, 25]. The distribution volume of hydrophilic medications (like morphine) is decreased, which increases the plasmatic concentrations and requires a lower dosing. Inversely, the distribution volume of lipophilic medications (like fentanyl) is increased, and this decreases their plasmatic concentrations and increases their half-life, often resulting in an accumulation of drugs [19]. Advanced age is also often associated with decreased serum albumin [36]: this is more frequent in the presence of chronic disease or malnutrition, and results in an increased free fraction of the medication. These changes are, however, only clinically significant for medications with a protein binding higher than 90%, a small distribution volume and a narrow therapeutic index [18].

Concerning the *metabolism* of drugs, liver mass and hepatic blood flow decrease with aging, which impairs drug clearance for flow-limited (high-clearance) drugs, and some authors suggest a 20–60% impairment of the intrinsic metabolic drug clearance [10]. The activity of phase I enzymatic reactions seems to be reduced, whereas activity of phase II enzymatic reactions is usually not modified [47]. Concerning *renal elimination*, renal mass and tubular secretion decrease significantly with age. There is a 30–50% decrease of glomerular filtration at 80 years old, which results in accumulation of renally excreted medications. Renal function and creatinine clearance can be estimated with the Cockroft–Gault formula, taking into account age, weight, serum creatinine, and gender [12]. In older malnourished patients with decreased muscle mass, this formula overestimates creatinine clearance.

Pharmacodynamic Changes

Age-related pharmacodynamic changes often result in increased sensitivity of older patients to medications and, consequently, increased occurrence of adverse effects (AEs) [34]. More specifically, increased sensitivity of cholinergic receptors makes older patients more sensitive to AEs from anticholinergic medications, including tricyclic antidepressants.

Decreased homeostasis can explain the delayed recovery of basal state following impairment of a physiological function in older patients, including development of acute renal failure or gastrointestinal bleeding with nonsteroidal anti-inflammatory drugs (NSAIDs) administration or sedation associated with opioids.

ANALGESICS AND RED FLAGS OF PAIN TREATMENT IN THE ELDERLY

Pain evaluation is particularly difficult in patients with dementia, and this central point is largely discussed in other chapters (see Chapters 9–11). Suspicion of pain in demented patients may be raised by behavioral changes like agitation and aggression, and assessment of the efficacy of an analgesic relies on a systematic reevaluation of pain and on the reliability of the scale. While agitation and aggression may be symptoms of pain in noncommunicative patients, they may also be symptoms of dementia. These Behavioural and Psychological Symptoms of Dementia (BPSD) may orientate treatment toward psychopharmacological rather than analgesic treatment or may increase the risk of serious side effects with analgesics.

In older patients with polymedication and age-related pharmacological changes, treatment of pain will bring an additional pharmacological burden and the choice of the analgesic should follow recommendations and be individualized. The frequent polypharmacy in older patients leads to an increased risk of drug–drug interactions and related toxicity [38].

Paracetamol is widely used in older patients because of the high prevalence of joint pathologies and recommended as the first-line oral analgesic [3, 4]. Adverse Effects (AEs) are rare, with hepatotoxicity being the main safety concern in the context of depleted glutathione stores associated with malnutrition, prolonged fasting, underweight, poor nutritional status or alcoholism, age-related changes of antioxidant status, or dehydration [39, 44, 45].

NSAIDs and the cyclooxygenase-II selective inhibitors (coxibs) have a proven efficacy but a well-defined toxicity profile (gastrointestinal, renal, and cardiovascular), and NSAIDs may only be considered rarely, and with extreme caution, in highly selected older patients who have failed other safer therapies [4]. Studies have demonstrated that there is a high prevalence of inappropriate NSAIDs and coxibs usage in the elderly population [1, 55, 56]. Inappropriate medication prescription (especially the type of drug rather than the dosage) is frequent in older patients, and patients taking NSAIDs should be reassessed on a regular basis to ensure ongoing benefits, absence of toxicity, and drug–drug or drug–disease interactions [4]. A systematic literature review has recently suggested that an increased risk for accidental falls is probable when older persons are exposed to NSAIDs [21]. Topical NSAIDs have demonstrated efficacy similar to oral NSAIDs, with a low incidence of adverse events [8].

Opioid analgesics are recommended for the treatment of chronic pain of moderate to severe intensity with pain-related functional impairment or diminished quality of life [4, 37]. A review on the use of opioids in chronic pain in the elderly, with a focus on buprenorphine, fentanyl, hydromorphone, methadone, morphine, and oxycodone, stresses that older patients respond to opioid treatment as well as younger patients, but tolerability is often a limiting factor. It is not possible to recommend the use of a specific opioid [37], and the benefit–risk ratio of each opioid should be considered as well as comorbidities and concomitant medications. The general rule, applied in geriatrics but very strongly with opioids, is to start with the lowest dose possible, and titrate according to the analgesic response and AEs. Over the last two decades, opioid prescription has exploded leading to an opioid epidemic with adverse consequences [32]. Elderly patients have not escaped this epidemic. It is linked to a number of causes including liberalization of laws governing the prescribing of opioids for the treatment of chronic noncancer pain, allegations of undertreatment of pain and underuse of opioids in the elderly, increased prevalence of chronic pain, and longer life expectancy. From 1997 to 2007, hydrodrocodone usage has increased by 280% whereas oxycodone usage has increased by 866% [32]. In older persons opioids are prescribed for cancer pain treatment but also for noncancer pain and osteoarthritis. Osteoarthritis is one of the most common diseases of old age and a leading cause of disability and of chronic pain worldwide. Benefits and harms of opioids in the elderly are largely reviewed in the literature and are associated with a much higher risk of fracture [51, 52] than other treatments [17, 29].

Neuropathic Pain Treatment

Neuropathic pain is common in older persons and remains a difficult area of pain care. Assessment of neuropathic pain is not easy especially in older persons with cognitive disorders. First-line medications of neuropathic pain include tricyclic antidepressants, selective serotonin and norepinephrine reuptake inhibitors (duloxetine and venlafaxine), calcium channel α_2-δ ligands (gabapentin and pregabalin), and topical lidocaine. The American

Geriatrics Society (AGS) revised some of the previous AGS recommendations on pharmacological treatment of persistent pain in older adults [3, 4] and strongly recommends that tertiary tricyclic antidepressants should be avoided in older adults because of the risk of anticholinergic cardiac and cognitive AEs [17, 46]. Antiepileptics have also a number of AEs including dizziness, somnolence, gait disturbance, falls, and reduction of doses are recommended [41]. The known AEs of the classic drugs used in neuropathic pain may preclude their use in the frail older person. Topical and noninvasive treatments may be useful alone or in combination with systemic treatments. In older patients suffering from postherpetic neuralgia, the 5% lidocaine-medicated plaster is allowed to reduce the use of antidepressants and opioids [11].

In conclusion, pharmacological treatment of pain in the older patient is challenging because of comorbidities that necessitate multiple medications (older patients are reported to take between 5 and 10 drugs every day) with potential interactions [29, 40] and with the risk of inappropriate medication prescription in approximately one in five prescriptions to elderly persons [35]. The challenges surrounding analgesic prescribing in older people are further amplified in the presence of frailty and impaired cognition [33]. Frailty and impaired cognition may impact on the pharmacokinetics and pharmacodynamics of analgesics in this population and increase further its heterogeneity. Adequate dosage finding of analgesics relies on an individualized approach of pain management. Frailty is also associated with pain [33] and patients with dementia often present neuropsychiatric symptoms, and these confusingly may also be symptoms of pain.

BEHAVIORAL OR PSYCHOLOGICAL SYMPTOMS AND THEIR TREATMENT

There is a large literature on neuropsychiatric symptoms, also called Behavioural and Psychological Symptoms of Dementia (BPSD) [7, 23, 26, 48, 50]. Although cognitive decline is the hallmark of dementia, these noncognitive symptoms, including agitation, aggression, delusions, hallucinations, repetitive vocalizations, wandering, depression, apathy, anxiety, disinhibition, etc., may also be due to pain or dehydration. This may be confusing in patients with dementia as pain is frequent but because of the patients' inability to communicate their discomfort, pain is difficult to suspect and evaluate. BPSD are common in patients with Alzheimer's disease, affect 40–60% of individuals living in care home settings [7], and have been observed in 60–98% of patients with dementia [50]. First-line treatment of BPSD is nonpharmacological management in a multidisciplinary team, with an important role played by occupational therapists [16]. There are no recommended medications, but it has been a common practice to use a number of drugs acting on the central nervous system despite little evidence of efficacy. Pain should always be considered as a common possible cause of agitation or aggression and should be adequately treated. A cluster randomized clinical trial with paracetamol 3 g/day in 352 patients showed a significant improvement in agitation [22]. Paracetamol has been shown to have a central mechanism of action on the serotonergic descending pathways, but with no deleterious central AEs [43], and it has been also demonstrated to be active on social "pain" and have a soothing impact in adverse situations [13].

Multiple classes of drugs are used for BPSD, including antipsychotics, anticonvulsants, antidepressants, anxiolytics, cholinesterase inhibitors, and N-methyl-D-aspartate–receptor modulators [7, 23, 26, 48, 50, 53].

Psychotropic medication is common in dementia patients with a prevalence ranging between 17% and 78% [26, 48]. Typical antipsychotics (i.e., haloperidol, thioridazine, droperidol, promazine), developed in the 1950–1960s to treat schizophrenia, have major AEs including dystonia, tardive dyskinesia, cognitive impairment, and cardiac arrhythmias. Haloperidol showed an improvement of aggression but not of agitation [28], and despite its negative safety profile is still used today.

Atypical antipsychotics are the second generation of antipsychotics developed in the 1990s (i.e., risperidone, olanzapine, aripiprazole, quetiapine) and have largely replaced the first-generation drugs because of their slightly better safety profile on tardive dyskinesia. However, the risk of delirium [7] because of anticholinergic effects and the increased mortality (because of oversedation, dehydration, and cardiac arrhythmias) have been highlighted in the literature. Risperidone and aripiprazole produce modest but significant improvement in aggression, and risperidone is the only recommended antipsychotic when other therapeutic approaches have failed, if there is extreme distress or risk and for a maximal period of 12 weeks. Antipsychotics have no other beneficial effect on BPSD apart from aggression. Long-term prescription increases AEs with no significant benefit, and there should be a judicious short-term prescription of antipsychotics.

Antidepressants show very limited evidence to improve agitation and other BPSD. Among serotonergic antidepressants (sertraline, fluoxetine, citalopram, and trazodone), only citalopram showed some benefit; but although antidepressants are well tolerated and effective in depression, they do not appear to be very effective in BPSD [50]. Anticonvulsants show some promise for pain alleviation with carbamazepine but not with valproate. Although there was a good tolerability in Alzheimer patients [50] in the clinical trials, carbamazepine presents severe hematologic and dermatological AEs, and many drug interactions [24] and is not recommended. Benzodiazepines are not recommended for BPSD, as they may increase agitation and have been shown to increase confusion and falls [20].

Cholinesterase inhibitors (donezepil, galantamine, rivastigmine) do not show benefit in agitation or aggression but present some evidence of a slight effect on depression, apathy, and anxiety [7].

Memantine, a N-methyl-D-aspartate–receptor antagonist, shows encouraging evidence. There are contradictory findings in the different trials: some of them show some benefit in the treatment of mild to moderate agitation and aggression [50], but more trials are needed. Likewise, prazosin, an α-adrenoceptor blocker, presents promising evidence but only one randomized clinical trial has been published so far [50].

In conclusion, BPSD treatment in dementia should encompass the treatment of underlying medical pathologies, pain symptoms alleviation, and use of nonpharmacological techniques. Short-term use of atypical antipsychotics should be second-line treatment.

CONCLUSION

In the elderly population, the right balance between efficacy and tolerance of drugs in pain treatment is always searched. The commonest side effect of all medications is neuropsychological symptoms especially in long-term care settings [15]. Evidence for AEs of some antipsychotics (antidepressants, neuroleptics, benzodiazepines, sedatives/hypnotics), for example, fall occurrence has been well documented [20, 27]. Beside the red flags that also have to be considered in the treatment of elderly individuals with analgesics, further specific challenges are associated with the pharmacological pain treatment of patients with dementia. The situation becomes indeed even more difficult when the patient is frail, with cognitive impairment, and has an increasing severity of dementia. Because of the difficulties in pain assessment, the titration of action and dosage finding are very cumbersome. The confusion of pain and BPSD may lead to an erroneous application of psychopharmacological medication like neuroleptics. Patients taking more than one CNS drug or suffering psychiatric illness need more professionals' attention. Polymedication should be hierarchized in order to avoid AEs and drug–drug interactions that are very common in the elderly. Delirium may occur in 60% of those hospitalized and in 45% of the cognitively impaired [28]. It may result from drug effects, and deliriogenic drugs, including antipsychotics, should be avoided in elderly patients [31]. The combination of being elderly and chronically cognitively impaired leads to a high risk of delirium with the associated increased risk of prolonged hospital stay, complications, and poor outcomes [28]. While pharmacological pain treatment needs to be optimized, nonpharmacological approaches should always be tried and combined for a synergistic therapeutic benefit.

REFERENCES

1. Abraham NS, El-Serag HB, Johnson ML. National adherence to evidence-based guidelines for the prescription of nonsteroidal anti-inflammatory drugs. J Gastroenterol 2005;129:1171–8.
2. American College of Rheumatology Ad Hoc Group on Use of selective and nonselective NSAI drugs. Recommendations for use: an American College of Rheumatology white paper. Arthritis Rheum 2008;59:1058–73.
3. American Geriatrics Society [AGS] Panel on Persistent Pain in Older Persons. The management of persistent pain in older persons. J Am Geriatr Soc 2002; 50:S205–24.
4. American Geriatrics Society Panel on the Pharmacological Management of Persistent Pain in Older Persons. Pharmacological management of persistent pain in older persons. J Am Geriatrics Soc 2009;57:1331–46.
5. Arnstein RN. Balancing analgesic efficacy with safety concerns in the older patient. Pain Manag Nurs 2010;11:S11–22.
6. Australian Pain Society. Pain in residential aged care facilities management strategies. Sydney: Australian Pain Society; 2005.
7. Ballard C, Corbett A. Agitation and aggression in people with Alzheimer's disease. Curr Opin Psychiatry 2013;26:252–9.
8. Baraf HS, Gloth FM, Barthel HR, Gold MS, Altman RD. Safety and efficacy of topical diclofenac sodium gel for knee osteoarthritis in elderly and younger patients: pooled data from three randomized, double-blind, parallel-group, placebo-controlled, multicenter trials. Drugs Aging 2011;28:27–40.
9. British Pain Society. The assessment of pain in older people. Concise guidance to good practice. A series of evidence-based guidelines for clinical management. Number 8. National guidelines. London: Royal College of Physicians of London; 2007.
10. Butler JM, Begg EJ. Free drug metabolic clearance in elderly people. Clin Pharmacokin 2008; 47:297–321.
11. Clère F, Delorme-Morin C, George B, Navez M, Rioult B, Tiberghien-Chatelain F, Ganry H. 5% lidocaine medicated plaster in elderly patients with postherpetic neuralgia: results of a compassionate use programme in France. Drugs Aging 2011;28:693–702.
12. Cockcroft DW, Gault MH. Prediction of creatinine clearance from serum creatinine, Nephron 1976;16:31–41.
13. Dewall CN, Macdonald G, Webster GD, Masten CL, Baumeister RF, Powell C, Combs D, Schurtz DR, Stillman TF, Tice DM, Eisenberger NI. Acetaminophen reduces social pain: behavioral and neural evidence. Psychol Sci 2010;21:931–7.
14. Fick DM, Cooper JW, Wade WE, Waller JL, Maclean JR, Beers MH. Updating the Beers criteria for potentially inappropriate medication use in older adults: results of a US consensus panel of experts. Arch Intern Med 2003;163:2716–24.
15. Field TS, Gurwitz JH, Avorn J, McCormick D, Jain S, Eckler M, Benser M, Bates DW. Risk factors for adverse drug events among nursing home residents. Arch Intern Med 2001;161:1629–34.
16. Fraker J, Kales HC, Blazek M, Kavanagh J, Gitlin LN. The role of the occupational therapist in the management of neuropsychiatric symptoms of dementia in clinical settings. Occup Ther Health Care 2014;28:4–20.

17. Gloth III FM. Pharmacological management of persistent pain in older persons: focus on opioids and nonopioids. J Pain 2011;1:S14–20.
18. Grandison MK, Boudinot FD. Age-related changes in protein binding of drugs: implications for therapy. Clin Pharmacokin 2000;38:271–90.
19. Hammerlein A, Derendorf H, Lowenthal DT. Pharmacokinetic and pharmacodynamic changes in the elderly: clinical implications. Clin Pharmacokin 1998;35:49–64.
20. Hartikainen S, Lonnroos E, Louhivuori K. Medication as a risk factor for falls: critical systematic review. J Gerontol A Biol Sci Med Sci 2007;62:1172–81.
21. Hegeman J, van den Bemt BJ, Duyses J, van Limbeek J. NSAIDs and the risk of accidental falls in the elderly: a systematic review. Drug Saf 2009;32:489–98.
22. Husebo BS, Ballard C, Sandvik R, Nilsen OB, Aarsland D. Efficacy of treating pain to reduce behavioural disturbances in residents of nursing homes with dementia: cluster randomised clinical trial. BMJ 2011;343:d4065
23. Kamble P, Chen H, Sherer JT, Aparasu RR. Use of antipsychotics among elderly nursing home residents with dementia in the US: an analysis of National Survey Data. Drugs Aging 2009;26:483–92.
24. Kim JY, Lee J, Ko YJ, Shin JY, Jung SY, Choi NK. Multi-indication carbamazepine and the risk of severe cutaneous adverse drug reactions in Korean elderly patients: a Korean health insurance data-based study. PLoS One 2013;8:e83849.
25. Kinirons MT, Crome P. Clinical pharmacokinetics considerations in the elderly: an update. Clin Pharmacokin 1997;33:302–12.
26. Kverno KS, Rabins PV, Blass DM, Hicks KL, Black BS. Prevalence and treatment of neuropsychiatric symptoms in advanced dementia. J Gerontol Nurs 2008;34:8–150.
27. Leipzig RM, Cumming RG, Tinetti ME. Drugs and falls in older people: a systematic review and meta-analysis: I. Psychotropic drugs. J Am Geriatr Soc 1999;47:30–9.
28. Lonergan E, Britton AM, Luxenberg J, Wyller T. Antipsychotics for delirium. Cochrane Database Syst Rev 2007;2:CD005594.
29. Lussier D, Pickering G. Pharmacology considerations in older patients. In Beaulieu P, Lussier D, Porreca F, Dickenson AH, editors. Pharmacology of pain. Seattle: IASP Press; 2010. p. 547–67.
30. Macintyre PE, Schug SA. Acute pain management: a practical guide, 3rd edition. Edinburgh: Saunders Elsevier; 2007.
31. Maclullich AM, Anand A, Davis DH, Jackson T, Barugh AJ, Hall RJ, Ferguson KJ, Meagher DJ. New horizons in the pathogenesis, assessment and management of delirium. Age Ageing 2013;42:667–74.
32. Manchikanti L, Helm S, Fellows B, Janata JW, Pampati V, Grider, JS, Boswell MV. Opioid epidemic in the United States. Pain Phys 2012;15:ES9–38.
33. McLachlan AJ, Bath S, Naganathan V, Hilmer SN, Le Couteur DG, Gibson SJ, Blyth FM. Clinical pharmacology of analgesic medicines in older people: impact of frailty and cognitive impairment. Br J Clin Pharmacol 2011;71:351–64.
34. Nolan L, O'Malley K. Prescribing for the elderly. Part I: sensitivity of the elderly to adverse drug reactions, J Amer Geriatr Soc 1988;32:142–9.
35. Opondo D, Eslami S, Visscher S, de Rooij SE, Verheij R, Korevaar JC, Abu-Hanna A. Inappropriateness of medication prescriptions to elderly patients in the primary care setting: a systematic review. PLoS One 2012;7:e43617
36. Paolisso G, Gambardella A, Balbi V, Ammendola S, D'Amore A, Varrichio M. Body composition, body fat distribution, and resting metabolic rate in healthy centenarians, Amer J Clin Nut 1995;62:746–50.
37. Pergolizzi J, Boger RH, Budd K, Dahan A, Erdine S, Hans G, Kress HG, Langford R, Likar R, Raffa RB, Sacerdote P. Opioids and the management of chronic severe pain in the elderly: consensus statement of an International Expert Panel with focus on the six clinically most often used World Health Organization Step III opioids (buprenorphine, fentanyl, hydromorphone, methadone, morphine, oxycodone). Pain Pract 2008;8:287–313.
38. Pickering G. Frail elderly, nutritional status and drugs. Arch Gerontol Geriatr 2004;38:174–80.
39. Pickering G. Paracetamol use in the elderly. J Pain Manag 2008;1:35–9.
40. Pickering G. Analgesic use in the older person. Curr Opin Support Palliat Care 2012;6:207–12
41. Pickering G. Antiepileptics for post-herpetic neuralgia: current and future prospects. Drugs Aging 2014;31:653–60.
42. Pickering G, Leplege A. Herpes Zoster, postherpetic neuralgia and quality of life. Pain Practice 2011;11: 397–402.
43. Pickering G, Loriot MA, Libert F, Eschalier A, Beaune P, Dubray C. Analgesic effect of acetaminophen in humans: first evidence of a central serotonergic mechanism. Clin Pharmacol Ther 2006;79:371–8.

44. Pickering G, Schneider E, Papet I, Pujos-Guillot E, Pereira B, Simen E, Dubray C, Schoeffler P. Acetaminophen metabolism after major surgery: a bigger challenge with increasing age. Clin Pharmacol Ther 2011; 90:707–11.
45. Pujos-Guillot E, Pickering G, Lyan B, Ducheix G, Brandolini-Bunlon M, Glomot F, Dardevet D, Dubray C, Papet I. Therapeutic paracetamol treatment in older persons induces dietary and metabolic modifications related to sulfuramino acids. Age (Dordr) 2012;34:181–93.
46. Reisner L. Pharmacological management of persistent pain in older persons. J Pain 2011;12:S21–S29.
47. Schmucker DL. Liver function and phase I drug metabolism in the elderly: a paradox, Drugs Aging 2001;18:837–51.
48. Schulze J, Glaeske G, van den Bussche H, Kaduszkiewicz H, Koller D, Wiese B, Hoffmann F. Prescribing of antipsychotic drugs in patients with dementia: a comparison with age-matched and sex-matched non-demented controls. Pharmacoepidemiol Drug Saf. 2013;22:1308–16.
49. Shi S, Mörike K, Klotz U. The clinical implications of ageing for rational drug therapy. Eur J Clin Pharmacol 2008;64:183–99.
50. Sink KM, Holden KF, Yaffe K. Pharmacological treatment of neuropsychiatric symptoms of dementia: a review of the evidence. JAMA 2005;293:596–608.
51. Solomon DH, Rassen JA, Glynn RJ, Garneau K, Levin R, Lee J, Schneeweiss S. The comparative safety of opioids for nonmalignant pain in older adults. Arch Intern Med 2010;170:1979–86.
52. Solomon DH, Rassen JA, Glynn RJ, Lee J, Levin R, Schneeweiss S. The comparative safety of analgesics in older adults with arthritis. Arch Intern Med 2012;170:1968–78.
53. Trinh NH, Hoblyn J, Mohanty S, Yaffe K. Efficacy of cholinesterase inhibitors in the treatment of neuropsychiatric symptoms and functional impairment in Alzheimer disease: a meta-analysis. JAMA 2003;289:210–6.
54. Tumer N, Scarpace PJ, Lowenthal DT. Geriatric pharmacology: basic and clinical considerations. Annu Rev Pharmacol Toxicol 1992;32:271–302.
55. Van Leen MWF, Van Der Eijk I, Schols JMGA. Prevention of NSAID gastropathy in elderly patients. An observational study in general practice and nursing homes. Age Ageing 2007;36:414–8.
56. Visser LE, Graatsma HH, Tricker BHC. Contraindicated NSAIDs are frequently prescribed to elderly patients with peptic ulcer disease. Br J Clin Pharmacol 2002;53:183–8.
57. Zhang W, Doherty M, Arden N, EULAR Standing Committee for International Clinical Studies Including Therapeutics (ESCISIT). EULAR evidence based recommendations for the management of hip osteoarthritis: report of a task force of the EULAR Standing Committee for International Clinical Studies Including Therapeutics (ESCISIT). Ann Rheum Dis 2005;64:669–81.

CHAPTER 19

Pain, Exercise, and Dementia

Steven M. Savvas and Stephen J. Gibson

To date, very few studies have systematically explored the triumvirate relationship between pain, dementia, and physical activity. Yet the evidence base shows that physical activity for the cognitively intact improves pain outcomes and is protective of cognitive functioning [32, 56, 74, 84]. Evidence is still limited but encouraging that physical activity is also important in supporting the cognitive ability of older adults with neurocognitive disorders [26]. In light of this, is there a dual benefit for promoting physical activity for individuals with cognitive impairment to improve both pain and cognition? Exercise is recommended for older people in general for its positive effects and will be discussed in the section on the relationship between pain and exercise, but a dual benefit would emphasize the added importance of exercise programs for those in pain and with cognitive deficits.

Promoting physical activity in people with cognitive impairment is not without difficulties. For example, older people with dementia have shown decreased levels of physical activity [80], especially those living with dementia in long-term care who are less engaged in physical activity than their peers without dementia [59]. Despite the decreased levels of physical activity in this cohort, studies highlight the benefits of physical exercise for people with dementia, including improvements in gait [71] and physical functioning [64]. The section on physical activity interventions for cognitive function will review the efficacy of activity programs and discuss some of the practical considerations when attempting to utilize these approaches in older people with cognitive impairments.

THE ROLE OF EXERCISE IN THE MANAGEMENT OF PAIN

Introduction

Chronic pain is a complex and challenging condition to treat, heterogeneous in its clinical presentation, and frequently comorbid with other exacerbating health problems. Chronic pain impacts the individual on multiple domains and is associated with emotional distress, disturbed mental state, sleep disturbance, cognitive impairment, movement dysfunction, social and occupational disability, impaired sexual function, financial impact, and overall diminished quality of life [5, 10, 25, 47, 51, 57, 67]. Multifactorial pain models that can address multiple dimensions of the pain experience are needed for comprehensive pain management, though the evidence of the effectiveness of such models on pain and pain-related disability is modest [83]. Nonetheless, these models have value as they target biological, psychological, and sociological components that are fundamentally involved in the development and prolongation of chronic pain.

Treatment for chronic pain includes both pharmacological and nonpharmacological approaches, with physical activity and exercise viewed as particularly important nonpharmacological therapies in any pain management framework. In this context, physical activity is a broad term for any muscle-related body movement that expends energy, whereas exercise is a form of structured physical activity aimed to improve or maintain physical fitness. Many barriers impede optimal utilization of physical therapies for chronic pain patients, with pain itself commonly cited as a principle reason for activity limitation. Still the benefits of physical therapies are clear, though the comparative benefits of specific forms of physical therapies remains equivocal, as does the effectiveness of such treatments in specific subgroups such as people with dementia and pain.

This section reviews the benefits of physical activity therapies for chronic pain management as well as associated barriers in older populations. These therapies will be discussed as they relate to conceptual pain models that are multifactorial in approach and that aim to address the physical, emotional, cognitive, and social components of chronic pain.

Multifactorial Chronic Pain Frameworks

Traditional biomedical models of pain are incomplete in their understanding and management of chronic pain, as these frameworks are often insufficient in either explaining patient pain-related problems, or accounting for the absence of pain in people with similar structural abnormalities as pain sufferers. More contemporary models are multidimensional and have expanded to include psychological and sociological components of pain, recognizing the role of central nervous system processes that may exacerbate and prolong pain and pain-related disability [54]. Within these models, psychological/behavioral factors have seen particular attention as contributors that promote chronic pain, with some emphasis on the concept of fear avoidance [76, 77].

Fear-avoidance models propose that pain may persist due to a patient adopting avoidant behaviors that are a consequence of an excessive fear of pain or injury. Though some of the basic tenets of these models have empirical support [46], recent evidence fails to support some aspects of the model [82], coupled with poorer-than-expected results from clinical interventions based on fear-avoidance principles [63]. Furthermore not all patients can be attributed to fear-avoidance behaviors, as some patients are better characterized as adopting avoidance-endurance behaviors that are considered contradictory to fear avoidance [31]. Finally, these behavioral models also do not address all dimensions of pain, for example, the sociological or environmental factors that contribute to pain and disability.

A unified biopsychosocial model for chronic pain is still needed, especially regarding the rehabilitation around social and environmental contributors to pain. Here, the International Classification of Functioning, Disability, and Health Framework (ICF) [81] can have utility in providing an expanded framework that recognizes the role of social factors and environment in the interaction between functioning and disability. A benefit of such a model in the context of chronic pain is the recognition of the importance of reframing treatment goals for older patients and those with dementia. Whereas goals may be centered on functional restoration and resumption of all physical activities for a younger patient, these goals may not be foremost considerations for older people or those with cognitive impairment. Appropriate goals may instead focus on sufficient improvement for increasing recreational pastimes, social interactions, or functional independence.

Barriers to Physical Therapies for Chronic Pain

Physical activity is a nonpharmacological treatment recommended in chronic pain management guidelines [1, 50]. However, pain itself is recognized as a substantial barrier in physical activity and exercise adherence [61]. This is particularly so with higher levels of pain that severely limits behaviors that typically promote increased physical activity. A further hindrance is that painful conditions often limit the ability for physical movement, and therefore, regardless of the etiology, a consequence of chronic pain is typically a generalized psychomotor slowing of movement with accompanying "stiffness." These sequelae are generally fatiguing as they are physiologically inefficient [62]. For example, Lee et al. [45] compared patients with and without lower back pain and reported that pain patients had poorer walking performance despite similar exertion levels. Therefore, the pain itself and the associated stiffness and fatigue are all identified barriers to exercise [61].

Other factors such as psychopathology can also impair physical performance. Depression, a common comorbidity of chronic pain, has been shown to compound on poor physical performance, with depressed chronic pain patients showing severely compromised movement speeds [72]. As lower physical activity levels are associated with higher depression levels [9], this suggests a reciprocal detrimental relationship between chronic pain, physical activity, and depression. So in response to barriers such as pain, stiffness, and fatigue, chronic pain patients decrease physical activity, in turn increasing the likelihood of depressive symptomatology, and thereby reinforcing poor physical performance. However, this picture is incomplete as research on survivors of breast cancer with pain suggests that physical activity is only a partial mediator, and that other pathways also explain the relationship between pain and depression [69].

Exercise and Pain

Despite these barriers, two streams of evidence emphasize the importance of exercise for pain management. The first are the limited experimental pain perception studies that suggest that exercise regimes can modify the sensory aspects of pain perception and tolerance. The other line of evidence is clinical outcome studies showing that exercise interventions can improve pain report and pain-related function. Together the evidence highlights the beneficial role of exercise on pain-related outcomes.

Exercise and Pain Perception

Some limited evidence suggests that different exercise modalities can have an analgesic effect on pain threshold and pain intensity. A review of two exercise types (acute isometric exercise for strength training and aerobic exercise for cardiovascular) in chronic pain patients suggests variable results [56], somewhat dependent on the chronic pain condition. For aerobic exercise, the induced analgesic effect size on pain threshold is small at 0.19 (SD = 0.52). Aerobic effect on pain intensity shows more moderate analgesic effects with $d = 0.42$ (SD = 1.53), but variability is high across studies. Isometric exercise results were mixed and may be dependent on the specific chronic pain condition. For example, there was increased pain perception in fibromyalgia patients while reduced pain perception for patients with shoulder myalgia. In conclusion, literature on the benefits of exercise on pain perception is small and still inconclusive, as compared to the much larger body of work on the benefits of exercise intervention programs on pain relief and other pain-related outcomes.

Exercise and Pain-Related Outcomes

An umbrella review of nine systematic reviews of exercise on fibromyalgia supports the conclusion that exercise training in multiple modalities can improve pain relief and physical function, typically showing small to moderate effects on both domains [11]. The majority of studies included in the reviews were exercise regimes performed two or three times per week, of moderate intensity (64–76% HR max), between 31 and 60 minutes in duration, and over a period of between 7 and 12 weeks. A review of just resistance training for fibromyalgia (exercise training performed against resistance, e.g., hand weights) showed that resistance exercise improves function, pain, muscle strength, and tenderness compared with controls [15]. However, evidence is mixed whether resistance training performs better or worse than other exercise regimens such as aerobics or flexibility exercise.

A review of aquatic exercise training for fibromyalgia also showed some modest improvements of aquatic exercise compared with controls on outcomes that included pain, stiffness, fatigue, function, and muscle strength [12]. However, only two outcomes were clinically significant with aquatic exercise improving stiffness by 27% and muscle strength by 37%. A comparison of aquatic- versus land-based exercise programs showed no significant differences on function, pain, or stiffness outcomes.

A separate systematic review and meta-analysis showed that exercise programs (strengthening, flexibility, or aerobics) for lower limb osteoarthritis were more beneficial for pain relief and improving functional limitations than no exercise [74]. Most of the studies in the analysis are related to knee osteoarthritis. A study that evaluated an integrated rehabilitation program combining self-management, coping and individually tailored exercise regime over 12 supervised sessions for 6 weeks has also shown longer-term benefits persist at 6 months with standardized effect sizes of 0.29 for function and 0.27 for pain, in favor of the rehabilitation group versus usual care [36].

Targeted exercise approaches are also shown to be effective with a systematic review on the effect of exercise therapy (exercise with varying levels of therapist supervision) on chronic low back pain showing modest pain score improvements with exercise therapy compared with low-intensity home exercise without supervision [32]. Eight of 11 studies reviewed showed no difference between exercise therapy and other forms of nonpharmacological treatment modalities. Routine exercise is also shown to improve pain outcomes in peripheral neuropathies. Animal studies (primarily on diabetic neuropathic pain) suggest that aerobic exercise improves degenerate peripheral nerve function [48] and can delay the onset of diabetic pain [17].

In conclusion, there is consensus that for chronic pain patients any type of exercise is better than none [56, 74], and that activity improves quality of life, promotes well-being, and reduces disability [40]. Therapy for chronic pain typically focuses on improving function and activity despite ongoing pain [3], and suggests that core beliefs may need to be challenged (such as fear-avoidance behaviors to exercise and activity) as well as motivational aspects that may be related to fatigue and depression. A study of exercise paired with a cognitive behavior treatment approach suggests that chronic painful osteoarthritis of the knee is amenable to such an integrated treatment approach [36]. Both pain and physical function improved after treatment, and persisted long term [35]. A review of multidisciplinary treatments that included physical exercise with at least one other biopsychosocial treatment approach showed moderate effectiveness of multidisciplinary treatment for reducing pain intensity in the short term, compared either to no treatment/waiting list controls, or other active nonpharmacological treatments [75]. However, the effect was extinguished by follow-up.

Targeting factors that contribute to pain is a foremost consideration. For example, a meta-analysis review of the effect of exercise on depression has shown that exercise has a moderate effect on depression compared with no treatment or control interventions [21], equivalent to a difference of about 5 points on the Beck Depression Inventory [20]. Likewise, another meta-analysis on the effect of exercise on general mood and well-being showed that acute aerobic exercise was associated with increased positive affect [68]. How these results translate to the effectiveness of exercise for chronic pain in people with dementia is still largely unknown. However, a meta-analysis of the general benefits of exercise programs for people with dementia showed evidence of improvements in depression [26]. Movement speed can be improved without increasing pain scores, by using sensory enhancement such as music and virtual reality [66]. Another study suggests that tailored physical activity pacing is more effective than general activity pacing in reducing fatigue [53] and stiffness [70] in osteoarthritis of the knee or hip.

Considerations of Physical Activity Treatment

Caution is needed with the clinical application of physical activity as although exercise is health promoting, its overuse may be harmful and pain promoting [30]. Evidence is also emerging that physical activity levels that are too high are linked with lower back pain [2], suggesting a U-shaped relationship between physical activity and pain with too-low or too-high activity both detrimental to pain outcomes. In comparison, moderate levels of activity are associated with less pain [29, 33]. Determining what constitutes an appropriate level of physical activity can be difficult, though identifying patients as fear avoidance or pain persistent using avoidance-endurance models of pain may be insightful in recommending either increased activity levels or appropriate pacing strategies, respectively [31].

The level of function of the patient should be a guide in recommending an appropriate exercise therapy. Obesity and cognitive impairment are both limiting factors in this regard. Adherence to an exercise regimen is also important, and due consideration is needed to choose an exercise program that is relevant and engaging for the chronic pain patient. As evidence is limited that one exercise program is better than all others, clinicians should consult with patients about their preferences as this may improve compliance and may well be a better predictor of a successful outcome than the choice of a particular exercise style. This is not to insist that specific therapies are without added purpose. Specific physical therapies that target specific physical impairments are appropriate and would be expected to be of particular benefit. For example, muscle weakness would more likely be targeted better with strengthening exercises than flexibility therapies.

Summary

Pain is a complex and challenging multidimensional condition. A multifactorial pain management framework that addresses the biological, psychological, cognitive, and sociological components that promote and prolong pain is therefore needed. Physical activity and exercise are considered central in any pain management framework, and the research base does not advocate any one form of exercise as preferential to another. Barriers in adherence to exercise programs may be substantial, but with due clinical consideration are not insurmountable.

PHYSICAL EXERCISE AS AN INTERVENTION FOR IMPROVING COGNITIVE FUNCTION

In addition to the noted benefits of physical exercise as an important part of pain management, and for improving general health and cardiovascular health in particular, recent studies also suggest that physical activity programs may also improve cognitive function and reduce the risk of dementia in older adults. As such, this type of therapy may be of potentially greater benefit and be especially suited when considering management options for persons with both dementia and bothersome pain. Consistent evidence in support of the notion that physical exercise and fitness improves or maintains the cognitive functioning of older persons has come from numerous cross-sectional and longitudinal studies [52]. The number of controlled studies examining physical exercise and activity programs as a lifestyle intervention for reducing cognitive decline in healthy older adults as well as in those with dementia has also grown exponentially in the past 15 years. Indeed, there are now available multiple systematic reviews of randomized controlled trials of physical exercise, although the potential benefits of exercise for improving cognitive function remains somewhat controversial [4, 6, 14, 26–28, 34, 42, 58, 78]. In persons with dementia, improvements in the performance of activities of daily living and reduction in falls have been noted as additional benefits of regular physical activity [16, 23, 79].

Cross-Sectional and Longitudinal Studies of Physical Activity and Cognition

There are multiple epidemiological studies investigating the association between levels of physical activity and risk of cognitive impairment or dementia in older age. Methods of monitoring physical activity and fitness include self-reported activity levels as well as more objective indices (motion sensors, pedometers, heart rate monitoring). The intensity and types of physical exercise being monitored also varies considerably between different studies, and this has been regarded as a methodological weakness of this literature [52]. Nonetheless, a comprehensive systematic review [65] of more than 120 observational studies conducted until 2010 concluded that leisure activity probably does reduce the risk of cognitive decline over 12 months follow-up when considered among a myriad of other potential risks and preventive factors. Other recent systematic reviews also confirm that moderately active individuals have a significantly lower risk of dementia or cognitive decline when compared to sedentary persons, and that the magnitude of effect varies between a 35% and 50% risk reduction dependent upon the intensity of regular exercise/activity [6, 37, 43, 60, 73]. These reviews do acknowledge that there are some negative studies, particularly when the sample size is relatively small (<1000 subjects), when the measures of cognitive function lack sensitivity, or when physical activity is operationalized over relatively short periods. It has been argued that aerobic fitness and consequent increased oxygen supply to neural tissues may be a major explanation for the observed association between physical activity and cognitive function, although increased brain volume and improved functional connectivity between various brain regions have also been suggested [6, 43]. Regardless of the exact reasons, most of the available longitudinal and cross-sectional studies consistently show a small but positive relationship between greater levels of physical activity and a lower risk of cognitive decline in older people.

Randomized Controlled Trials of Physical Activity and Cognitive Function

Many randomized controlled trials have investigated the potential benefits of physical exercise on cognitive functioning, and these can be demarcated into those in subjects with normal cognition, cognitively impaired older adults, and those with dementia. The exact types of physical exercise or activity program vary widely between different studies, thus making it difficult to directly compare findings. Some examples of moderate-intensity physical activities include walking, swimming, aquarobics, resistance training, circuit weight training, dance, Tai Chi, and recreational sports (golf, tennis, cycling, team sports). The intensity of intervention also varies widely between different studies lasting from a few minutes of moderate exercise to several hours per week. This variance makes it difficult to evaluate the potential benefits of any particular type of activity/exercise program on cognitive function as well as the ability to generate firm conclusions about the efficacy of this generic mode of therapy. Nonetheless, as outlined below there is now growing evidence in support of physical activity/exercise as an effective treatment for the prevention of cognitive decline and for ameliorating the risk of developing dementia.

In older adults with intact cognitive function, a meta-analysis of 18 randomized trials by Colcombe and Kramer [19] showed that aerobic fitness training had a robust effect on improving cognitive function and particularly executive-control processes in previously sedentary individuals. The magnitude of effect was found to be dependent on the length of training intervention, the type of intervention and gender of participants (females doing better). Subsequent trials have reinforced these findings [39, 55], including long-term studies of cognitive aging in those who stay physically active versus those who do not [4, 28, 42]. The most recent systematic review [86] of 12 randomized trials, however, suggested that aerobic exercise may not be the "magic bullet" for enhancing *overall* cognitive function in healthy older adults, although specific elements may benefit.

A few randomized trials of physical exercise in persons with mild cognitive impairment but not dementia were conducted recently. The Fitness for the Ageing Brain study (FABS) examined a 24-week, home-based, graded walking program (at least 150 minutes per week) on cognitive health [44]. Advanced strategies were used to facilitate compliance with the exercise program and persons were encouraged to continue with their activity program beyond 24 weeks, but without any further structured support from the research team. Adults aged 50 years and older were followed up over 18 months and cognitive performance was monitored using the ADAS-Cog. A significant improvement in scores was noted immediately following the 24-week exercise program, and this improvement was maintained at 12 and 18 months postintervention. Subject selection did not specifically target sedentary individuals, yet a more recent trial suggests that the greatest benefits of exercise may be seen in these individuals [7]. Lam et al. [41] examined a Tai Chi intervention in 389 older adults with a diagnosis of mild cognitive impairment (not dementia). Participants were required to practice Tai Chi in a group setting at least three times per week for 30 minutes per occasion for 8 to 12 weeks and a control group practiced stretching exercises of similar duration. Both groups showed significant improvement in subjective memory complaints and cognitive performance (as measured by the ADAS-cog, MMSE, and various neuropsychological cognitive tasks), while the intervention group showed greater levels of improvement in balance, visual attention, and scores on the Clinical Dementia Rating scale. This might suggest that activities which include a strong cognitive element may have a greater effect than exercise alone, and this agrees with a recent meta-analysis on the effects of Tia Chi [78].

The potential cognitive benefit of exercise in persons with dementia has also been demonstrated across a number of randomized trials. A systematic review by Heyn et al. [34] of 30 randomized controlled trials concluded that exercise can improve fitness, physical function, and cognitive performance in people with dementia and cognitive impairment. Many studies were quite small, of poor–moderate quality and used a diverse range of physical activities and cognitive measures, but the overall effect size for cognitive improvement was 0.57. A more recent French study of nursing home residents with Alzheimer's disease also demonstrated positive cognitive outcomes after 15 weeks of three 60 minute classes per week [38], and this is consistent with other available studies [85]. However, the most recent systematic reviews of physical exercise and cognitive improvements in persons with dementia have raised some doubt about the efficacy of this mode of treatment [26, 58]. Both reviews comment that further studies are needed, but note that the current evidence for positive treatment effects of exercise on cognitive performance in persons with Alzheimer's disease and other forms of dementia is equivocal at best. This seemingly contrasts with the noted postexercise training improvements in fitness, physical functioning, and cardiovascular factors regardless of the stage of dementia [13].

In aggregate, there is strong evidence to support the efficacy of exercise programs for improving cognitive function in the healthy elderly and in older persons with mild cognitive impairment (not dementia), but not yet in those with a diagnosed dementia, despite some positive trials. Selection of participants may be an important consideration as already active adults are likely to benefit less from standard walking programs or moderate aerobic exercise when compared to the improvements seen in persons who are sedentary. The duration, intensity, and exact type of physical exercise may also be a relevant issue that contributes to the success of the intervention.

Program Selection and Practical Considerations

Many considerations when advising and encouraging older adults with cognitive impairment on how to increase their physical activity are present. These include individual needs, health and medical conditions including falls history, their level of fitness and physical skill, past and current physical activity, living environment, support network, and perceived preferences. The choice of a suitable program may vary in people with cognitive impairment due to issues with orientation and sense of direction, impaired concentration, and planning skills. For example, for someone at risk of falls and with reduced orientation, an unsupervised walking program may be inappropriate. A supervised walking program three times a week starting at 15 minutes of slow walking in week 1 would be the least complicated program meeting current aerobic physical activity guidelines. Increase the slow walking by 5 minutes each week for 8 weeks to reach 150 minutes a week. At the same time, intensity can also be increased by gradually increasing the walking speed, as the person becomes more accustomed to the program.

Promoting physical activity in older adults is a complex area of research based on several theories of behavior change, including stages of change theory [49]. Participants with cognitive impairment may have difficulty with these complex processes, so it is recommended that if used, these approaches should be tailored to the participant's level of understanding and ability to use them. To maximize the chances of success, the less-complex tasks of rewarding oneself, exercising with a partner, and using a variety of meaningful physical activities matched to the person's capabilities should be utilized. Family and friends or significant others such as care staff or clinicians can all provide social support for physical activity and improve adherence with an exercise program. Goal setting is also an important component for ensuring continued physical activity, and all goals should be specific, measureable, achievable, realistic, and timely. For Alzheimer's disease patients in cognitive rehabilitation programs, goal-setting has been demonstrated as an effective approach [18].

Adherence to physical exercise programs can be difficult, although achievable. Reported retention rates to physical activity programs involving participants with cognitive impairment range from 92% [24] to 85% [22] to 79% [8] at 6 months duration. Reasons for dropout from these programs include participant/family illness, time commitments, or personal reasons [8, 22, 24]. Activity/exercise programs also appear to be quite safe for participants with cognitive impairment, as adverse events possibly related to physical activity are at around 6% to 7% [8, 24].

Overall, the increasing numbers of clinical trials as well as systematic and nonsystematic reviews reflect the recommendation of physical activity as a healthy behavior for older adults with cognitive impairment. This is considered an important emerging topic when considering best practice management approaches for cognitive impairment, though the literature on how to best translate this evidence into routine clinical practice is much less developed. Despite many existing knowledge gaps, the multiple benefits of physical activity justify that community services and clinical settings update their management approaches with the aim to routinely offer participation in physical activity to people with cognitive impairment.

CONCLUSIONS

This chapter has provided an overview of the literature on using physical activity programs in older adults with pain and in those with cognitive impairments. Quantifying the benefits of exercise on pain outcomes for people with dementia has been little explored in the research literature, though it is reasonable to assume that as exercise is beneficial for pain in the cognitively intact and is somewhat protective of cognitive function, there may a dual benefit of exercise as a pain management strategy and a way to help protect or improve cognitive function in older people. Therefore, targeted physical activity programs are highly recommended for this vulnerable group. Major challenges ahead include how to best integrate a targeted physical exercise program in a cost-effective intervention, and developing strategies to overcome sedentary behavior.

REFERENCES

1. Abdulla A, Adams N, Bone M, Elliott AM, Gaffin J, Jones D, Knaggs R, Martin D, Sampson L, Schofield P, British Geriatric Society. Guidance on the management of pain in older people. Age Ageing 2013;42:i1–57.
2. Abenhaim L, Rossignol M, Valat JP, Nordin M, Avouac B, Blotman F, Charlot J, Dreiser RL, Legrand E, Rozenberg S, Vautravers P. The role of activity in the therapeutic management of back pain. Report of the International Paris Task Force on Back Pain. Spine 2000;25:1S–33S.
3. Airaksinen O, Brox JI, Cedraschi C, Hildebrandt J, Klaber-Moffett J, Kovacs F, Mannion AF, Reis S, Staal JB, Ursin H, Zanoli G. Chapter 4 European guidelines for the management of chronic nonspecific low back pain. Eur Spine J 2006;15:s192–300.
4. Almeida OP, Khan KM, Hankey GJ, Yeap BB, Golledge J, Flicker L. 150 minutes of vigorous physical activity per week predicts survival and successful ageing: a population-based 11-year longitudinal study of 12 201 older Australian men. Br J Sports Med 2014;48:220–5.
5. Ambler N, Williams AC, Hill P, Gunary R, Cratchley G. Sexual difficulties of chronic pain patients. Clin J Pain 2001;17:138–45.

6. Antunes HKM, Santos RF, Cassilhas R, Santos RV, Bueno OF, de Mello MT. Reviewing on physical exercise and the cognitive function. Rev Bras Med Esporte 2006;12:108–14.
7. Baker LD, Frank LL, Foster-Schubert K, Green PS, Wilkinson CW, McTiernan A, Plymate SR, Fishel MA, Stennis Watson G, Cholerton BA, et al. Effects of aerobic exercise on mild cognitive impairment. Arch Neurol 2010;67:71–9.
8. Barnes D, Santos-Modesitt W, Poelke G, Kramer A, Castro C, Middleton L, Yaffe K. The mental activity and exercise (max) trial: a randomized controlled trial to enhance cognitive function in older adults. JAMA Intern Med 2013;173:797–804.
9. Battaglini CL, Mills RC, Phillips BL, Lee JT, Story CE, Nascimento MG, Hackney AC. Twenty-five years of research on the effects of exercise training in breast cancer survivors: a systematic review of the literature. World J Clin Oncol 2014;5:177–190.
10. Berryman C, Stanton TR, Bowering KJ, Tabor A, McFarlane A, Moseley GL. Do people with chronic pain have impaired executive function? A meta-analytical review. Clin Psychol Rev 2014;34:563–79.
11. Bidonde J, Busch AJ, Bath B, Milosavljevic S. Exercise for adults with fibromyalgia: an umbrella systematic review with synthesis of best evidence. Curr Rheumatol Rev 2014;10:45–79.
12. Bidonde J, Busch AJ, Webber SC, Schachter CL, Danyliw A, Overend TJ, Richards RS, Rader T. Aquatic exercise training for fibromyalgia. Cochrane Database Syst Rev 2014;10:CD011336.
13. Blankevoort CG, van Heuvelen MJG, Boersma F, Luning H, de Jong J, Scherder EJA. Review of effects of physical activity on strength, balance, mobility and ADL performance in elderly subjects with dementia. Dement Geriatr Cogn Disord 2010;30:392–402.
14. Bullo V, Bergamin M, Gobbo S, Sieverdes JC, Zaccaria M, Neunhaeuserer D, Ermolao A. The effects of Pilates exercise training on physical fitness and wellbeing in the elderly: A systematic review for future exercise prescription. Prev Med 2015;75:1–11.
15. Busch AJ, Webber SC, Richards RS, Bidonde J, Schachter CL, Schafer LA, Danyliw A, Sawant A, Dal Bello-Haas V, Rader T, Overend TJ. Resistance exercise training for fibromyalgia. Cochrane Database Syst Rev 2013;12:CD010884.
16. Chan WC, Fai Yeung JW, Man Wong CS, Wa Lam LC, Chung KF, Hay Luk JK, Wah Lee JS, Kin Law AC. Efficacy of physical exercise in preventing falls in older adults with cognitive impairment: a systematic review and meta-analysis. J Am Med Dir Assoc 2015;16:149–54.
17. Chen Y-W, Hsieh P-L, Chen Y-C, Hung C-H, Cheng J-T. Physical exercise induces excess hsp72 expression and delays the development of hyperalgesia and allodynia in painful diabetic neuropathy rats. Anesth Analg 2013;116:482–90.
18. Clare L, Evans S, Parkinson C, Woods R, Linden D. Goal-setting in cognitive rehabilitation for people with early-stage Alzheimer's disease. Clin Gerontol 2011;34:220–36.
19. Colcombe S, Kramer AF. Fitness effects on the cognitive function of older adults: a meta-analytic study. Psychol Sci 2003;14:125–30.
20. Cooney G, Dwan K, Mead G. Exercise for depression. JAMA 2014;311:2432–3.
21. Cooney GM, Dwan K, Greig CA, Lawlor DA, Rimer J, Waugh FR, McMurdo M, Mead GE. Exercise for depression. Cochrane Database Syst Rev 2013;9:CD004366. Accessed October 13, 2015 at http://onlinelibrary.wiley.com.ezp.lib.unimelb.edu.au/doi/10.1002/14651858.CD004366.pub6/abstract
22. Cox KL, Flicker L, Almeida OP, Xiao J, Greenop KR, Hendriks J, Phillips M, Lautenschlager NT. The FABS trial: a randomised control trial of the effects of a 6-month physical activity intervention on adherence and long-term physical activity and self-efficacy in older adults with memory complaints. Prev Med 2013;57:824–30.
23. El-Khoury F, Cassou B, Charles M-A, Dargent-Molina P. The effect of fall prevention exercise programmes on fall induced injuries in community dwelling older adults: systematic review and meta-analysis of randomised controlled trials. BMJ 2013;347:f6234.
24. Fiatarone Singh MA, Gates N, Saigal N, Wilson GC, Meiklejohn J, Brodaty H, Wen W, Singh N, Baune BT, Suo C, et al. The Study of Mental and Resistance Training (SMART) Study—resistance training and/or cognitive training in mild cognitive impairment: a randomized, double-blind, double-sham controlled trial. J Am Med Dir Assoc 2014;15:873–80.
25. Finan PH, Goodin BR, Smith MT. The association of sleep and pain: an update and a path forward. J Pain 2013;14:1539–52.
26. Forbes D, Forbes SC, Blake CM, Thiessen EJ, Forbes S. Exercise programs for people with dementia. Cochrane Database Syst Rev 2015;4:CD006489.

27. Gates N, Fiatarone Singh MA, Sachdev PS, Valenzuela M. The effect of exercise training on cognitive function in older adults with mild cognitive impairment: a meta-analysis of randomized controlled trials. Am J Geriatr Psychiatry 2013;21:1086–97.
28. Hamer M, Lavoie KL, Bacon SL. Taking up physical activity in later life and healthy ageing: the English longitudinal study of ageing. Br J Sports Med 2014;48:239–43.
29. Hasenbring MI, Hallner D, Klasen B, Streitlein-Böhme I, Willburger R, Rusche H. Pain-related avoidance versus endurance in primary care patients with subacute back pain: psychological characteristics and outcome at a 6-month follow-up. Pain 2012;153:211–7.
30. Hasenbring MI, Lundberg M, Parker R, Söderlund A, Bolton B, Smeets RJEM, Ljutov A, Simmonds MJ. Pain, mind, and movement in musculoskeletal pain: is physical activity always health-promoting or are there detrimental aspects? Clin J Pain 2015;31:95–6.
31. Hasenbring MI, Verbunt JA. Fear-avoidance and endurance-related responses to pain: new models of behavior and their consequences for clinical practice. Clin J Pain 2010;26:747–53.
32. Hayden JA, van Tulder MW, Tomlinson G. Systematic review: strategies for using exercise therapy to improve outcomes in chronic low back pain. Ann Intern Med 2005;142:776–85.
33. Heneweer H, Vanhees L, Picavet HSJ. Physical activity and low back pain: a U-shaped relation? Pain 2009;143:21–5.
34. Heyn P, Abreu BC, Ottenbacher KJ. The effects of exercise training on elderly persons with cognitive impairment and dementia: a meta-analysis. Arch Phys Med Rehabil 2004;85:1694–704.
35. Hurley MV, Walsh NE, Mitchell H, Nicholas J, Patel A. Long-term outcomes and costs of an integrated rehabilitation program for chronic knee pain: a pragmatic, cluster randomized, controlled trial. Arthritis Care Res 2012;64:238–47.
36. Hurley MV, Walsh NE, Mitchell HL, Pimm TJ, Patel A, Williamson E, Jones RH, Dieppe PA, Reeves BC. Clinical effectiveness of a rehabilitation program integrating exercise, self-management, and active coping strategies for chronic knee pain: a cluster randomized trial. Arthritis Rheum (Arthritis Care Res) 2007;57:1211–9.
37. Jedrziewski MK, Ewbank DC, Wang H, Trojanowski JQ. Exercise and cognition: results from the National Long Term Care Survey. Alzheimers Dement 2010;6:448–55.
38. Kemoun G, Thibaud M, Roumagne N, Carette P, Albinet C, Toussaint L, Paccalin M, Dugué B. Effects of a physical training programme on cognitive function and walking efficiency in elderly persons with dementia. Dement Geriatr Cogn Disord 2010;29:109–14.
39. Klusmann V, Evers A, Schwarzer R, Schlattmann P, Reischies FM, Heuser I, Dimeo FC. Complex mental and physical activity in older women and cognitive performance: a 6-month randomized controlled trial. J Gerontol A Biol Sci Med Sci 2010;65:680–8.
40. Koes BW, van Tulder MW, Thomas S. Diagnosis and treatment of low back pain. BMJ 2006;332:1430–4.
41. Lam LCW, Chau RCM, Wong BML, Fung AWT, Lui VWC, Tam CCW, Leung GTY, Kwok TCY, Chiu HFK, Ng S, Chan WM. Interim follow-up of a randomized controlled trial comparing Chinese style mind body (Tai Chi) and stretching exercises on cognitive function in subjects at risk of progressive cognitive decline. Int J Geriat Psychiatry 2011;26:733–40.
42. Larson EB, Wang L, Bowen JD, McCormick WC, Teri L, Crane P, Kukull W. Exercise is associated with reduced risk for incident dementia among persons 65 years of age and older. Ann Intern Med 2006;144:73–81.
43. Lautenschlager NT, Cox K, Cyarto EV. The influence of exercise on brain aging and dementia. Biochim Biophys Acta 2012;1822:474–81.
44. Lautenschlager NT, Flicker L, Cox KL, Foster JK, Almeida OP, van Bockxmeer FM, Greenop KR, Xiao J. Effect of physical activity on cognitive function in older adults at risk for Alzheimer disease: a randomized trial. JAMA 2008;300:1027–37.
45. Lee CE, Simmonds MJ, Novy DM, Jones SC. Functional self-efficacy, perceived gait ability and perceived exertion in walking performance of individuals with low back pain. Physiother Theory Pract 2002;18:193–203.
46. Leeuw M, Goossens MEJB, Linton SJ, Crombez G, Boersma K, Vlaeyen JWS. The fear-avoidance model of musculoskeletal pain: current state of scientific evidence. J Behav Med 2007;30:77–94.
47. Liu X, Li L, Tang F, Wu S, Hu Y. Memory impairment in chronic pain patients and the related neuropsychological mechanisms: a review. Acta Neuropsychiatr 2014;26:195–201.
48. Malysz T, Ilha J, do Nascimento PS, De Angelis K, Schaan BD, Achaval M. Beneficial effects of treadmill training in experimental diabetic nerve regeneration. Clinics 2010;65:1329–37.
49. Marcus BH, Banspach SW, Lefebvre RC, Rossi JS, Carleton RA, Abrams DB. Using the stages of change model to increase the adoption of physical activity among community participants. Am J Health Promot 1992;6:424–9.

50. Marley J, Tully MA, Porter-Armstrong A, Bunting B, O'Hanlon J, McDonough SM. A systematic review of interventions aimed at increasing physical activity in adults with chronic musculoskeletal pain—protocol. Syst Rev 2014;3:106.
51. McCarberg BH, Nicholson BD, Todd KH, Palmer T, Penles L. The impact of pain on quality of life and the unmet needs of pain management: results from pain sufferers and physicians participating in an Internet survey. Am J Ther 2008;15:312–20.
52. Miller DI, Taler V, Davidson PSR, Messier C. Measuring the impact of exercise on cognitive aging: methodological issues. Neurobiol Aging 2012;33:622.e29–43.
53. Murphy SL, Lyden AK, Smith DM, Dong Q, Koliba JF. Effects of a tailored activity pacing intervention on pain and fatigue for adults with osteoarthritis. Am J Occup Ther 2010;64:869–76.
54. Murphy SL, Phillips K, Williams DA, Clauw DJ. The role of the central nervous system in osteoarthritis pain and implications for rehabilitation. Curr Rheumatol Rep 2012;14:576–82.
55. Muscari A, Giannoni C, Pierpaoli L, Berzigotti A, Maietta P, Foschi E, Ravaioli C, Poggiopollini G, Bianchi G, Magalotti D, et al. Chronic endurance exercise training prevents aging-related cognitive decline in healthy older adults: a randomized controlled trial. Int J Geriatr Psychiatry 2010;25:1055–64.
56. Naugle KM, Fillingim RB, Riley JL. A meta-analytic review of the hypoalgesic effects of exercise. J Pain 2012;13:1139–50.
57. Ohayon MM, Schatzberg AF. Using chronic pain to predict depressive morbidity in the general population. Arch Gen Psychiatry 2003;60:39–47.
58. Öhman H, Savikko N, Strandberg TE, Pitkälä KH. Effect of physical exercise on cognitive performance in older adults with mild cognitive impairment or dementia: a systematic review. Dement Geriatr Cogn Disord 2014;38:347–65.
59. Paavilainen P, Korhonen I, Lötjönen J, Cluitmans L, Jylhä M, Särelä A, Partinen M. Circadian activity rhythm in demented and non-demented nursing-home residents measured by telemetric actigraphy. J Sleep Res 2005;14:61–8.
60. Paterson DH, Warburton DE. Physical activity and functional limitations in older adults: a systematic review related to Canada's Physical Activity Guidelines. Int J Behav Nutr Phys Act 2010;7:38.
61. Petursdottir U, Arnadottir SA, Halldorsdottir S. Facilitators and barriers to exercising among people with osteoarthritis: a phenomenological study. Phys Ther 2010;90:1014–25.
62. Pierrynowski MR, Tiidus PM, Galea V. Women with fibromyalgia walk with an altered muscle synergy. Gait Posture 2005;22:210–8.
63. Pincus T, Smeets RJEM, Simmonds MJ, Sullivan MJL. The fear avoidance model disentangled: improving the clinical utility of the fear avoidance model. Clin J Pain 2010;26:739–46.
64. Pitkälä KH, Pöysti MM, Laakkonen M, Tilvis RS, Savikko N, Kautiainen H, Strandberg TE. Effects of the Finnish Alzheimer disease exercise trial (FINALEX): a randomized controlled trial. JAMA Intern Med 2013;173:894–901.
65. Plassman BL, Williams JW, Burke JR, Holsinger T, Benjamin S. Systematic review: factors associated with risk for and possible prevention of cognitive decline in later life. Ann Intern Med 2010;153:182–93.
66. Powell W, Simmonds MJ. Virtual reality and musculoskeletal pain: manipulating sensory cues to improve motor performance during walking. Cyberpsychol Behav Soc Netw 2014;17:390–6.
67. Ratcliffe GE, Enns MW, Belik S-L, Sareen J. Chronic pain conditions and suicidal ideation and suicide attempts: an epidemiologic perspective. Clin J Pain 2008;24:204–10.
68. Reed J, Ones DS. The effect of acute aerobic exercise on positive activated affect: a meta-analysis. Psychol Sport Exercise 2006;7:477–514.
69. Sabiston CM, Brunet J, Burke S. Pain, movement, and mind: does physical activity mediate the relationship between pain and mental health among survivors of breast cancer? Clin J Pain 2012;28:489–95.
70. Schepens SL, Braun ME, Murphy SL. Effect of tailored activity pacing on self-perceived joint stiffness in adults with knee or hip osteoarthritis. Am J Occup Ther 2012;66:363–7.
71. Schwenk M, Zieschang T, Englert S, Grewal G, Najafi B, Hauer K. Improvements in gait characteristics after intensive resistance and functional training in people with dementia: a randomised controlled trial. BMC Geriatr 2014;14:73.
72. Simmonds M, Turner B. Long term, high dose opioids in veterans with chronic pain: are there benefits or just burdens? J Pain 2014;15:S101.
73. Sofi F, Valecchi D, Bacci D, Abbate R, Gensini GF, Casini A, Macchi C. Physical activity and risk of cognitive decline: a meta-analysis of prospective studies. J Intern Med 2011;269:107–17.

74. Uthman OA, van der Windt DA, Jordan JL, Dziedzic KS, Healey EL, Peat GM, Foster NE. Exercise for lower limb osteoarthritis: systematic review incorporating trial sequential analysis and network meta-analysis. Br J Sports Med 2014;48:1579.
75. van Middelkoop M, Rubinstein SM, Kuijpers T, Verhagen AP, Ostelo R, Koes BW, van Tulder MW. A systematic review on the effectiveness of physical and rehabilitation interventions for chronic non-specific low back pain. Eur Spine J 2011;20:19–39.
76. Vlaeyen JW, Kole-Snijders AM, Boeren RG, van Eek H. Fear of movement/(re)injury in chronic low back pain and its relation to behavioral performance. Pain 1995;62:363–72.
77. Waddell G, Newton M, Henderson I, Somerville D, Main CJ. A Fear-Avoidance Beliefs Questionnaire (FABQ) and the role of fear-avoidance beliefs in chronic low back pain and disability. Pain 1993;52:157–68.
78. Wayne PM, Walsh JN, Taylor-Piliae RE, Wells RE, Papp KV, Donovan NJ, Yeh GY. Effect of Tai Chi on cognitive performance in older adults: systematic review and meta-analysis. J Am Geriatr Soc 2014;62:25–39.
79. Weening-Dijksterhuis E, de Greef MHG, Scherder EJA, Slaets JPJ, van der Schans CP. Frail institutionalized older persons: a comprehensive review on physical exercise, physical fitness, activities of daily living, and quality-of-life. Am J Phys Med Rehabil 2011;90:156–68.
80. Westerterp KR, Meijer EP. Physical activity and parameters of aging: a physiological perspective. J Gerontol A Biol Sci Med Sci 2001;56:7–12.
81. WHO. International Classification of Functioning, Disability and Health (ICF). Accessed October 13, 2015 at http://www.who.int/classifications/icf/en/
82. Wideman TH, Asmundson GGJ, Smeets RJEM, Zautra AJ, Simmonds MJ, Sullivan MJL, Haythornthwaite JA, Edwards RR. Rethinking the fear avoidance model: toward a multidimensional framework of pain-related disability. Pain 2013;154:2262–5.
83. Williams AC de C, Eccleston C, Morley S. Psychological therapies for the management of chronic pain (excluding headache) in adults. Cochrane Database Syst Rev 2012;11:CD007407.
84. Williamson JD, Espeland M, Kritchevsky SB, Newman AB, King AC, Pahor M, Guralnik JM, Pruitt LA, Miller ME. Changes in cognitive function in a randomized trial of physical activity: results of the lifestyle interventions and independence for elders pilot study. J Gerontol A Biol Sci Med Sci 2009;64A:688–94.
85. Yágüez L, Shaw KN, Morris R, Matthews D. The effects on cognitive functions of a movement-based intervention in patients with Alzheimer's type dementia: a pilot study. Int J Geriatr Psychiatry 2011;26:173–81.
86. Young J, Angevaren M, Rusted J, Tabet N. Aerobic exercise to improve cognitive function in older people without known cognitive impairment. Cochrane Database Syst Rev 2015;4:CD005381.

CHAPTER 20

Psychological Approaches to Therapy

Rachel Bieu, Joseph Kulas, and Robert Kerns

PAIN

Pain is endemic to the human experience and advantageous when understood as manifesting as a signal indicating harm. Conceptualized in this way, pain is transitory, the expected result of an acute injury, illness, or surgery and resolving with removal of the source of pain and healing [39, 40]. Conversely, the experience of chronic or persistent pain is not consistent with this conceptualization. Understandably so, chronic pain can be devastating to individual well-being (physical, social, emotional, financial) as this pain serves little or no purpose in persisting beyond the expected window of healing or the understood resolution of the source of pain [39, 40, 64]. Persisting pain is increasingly becoming a global health problem with estimates suggesting that 20% of adults suffer from pain and 10% are newly diagnosed with chronic pain yearly [23]. Average length of suffering for those experiencing chronic pain is 7 years [23].

Demographically speaking, pain is not equally distributed, such that the risk for experiencing chronic pain increases as one ages, with high rates in the elderly and the highest rates of chronic pain experienced by the oldest of the old [1, 2, 59]. Epidemiological studies estimate that between 25% and 65% of the elderly living in the community and up to 80% living in an institutionalized setting experience chronic pain [47]. In the elderly, most commonly occurring pain is musculoskeletal and neuropathic which can restrict an individual's ability to carry out activities of daily living (ADLs), result in poor sleep, and increase susceptibility to other chronic disabling conditions, psychiatric, or otherwise. Further, pain coping is often complicated by stressful events unique to aging, including losses, bereavement, and a change in socializing and available supports [20, 29, 47, 56].

Despite an increase in prevalence as persons age, pain is consistently undertreated in the elderly [47]. This has been attributed to multiple factors including reporting habits of older persons, acceptance of these reports by caregivers, ability of caregivers to identify pain, and assessment variables. Additional contributors include reluctance to provide pharmacological agents given increased risk (e.g., polypharmacy, adverse side effects, and intoxication), insufficient training in pain management, and misconception with regard to nonpharmacological pain interventions [47].

DEMENTIA AND PAIN

In addition to chronic pain, age is also the principal risk factor for dementia, and therefore, it is likely that pain is similarly common in those who are experiencing cognitive decline. Presently, 5% of persons over the age of 65 carry a dementia diagnosis, rising to 50% in those aged over 90 years [1, 16].

Dementia is a nonspecific, umbrella term generally understood to mean that one's cognition is impaired to the extent that functional ability is affected. Dementia is subdivided into numerous diagnostic entities with varying course and prognosis. However, most require significant levels of care with estimates of 50–90% of long-term care residents suffering from dementia [11]. Cognitive deficits in those who are diagnosed with dementia are varied and include impairments in memory, language, executive functioning, visuospatial skill, and other neurocognitive domains. The impairments observed in those afflicted with dementia can also include psychological problems and behavioral disturbance [1, 14]. While memory dysfunction is most often described as impactful on the functioning of individuals with dementia, the behavioral and psychological symptoms of dementia, often termed "BPSD" [1], along with physical disability, have the greatest impact on quality of life, also leading to greater requirements of assistance and institutionalization [1].

Pain management is particularly daunting in the presence of dementia [1, 59]. Because pain is an experiential phenomenon, its assessment is typically completed through verbal description by the individual. However, the cognitive impairments associated with dementia often limit an individual's ability to express his or her pain. Depending on the level of impairment and complexity of cognitive skills required, individuals may struggle to use existing self-report pain scales. Persons with a more advanced dementia may be able to report pain either spontaneously or in response to questioning but may be unable to qualify pain, while there is a subset who will be unable to offer a yes-or-no response when prompted and thus cannot report pain [14]. Institutionalized residents with significant cognitive impairment have been found to report less pain despite more physical and functional disability than their cognitively intact counterparts [14, 53]. Unfortunately, this is further complicated by the reluctance of caregivers to accept the reports of pain from those with cognitive impairment and a lack of appropriate pain assessment tools. Furthermore, pain is often expressed via behavioral disturbance and is thought to be one of the chief causal factors of BPSD [12]. In such cases, expressions of pain may be perceived as nonspecific agitation, anxiety, or emotional distress. Interpretation of these behaviors by caregivers may not always result in the consideration of pain as causal and as such can leave pain untreated.

In the context of our aging world, given increasing incidence of chronic pain and dementia as persons age, it will be important to understand and appreciate effective alternative opportunities for intervention that have the potential to reduce other increasing risks accompanying age (e.g., polypharmacy, decreasing supports).

PSYCHOLOGICAL INTERVENTIONS FOR PAIN

The traditionally accepted biomedical model of pain assumes that a person's pain report is directly correlated to a specific disease state with diagnosis confirmed via objective tests substantiating physical damage [63]. Treatment utilizing this model would by extension focus on the physical aspects of the pain experience and thus suggests medical intervention.

However, this model has been criticized for its failure to recognize psychological and psychosocial factors, particularly their interaction with physiological factors. This shortcoming is most often highlighted when the presence and extent of pathology are not sufficient to account for reported symptoms; this often is the case in chronic pain.

Conversely, the biopsychosocial model focuses on the interaction of biological, psychological, and social variables asserting that the diversity in the expression of illness (severity, duration, manifested consequences) is better accounted for by the complex interrelationships between pathological changes, psychological status, and social and cultural contexts [63]. From this perspective, persistent pain may have less to do with observable pathology. Considering chronic pain and thinking longitudinally, what was initiated due to biological factors may be maintained or complicated as a result of related physical anxieties, psychological judgments, and interpretations of internal physiological signs, social factors affecting behavioral responses, interpretations of physical anxieties, or perceived internal psychological signs. Thus, treatment of pain should benefit from the amelioration of these maintaining factors. Psychological treatments have been developed that are useful in addressing the role of cognitive, behavioral, and emotional factors in the development and maintenance of chronic pain. These interventions have included cognitive–behavioral, mindfulness, and self-regulatory approaches.

Cognitive Behavioral Therapy

Cognitive Behavioral Therapy (CBT) incorporates both cognitive and behavioral techniques in an effort to alter behavior [62, 65]. Given the long history of CBT, there is a diversity of approaches to its implementation. While approaches are distinct to varying degrees, they are also overlapping, having in common three fundamental assumptions (1) that cognition(s) or thought (e.g., appraisals) affects behavior; (2) that cognition(s) can be tracked and modified, this requiring some interim assessment of cognitive activity and; (3) that a desired behavior(s) may be achieved following cognitive change [17]. Beyond these core assumptions five dimensions have been suggested in characterizing CBT approaches including the theoretical orientation of the therapeutic approach and the theoretical target of change, aspects of the client–therapist relationship, the cognitive target for change, the type of evidence use for cognitive assessment, and the degree of client emphasized self-control. CBT was originally designed for the treatment of more traditional psychological disorders, such as depression and anxiety, but has since been successfully applied in the treatment of a number of psychophysiological conditions including pain.

The evolution of CBT for pain management is engendered in the larger developing CBT model such that the initial intervention pioneered in multidisciplinary pain management [19] focused on operant conditioning using reinforcement for self-management techniques such as involvement in progressive relaxation [40]. Using operant conditioning, behavioral responses to pain were modified given the consequences of the environment in which the behavior occurred (e.g., behavior that is reinforced is increased). The cognitive aspects of CBT, more prominent as the treatment has evolved, have been found to be useful in both the reduction of pain, benefiting functional ability, as well as in the stabilizing of mood and reduction of disability [40, 41]. Cognitive interventions include the identification of negative automatic thoughts and ideally the replacement of maladaptive thoughts with those which are adaptive. Important to treatment rationale is an individual understanding of how one's cognitions and behaviors affect the pain experience, highlighting individual utility in controlling pain. Skills training or pain-coping strategies tailored to an individual's needs, can include a variety of techniques such as self-regulatory strategies (e.g., relaxation techniques), pleasant activity scheduling, distraction methods, and cognitive restructuring. In cognitive restructuring, negative pain thoughts are identified and challenged so that they can be substituted with tractable and malleable coping thoughts. Finally, learned coping skills are applied and maintained. Applying skills to an expanding variety of situations, persons are counseled in problem-solving so that they can effectively deal with challenging situations as they arise. Self-monitoring and behavioral contracting is used to prompt and reinforce coping skills practice.

Mindfulness Approaches

It has been argued that the evolution of CBT can be divided into three distinct and overlapping generations with mindfulness approaches representing the third wave, following traditional behavioral and CBT [25]. Mindfulness is a way of directing one's attention, generally described as an intentional focus on the present moment without judgment [6]. Mindfulness-based treatment approaches, including mindfulness-based stress reduction (MBSR), mindfulness-based cognitive therapy (MBCT), and acceptance and commitment therapy (ACT), access a variety of methods for teaching attention to the present moment or mindful awareness. Briefly, MBSR and MBCT include both formal meditation and informal practices, while ACT highlights largely shorter and less-formal activities practicing constituent skills of mindfulness. Variations aside, common to formal and informal mindfulness practices are two general instructions [6]. Persons are encouraged to focus their attention directly on an activity. Observing carefully if their attention wanders, they are to note this subsequently returning their focus to their target. The same is applied to bodily sensations or emotions that should arise [6].

Mindfulness-Based Stress Reduction (MBSR)

MBSR was developed in a behavioral medicine setting with individuals with chronic pain and stress-related conditions and is based on intensive training in mindfulness meditation [6, 36, 37]. In its standard form, MBSR is relayed as an 8-week class with weekly sessions lasting 2.5–3 hours and an all-day intensive session held in week 6. Classes or group sessions are experiential, with a large portion of time devoted to practice exercises and discussion of members' experiences with the like. A variety of exercises are taught with didactic information about stress incorporated into most sessions [6]. Additionally, participants are required to engage in extensive homework (at least 45 minutes/day for 6 days/week) consisting of practice of mindfulness exercises.

Mindfulness-Based Cognitive Therapy (MBCT)

MBCT is based on MBSR and therefore relies on many of the same components. In addition, MBCT includes the monitoring of pleasant and unpleasant events. Like MBSR, MBCT is often conducted in an 8-week group with 2-hour weekly sessions. The nature of group discussion and importance of homework still applies. MBCT does not include traditional CBT exercises designed to change thoughts but does integrate several exercises based on elements of cognitive therapy meant to deemphasize internal experience. Examples of exercises include the thoughts and feelings exercise or the moods, thoughts, and alternative viewpoints exercise. In MBCT participants practice mindfulness of thoughts, letting them come and go, working in the knowledge that thoughts are not facts.

Acceptance and Commitment Therapy

ACT highlights the manner in which persons maintain their difficulties through language and psychological inflexibility [26–28]. Common to ACT is the perspective that the tendency to avoid unpleasant thoughts and feelings is at the core of suffering and that psychological flexibility is found in learning to experience both pleasant and unpleasant internal states rather than in attempting to control or eliminate them. Thus in ACT, individuals are taught to notice their thoughts without judgment or engagement, fostering a continued respect for self and one's core values [26–28, 40].

ACT as applied to chronic pain management suggests that while pain is unpleasant it is not pain itself but rather an individual's persistent struggle with pain that causes distress. From this perspective, continuing attempts to control chronic pain are maladaptive [15]. Failure to accept pain results in avoidance and the seeking of alleviating interventions. Though, if no reduction in pain is found, activity is avoided and disability maintained; therefore, such an intervention is not in the best interest of the client. As such ACT argues that individuals may receive better outcomes in reducing avoidance and other attempts at control, fostering acceptance and focusing on achievable goals (e.g., change language and way of thinking and therefore implementing a sense of control over one's responses to emotions as opposed to decreasing the occurrence of unwanted internal stimuli or events) [18]. Methods used in ACT are not entirely unique to this approach and may include exposure therapies, written exercises focusing on core values, and experiential exercises including breathing techniques highlighting awareness, focus, and the present moment [26].

Self-Regulatory Approaches

Pain is conceptualized as a psychophysiological condition wherein biological and psychological factors interact to influence perception. Self-regulatory techniques are designed to exploit this mind–body connection in order to increase sense of control over physiological or emotional states thereby impacting the pain experience. Self-regulatory approaches may include biofeedback and relaxation training [40].

Biofeedback

Biofeedback is a technique of providing person's biological information in real time, the goal being to increase awareness of changing physiological processes so that individuals can learn to gain control over bodily reactions associated with a perceived automatic response [22, 40]. In pain management, physiological targets are factors directly related to pain exacerbations and emotional responses to pain [40].

Relaxation Training

Relaxation training focuses on the identifying of tension within the mind and body and the subsequent application of techniques including deep breathing, progressive muscle relaxation (PMR), and visualization to both lessen tension and modify pain perception [40].

Relaxation training educates persons about the bidirectional relationship between emotional (stress) and physiological (muscle tension) states. These techniques are often used in support of or to supplement other treatment regimens [40].

Hypnotherapy

Hypnosis is generally understood as an altered state of consciousness. It can be combined with any type of therapy and when combined is termed hypnotherapy [9]. Thus, hypnosis can be operationalized in various ways depending on the therapeutic perspective employed. Generally, hypnosis relies heavily on attention. Related to the careful focus of attention, is the ability to resist or shut out distraction from internal and external stimuli [9]. Individuals are taught to delve into this state whenever wanted or needed utilizing behavioral cues. In the context of pain management, persons are taught to focus their attention in such a way to alter their subjective pain experience [40].

EVALUATION OF PSYCHOLOGICAL TREATMENTS FOR PAIN IN ADULTS

Evaluation of the efficacy of psychosocial interventions for pain in adults has suggested a good response through the use of these methods. Morley et al. [49] conducted a meta-analysis of randomized controlled trials (RCTs) of CBT, behavioral treatment, and self-regulatory (biofeedback, relaxation training) interventions applied to various chronic pain conditions and found that for all outcome measures (pain expression, activity level) any of the psychological interventions studied was more effective than a wait-list control condition [39, 49]. When compared to active treatment controls, CBT and behavioral treatment were found to be effective [39]. Hoffman et al. [32] conducted a meta-analysis of psychological interventions for chronic low back pain. Here a total of 205 effect sizes from 22 studies were pooled in 34 analyses. Overall, results yielded positive effects of psychological treatments of CLBP for pain intensity, pain-related interference, health-related quality of life, and depression [32]. When interventions were compared to wait-list controls, moderate effect sizes were found for pain intensity and health-related quality of life. When compared to active controls, small effects were found for reducing pain interference and moderate effects for lowering work-related disability [32]. Cognitive–behavioral and self-regulatory interventions were most efficacious.

PSYCHOLOGICAL INTERVENTIONS FOR PAIN IN THE ELDERLY

Cognitive and behavioral interventions for elderly chronic pain patients continue to be relatively unstudied; however, available (see Table 20-1) and accumulating support suggests that the elderly benefit from these approaches in the same way as their younger counterparts [47, 66]. Moreover, it has been suggested that first-line pharmacological treatment for chronic pain in the aged is most effective when combined with nonpharmacological intervention [21, 47].

TABLE 20-1 Studies Investigating Psychological Intervention in the Treatment of Pain in the Aged

Study	Mean Age	N	Treatment
Cook [13]	77.0	22	Cognitive–behavioral pain management
Reid et al. [58]	77.4	14	Cognitive–behavioral therapy
Andersson et al. [2]	72.0	21	Cognitive–behavioral group Intervention
Morone et al. [50]	74.9	37	Mindfulness meditation/mindfulness-based stress reduction (MBSR)
Arena et al. [4]	69.0	10	Progressive muscle relaxation (PMR) therapy
Arena et al. [3]	65.0	8	Electromyographic biofeedback training
McBee et al. [48]	85.0	14	Psychoeducational relaxational group
Nicholson and Blanchard [51]	66.7	14	Combined relaxation training, cognitive therapy, and biofeedback
Kabela et al. [38]	Range 66–77	16	Various combinations of relaxation (e.g., PMR, breathing), cognitive stress coping, and biofeedback

Cognitive Behavioral Therapy in Elderly Populations

Cook [13] implemented a cognitive behavioral pain management program for elderly nursing home residents with chronic pain. Specifically, a randomized group design was used comparing a CBT intervention to an attention/support control intervention. Both interventions were relayed in weekly group sessions lasting 10 weeks. Participants were 13 men and 9 women from two nursing homes, ranging in age from 61 to 98 ($M = 72$). While the programs were perceived as equally credible both before and after intervention, results found that individuals who received CBT reported less pain and pain-related disability. More treatment effects were maintained at 4-month follow-up, despite an overall increase in reported pain. There were no significant treatment effects for depression or medication ratings. Similarly, Reid et al. [58] administered CBT to largely female (86%) senior housing residents with chronic pain aged 65 or older ($M = 77.4$). CBT was administered in 10 weekly individual sessions, with participants phoned 5 days on average after each session to gauge comprehension, usefulness of materials, and adherence to assigned homework exercises. Comprehension of CBT exceeded 97% and mean rating for usefulness of treatment sessions ranged from 7.5 to 9.4. The mean number of days per week that individuals completed homework exercises ranged from 1.8 to 4.0. At 2 weeks, posttreatment versus pretreatment assessment [58] found significant reductions in pain intensity and pain-related disability scores. While treatment effects were noted to decrease over time, they did not return to pretreatment levels as of 24 weeks.

Mindfulness

Morone et al. [50] looked at a mindfulness-based intervention for chronic pain in the elderly. Community-dwelling adults aged 65 and older ($M = 74.9$) were randomized to either an 8-week mindfulness-based meditation group or a wait-list control group. Overall, 37 participants were randomized within a 6-month period. The intervention was well tolerated as the study evidenced a high overall completion rate with 68% (13/19) of the intervention group and 78% (14/18) of the wait-list control group after they crossed over to the intervention finishing all aspects of the intervention. Of the 13 participants in the intervention group who completed the 8-week program, 12 were available for 3-month follow-up with no significant difference found in 8-week versus 2-month scores. Participants were found to have meditated an average of 4.3 days/week for an estimated 31.6 minutes/day. Compared to the wait-list control group, the mindfulness group showed significant improvement in pain acceptance, activities engagement, and physical function. Further speaking to long-standing benefit and ease of maintenance, most participants continued to meditate of their own accord at 3-month follow-up.

Self-Regulatory

Arena et al. [3] evaluated a self-regulatory intervention in the elderly. Here the effects of a 12-session frontal electromyographic biofeedback training regimen on headache in eight elderly tension headache sufferers ($N = 8$, $M = 65$ years) was studied. Biofeedback sessions were modified slightly in an effort to increase comprehension, learning, and recall of purpose and instructions. Results of a 3-month posttreatment assessment showed significant decreases in overall headache activity in 50% or greater of the subjects with moderate improvement (35–45%) in three of the four remaining subjects. Significant pre–post difference was also found for number of headache free days, peak headache activity, and medication index.

A prior study by Arena et al. [4] applied relaxation therapy to tension headache in the elderly ($N = 10$, $M = 69$ years). Subjects received an 8-week progressive muscle-relaxation therapy regimen. Similar to Arena et al. [3], results posttreatment showed significant reductions in overall headache activity (50% or greater) in seven subjects. Significant pre–post differences were also seen for number of headache-free days, peak headache activity, and medication index.

Meta-Analytic Studies Reviewing Cognitive and Behavioral Interventions

Lunde et al. [47] conducted a meta-analysis reviewing cognitive and behavioral interventions for chronic pain in the elderly. Overall, Lunde et al. [47] found that cognitive and behavioral interventions (including CBT, mindfulness, and self-regulatory interventions) produce improvement in self-reported pain experience in the elderly with an overall mean effect size for treatment versus pretreatment or control condition of 0.47 at posttreatment and 0.56 at follow-up. Effect sizes were consistent with the Morley et al. [49] meta-analysis of cognitive and behavioral treatment of chronic pain in adults. Further, meta-analyses for psychological treatments of depression and anxiety in the elderly [52, 61] find overall effect sizes of 0.55 and 0.78. Therefore, in applying nonpharmacological interventions in older persons, overall effect sizes for pain are consistent with effects obtained in younger cohorts and for more traditional psychological disorders.

PSYCHOLOGICAL TREATMENT OF PAIN IN COGNITIVELY IMPAIRED POPULATIONS

As noted above, pain is highly comorbid with dementia and consistently undertreated. Research indicates that both pharmacological and nonpharmacological interventions are underutilized in cognitively impaired populations. In the context of a progressive process whereby ability to effectively communicate needs deteriorates, treatment opportunity is lost when behavioral symptoms are unnoticed, dismissed, or not understood and acknowledged as arising from physiological or psychosocial unmet needs [42].

Individuals with dementia report pain less often, less spontaneously, and at a lower intensity than their cognitively intact counterparts with ability to verbally communicate pain or discomfort generally decreasing as dementia severity increases [7, 42, 56]. For those who are cognitively impaired, behaviors such as vocalizations (e.g., sighing, moaning, calling out, verbal abuse, repetitive vocalizations, noisy breathing), facial expressions (e.g., grimacing or frowning), restless or strained body expressions (e.g., fidgeting, increased pacing, or rocking), or agitation and resistance to care may represent the most prominent or the only feature of pain. Unfortunately, it is often the case that such symptoms are disregarded or interpreted as characteristic of dementia rather than recognized as a symptom of pain [56]. Recognition of pain when information is less readily available to caregivers calls for more thorough evaluation, this then potentiating opportunities for intervention, both in the treatment of pain and behavioral symptoms. However, in the absence of comprehensive assessment, individuals with dementia are unfortunately more likely to receive psychotropic medications rather than appropriate pain treatment [7, 42, 56].

In light of the possibility of pain serving as a causative factor in the presentation of BPSD, it is important that the control of pain in those suffering from dementia is clear. Research demonstrating the efficacy of pain treatment in reducing behavioral symptoms in dementia has largely focused on pharmacological intervention [10, 33, 34]. As an example, Chibnall et al. [10] investigated the effect of regularly scheduled analgesic medication on behavior, emotional well-being, and use of psychotropic medication. Here, 25 nursing home residents with moderate to severe dementia received 4 weeks of treatment with acetaminophen and 4 weeks of a placebo. Results showed that those receiving acetaminophen spent more time in social interaction, engaged with media, talking to themselves, engaged in work-like activity, and experiencing unattended distress. They also spent less time in their rooms, less time removed from the unit, and less time in personal care activities. However, despite increased activity and socialization, no effect was seen for agitation, emotional well-being, or need for psychotropic medication.

In contrast to primary pharmacological intervention, there is increasing research available showing the efficacy of psychosocial and behavioral interventions in the reduction of neuropsychiatric symptoms manifesting in behavioral symptoms [5, 8, 44–46]. Ayalon et al. [5] conducted an investigation of the available research on the effect of nonpharmacologic interventions for neuropsychiatric symptoms among persons with dementia. Three RCTs and six single case designs (SCDs) met criteria and were included in the review. Intervention type included unmet needs interventions (one SCD), behavioral interventions (four SCDs), caregiving interventions (three RCTs), and bright-light therapy (one SCD). The results of the review suggested variable efficacy dependent on the type of intervention used. Approaches that utilized an unmet needs intervention that focused on assessing the motivation driving neuropsychiatric symptoms and designing an intervention to reduce those symptoms or their intensity found moderate reductions in problem behaviors. Comparatively, behavioral interventions treating neuropsychiatric symptoms via contingency management (e.g., reward removal) were found to result in a relative reduction of 50–100% in neuropsychiatric symptoms. Examination of the above approaches when taught to caregivers yielded mixed results with one RCT finding a reduction in four neuropsychiatric symptoms subscales including ideation disturbance, irritability, verbal agitation, and physical aggression at 6-month follow-up, a second RCT finding significant improvement in frequency and severity of intervention-associated target behaviors, and a third finding no effect. Finally, examination of available studies of bright-light therapy where exposure to direct bright light is provided to engender a calming effect on an agitated patient found short-lived improvements in agitated behavior. Overall, findings from this review suggest that nonpharmacological interventions targeting neuropsychiatric symptoms in persons with dementia may be effective.

Despite these inroads in understanding nonpharmacological intervention, particularly those based on the biopsychosocial model, there appears a disconnect in treatment approach and lack of understanding between the relationship between pain and behavioral symptoms, how they co-occur, and which interventions are effective at lessening both pain and behavioral symptoms [56]. The bridging of this disconnect then, as described by Piper et al. [56], may lie in the appropriate modification of psychological treatments to meet the needs of a cognitively impaired population. Although limited research is available to support such modifications with regard to pain, a relatively larger body of literature exists supporting their modification in the treatment of neuropsychiatric symptoms including depression and anxiety.

As an example of this approach Kraus et al. [43] discuss a modified version of CBT for anxiety in dementia (CBT-AD), this protocol developed, piloted, and modified over two years with seven mildly demented participants [43]. Modifications were made to the content, structure, and learning strategies of CBT in an effort to adapt to the cognitive limitations of the patients, for example, adapting simplified checklists such that they mainly required recognition skills. Psychoeducation and skills including diaphragmatic breathing, coping self-statements, exposure, and behavioral activation were simplified. For example, breathing was introduced with simplified procedures including breathing deeply and slowly. This contrasted with a traditional multistep diaphragmatic breathing technique. Collaterals (e.g., caregivers such as spouses and children) were trained as coaches (e.g., encouraging participants to breathe slowly and praising effort). Practice was done daily and encouraged in the context of distress. In later sessions participants were encouraged to practice when they had difficulty sleeping at night. This was reinforced with prompting and practicing appropriate responses. Furthermore, sessions were shortened to accommodate for attention and fatigue and were limited to the teaching of one or two skills. In these sessions patients were encouraged to repeat information to facilitate learning and to actively participate in the creating of reminder cues serving retrieval. Finally, therapists relied on spaced retrieval, an evidence-based method for improving learning and retrieval, relying on procedural memory. In their protocol, patients and their collaterals participated in nine sessions over 10 weeks, with sessions lasting 30–45 minutes. The first sessions focused on monitoring and deep breathing with further sessions focusing on the use of coping self-statements (fourth) and behavioral activation (seventh). During each session, participants were provided with simplified written instructions and a concrete homework plan to be completed. In addition, brief phone calls with the patient occurred once a week between sessions to test for comprehension and difficulties using the skills learned in the previous session. These phone calls also encouraged practice. Posttreatment, during a subsequent 3-month period weekly and then bi-weekly phone calls were made to continue to facilitate the use of skills. The results of this early pilot suggested that a modified CBT protocol may be advantageous in a dementia population as clinically meaningful reductions in anxiety were found. Patient one's posttreatment assessment indicated a decrease in anxiety according to the Rating Anxiety in Dementia Scale (RAID; pre-RAID = 19, post-RAID = 10). Collateral informant also reported decreased restlessness, improved mood, and increased participation in pleasurable activities. Caregiver distress decreased minimally as measured by the Neuropsychiatric Inventory (NPI) (pre = 3, post = 2), and the NPI anxiety subscale remained stable at 4. At 6-month follow-up the RAID dropped to 7, caregiver distress returned to baseline at 3, and NPI anxiety remained at 4. Individual successes were more pronounced. For instance, Patient two's posttreatment assessment showed a decrease in RAID (pre = 12, post = 8) and NPI anxiety scores (pre = 8, post = 1) and Patient two's caregiver distress dropped from 1 to 0.

Further research has supported this early work in suggesting the benefit of psychological approaches in the treatment of psychiatric symptoms in cognitively impaired populations. Regan and Varanelli [57] conducted a systematic review looking at community-based intervention studies aiming to improve depression, anxiety, or adjustment. For the purposes of the review, participants met published Mild Cognitive Impairment (MCI) criteria [55] or were described as having mild–moderate dementia. Studies used psychological and social interventions designed to improve mood, or adjustment and quality of life for individuals diagnosed with MCI or dementia. Sixteen of 921 studies identified met inclusion criteria. A wide range of psychotherapeutic approaches (e.g., problem-solving, CBT) and formats (e.g., individual, group) were found across studies. Overall, five different psychotherapeutic approaches were used. Both recovery-oriented therapy and brief psychodynamic therapy were individual based; CBT and exploratory psychotherapy were group based; and a mixed program included both individual and group aspects. Results found positive improvements in well-being and adjustment in studies utilizing recovery-oriented [35] and CBT approaches [54, 60]; however, no evidence was apparent for constructivist, brief psychodynamic, or exploratory approaches. The extent to which approaches were modified varied across studies. For example, in Jha et al. [35], utilizing a recovery-based intervention, no modification is described. While in CBT interventions [54, 60] multiple modifications are discussed including introduction of one skill at a time, fewer total skills with extra time spent on practice and repetition, regular summation of material, involvement of a friend or family member in implementation, use of telephone follow-up to reinforce concepts, among others. Overall, several studies, using problem-solving and modified CBT approaches showed promise.

Finally, a single study (see Table 20-2) is found acknowledging a comprehensive modified non-pharmacological intervention, speaking to co-existing problems, including pain, mood, and behavioral dysfunction, in a cognitively impaired population [11]. Cipher, Clifford, and Roper conducted a two-part study in an effort to investigate the efficacy of multimodal cognitive behavioral therapy (MCBT) for the treatment of pain, depression, behavioral dysfunction, and health-care utilization in a sample of cognitively impaired long-term care residents with chronic pain. Initially, 44 consecutive patients (mean age = 82 years) received eight sessions of MCBT over a 5-week period. The patients initially underwent a thorough initial evaluation assessing for presenting problems, medical and psychosocial histories, current dysfunctional behaviors, level of dementia or cognitive impairment,

TABLE 20-2 **Studies Investigating Psychological Intervention in the Treatment of Pain in Dementia**

Study	Mean Age	N	Treatment
Cipher et al. [11]	82.0	44	Multimodal Cognitive–behavioral therapy (CBT)

level of cooperation with ADLs, emotional distress, pain, current social support systems, patient's perceptions of self, situation, future and most imminently their historical motivational themes, and current desired outcomes. Subsequent early treatment sessions focused on establishing motivating themes and values congruent with assessed history. These historically congruent themes were used repeatedly to facilitate the patients' reassessments of their situations which resulted in pain, mood disturbance, and interpersonal difficulty, among other problems. The more advanced the dementia, the more overtly behavioral and directive the therapy used. Collaterals such as family members or other health providers were included in the process as appropriate. The MCBT model was self-correcting and depended on continued assessment and flexibility. If one technique didn't work another was tried with adjusting techniques added to the patient's treatment plan. Pre- and postanalyses showed that following intervention, patients exhibited significant reductions in pain, activity interference and emotional distress secondary to pain, and significant increases in most ADLs. They also showed significant reductions in the intensity, frequency, and duration or behavioral disturbances but not number of disturbances. A follow-up study compared the MCBT treatment group with a matched control group looking at health-care utilization. Group comparisons revealed that the treatment group required significantly fewer physician visits and change orders than the control group. The groups did not significantly differ on number of hospital stays or number of emergency department visits since last assessment [11]. Considering cognitively impaired populations, findings from Cipher, Clifford, and Roper offers support for continued interdisciplinary assessment and management of comorbidities with modified flexible nonpharmalogical intervention.

IMPLICATIONS FOR TREATMENT/INTERVENTION

In light of limited availability of description let alone empirical evidence of efficacious psychological interventions, the following section provides an overview and brief description of key issues and intervention in the treatment of pain in cognitively impaired populations.

Dementia exists along a continuum and is often progressive. This argues first for a system of continuous assessment. The initial assessment should be comprehensive and include evaluation of an individual's medical and psychosocial history, current dysfunctional behaviors (e.g., BPSD, disruptive behavior), cognitive and functional status, pain, emotional distress, current social support system, and in considering treatment, motivational themes, or desired outcomes. Providers should be familiar with recommendations tailored to the assessment of pain in older adults including those with advanced dementia, or the nonverbal patient. Recommendations have been summarized for the consumer in a consensus document and guiding principles [24, 30, 31] (see Chapters 9 to 15). Briefly, experts compiling these documents advise the following when assessing pain in this population (1) taking into account patient history, interview information, and results of physical examinations; (2) use of assessment approaches that include both self-report and observational measures; (3) the utilization of movement-based tasks as these are more likely to identify persistent pain and can offer enhanced sensitivity and specificity; (4) the implementation of an analgesic trial and investigation as to the extent to which this abates behavioral indicators of pain; (5) comprehensive assessment should further include evaluation of related contributors to pain and patient functioning such as mood, social supports, and coping; (6) collateral information should be gathered from knowledgeable informants (e.g., caregivers); and (7) following the establishment of a baseline individuals, should be monitored frequently over time and should assessment tools be used, they should be used appropriately and under consistent circumstances [24, 30, 31]. Consistent with many areas of medicine, a team-based approach to treatment of both pain and BPSD will be most effective, particularly as it relates to effective communication of changes in the patient's status. Furthermore, ongoing reminders to all staff involved in a patient's care for the potential presence of pain as a precipitant factor will reinforce the need for its continuous assessment.

When considering a population with dementia, assessment of cognitive abilities will be paramount. The assessment of cognitive status will, to a large degree, determine how treatment is disseminated to the patient and guide how it will need to be modified with potential disease progression. Ongoing assessment of cognitive status can be operationalized via the use of brief, repeatable cognitive assessments or batteries which will allow for accurate longitudinal comparisons that can provide information concerning how effective the current approach will be. Assessment in the earlier stages of decline will incorporate tests that would be similar to those used with cognitively intact individuals. However, the assessment of the patients functioning will change as their cognitive skills deteriorate. In very late stages, this assessment will focus more on an individual's functional ability and ability to communicate their needs and understand questions posed to them, rather than their absolute cognitive level in comparison to peers. Ongoing consultation with neuropsychologists familiar with geropsychiatric patients should be considered.

Given base rates for chronic pain in the aging population, the assumption that the patient is in pain should be the rule rather than the exception [47]. Continued assessment of pain symptoms should occur frequently, with daily assessment in the presence of disruptive or dysfunctional behaviors regardless of injury status. Assessment of pain is closely tied to one's cognitive status and will need to be increasingly simplified depending on the cognitive abilities of a given individual. Those providing care are encouraged to bear in mind that individuals who are more impaired report pain less often, less spontaneously, and at a lower intensity than their cognitively intact counterparts. Further, increasingly lacking the ability to communicate pain with disease progression, pain in more advanced stages of cognitive decline is often expressed via behavioral disturbance. Thus, depending on ability level, pain may be gauged by an appropriate self-report measure or conversely by staff observation and measurement or rating such as frequency and intensity of BPSD (e.g., vocalizations such as sighing, moaning, calling out, verbal abuse, repetitive utterances, nosy breathing, facial expressions such as grimacing or frowning, restless or strained body expressions such as fidgeting or increased pacing or rocking, or agitation and resistance to care; [56]). The use of standardized assessment measures to document increases and decreases in the presence of BPSD will at this stage guide treatment and track its effectiveness.

In the absence of an accurate verbal self-report, combined pharmacological and non-pharmacological intervention is advised, as it has been suggested that first-line pharmacological treatment for chronic pain in the aged is most effective when combined with nonpharmacological intervention [21, 47]. In a demented population, regularly scheduled nonopioid analgesic medication (acetaminophen) has been found to have a positive effect on activity and socialization with no effect seen for agitation, emotional well-being, or the need for psychotropic medication [10]. Thus, the combination of a medically appropriate analgesic (acetaminophen, ibuprofen; preferably nonopioid given numerous risks including intoxication and falls) with a first-line psychological intervention may be a useful treatment approach in populations unable to verbalize the source of their distress effectively.

In this way, improvement in pain can be addressed simultaneously while treating other potential problems including emotional and psychosocial well-being. This is likely to be more effective than more commonly observed approaches in the presence of BPSD where psychotropic medications are provided as a first-line treatment [7, 42, 56]. However, when pain is thought to be a potential precipitant it is thought that that first-line analgesics which have a prompter response combined with nonpharmacological intervention already proven, efficacious in treating a greater number of symptoms common to individuals with dementia, will have a greater positive impact.

With regard to choosing a psychological intervention, a modified CBT protocol is suggested [11, 43, 54, 57, 60]. CBT incorporates both cognitive and behavioral techniques in an effort to alter behavior [65]. This modality is designed to increase individual understanding of how one's cognitions and behaviors affect experience, highlighting individual utility in controlling pain. Skills training or pain-coping strategies, tailored to needs, may include a variety of techniques such as simplified self-regulatory strategies (e.g., breathing), pleasant activities scheduling, and distraction methods, among others. Overall, the more advanced the dementia, the more overtly behavioral and directive the therapy need be. Intervention will necessitate continued assessment and flexibility such that if one strategy is not working, the technique is adjusted. Intervention may be done in an individual or small group format with the involvement of caregivers encouraged. This will be important for facilitating practice outside of sessions. Intervention length may vary, from five to ten weeks depending on resources and patient need with patients attending weekly. Sessions should be shortened (30–45 minutes) to accommodate for fatigue with skills introduced one at a time, two skills maximum per session with fewer skills total overall. Across sessions staff should promote repeated exposure with regular summation of material, the patient's active involvement in the establishment of cues or prompts serving retrieval, and extra time spent practicing new skills. Homework will also be included. Patients should be provided with simplified written instructions during each session and a short concrete homework plan to be completed outside of session. Traditional CBT activity forms to be used can be easily altered. As an example, checklists may be simplified to require majority recognition skills. Brief check-in, via phone or in person, depending on the circumstance, should be done once a week between sessions to test for comprehension and any trouble in using the skill(s) learned in the previous session; check-in should also reinforce practice outside of sessions. Following the conclusion of the intervention, check-in should continue if possible for approximately 3 months, transitioning from weekly to bi-weekly and continuing to encourage the use and practice of learned skills. In the presence of severe cognitive deterioration, much of the treatment will focus on the training of caregivers to recognize BPSD and to utilize appropriate behavioral approaches to dealing with those symptoms. Support provided to the caregivers, particularly as it relates to treatment fidelity and understanding the limits imposed by the patient's cognitive status, will be important to assure that the caregiver has confidence in the treatment.

CONCLUSION

In conclusion, the presence of underreported or undertreated pain continues to be an ongoing problem that often leads to ineffective treatment. Paramount to the problem is the frequent misappropriation of BPSD as a dementia by-product leading to treatment with ineffective psychotropic agents. Given the size and scope of the issue, the development and application of a successful comprehensive pain management intervention for individuals with cognitive impairment is a pressing need as the number of individuals with dementia is expected to climb dramatically. The first step will understandably be to provide adequate and ongoing training to the treating staff and clinicians as to the prevalence and impact of pain. As with many interventions for broad or multifaceted problems, the best treatment can often be achieved via a change in staff awareness as to the nature of the problem. Beyond these improvements in staff knowledge, a program that aims to treat the many factors, both medical and psychological that can impact pain in conjunction with an approach that understands the many complicated factors associated with assessment and the dissemination of a multimodal intervention will ultimately lead to a better patient result, ideally lesser physical disability and a greater quality of life.

REFERENCES

1. Achterberg WP, Pieper MJ, van Dalen-Kok AH, de Waal MW, Husebo BS, Lautenbacher S, Kunz M, Scherder EJ, Corbett A. Pain management in patients with dementia. Clin Interv Aging 2013;8:1471–82.
2. Andersson G, Johansson C, Nordlander A, Asmundson GJ. Chronic pain in older adults: a controlled pilot trial of a brief cognitive-behavioural group treatment. Behav Cogn Psychother 2012;40:239–44.
3. Arena JG, Hannah SL, Bruno GM, Meador KJ. Electromyographic biofeedback training for tension headache in the elderly: a prospective study. Biofeedback Self Regul 1991;16:379–90.
4. Arena JG, Hightower NE, Chong GC. Relaxation therapy for tension headache in the elderly: a prospective study. Psychol Aging 1988;3:96–8.
5. Ayalon L, Gum AM, Feliciano L, Arean PA. Effectiveness of nonpharmacological interventions for the management of neuropsychiatric symptoms in patients with dementia: a systematic review. Arch Intern Med 2006;166:2182–88.
6. Baer RA. Mindfulness-based treatment approaches: clinician's guide to evidence base and applications. Boston: Academic Press; 2006.
7. Bharani N, Snowden M. Evidence-based interventions for nursing home residents with dementia-related behavioral symptoms. Psychiatr Clin North Am 2005;28:985–1005.
8. Brodaty H, Arasaratnam C. Meta-analysis of nonpharmacological interventions for neuropsychiatric symptoms of dementia. Am J Psychiatry 2012;169:946–53.
9. Brown DP, Fromm E. Hypnotherapy and hypnoanalysis. Hillsdale, NJ: L. Erlbaum Associates; 1986.
10. Chibnall JT, Tait RC, Harman B, Luebbert RA. Effect of acetaminophen on behavior, well-being, and psychotropic medication use in nursing home residents with moderate-to-severe dementia. J Am Geriatr Soc 2005;53:1921–9.
11. Cipher DJ, Clifford PA, Roper KD. The effectiveness of geropsychological treatment in improving pain, depression, behavioral disturbances, functional disability, and health care utilization in long-term care. Clin Gerontol 2007;30:23–40.
12. Cohen-Mansfield J. Use of patient characteristics to determine nonpharmacologic interventions for behavioral and psychological symptoms of dementia. Int Psychogeriatr 2000;12:373–80.
13. Cook AJ. Cognitive-behavioral pain management for elderly nursing home residents. J Gerontol B Psychol Sci Soc Sci 1998;53:51–9.
14. Cook AK, Niven CA, Downs MG. Assessing the pain of people with cognitive impairment. Int J Geriatr Psychiatry 1999;14:421–5.
15. Dahl J, Lundgren T. Acceptance and commitment therapy (ACT) in the treatment of chronic pain. In: Baer RA, editor. Mindfulness-based treatment approaches clinician's guide to evidence base and applications. San Diego: Academic Press; 2006.
16. Davis LL, Buckwalter K, Burgio LD. Measuring problem behaviors in dementia: developing a methodological agenda. ANS Adv Nurs Sci 1997;20:40–55.
17. Dobson KS, Dozios DJ. Historical and philosophical bases of the cognitive-behavioral therapies. In: Dobson KS, editor. Handbook of cognitive-behavioral therapies, 3rd edition. New York: Guilford Press; 2010.
18. Esteve R, Ramirez-Maestre C, Lopez-Marinez AE. Adjustment to chronic pain: the role of pain acceptance, coping strategies, and pain-related cognitions. Ann Behav Med 2007;33:179–88.

19. Fordyce WE. Behavioral methods for chronic pain and illness. Saint Louis: Mosby; 1976.
20. Gibson SJ. Pain and aging: a comparison of the pain experience over the adult lifespan. In: Dostrovsky JO, Carr DB, Koltzenburg M, editors. Proceedings of the 10th World Congress on Pain Progress in pain research and management. Seattle: IASP Press; 2003.
21. Gibson SJ. Older person's pain. Pain: Clin Updat 2006;14:1–4.
22. Giggins OM, Persson UM, Caulfield B. Biofeedback in rehabilitation. J Neuroeng Rehabil 2013;10:60.
23. Goldberg DS, McGee SJ. Pain as a global public health priority. BMC Public Health 2011;11:770.
24. Hadjistavropoulos T, Herr K, Turk DC, Fine PG, Dworkin RH, Helme R, Jackson K, Parmelee PA, Rudy TE, Lynn Beattie B, et al. An interdisciplinary expert consensus statement on assessment of pain in older persons. Clin J Pain 2007;23:S1–43.
25. Hayes SC, Luoma JB, Bond FW, Masuda A, Lillis J. Acceptance and commitment therapy: model, processes and outcomes. Behav Res Ther 2006;44:1–25.
26. Hayes SC, Strosahl K. A practical guide to acceptance and commitment therapy. New York, NY: Springer; 2004.
27. Hayes SC, Strosahl K, Wilson KG. Acceptance and commitment therapy: an experiential approach to behavior change. New York: Guilford Press; 1999.
28. Hayes SC, Strosahl K, Wilson KG. Acceptance and commitment therapy: the process and practice of mindful change. New York: Guilford Press; 2012.
29. Helme RD, Gibson SJ. The epidemiology of pain in elderly people. Clin Geriatr Med 2001;17:417–31.
30. Herr K, Coyne PJ, Key T, Manworren R, McCaffery M, Merkel S, Pelosi-Kelly J, Wild L. Pain assessment in the nonverbal patient: position statement with clinical practice recommendations. Pain Manag Nurs 2006;7:44–52.
31. Herr K, Coyne PJ, McCaffery M, Manworren R, Merkel S. Pain assessment in the patient unable to self-report: position statement with clinical practice recommendations. Pain Manag Nurs 2011;12:230–50.
32. Hoffman BM, Papas RK, Chatkoff DK, Kerns RD. Meta-analysis of psychological interventions for chronic low back pain. Health Psychol 2007;26:1–9.
33. Husebo BS, Ballard C, Aarsland D. Pain treatment of agitation in patients with dementia: a systematic review. Int J Geriatr Psychiatry 2011;26:1012–8.
34. Husebo BS, Ballard C, Sandvik R, Nilsen OB, Aarsland D. Efficacy of treating pain to reduce behavioural disturbances in residents of nursing homes with dementia: cluster randomised clinical trial. BMJ 2011;343:d4065.
35. Jha A, Jan F, Gale T, Newman C. Effectiveness of a recovery-orientated psychiatric intervention package on the wellbeing of people with early dementia: a preliminary randomised controlled trial. Int J Geriatr Psychiatry 2013;28:589–96.
36. Kabat-Zinn J. An outpatient program in behavioral medicine for chronic pain patients based on the practice of mindfulness meditation: theoretical considerations and preliminary results. Gen Hosp Psychiatry 1982; 4:33–47.
37. Kabat-Zinn J. Full catastrophe living : using the wisdom of your body and mind to face stress, pain, and illness. New York, NY: Delacorte Press; 1990.
38. Kabela E, Blanchard EB, Appelbaum KA, Nicholson N. Self-regulatory treatment of headache in the elderly. Biofeedback Self Regul 1989;14:219–28.
39. Kerns RD, Morley S, Vlaeyen JWS. Psychological Interventions for Chronic Pain. In: Castro-Lopes J, Raja S, Schmetz M, editors. Pain 2008—an updated review. Washington, DC: IASP Press; 2008.
40. Kerns RD, Sellinger J, Goodin BR. Psychological treatment of chronic pain. Annu Rev Clin Psychol 2011; 7:411–34.
41. Kerns RDJ, Turk DC, Holzman AD, Rudy TE. Comparison of cognitive-behavioral and behavioral approaches to the outpatient treatment of chronic pain. Clin J Pain 1985;1:195–203.
42. Kovach CR, Logan BR, Noonan PE, Schlidt AM, Smerz J, Simpson M, Wells T. Effects of the Serial Trial Intervention on discomfort and behavior of nursing home residents with dementia. Am J Alzheimers Dis Other Demen 2006;21:147–55.
43. Kraus CA, Seignourel P, Balasubramanyam V, Snow AL, Wilson NL, Kunik ME, Schulz PE, Stanley MA. Cognitive-behavioral treatment for anxiety in patients with dementia: two case studies. J Psychiatr Pract 2008;14:186–92.
44. Kverno KS, Black BS, Nolan MT, Rabins PV. Research on treating neuropsychiatric symptoms of advanced dementia with non-pharmacological strategies, 1998–2008: a systematic literature review. Int Psychogeriatr 2009;21:825–43.
45. Kverno KS, Rabins PV, Blass DM, Hicks KL, Black BS. Prevalence and treatment of neuropsychiatric symptoms in advanced dementia. J Gerontol Nurs 2008;34:8–15.

46. Livingston G, Johnston K, Katona C, Paton J, Lyketsos CG. Systematic review of psychological approaches to the management of neuropsychiatric symptoms of dementia. Am J Psychiatry 2005;162:1996–2021.
47. Lunde LH, Nordhus IH, Pallesen S. The effectiveness of cognitive and behavioural treatment of chronic pain in the elderly: a quantitative review. J Clin Psychol Med Settings 2009;16:254–62.
48. McBee L, Westreich L, Likourezos A. A psychoeducational relaxation group for pain and stress management in the nursing home. J Soc Work Long-Term Care 2004;3:15–28.
49. Morley S, Eccleston C, Williams A. Systematic review and meta-analysis of randomized controlled trials of cognitive behaviour therapy and behaviour therapy for chronic pain in adults, excluding headache. Pain 1999;80:1–13.
50. Morone NE, Greco CM, Weiner DK. Mindfulness meditation for the treatment of chronic low back pain in older adults: a randomized controlled pilot study. Pain 2008;134:310–9.
51. Nicholson NL, Blanchard EB. A controlled evaluation of behavioral treatment of chronic headache in the elderly. Behav Ther 1993;24:395–408.
52. Nordhus IH, Pallesen S. Psychological treatment of late-life anxiety: an empirical review. J Consult Clin Psychol 2003;71:643–51.
53. Parmelee PA, Smith B, Katz IR. Pain complaints and cognitive status among elderly institution residents. J Am Geriatr Soc 1993;41:517–22.
54. Paukert AL, Calleo J, Kraus-Schuman C, Snow L, Wilson N, Petersen NJ, Kunik ME, Stanley MA. Peaceful mind: an open trial of cognitive-behavioral therapy for anxiety in persons with dementia. Int Psychogeriatr 2010;22:1012–21.
55. Petersen RC, Negash S. Mild cognitive impairment: an overview. CNS Spectr 2008;13:45–53.
56. Pieper MJ, van Dalen-Kok AH, Francke AL, van der Steen JT, Scherder EJ, Husebo BS, Achterberg WP. Interventions targeting pain or behaviour in dementia: a systematic review. Ageing Res Rev 2013;12:1042–55.
57. Regan B, Varanelli L. Adjustment, depression, and anxiety in mild cognitive impairment and early dementia: a systematic review of psychological intervention studies. Int Psychogeriatr 2013;25:1963–84.
58. Reid MC, Otis J, Barry LC, Kerns RD. Cognitive-behavioral therapy for chronic low back pain in older persons: a preliminary study. Pain Med 2003;4:223–30.
59. Scherder EJ, Eggermont L, Plooij B, Oudshoorn J, Vuijk PJ, Pickering G, Lautenbacher S, Achterberg W, Oosterman J. Relationship between chronic pain and cognition in cognitively intact older persons and in patients with Alzheimer's disease. The need to control for mood. Gerontology 2008;54:50–8.
60. Scholey KA, Woods BT. A series of brief cognitive therapy interventions with people experiencing both dementia and depression: a description of techniques and common themes. Clin Psychol Psychother 2003;10:175–85.
61. Scogin F, McElreath L. Efficacy of psychosocial treatments for geriatric depression: a quantitative review. J Consult Clin Psychol 1994;62:69–74.
62. Turk DC, Meichenbaum D, Genest M. Pain and behavioral medicine: a cognitive-behavioral perspective. New York: Guilford Press; 1983.
63. Turk DC, Monarch ES. Biopsychosocial perspectives on chronic pain. In: Turk DC, Gatchel RJ, editors. Psychological approaches to pain management: a practitioner's handbook. New York: The Guilford Press; 2002.
64. Turner JA, Chapman CR. Psychological interventions for chronic pain: a critical review. I. Relaxation training and biofeedback. Pain 1982;12:1–21.
65. Veehof MM, Oskam MJ, Schreurs KM, Bohlmeijer ET. Acceptance-based interventions for the treatment of chronic pain: a systematic review and meta-analysis. Pain 2011;152:533–42.
66. Waters SJ, Woodward JT, Keefe FJ. Cognitive-behavioral therapy for pain in older adults. In: Gibson SJ, Weiner DK, editors. Pain in older persons progress in pain research and management. Seattle: IASP Press; 2005.

CHAPTER 21

Placebo Analgesia in Dementia

Martina Amanzio and Fabrizio Benedetti

The psychosocial context surrounding the patient and the psychobiological model offer interesting perspectives from which to study the placebo analgesic response. Some authors use the term placebo response to mean any type of improvement that may take place in a placebo group of a clinical trial, even if that improvement is related to statistical artifacts such as sampling bias and regression to the mean, or to the natural history of a clinical condition. Importantly, the term placebo response should only be reserved for an active neurobiological process that occurs as a result of a dummy treatment. Indeed, brain activity changes related to the psychosocial context in the form of a procedure to elicit placebo analgesia (PA) allow us to describe, through a variety of approaches, the specific neurophysiological effect. The interesting aspect of studying PA lies in the fact that the specific effects of a drug are removed to collect the effects of a positive psychosocial context on the patient's responses. Likewise, the open–hidden paradigm allows us to differentiate the specific effects of an active drug from those of a positive psychosocial context [5, 7, 14]. Indeed, through this, it is possible to dissociate the benefit of the psychosocial context where the treatment is overtly given from the pharmacodynamics effect of the treatment itself. Interestingly, the results obtained through these studies demonstrate that the same drug at the same dosage and with the same infusion time is more effective when it is administered overtly rather than covertly.

Contextual information leading to placebo responses arises either from conscious expectancies about a positive anticipated treatment effect or from prior learning in the form of conditioning with active treatments [1]. The context surrounding the administration of a placebo may lead individuals to expect improvement and positive outcomes. On the opposite side, negative contextual information can lead individuals to expect a worsening of symptoms, which in turn can produce a nocebo effect. One way to identify nocebo effects is the analysis of side effects in placebo groups of randomized double-blind placebo-controlled trials [4].

The importance of these studies in medical practice is represented by the possible exploitation to the patient's advantage, so that the placebo component of a therapy can be maximized and nocebo side effects minimized. This aspect should be, for example, considered in patients with cognitive impairment related to dementia who, compared with mild cognitive impaired patients, are more vulnerable to feel adverse events of symptoms even during a placebo treatment [3]. Another crucial aspect is represented by the disruption of placebo mechanisms, which may require increased therapeutic doses of drugs to compensate for the loss of the placebo response, as described below [8, 10].

In this chapter, we try to answer specific questions regarding patients with cognitive impairment, even though we have only a limited understanding of the neurocognitive factors that influence patients' response to placebo. We first analyze the role of the prefrontal cortex in the placebo analgesic response; then, we describe some recent studies that investigated PA when an impairment of prefrontal functioning occurs.

THE PREFRONTAL AREAS IN PLACEBO ANALGESIA

Modern brain imaging techniques have been fundamental in the understanding of PA, and many brain imaging studies have been carried out to describe the functional neuroanatomy of the placebo analgesic effect [11, 16, 17, 20, 22, 26, 28, 30, 34, 35, 40, 41, 45, 46, 48, 49, 51, 52].

The first imaging study of PA showed that a subset of brain regions is similarly affected by either a placebo or a μ-opioid agonist [34]. In particular, the administration of a placebo induced the activation of the rostral anterior cingulate cortex, the orbitofrontal cortex, and the anterior insula, and there was a significant co-variation in activity between the rostral anterior cingulate cortex and the lower pons/medulla, and a subsignificant co-variation between the rostral anterior cingulate cortex and the periaqueductal gray, suggesting that a descending pain-modulating circuit is involved in PA. Experimental evidence shows that this modulating descending circuit, as described by Fields and Basbaum [18], involves the spinal cord [17, 19, 29].

In a functional magnetic resonance imaging study of experimentally induced pain in healthy subjects, Wager et al. [48] found that PA was related to decreased neural activity in pain-processing areas of the brain. Pain-related neural activity was reduced within the thalamus, anterior insular cortex, and anterior cingulate cortex during the placebo condition as compared with the baseline condition. The magnitudes of these decreases were correlated with reductions in pain ratings. Wager et al. [48] did analyze not only the time period of pain, but also the time period of the anticipation of pain. They hypothesized increases in neural activity within brain areas involved in expectation, and indeed, they found significant positive correlations between increases in brain activity in the anticipatory period and decreases in pain and pain-related neural activity during stimulation within the placebo condition. The brain regions showing positive correlations during the anticipatory phase included the orbitofrontal cortex, dorsolateral prefrontal cortex, rostral anterior cingulate cortex, and midbrain periaqueductal gray. The dorsolateral prefrontal cortex is a region that has been associated with the representation and maintenance of information needed for cognitive control, consistent with a role in expectation [32]. On the other hand, the orbitofrontal cortex is associated with functioning in the evaluative and reward information relevant to allocation of control, consistent with a role in affective or motivational responses to anticipation of pain [15].

The anterior cingulate cortex is often reported to be involved in PA, although some discordant results have been obtained. For example, it was found to have increased activity in a study by Petrovic et al. [34] and decreased activity in a study by Wager et al. [48], which might be explained on the basis of the different experimental settings.

Most of the brain imaging studies aiming at investigating PA have been performed in experimental settings using healthy volunteers. By contrast, Price et al. [35] conducted a functional magnetic resonance imaging study in which brain activity of irritable bowel syndrome (IBS) patients was measured in response to rectal distension by a balloon barostat (a tonic pain stimulus). In particular, the patients were placed in the scanner and the experimenter applied the same agent to the balloon for each condition (saline jelly), just before the balloon was inserted. However, in the rectal placebo (RP) condition, the experimenter told the patients, "The agent that you have just received is known to powerfully reduce pain in some patients." This suggestion is identical to that used in previous studies by the same group and is one that could be ethically applied during some active treatments. A large placebo effect was produced in the RP condition and accompanied by large reductions in neural activity in the thalamus, the primary and secondary somatosensory cortices, the insula, and the anterior cingulate cortex during the period of stimulation. It was accompanied by increases in neural activity in the rostral anterior cingulate cortex, bilateral amygdala, and periaqueductal gray [36]. This study is quite important and informative, as it shows that placebos act on the brain in a clinically relevant condition (indeed IBS is considered a clinically relevant model of PA) in the same way as they do in the experimental setting. Therefore, the involvement of key areas in PA, such as the anterior cingulate cortex, not only is limited to experimental noxious stimuli, but also extends to clinical pain. The study by Price et al. [35] is also interesting because reductions in brain activity occurred during the stimulus presentation itself, not just when subjects reported pain. In fact, it has been argued that the length of the painful stimulation may be critical for the measurement of placebo effects, as most studies used short heat or electric shock as pain stimuli and recorded activity decreases during periods extending after the stimulus offset, thus possibly including a later cognitive reappraisal of the significance of pain and/or late neural activity influenced by report bias.

To determine whether expectation of analgesia exerts its psychophysical effect through changes of the perceptual sensitivity of early cortical processes (in the primary and secondary somatosensory areas) or on later cortical elaborations, such as stimulus identification and response selection in the anterior cingulate cortex, Lorenz et al. [27] used high temporal resolution techniques (magnetoencephalography). They found that activity in the secondary somatosensory cortex was highly correlated with the extent of influence of the subjective pain rating by prestimulus expectation, while anterior cingulate cortex activity seemed to be associated only to stimulus intensity and related attentional engagement. In another study on laser-evoked potentials by Wager et al. [47], early nociceptive components were found to be affected by placebos. Therefore, later cognitive reappraisal of the significance of pain and/or late neural activity influenced by report bias cannot be responsible for this early modulation. This indicates that the very early sensory components are affected by placebo manipulation.

Overall, all these brain imaging data have been summarized by using a meta-analysis approach with the activation likelihood estimation method [2]. Nine functional magnetic resonance studies and two positron emission tomography studies were selected for the analysis. In particular, we analyzed the data through the model of three temporal stages of PA by Kong et al. [23].

- Stage 1, named expectation/anticipation-phase. Before the pain starts, expectation or anticipation of pain relief could modulate perception of the subsequent pain stimuli.
- Stage 2, expressed as the phase of noxious stimuli administration. During administration of painful stimuli, placebo treatment can inhibit the incoming nociceptive signals.
- Stage 3, the appraisal phase of subjective pain rating. When the pain stimulus is over, previous knowledge of treatment effect may unconsciously distort subjective pain rating.

Since only two out of eleven studies assessed the third stage, we analyzed only the first two stages [2]. During the expectation phase of analgesia, areas of activation were found in the left anterior cingulate, in the right precentral and lateral prefrontal cortex, and in the left periaqueductal gray. In the phase during pain stimulation, activations were found in the anterior cingulate and medial and lateral prefrontal cortices, left inferior parietal lobule and postcentral gyrus, anterior insula, thalamus, hypothalamus, periaqueductal gray, and pons. Conversely, deactivations were found in the left mid- and posterior cingulate cortex, in the superior temporal and precentral gyri, in the left anterior and right posterior insula, in the claustrum and putamen, and in the right thalamus and caudate body.

These meta-analytic data summarize all brain imaging studies and give a global figure of the sequence of events following placebo administration: After the activation of a pain modulatory network during the expectation phase and the early pain phase, several deactivations occur in different areas involved in pain processing.

Interestingly, these results revealed a special role of the midcingulate and anterior insula cortices, whose joint activity is based on the engagement of attentional resources that are allocated to perceptual processes based on the salience of the incoming information as well as the relevance of the information for prioritized goals [25]. Bottom–up attentional processes have mainly been related to the anterior insula and midcingulate cortex and the salience network. Once a stimulus has been detected as salient, the anterior insula activates the cognitive control network [42], thereby facilitating task-related information processing. In this way, the experimental stimuli under investigation will have preferential access to the brain attentional resources [31]. The anterior insula also decreases activity in the *default mode network* [42] that shows decreased activation during sensory or cognitive processing. Interestingly, we found two regions of the default mode network that are deactivated during PA, namely, the posterior cingulate cortex (BA 31) and the lateral temporal cortex (BA 21) [2]. Although the relevance of default mode network modulation for selective attention is less well understood, there is evidence showing that the failure of this network regulation through the anterior insula leads to inefficient cognitive control [12]. The link between salience network abnormality and default mode network function is in keeping with some studies showing that salience network dysfunction in patients with frontotemporal dementia is associated with abnormalities in the default mode network [50]. The most compelling evidence of a link between clinical disease and disruption of the default network has been found in Alzheimer disease. Earliest studies found a hypometabolism in some regions of the default network, including the posterior cingulated cortex, inferior parietal lobule, and lateral temporal cortex [13]. Hypometabolism in Alzheimer disease progresses with the disease and correlates with mental status [21, 33]. Importantly, understanding PA in patients with dementia by studying the neurophysiological elements modulated by expectation is an important endeavor that has strong clinical implications. Indeed, a patient's expectancy of improvement may influence outcomes in placebo response, representing a promising new strategy of pain treatment.

IF THERE IS NO PREFRONTAL CONTROL, THERE IS NO PLACEBO RESPONSE

A common finding across different neuroimaging studies is represented by the involvement of the prefrontal areas in the placebo response (e.g., the dorsolateral prefrontal cortex). As in Alzheimer disease, the frontal lobes are severely affected with marked neuronal degeneration in the dorsolateral prefrontal cortex, the orbitofrontal cortex, and the anterior cingulate cortex [44], and the prefrontal lobes are responsible for complex mental functions; it is reasonable to expect a disruption of placebo responsiveness in these patients.

On the basis of these considerations, Benedetti et al. [8] studied Alzheimer patients at the initial stage of the disease and after one year, in order to see whether the placebo component of the therapy was affected by the disease. The placebo component of the analgesic therapy was found to be correlated with both cognitive status and functional connectivity among different brain regions, according to the rule "the more impaired the prefrontal connectivity, the smaller the placebo response." In a more recent study, Stein et al. [43] used diffusion tensor magnetic resonance imaging to test the hypothesis of the role of white matter integrity in placebo responsiveness. In this study, the integrity of white matter tracts was quantified by fractional anisotropy. First, correlations of fractional anisotropy with the analgesic placebo effect were computed voxel-wise within key regions of the descending pain modulatory system. In addition, the authors used the local orientation information obtained by diffusion imaging to trace white matter pathways that connect the top-down pain modulatory regions with the PAG. Interestingly, Stein et al. [43] hypothesized that higher fractional anisotropy values within key regions of the descending pain modulatory system are positively correlated with the individual placebo analgesic response. The results showed that the individual placebo analgesic effect was indeed found to be correlated with white matter integrity indexed by fractional anisotropy, particularly in the right dorsolateral prefrontal cortex, left rostral anterior cingulate cortex, and the periaqueductal gray. Probabilistic tractography seeded in these regions showed that stronger placebo analgesic responses were associated with increased mean fractional anisotropy values within white matter tracts connecting the periaqueductal gray with the rostral anterior cingulate cortex and the dorsolateral prefrontal cortex. Therefore, the study both on Alzheimer patients [8] and on white matter integrity in normal subjects [43] demonstrates the importance of prefrontal functioning and connectivity in the placebo response.

To support the crucial role of the prefrontal cortex in the occurrence of placebo responses, Krummenacher et al. [24] used repetitive transcranial magnetic stimulation (rTMS) to inactivate the prefrontal cortex during PA. These investigators inactivated the left and right dorsolateral prefrontal cortex during a procedure inducing PA and found that rTMS completely blocked the analgesic placebo response. Therefore, the inactivation of the prefrontal lobes has the same effects as those observed in prefrontal degeneration in Alzheimer disease and reduced integrity of prefrontal white matter.

Interestingly, Eippert et al. [16] found that the opioid antagonist naloxone blocks PA, along with a reduction in the activation of the dorsolateral prefrontal cortex, suggesting that a prefrontal opioidergic mechanism is crucial in the placebo analgesic response. Thus, a disruption of prefrontal control is associated with a loss of placebo response [6].

CLINICAL IMPLICATIONS

At least two important clinical implications emerge from the disruption of placebo mechanisms in Alzheimer disease. First, the reduced efficacy of an analgesic treatment underscores the need of considering a possible revision of some therapies in Alzheimer patients to compensate for the loss of placebo-related and expectation-related mechanisms. The affective–emotional component of pain is impaired in Alzheimer disease, whereas the sensory–discriminative component is maintained, indicating that Alzheimer patients can distinguish a painful from a tactile stimulus [9, 10]. Although people with Alzheimer disease can perceive pain, there is a lower consumption of analgesics among them compared with controls, which can be due to their inability to communicate their suffering [37, 38]. By considering that many of these patients are likely to show severe impairment of the prefrontal lobes and thus a loss of placebo- and expectation-related mechanisms, low doses of analgesics can be totally inadequate to relieve any kind of pain. Therefore, the analgesic treatments should be increased to compensate for the loss of these mechanisms. Second, as the prefrontal cortex can also be severely affected in other neurodegenerative conditions such as frontotemporal dementia and vascular dementia [38, 39], the neuroanatomical localization of placebo- and expectation-related mechanisms should alert us to the potential disruption of placebo mechanisms in all those conditions; whereby, the prefrontal lobes are involved.

Alzheimer patients who receive placebo treatment have also been found to report a high frequency of adverse events. Amanzio et al. [3] analyzed the rates of adverse events in patients with mild cognitive impairment and Alzheimer disease in the placebo arms of donepezil trials. An overall comparison of 81 categories of adverse events in the placebo arm of mild cognitive impairment versus Alzheimer disease trials showed that Alzheimer patients experienced a significantly higher number of adverse events than did mildly impaired patients. The fact that Alzheimer patients are at a greater risk of developing adverse events than are mild cognitive impairment patients may be related to a greater presence of somatic comorbidity, predisposing them to express emotional distress as physical symptoms and/or to Alzheimer patients being frailer and therefore more susceptible to adverse events.

FUTURE DIRECTIONS

In this chapter, we address some questions with important far-reaching implications for patients with primary dementia and especially with Alzheimer disease. However, our limited understanding of the factors that influence patients' response to a placebo treatment leads to a number of questions that need clarification in future research: (1) Do patients with cognitive impairment experience placebo responses differently from the general population? (2) Does disruption of different prefrontal areas produce different effects on placebo responses? (3) Is a higher degree of cognitive impairment and its diagnosis (e.g., Mild Cognitive Impairment versus Alzheimer Disease) related to more negative symptom outcomes and nocebo effects? Understanding of these questions will allow us to develop specific approaches of personalized medicine that takes patients with primary dementia into account.

REFERENCES

1. Amanzio M, Benedetti F. Neuropharmacological dissection of placebo analgesia: expectation-activated opioid systems versus conditioning-activated specific sub-systems. J Neurosci 1999;19:484–94.
2. Amanzio M, Benedetti F, Porro CA, Palermo S, Cauda F. Activation likelihood estimation meta-analysis of brain correlates of placebo analgesia in human experimental pain. HBM 2013;34:738–52.
3. Amanzio M, Benedetti F, Vase L. A systematic review of adverse events in the placebo arm of donepezil trials: the role of cognitive impairment. Int Psychogeriatr 2012;24:698–707.
4. Amanzio M, Latini Corazzini L, Vase L, Benedetti F. A systematic review of adverse events in placebo groups of anti-migraine clinical trials. Pain 2009;146:261–9.
5. Amanzio M, Pollo A, Maggi G, Benedetti F. Response variability to analgesics: a role for non-specific activation of endogenous opioids. Pain 2001;90:205–15.

6. Benedetti F. No prefrontal control, no placebo response. Pain 2010;148:357–58.
7. Benedetti F, Amanzio M, Maggi G. Potentiation of placebo analgesia by proglumide. Lancet 1995;346:1231.
8. Benedetti F, Arduino C, Costa S, Vighetti S, Tarenzi L, Rainero I, Asteggiano G. Loss of expectation-related mechanisms in Alzheimer's disease makes analgesic therapies less effective. Pain 2006;121:133–44.
9. Benedetti F, Arduino C, Vighetti S, Asteggiano G, Tarenzi L, Rainero I. Pain reactivity in Alzheimer patients with different degrees of cognitive impairment and brain electrical activity deterioration. Pain 2004;111:22–9.
10. Benedetti F, Vighetti S, Ricco C, Lagna E, Bergamasco B, Pinessi L, Rainero I. Pain threshold and tolerance in Alzheimer's disease. Pain 1999;80:377–82.
11. Bingel U, Lorenz J, Schoell E, Weiller C, Büchel C. Mechanisms of placebo analgesia: rACC recruitment of a subcortical antinociceptive network. Pain 2005;120:8–15.
12. Bonnelle V, Ham TE, Leech R, Kinnunen KM, Mehta MA, Greenwood RJ, Sharp DJ. Salience network integrity predicts default mode network function after traumatic brain injury. Proc Natl Acad Sci USA 2012;109:4690–5.
13. Buckner RL, Snyder AZ, Shannon BJ, LaRossa, G, Sachs R, Fotenos AF, Sheline YI, Klunk WE, Mathis CA, Morris JC, Mintun MA. Molecular, structural, and functional characterization of Alzheimer's disease: evidence for a relationship between default activity, amyloid and memory. J Neurosci 2005;25:7709–17.
14. Colloca L, Lopiano L, Lanotte M, Benedetti F. Overt versus Covert treatment for pain, anxiety and Parkinson' disease. Lancet Neurol 2004;3:679–84.
15. Dias R, Robbins TW, Roberts AC. Dissociation in prefrontal cortex of affective and attentional shifts. Nature 1996;380:69–72.
16. Eippert F, Bingel U, Schoell ED, Yacubian J, Klinger R, Lorenz J, Buchel C. Activation of the opioidergic descending pain control system underlies placebo analgesia. Neuron 2009;63:533–43.
17. Eippert F, Finsterbusch J, Bingel U, Büchel C. Direct evidence for spinal cord involvement in placebo analgesia. Science 2009;326:404.
18. Fields HL, Basbaum AI. Central nervous system mechanisms of pain modulation. In: Wall PD, Melzack R, editors. Textbook of pain Livingstone. Edinburgh: Churchill; 1999. p. 309–29.
19. Goffaux P, Redmond WJ, Rainville P, Marchand S. Descending analgesia—when the spine echoes what the brain expects. Pain 2007;130:137–43.
20. Hashmi JA, Baria AT, Baliki MN, Huang L, Schnitzer TJ, Apkarian AV. Brain networks predicting placebo analgesia in a clinical trial for chronic back pain. Pain 2012;153:2393–402.
21. Herholz K, Salmon E, Perani D, Baron JC, Holthoff V, Frolich L, Schonknecht P, Ito K, Mielke R, Kalbe E, et al. Discrimination between Alzheimer dementia and controls by automated analysis of multicenter FDG PET. Neuroimage 2002;17:302–16.
22. Kong J, Gollub RL, Rosman IS, Webb JM, Vangel MG, Kirsch I, Kaptchuk TJ. Brain activity associated with expectancy-enhanced placebo analgesia as measured by functional magnetic resonance imaging. J Neurosci 2006;26:381–88.
23. Kong J, Kaptchuk TJ, Polich G, Kirsch I, Gollub I. Placebo analgesia: findings from brain imaging studies and emerging hypotheses. Rev Neurosci 2007;18:173–190.
24. Krummenacher P, Candia V, Folkers G, Schedlowski M, Schönbächler G. Prefrontal cortex modulates placebo analgesia. Pain 2010;148:368–74.
25. Legrain V, Damme SV, Eccleston C, Davis KD, Seminowicz DA, Crombez G. A neurocognitive model of attention to pain: behavioral and neuroimaging evidence. Pain 2009;144:230–2.
26. Lieberman MD, Jarcho JM, Berman S, Naliboff BD, Suyenobu BY, Mandelkern M, Mayer EA. The neural correlates of placebo effects: a disruption account. Neuroimage 2004;22:447–55.
27. Lorenz J, Hauck M, Paur RC, Nakamura Y, Zimmermann R, Bromm B, Engel AK. Cortical correlates of false expectations during pain intensity judgments—a possible manifestation of placebo/nocebo cognitions. Brain Behav Immun 2005;19:283–95.
28. Lui F, Colloca L, Duzzi D, Anchisi D, Benedetti F, Porro CA. Neural bases of conditioned placebo analgesia. Pain 2010;151:816–24.
29. Matre D, Casey KL, Knardahl S. Placebo-induced changes in spinal cord pain processing. J Neurosci 2006;26:559–63.
30. Meissner K, Bingel U, Colloca L, Wager TD, Watson A, Flaten MA. The placebo effect: advances from different methodological approaches. J Neurosci 2011;31:16117–24.
31. Menon V, Uddin LQ. Saliency, switching, attention and control: a network model of insula function. Brain Struct Funct 2010; 214:655–67.
32. Miller EK, Cohen JD. An integrative theory of prefrontal cortex function. Annu Rev Neurosci 2001; 24:167–202.

33. Minoshima S, Giordani B, Berent S, Frey KA, Foster NL, Kuhl DE. Metabolic reduction in the posterior cingulate cortex in very early Alzheimer's disease. Ann Neurol 1997;42:85–94.
34. Petrovic P, Kalso E, Petersson KM, Ingvar M. Placebo and opioid analgesia-imaging a shared neuronal network. Science 2002;295:1737–40.
35. Price DD, Craggs J, Verne GN, Perlstein WM, Robinson ME. Placebo analgesia is accompanied by large reductions in pain-related brain activity in irritable bowel syndrome patients. Pain 2007;127:63–72.
36. Price DD, Finniss DG, Benedetti F. A comprehensive review of the placebo effect: recent advances and current thought. Annu Rev Psychol 2008;59:565–90.
37. Scherder EJ. Low use of analgesics in Alzheimer's disease: possible mechanisms. Psychiatry 2000;63:1–12.
38. Scherder EJ, Oosterman J, Swaab D, Herr K, Ooms M, Ribbe M, Sergeant J, Pickering G, Benedetti F. Recent developments in pain in dementia. BMJ 2005;330:461–4.
39. Scherder EJA, Sergeant JA, Swaab DF. Pain processing in dementia and its relation to neuropathology. Lancet Neurol 2003;2:677–86.
40. Scott DJ, Stohler CS, Egnatuk CM, Wang H, Koeppe RA, Zubieta JK. Individual differences in reward responding explain placebo-induced expectations and effects. Neuron 2007;55:325–36.
41. Scott DJ, Stohler CS, Egnatuk CM, Wang H, Koeppe RA, Zubieta JK. Placebo and nocebo effects are defined by opposite opioid and dopaminergic responses. Arch Gen Psychiatry 2008;65:220–31.
42. Sridharan D, Levitin, DJ, Menon V. A critical role for the right fronto-insular cortex in switching between central executive and default mode networks. Proc Natl Acad Sci USA 2008;105:12569–74.
43. Stein N, Sprenger C, Scholz J, Wiech K, Bingel U. White matter integrity of the descending pain modulatory system is associated with interindividual differences in placebo analgesia. Pain 2012;153:2210–17.
44. Thompson PM, Hayashi KM, de Zubicaray G, Janke AL, Rose SE, Semple J, Herman D, Hong MS, Dittmer SS, Doddrell DM, Toga AW. Dynamics of gray matter loss in Alzheimer's disease. J Neurosci 2003;23:994–1005.
45. Tracey I. Getting the pain you expect: mechanisms of placebo, nocebo and reappraisal effects in humans. Nat Med 2010;16:1277–83.
46. Wager TD, Atlas LY, Leotti LA, Rilling JK. Predicting individual differences in placebo analgesia: contributions of brain activity during anticipation and pain experience. J Neurosci 2011;31:439–52.
47. Wager TD, Matre D, Casey KL. Placebo effects in laser-evoked pain potentials. Brain Behav Immun 2006;20:219–30.
48. Wager TD, Rilling JK, Smith EE, Sokolik A, Casey KL, Davidson RJ, Kosslyn SM, Rose RM, Cohen JD. Placebo-induced changes in FMRI in the anticipation and experience of pain. Science 2004;303:1162–7.
49. Wager TD, Scott DJ, Zubieta JK. Placebo effects on human (micro)-opioid activity during pain. Proc Natl Acad Sci USA 2007;104:11056–61.
50. Zhou J, Greicius MD, Gennatas ED, Growdon ME, Jang JY, Rabinovici GD, Kramer JH, Weiner M, Miller BL, Seeley WW. Divergent network connectivity changes in behavioural variant frontotemporal dementia and Alzheimer's disease. Brain 2010;133:1352–1367.
51. Zubieta JK, Bueller JA, Jackson LR, Scott DJ, Xu Y, Koeppe RA, Nichols TE, Stohler CS. Placebo effects mediated by endogenous opioid activity on mu opioid receptors. J Neurosci 2005;25:7754–62.
52. Zubieta JK, Stohler CS. Neurobiological mechanisms of placebo responses. Ann NY Acad Sci 2009;1156:198–210.

CHAPTER 22

Palliative Care of Patients with Dementia and Pain

Elizabeth L. Sampson, Nele van den Noortgate, and J. T. van der Steen

The commonly used definition of pain is that it is "an unpleasant sensory and emotional experience associated with actual or potential tissue damage, or described in terms of such damage" [2]. Palliative care employs a very broad definition of pain, highlighting how it is not just a physical symptom and encompassing unpleasant emotional and even spiritual distress. The management of these forms of pain in people with dementia who are approaching the end of life is complex and requires great compassion and skill. We begin by defining palliative care and exploring how dementia can be thought of as a terminal illness and the types of setting in which people with dementia die. We then outline the important concepts of personhood and person-centered care. In addition to pain, other symptoms such as dyspnea (difficulty in breathing) are common at the end of life, and these are key causes of discomfort. Pain and discomfort are often thought of as similar concepts, but they are different. At the end of life, it may be more clinically relevant to consider comfort, which is more than just the absence of pain. We discuss how pain and discomfort tools may examine different aspects of the person with dementia's experience and how it is important to maintain this distinction. Work in this area of palliative care is still in its infancy, and thus many controversies remain, for example, around the use of strong opioids as death approaches and palliative sedation. We discuss these briefly at the end of the chapter.

INTRODUCTION TO PALLIATIVE CARE

The World Health Organization (WHO) defines palliative care as:

> An approach that improves the quality of life of patients and their families facing the problems associated with life threatening illness, through the prevention and relief of suffering by means of early identification and impeccable assessment and treatment of pain and other problems, physical, psychosocial and spiritual. [60]

All definitions of palliative care encompass a common philosophy, taking a holistic approach and taking into consideration the personhood of patients and their families, with a focus on dignity; a collaborative relationship between health care professionals, patients, and their families; good communication; and a central goal to maintain the *quality* of life.

The terms *end-of-life care* and *palliative care* are often used interchangeably. However, in some countries, for example, the United States, end-of-life care is favored because palliative care is sometimes associated only with dying from cancer whereas end-of-life care refers to all patients with life-limiting illnesses [34]. Whatever terminology is used, the WHO definition highlights how the management of pain is of paramount importance in palliative care. It is vital to anticipate that pain may occur and seek this using appropriate pain tools so that appropriate treatment can be given. This is of even more importance in people with advanced dementia who may not be able to verbally express that they are in pain.

Palliative care is sometimes mistakenly believed to involve the withdrawal or limitation of care, whereas the palliative care model takes an active approach with a clear focus on maintaining quality of life where the thoughtful management of symptoms such as pain is key. It is also important to acknowledge that end-of-life care seeks neither to hasten death nor to postpone it [34].

The word palliative comes from the Latin word *palliare*—to cloak. Palliative care developed from the hospice movement of the late 19th century where religious orders established places of care for the poor and dying in London, Dublin, Adelaide, and New York [6]. The modern hospice movement was founded at St Christopher's Hospice in South London by Dame Cicely Saunders in the 1960s. Since then, end-of-life care provision has expanded rapidly in many countries, but until recently, patients with cancer have remained the main focus for palliative care services. That this does not reflect the needs of the dying population is increasingly being acknowledged; while cancer remains the leading cause of death in those aged between 15 and 64 years, the proportion of deaths attributable to cancer then decreases, with diseases of the circulatory system (ischaemic heart disease and stroke) and respiratory diseases (chronic obstructive pulmonary diseases and pneumonia) becoming much more common. In high-income countries, 75% of people will die from chronic conditions, with a ratio of cancer to noncancer deaths of 1:2 [32]. Direct measurement of palliative care needs in the population has demonstrated how frailty and dementia are the most prevalent conditions, followed by cancer and organ failure. However, palliative care services have not reflected this. A clear dissonance can be seen between the focus on cancer of most specialist palliative care services and deaths from other nonmalignant causes [15].

CONCEPTUALIZING DEMENTIA AS A *TERMINAL* ILLNESS

Dementia is increasingly recognized as a life-limiting illness. A recent population study from the United Kingdom gave a median survival time from diagnosis of dementia to death of 4.1 years [61]; this is strongly influenced by age, with those aged 65–69 years surviving for a median 10.7 years and those aged 90 years and above surviving for 3.8 years [61]. This is approximately half the expected survival years when compared with standard actuarial tables.

However, identifying when frail older people with dementia are reaching the end of their life can be challenging. Medical and nursing home staff members consistently overestimate prognosis in advanced dementia. At nursing home admission, only 1.1% of residents were perceived to have life expectancy of less than 6 months; however, 71% died within that period [28]. Numerous studies have attempted to identify prognostic indicators or indices that may guide physicians to adopting a more palliative approach to care, but these tools are more reliable at identifying people with dementia at *low* risk of death rather than those at *higher* risk of death [49]. Clinical judgment, discussion with families and carers, and taking the opportunity to reassess or shift the goals of management towards palliative care at times of intercurrent illness or transition may be a more practical and reliable approach [48] than attempting to quantify a specific prognosis or survival time using survival indices.

WHERE DO PEOPLE WITH DEMENTIA DIE?

Up to 80% of care home residents have dementia, and residents of care homes are highly likely to die there, making good palliative care and pain management vital in these settings [12]. A number of barriers challenge the provision of good quality care and management of pain in these settings. These include high rates of staff turnover, lack of access to medical support, appropriate medications, and specialist palliative care resources when required. In addition, differences in funding arrangements and health care provision between countries influence how and where palliative care is delivered to people with severe dementia or those with dementia who are dying from other causes.

For example, in the United States, there is a focus on hospice appropriateness; whereby, Health Management Organizations will fund palliative care for people with dementia once it has been agreed that they have a likely survival time of less than 6 months [41]. In the Netherlands, care homes are served by their own dedicated specialist elderly care physicians (formerly called nursing home physicians) who are responsible for care in the last phase of life [38], whereas in the United Kingdom, care is coordinated mainly through primary care (general practitioner) services.

THE ROLE OF A PALLIATIVE CARE APPROACH IN PEOPLE WITH DEMENTIA

The course of dementia is often unpredictable; patients may live to and die in the advanced stages of the disease "dying from" dementia, or they may be in the early or moderate stages of dementia and die from other causes such as cardiovascular disease or cancer [16]. Thus, a palliative or supportive care approach to managing dementia is helpful because it allows a focus on management of comfort, specific symptoms such as behavioral problems or pain, anticipation of future needs, quality of life, and psychological and spiritual aspects of care rather than just prognosis [54]. This model of care may be just as applicable at the beginning of the earliest stages of dementia as in the advanced stages; it takes into account the complexities of caring for someone with dementia who, in contrast to other life-limiting illnesses, may lack the capacity to make treatment decisions for themselves and may experience a slow prolonged *dwindling* disease course interspersed with periods of acute illness such as urinary tract infection or pneumonia. Thus, another key aspect of a palliative care approach to managing dementia is the fact that it acknowledges uncertainty and supports clinicians in focusing on quality of life *and dying* [16].

An example of this type of model is given in Fig. 22-1 (adapted from van der Steen et al. [54]). It depicts changing care goals and priorities throughout the disease course. It suggests how more than one care goal can be important at any one time, for example, in the moderate stages of dementia; all three care goals may be important, but should, for example, an acute physical illness occur such as a myocardial infarction, then priorities of care may shift from prolongation of life to maximization of comfort [54]. As with the WHO definition of palliative care given earlier, this model also highlights how families, friends, and even

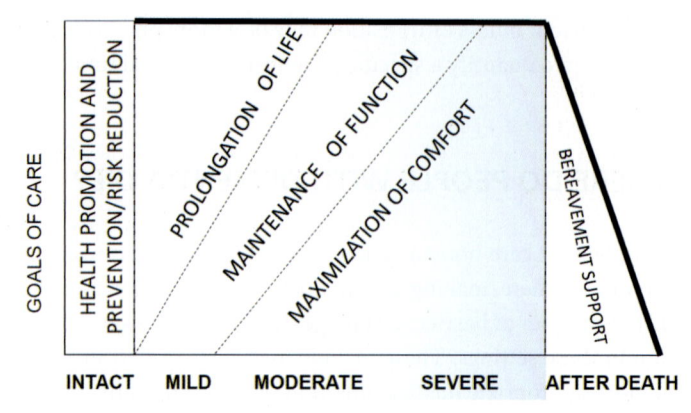

FIGURE 22-1 Dementia progression and suggested prioritization of care goals.

staff may need support in bereavement, although it is important to note that in dementia, where the person may undergo personality changes, a loss of autonomy, cognitive capacity, and the ability to communicate, carers may experience grief that is *anticipatory*—losing the person they love before they actually die [3].

Informal carers of people with dementia often suffer from significant levels of distress and burden [10]. They are frequently expected to act as proxies and may have to make difficult and emotionally demanding choices at the end of life, for example, whether or not their relative should be transferred to hospital [1]. These decisions can be a significant source of stress [14]. They may have to act as advocates for their relative or friend, or assist professionals in communicating with the person with dementia, for example, interpreting an individual's symptoms and signs of pain or other symptoms. Distinguishing between sources of discomfort (e.g., pain or being cold) in severe dementia by integrating the views of a range of caregivers was a key finding and one of the most widely agreed upon recommendations from the European Association for Palliative Care (EAPC) expert consultation (personal communication—van der Steen, 2014). Informal carers who feel competent or who rate themselves as having high levels of self-efficacy tend to cope better and have fewer mental health problems or depressive symptoms [47]. It has also been found that people with dementia die more comfortably when their families accept that this is a life-limiting illness; this association is mediated by better patient–family relationships [52]. Thus, a palliative care approach, which emphasizes the role of families and other friends or unpaid informal carers, may, by providing support and information, improve outcomes for both people with dementia and their carers.

A HOLISTIC APPROACH TO PAIN MANAGEMENT AND PALLIATIVE CARE IN DEMENTIA—PERSONHOOD AND TOTAL PAIN

Person-centered care is a principle philosophy in dementia care. It is a term synonymous with treating people as individuals, respecting their rights as a person, and (from a professional carer's perspective) building therapeutic relationships [26]. Kitwood [22] extended the concept of person-centered care to consider personhood and the status of being a person, and developed a definition of personhood: "A standing or status that is bestowed upon one human being by others, in the context of relationship and social being", which established the concept of person-centered care within relationships with others. People with dementia, particularly those in the advanced stages, are reportedly often denied care that is person centered, and some authors have argued that it is not possible to suffer if we are not sentient [4]. But, the relief of suffering is central to palliative care, and good pain management is an essential part of this. However, as we described earlier in this chapter, in palliative care, we also consider the broader definition—that of "total pain."

The "total pain" model of suffering highlights how, in all people reaching the end of life, pain is more than a physical and nociceptive experience. First conceptualized by Dame Cicely Saunders, it broadens the definition of pain and includes physical, psychological, social, emotional, and spiritual elements [5]. Psychological distress, including depression and anxiety, is common in people with dementia, even at the advanced stages [28]. Although there has been little research in this area, people with dementia, particularly in the earlier stages, may still experience existential distress—feelings of hopelessness, meaninglessness, disappointment, disrupted personality, or anxiety over dying [39]. Thus, some approaches to palliative care for people with advanced dementia, such as Namaste care (see below), which offers meaningful activities that provide social interaction and physical and spiritual care, may be very therapeutic in addressing aspects of "total pain".

CAUSES OF PAIN, DISTRESS, AND DISCOMFORT AT THE END OF LIFE OF PEOPLE WITH DEMENTIA

A number of studies from the European Union, the United States, and Israel have reported on the prevalence of physical, psychosocial, and spiritual symptoms at the end of life, enhancing our knowledge on the quality of end-of-life care for people with dementia [18, 28, 44, 50, 55]. From these studies, the most commonly reported clinical care problems at the end of life are eating and swallowing disorders (45.9–85.8% of the studied population), pressure ulcers (14.7–62.3%), urinary incontinence (89.2%), fever due to different types of infection (13.4–52.6%), and the development of pneumonia (10.8–50%).

The commonest reported physical symptoms at the end of life in the population with advanced dementia are pain in 12–76%, shortness of breath in 8–80%, and agitation in about 55%. Physical pain is often due to comorbid diseases such as arthritis, osteoporosis, dental damage, peripheral neuropathy, pressure sores, and shortness of breath (dyspnea) as a result of heart failure, chronic obstructive pulmonary disease, and pneumonia. Psychological symptoms such as behavioral disturbances occur in between 27% and 66%, with fear and anxiety seen in about 33% and 40% of the studied population, respectively. Resistance to care is also frequently reported (up to 42% of patients with advanced dementia) [18, 28, 44, 50, 55]. Spiritual concerns such as the meaning of suffering and life or thoughts such as "I am not yet finished here, I have still things to achieve" are rarely studied in patients with advanced dementia, and spiritual care may be neglected [36]. One recent study found that only 56% of the residents with dementia die peacefully, as perceived by relatives [9].

Differences in reported symptoms in population-based studies may be due to the use of different measures (dichotomous variables, frequency, intensity) and the use of different time frames (last days, week, or month) to register symptoms. Previous research shows that there is a considerable difference between what is observed by nurses and families on an individual level and what is found at a population-based level where the mean scores on evaluation tools correspond better than the individual scores [50]. In addition, there are regional variations; for example, family reports on comfort in the last week of life in the

United States are more favorable compared with Dutch reports [7] and also indicate a better quality of dying.

CLINICAL ASSESSMENT AND PRACTICAL APPROACH OF PEOPLE DYING WITH DEMENTIA

Undertreatment of pain and other symptoms (shortness of breath and agitation) in patients with advanced dementia during the last week of life is common, as recently shown by Hendriks et al. [18]. However, the recent white paper from the EAPC highlights optimal treatment of symptoms and providing comfort as the top priority for palliative care in dementia, stressing the importance of optimal detection and management of symptoms in patients with dementia [54].

The first step for adequate symptom management in our population is the detection of discomfort including pain. Moreover, dementia is principally a disease of older people, and holistic care of these patients will have to incorporate challenges such as dealing with disabilities, comorbidities, and age-related problems such as urinary retention, constipation, hearing, and visual impairment. Because of a higher risk of adverse drug reactions and iatrogenic illness in the older population, end-of-life care should always start with a medication review, eliminating those drugs that are no longer necessary and carefully starting those necessary for the comfort of the patient.

Pain

No specific evidence-based guidelines are available on the management of pain in patients with dementia at the end of life. Treatment of pain starts with an optimal assessment of pain; this is often complicated by communication problems in patients with advanced dementia. For guidelines concerning assessment of pain in patients with advanced dementia, see Chapter 13.

The basic principles of pain treatment (nonpharmacological and pharmacological) in older patients are also applicable to the older patients with advanced dementia [17]. However, pharmacological treatment is often complicated by swallowing disorders, and so other routes of delivery than oral should be considered. Patches may be used for patients with an expected survival of longer than a few weeks and relatively constant level of pain. However, as it takes a week to obtain a stable plasma level with fentanyl or buprenorphine, treatment with morphine (via a syringe driver) is often the first choice during the last days of life or during a period of unstable pain experience. Because of changes in pharmacokinetics and dynamics, plasma levels of morphine are usually higher in the older patient population, and so the starting dose of morphine should be low; for example, in a naive patient, 2.5 mg every 4–6 hours or 10 mg over 24 hour subcutaneously with 2.5 mg PRN Pro re nata, "as needed" could be considered as a starting dose: We strongly recommend that clinicians follow established guidelines where possible [17]. Pain treatment should be evaluated and adapted at least every 24 hours at the end of life (see also Chapter 18).

Shortness of Breath and Death Rattle

Dyspnea is an objective feeling of difficulty in breathing. It is important to look for possible causes as they can sometimes be actively treated. However, lower respiratory tract infections often occur in patients with advanced dementia and are associated with a high mortality rate (6-month mortality ranging from 36% up to 74%) despite antibiotic treatment [51], and high levels of discomfort [53]. Therefore, a management focus on symptom relief is vital to ensure quality of life.

Nonpharmacological support is important as severe dyspnea is often frightening and the anxiety induced can exacerbate symptoms. Listening to patients and family, careful explanation, and reassurance can be helpful for the patient. Simple measures such as a fan, a back rest in the bed, and an open window can help. Relaxation, breathing exercises, and help with expectoration of secretions by the physiotherapist are an important aid. The use of oxygen is often controversial; oxygen is only necessary if hypoxia can be demonstrated.

In pharmacological treatment, three classes of drugs may be useful, namely the opioids, corticosteroids, and benzodiazepines. A Cochrane review has shown evidence for the use of oral and parenteral morphine in the relief of dyspnea [20]. Corticosteroids are especially used for their anti-inflammatory effects. Benzodiazepines are important drugs in controlling anxiety aggravating the dyspnea. In the older persons, the use of short-acting benzodiazepines is preferred and may be beneficial. A possible choice is the use of sublingual lorazepam 1–2.5 mg orally or midazolam subcutaneously in low dose (2.5 mg in bolus, followed by 5 or 10 mg over 24 hours) [43].

Death rattle often appears the last 48 hours of life and is caused by respiratory secretions, which can no longer be cleared. This noisy breathing may be more distressing for the family than for the patient. Informing families about the origin of the death rattle is the first step in management. The use of anticholinergic medication, to diminish the production of respiratory secretions, is highly controversial in older populations especially those suffering from dementia.

Pressure Sores

The focus of the management of pressure sores at the end of life is to reduce or eliminate pain, to avoid odor, to reduce infection, and to allow an environment that can promote wound healing. In the case of severe wound infection, antimicrobial agents should be considered. To avoid odor, topical or systemic metronidazole, dressings with silver or medical-grade honey, and charcoal or activated charcoal dressings could be considered [33].

Nutrition and Hydration Needs at the End of Life: Is There Place for Tube Feeding?

As swallowing disorders and weight loss are one of the most prevalent symptoms at the end of life, the question of artificial nutrition and hydration is often raised. No clear evidence is available on the benefit of gastric tube feeding for survival, nutritional status, the development of pressure sores, or the risk of aspiration pneumonia in populations with severe dementia [11, 13]. The most important reason that no benefit is seen in this population is the natural courses of the underlying disease where the anorexia–cachexia syndrome and swallowing problems are an important sign of functional decline and the start of the dying process.

However, many family members and caregivers have difficulty with the perception that they are letting their loved one starve to death [11]. It is very important to pay careful attention to the process of communication and the early involvement of patients and family members before the point that the patient is not able to take food or fluids. Patients and families often start from the concept that "she/he won't eat and therefore she/he will die." This concept should be translated into the concept that "she/he is dying and therefore she/he will not eat." If the family can accept the patient is dying, there is less need to discuss withholding or withdrawing of the artificial nutrition and fluids. However, health care workers should be aware that giving food in our culture is often the first and last sign of caring for the loved ones. If feeding is not possible anymore, other ways of caring such as participating in mouth care, toileting, and positioning should be offered to the family.

DETECTING DISCOMFORT AND PAIN IN ADVANCED DEMENTIA AND AT THE END OF LIFE

As with quality of life, in principle, pain, comfort, or discomfort or distress forms subjective and personal experiences. Kolcaba's theory of comfort [23] refers to three types of comfort: relief—the state of having had a specific need met or mediated; ease—the state of calm and contentment; and transcendence—the state in which one rises above problems or pain. In patients with advanced dementia or at the end of life, comfort may comprise the same three types, although we know little about transcendence, and this might require a level of reflection that may not always be achieved. Nevertheless, comfort is an important goal of care for people with advanced dementia [54]. Pain at the end of life may be conceptualized as contributing to a lack of comfort, which affects quality of life and dying [45]. This is consistent with pain included as an item in a measure of comfort (or lack of it, discomfort) at the end of life with dementia [57]. Significant pain can be perceived as usually resulting in discomfort, but vice versa, pain is just one of more possible causes of discomfort with other causes, for example, being cold, constipated, anxious, or disturbed by others [8, 21]. In the development of the classical Discomfort Scale—Dementia of Alzheimer Type (DS-DAT), discomfort was, therefore, defined more broadly as a negative emotional or physical state subject to variation in magnitude in response to internal or environmental conditions [19].

Detection of pain is especially difficult in the advanced stages and at the end of life when people may also suffer from acute health problems that alter their usual behavior. Yet, a pain assessment tool assumes pain as the cause of observed behavior, unlike a tool that assesses discomfort. Therefore, the assessment of discomfort in clinical practice more clearly points to the necessity for further examination of possible causes. On the other hand, as we have seen the chance that a patient with dementia is in pain at the end of life is very high, and there may also be little time to act, it may be appropriate to use a validated pain assessment tool at the end of life. This approach may be even more effective if a detailed physical examination is carried out at the same time.

Pain and (dis)comfort tools share many items in common, including rather nonspecific items such as those referring to negative vocalization or agitation. Pain tools may even include positive qualifications that increase the odds of calculating a total score that indicates "no pain," such as a relaxed body language in the Pain Assessment in Advanced Dementia (PAINAD) [59]. Agitation is a difficult item as it frequently occurs in dementia even at the end of life [18], it may be confused with rejection of care [56], the presence of agitation complicates pain assessment [40], and some studies (although few longitudinal or intervention studies) found some association between pain and agitation in dementia [35]. Nevertheless, because pain in dementia may be expressed in different ways, inclusion of some nonspecific items may help detect pain, especially when a certain cut-off value indicates likely pain (such that pain is not concluded from endorsing one nonspecific item). However, pain and discomfort tools developed by the same group (e.g., the PAINAD and DS-DAT) may be more similar than two pain tools or two discomfort tools, such as the DS-DAT and the individual mapping and comparison to the person's usual presentation for the Disability Distress Assessment Tool (DisDAT) [21]. This points to the need for further psychometric work on optimal combinations of items for pain and discomfort tools.

Assessing and monitoring symptoms is central to a palliative approach. The development of tools to assess pain and discomfort was also triggered by concerns about treatment. More recently, with increasing use of opioids, concerns have been raised about overtreatment, or unselective treatment if it is readily assumed that pain is invariably a cause of behavioral symptoms [21]. However, although recent research often detects no difference between patients with dementia and no dementia in pain, undertreatment of pain persists at least in some places [29]. This is shown, for example, by research in patients with dementia and terminal cancer, where the most cognitively impaired patients were the least likely to receive opioids [30]. Even though there is little evidence for use of tools in clinical practice to decrease pain and increase comfort, multifaceted efforts and awareness raising may help achieve more comfort and less pain in advanced dementia and at the end of life [42].

COMPLEXITIES AND POTENTIAL CONTROVERSIES IN PALLIATIVE CARE FOR PEOPLE WITH DEMENTIA

Dementia has not always been viewed as a life-limiting illness, and the concept that a palliative care approach may be warranted for people with dementia has developed slowly since the 1980s when Volicer introduced the concept of hospice care for people with dementia [58]. Since then, research has mainly focused on specific symptoms and the management of these such as feeding problems or the management of pneumonia [37]. Research in palliative care is challenging, and therefore, although this approach appears to be a humane and worthy one, there is still relatively little robust evidence of its effectiveness in improving quality of death for people with dementia and outcomes for families and other carers [48].

The point at which health and social care staff should adopt a palliative approach to management is also not clearly defined or accepted; in developing the EAPC statement on palliative care for dementia, there was some disagreement among experts on at which stage a palliative care approach should be taken. Certainly in the earlier stages of dementia, prolongation of life may be appropriate, both clinically and in terms of maintaining quality of life [54]. Even in the moderate or severe stages of dementia, it may be appropriate to treat pneumonia or, for example, cancer if this is in keeping with the wishes of the person with dementia and their family and may relieve suffering. Professionals vary in their opinions as to whether a palliative care approach is warranted or beneficial, particularly in the earlier stages of dementia; research has found that younger experts and those with predominantly expertise in dementia are the most critical regarding applicability of palliative care in dementia earlier in the disease trajectory.

The use of opioid analgesia in frail older people has also caused some controversy. This has mainly centered on the potential double effect of these medications; doses required to relieve pain and suffering may also shorten life by causing respiratory depression. In these circumstances, the doctrine of double effect is often quoted [24]. This states that a harmful effect of treatment, even resulting in death (i.e., respiratory depression), is permissible if it is not intended and occurs as a side effect of a beneficial action (the relief of pain). Little research has been done on this aspect of palliative care in dementia; however, if anything, previous research suggested that opioid analgesia was under prescribed in people with dementia [31], but we have little recent information to inform us whether this is still the case. In people dying with cancer, a recent systematic review has found that the use of opioids for symptom control in the advanced disease stages or in the last days of life does not have any effect on patient survival [25].

In the Netherlands, about one of five patients with dementia die with continuous deep sedation maintained until death, according to their physician [18]. Although not specific to dementia, recent research indicated that along with physical symptoms, psychological and existential suffering may contribute to a clinical and emotional state in the patients where other treatment options are not helpful, and both patient and family preferences influenced the decision to use palliative sedation [46]. Research in six European countries showed that older people and those with nonmalignant disease were less likely to receive palliative sedation [27]. These research findings suggest that in addition to medical issues, ethical aspects are highly relevant in the decision making on palliative sedation in dementia, to promote comfort in dying and a state of (un)consciousness in keeping with patient and family wishes.

CONCLUSIONS

A palliative care approach has much to offer the person with dementia, their family, and other caregivers. Pain management is of primary importance, but the maintenance of comfort and the minimization of distress through the careful assessment and treatment of other symptoms such as dyspnea and swallowing problems is vital. Although there are controversies around the stage of dementia at which a palliative care model should be adopted, many of its principles, such as taking a holistic approach to suffering and involving families, are also features of good quality dementia care.

REFERENCES

1. Adelman RD, Tmanova LL, Delgado D, Dion S, Lachs MS. Caregiver burden: a clinical review. JAMA 2014;311:1052–60.
2. Bonica JJ. The need of a taxonomy. Pain 1979;6:247–8.
3. Chan D, Livingston G, Jones L, Sampson EL. Grief reactions in dementia caregivers: a systematic review. Am J Geriatr Psychiatry 2011;28:1–17.
4. Cherny NI, Coyle N, Foley KM. Suffering in the advanced cancer patient: a definition and taxonomy. J Palliat Care 1994;10:57–70.
5. Clark D. 'Total pain', disciplinary power and the body in the work of Cicely Saunders, 1958–1967. Soc Sci Med 1999;49:727–36.
6. Clark D. From margins to centre: a review of the history of palliative care in cancer. Lancet Oncol 2007;8:430–8.
7. Cohen LW, van der Steen JT, Reed D, Hodgkinson JC, van Soest-Poortvliet MC, Sloane PD, Zimmerman S. Family perceptions of end-of-life care for long-term care residents with dementia: differences between the United States and the Netherlands. J Am Geriatr Soc 2012;60:316–22.
8. Cohen-Mansfield J, Thein K, Marx MS, Dakheel-Ali M, Jensen B. Sources of discomfort in persons with dementia. JAMA Intern Med 2013;173:1378–9.
9. De Roo ML, van der Steen JT, Galindo GF, Van Den Noortgate N, Onwuteaka-Philipsen BD, Deliens L, Francke AL. When do people with dementia die peacefully? An analysis of data collected prospectively in long-term care settings. Palliat Med 2014;28:210–9.

10. Dunkin JJ, Anderson-Hanley C. Dementia caregiver burden: a review of the literature and guidelines for assessment and intervention. Neurology 1998;51:S53–60.
11. Finucane TE, Christmas C, Travis K. Tube feeding in patients with advanced dementia: a review of the evidence [comment; Review] [77 refs]. JAMA 1999;282:1365–70.
12. Froggatt KA, Wilson D, Justice C, Macadam M, Leibovici K, Kinch J, Thomas R, Choi J. End-of-life care in long-term care settings for older people: a literature review. Int J Older People Nurs 2006;1:45–50.
13. Gillick MR. Rethinking the role of tube feeding in patients with advanced dementia. N Engl J Med 2000;342:206–10.
14. Givens JL, Lopez RP, Mazor KM, Mitchell SL. Sources of stress for family members of nursing home residents with advanced dementia. Alzheimer Dis Assoc Disord 2012;26:254–9.
15. Gomez-Batiste X, Martinez-Munoz M, Blay C, Amblas J, Vila L, Costa X, Espaulella J, Espinosa J, Constante C, Mitchell GK. Prevalence and characteristics of patients with advanced chronic conditions in need of palliative care in the general population: a cross-sectional study. Palliat Med 2014;28:302–11.
16. Goodman C, Evans C, Wilcock J, Froggatt K, Drennan V, Sampson E, Blanchard M, Bissett M, Iliffe S. End of life care for community dwelling older people with dementia: an integrated review. Int J Geriatr Psychiatry 2010;25:329–37.
17. Hanlon JT, Backonja M, Weiner D, Argoff C. Pharmacological management of persistent pain in older persons. J Am Geriatr Soc 2009;57:1331–46.
18. Hendriks SA, Smalbrugge M, Hertogh CM, van der Steen JT. Dying with dementia: symptoms, treatment, and quality of life in the last week of life. J Pain Symptom Manag 2013;47:710–20.
19. Hurley AC, Volicer BJ, Hanrahan PA, Houde S, Volicer L. Assessment of discomfort in advanced Alzheimer patients. Res Nurs Health 1992;15:369–77.
20. Jennings AL, Davies AN, Higgins JP, Gibbs JS, Broadley KE. A systematic review of the use of opioids in the management of dyspnoea. Thorax 2002;57:939–44.
21. Jordan A, Regnard C, O'Brien JT, Hughes JC. Pain and distress in advanced dementia: choosing the right tools for the job. Palliat Med 2012;26:873–8.
22. Kitwood T. The experience of dementia. Ageing Ment Health 1997;1:13–22.
23. Kolcaba K. Evolution of the mid range theory of comfort for outcomes research. Nurs Outlook 2001;49:86–92.
24. Lo B, Rubenfeld G. Palliative sedation in dying patients: "we turn to it when everything else hasn't worked". JAMA 2005;294:1810–6.
25. Lopez-Saca JM, Guzman JL, Centeno C. A systematic review of the influence of opioids on advanced cancer patient survival. Curr Opin Support Palliat Care 2013;7:424–30.
26. McCormack B, Dewing J, McCance T. Developing person-centred care: addressing contextual challenges through practice development. Online J Issues Nurs 2011;16:3.
27. Miccinesi G, Rietjens JA, Deliens L, Paci E, Bosshard G, Nilstun T, Norup M, van der Wal G. Continuous deep sedation: physicians' experiences in six European countries. J Pain Symptom Manag 2006;31:122–9.
28. Mitchell SL, Kiely DK, Hamel MB. Dying with advanced dementia in the nursing home. Arch Intern Med 2004;164:321–6.
29. Mitchell SL, Kiely DK, Miller SC, Connor SR, Spence C, Teno JM. Hospice care for patients with dementia. J Pain Symptom Manag 2007;34:7–16.
30. Monroe TB, Carter MA, Feldt KS, Dietrich MS, Cowan RL. Pain and hospice care in nursing home residents with dementia and terminal cancer. Geriatr Gerontol Int 2013;13:1018–25.
31. Morrison RS, Siu AL. A comparison of pain and its treatment in advanced dementia and cognitively intact patients with hip fracture. J Pain Symptom Manag 2000;19:240–8.
32. Murray CJ, Lopez AD. Alternative projections of mortality and disability by cause 1990–2020: Global Burden of Disease Study. Lancet 1997;349:1498–504.
33. Nenna M. Pressure ulcers at end of life: an overview for home care and hospice clinicians. Home Healthc Nurse 2011;29:350–65.
34. Payne S, Radbruch L, Payne. White Paper on standards and norms for hospice and palliative care in Europe: part 1—recommendations from the European Association for Palliative Care. Eur J Palliat Care 2009; 16:278–89.
35. Pieper MJ, van Dalen-Kok AH, Franke AL, van der Steen JT, Scherder EJ, Husebo BS, Achterberg WP. Interventions targeting pain or behaviour in dementia: a systematic review. Ageing Res Rev 2013;12:1042–55.
36. Sampson EL, Gould V, Lee D, Blanchard MR. Differences in care received by patients with and without dementia who died during acute hospital admission: a retrospective case note study. Age Ageing 2006; 35:187–9.

37. Sampson EL, Ritchie CW, Lai R, Raven PW, Blanchard MR. A systematic review of the scientific evidence for the efficacy of a palliative care approach in advanced dementia. Int Psychogeriatr 2005;17:31–40.
38. Schols JM, Crebolder HF, van WC. Nursing home and nursing home physician: the Dutch experience. J Am Med Dir Assoc 2004;5:207–12.
39. Schulz R, McGinnis KA, Zhang S, Martire LM, Hebert RS, Beach SR, Zdaniuk B, Czaja SJ, Belle SH. Dementia patient suffering and caregiver depression. Alzheimer Dis Assoc Disord 2008;22:170–6.
40. Shega JW, Hougham GW, Stocking CB, Cox-Hayley D, Sachs GA. Pain in community-dwelling persons with dementia: frequency, intensity, and congruence between patient and caregiver report. J Pain Symptom Manag 2004;28:585–92.
41. Shega JW, Levin A, Hougham GW, Cox-Hayley D, Luchins D, Hanrahan P, Stocking C, Sachs GA. Palliative excellence in Alzheimer care efforts (PEACE): a program description. J Palliat Med 2003;6:315–20.
42. Simard J, Volicer L. Effects of Namaste Care on residents who do not benefit from usual activities. Am J Alzheimers Dis Other Demen 2010;25:46–50.
43. Simon ST, Higginson IJ, Booth S, Harding R, Bausewein C. Benzodiazepines for the relief of breathlessness in advanced malignant and non-malignant diseases in adults. Cochrane Database Syst Rev 2010; CD007354.
44. Sternberg S, Bentur N, Shuldiner J. Quality of care of older people living with advanced dementia in the community in Israel. J Am Geriatr Soc 2014;62:269–75.
45. Stewart AL, Teno J, Patrick DL, Lynn J. The concept of quality of life of dying persons in the context of health care. J Pain Symptom Manag 1999;17:93–108.
46. Swart SJ, van der Heide A, van ZL, Perez RS, Zuurmond WW, van der Maas PJ, van Delden JJ, Rietjens JA. Continuous palliative sedation: not only a response to physical suffering. J Palliat Med 2014;17:27–36.
47. van der Lee J, Bakker TJ, Duivenvoorden HJ, Droes RM. Multivariate models of subjective caregiver burden in dementia: a systematic review. Ageing Res Rev 2014;15C:76–93.
48. van der Steen JT. Dying with dementia: what we know after more than a decade of research. J Alzheimers Dis 2010;22:37–55.
49. van der Steen JT, Albers G, Licht-Strunk E, Muller MT, Ribbe MW. A validated risk score to estimate mortality risk in patients with dementia and pneumonia: barriers to clinical impact. Int Psychogeriatr 2011;23:31–43.
50. van der Steen JT, Gijsberts MJ, Knol DL, Deliens L, Muller MT. Ratings of symptoms and comfort in dementia patients at the end of life: comparison of nurses and families. Palliat Med 2009;23:317–24.
51. van der Steen JT, Lane P, Kowall NW, Knol DL, Volicer L. Antibiotics and mortality in patients with lower respiratory infection and advanced dementia. J Am Med Dir Assoc 2012;13:156–61.
52. van der Steen JT, Onwuteaka-Philipsen BD, Knol DL, Ribbe MW, Deliens L. Caregivers' understanding of dementia predicts patients' comfort at death: a prospective observational study. BMC Med 2013;11:105.
53. van der Steen JT, Pasman HR, Ribbe MW, van der WG, Onwuteaka-Philipsen BD. Discomfort in dementia patients dying from pneumonia and its relief by antibiotics. Scand J Infect Dis 2009;41:143–51.
54. van der Steen JT, Radbruch L, Hertogh CM, de Boer ME, Hughes JC, Larkin P, Francke AL, Junger S, Gove D, Firth P, Koopmans RT, Volicer L. White paper defining optimal palliative care in older people with dementia: a Delphi study and recommendations from the European Association for Palliative Care. Palliat Med 2014;28:197–209.
55. Vandervoort A, Van den Block L, van der Steen JT, Volicer L, Vander SR, Houttekier D, Deliens L. Nursing home residents dying with dementia in Flanders, Belgium: a nationwide postmortem study on clinical characteristics and quality of dying. J Am Med Dir Assoc 2013;14:485–92.
56. Volicer L, Bass EA, Luther SL. Agitation and resistiveness to care are two separate behavioral syndromes of dementia. J Am Med Dir Assoc 2007;8:527–32.
57. Volicer L, Hurley AC, V, Blasi ZV. Scales for evaluation of end-of-life care in dementia. Alzheimer Dis Assoc Disord 2001;15:194–200.
58. Volicer L, Rheaume Y, Brown J, Fabiszewski K, Brady R. Hospice approach to the treatment of patients with advanced dementia of the Alzheimer type. JAMA 1986;256:2210–3.
59. Warden V, Hurley AC, Volicer L. Development and psychometric evaluation of the Pain Assessment in Advanced Dementia (PAINAD) scale. J Am Med Dir Assoc 2003;4:9–15.
60. World Health Organisation. Cancer pain relief and palliative care, Vol. Technical Report Series 804. Geneva: WHO; 1990.
61. Xie J, Brayne C, Matthews FE. Survival times in people with dementia: analysis from population based cohort study with 14 year follow-up. BMJ 2008;336:258–62.

CHAPTER 23

Multidisciplinary and Multiprofessional Treatments

Benny Katz

The population aged over 60 years is growing faster than any other age group. People are not only living longer and remaining healthy into old age, but also more people than ever before are living with age-related degenerative diseases [25]. By 2050, one in five of the world's population will be aged 60 years or older and the number of people aged 80 years and older will quadruple between 2000 and 2050 [32]. Advanced age is associated with an increased prevalence of both pain and dementia. Painful conditions are among the major reasons for older people accessing the health-care system [27]. About one in four people aged over 85 years is affected by dementia, and one in two nursing home residents [4, 9]. About 50% of people with dementia regularly experience pain. Nursing home residents often have more severe diseases and more advanced dementia. The prevalence of pain in nursing homes is as high as 80% [6]. The neurocognitive features of dementia make the identification, assessment, and management of pain more challenging.

Analgesics are the mainstay of pain treatment in the aged population [3]. This is on the basis of accessibility and efficacy. Analgesics may be effective as a single modality; however, any benefit must be balanced against the increased risk of adverse effects and drug interactions in older people. Alternate strategies should be sought when this balance is unacceptable. Pain management guidelines usually advocate a multidisciplinary approach, combining pharmacological with nonpharmacological strategies. This is based on a consensus of experts, as the evidence to support this recommendation is sparse, especially for people with dementia [1, 3]. Reasons for considering a multidisciplinary approach for the management of persistent pain in older adults with dementia include the following:

PUBLICATION BIAS

The treatment of older people is often based on research undertaken in younger subjects. By the nature of this research, the results may not be generalizable to the older patient seen in daily practice. The rigorous selection criteria for randomized controlled trials (RCTs) aimed at ensuring internal validity has the effect of excluding older people, particularly those with comorbid conditions such as cognitive impairment and dementia. This methodology is more suited for pharmacological studies. The results do not capture the other physical and mental health benefits of nonpharmacological approaches such as physical and cognitive–behavioral therapies.

The systematic exclusion of older people from studies of common age-related conditions is highlighted in the Cochrane review of exercise for osteoarthritis of the knee [12]. This systematic review included 32 RCTs involving almost 3800 subjects. In only three of these studies, involving 354 subjects, was the mean age of the participants >70 years. There were no studies where the mean age was ≥75 years.

The exclusion of older subjects from RCTs published in high-impact medical journals was examined by Van Spall and colleagues, reporting that 38.5% of trials excluded subjects on age criteria alone, usually over 65 years, and in 47% of trials on the presence of common age-related medical conditions. In less than half the trials was there strong justification for the exclusion criteria [31]. Taylor and colleagues [30] investigated the exclusion criteria in 434 RCTs published in an influential geriatric medical journal. Cognitive impairment was an explicit exclusion criterion in 29% and a further 16% of studies used methods that were likely to effectively exclude participation by cognitively impaired individuals, such as recruitment by telephone or mail outs.

In the absence of strong evidence on which to base treatment from studies that include older people including those with dementia, the safety of nonpharmacological approaches and the general physical and mental health benefits of multidisciplinary approaches makes them attractive options.

Multidisciplinary Approach to Pain Management

John Bonica established the world's first pain clinic at the University of Washington in 1961. Despite the advances that have occurred in medical knowledge and therapeutic options over time, the multidisciplinary biopsychosocial approach remains the preferred option for the management of chronic pain that has not responded to standard treatments. Substantial evidence exists to support the effectiveness of this approach [13, 19]. There is some evidence that older patients also benefit [7, 20].

Multidisciplinary Approach in Geriatric Medicine

The multidisciplinary process known as Comprehensive Geriatric Assessment (CGA) has been shown to improve health outcomes when compared with usual care across a range of health-care settings. CGA adopts a multidisciplinary approach to identify medical, psychological, functional, and social issues affecting an older person in order to develop a coordinated plan aimed at improving health status, function, and long-term outcomes [8, 29]. CGA does take into consideration the impact of dementia. It has been successfully integrated into range of health-care settings including Pain Management Clinics for Older People [17].

This chapter describes a Pain Management Clinic for Older People that manages older patients with persistent pain including many with impaired cognition and dementia. The operation of the clinic is described, with specific emphasis on the features of the clinic designed to service the needs of this population.

PAIN MANAGEMENT CLINIC FOR OLDER PEOPLE

The Pain Clinic for Older People was established in 2012 within a university-affiliated teaching hospital in Melbourne Australia. It complements a range of pain services within the hospital covering acute, chronic, and cancer-related pains. The Pain Clinic for Older People employs a geriatrician/pain specialist, senior nurse, physiotherapist, clinical psychologist, and administrative staff. Access to other disciplines including interpreters, social work, occupational therapy, dietetics, and psychiatry is available on referral. Prior to joining the clinic, the staff had more than 50 years' collective experience in pain management [14, 17].

Initial contact with the clinic may come from a family member or health-care professional; however, the clinic requires referral by the patient's primary care physician who plays an important role in delivery of the pain management plan. To be eligible to attend the clinic, a person must have pain and other significant age-related conditions likely to affect management, such as cognitive impairment, mobility impairment, falls, frailty, or multi-morbidity. Residents of aged care facilities are not excluded. There are no out-of-pocket expenses for patients attending this clinic under Australia's universal health insurance scheme.

Appointments are usually offered within 4–8 weeks of referral. Patients are encouraged to attend with a family member or other close person. The initial assessment takes approximately 3 hours. Most patients opt for this to take place in a single attendance, although there is an option for the assessment to be divided over two visits. The pace of the assessment is adjusted according to the individual's ability. Regular refreshment and bathroom breaks are incorporated into the visit. Once commenced, it is unusual for a patient not to complete the assessment in a single visit. The features of this clinic designed to cater for the special needs of frail older people are outlined in Table 23-1.

The pain clinic team works in pairs to avoid the inconvenience for the patient having to repeat the history and undergo examinations by different health professionals. Working together, the nurse and clinical psychologist undertake the comprehensive geriatric screen, social and psychological assessments. The physician and physiotherapist undertake the medical and musculoskeletal assessments together. The paired approach enables the patient to go through the assessment quicker and with less stress, but it is more time consuming for the staff. The multidisciplinary assessment is followed by a case conference and patient feedback session. See Table 23-2.

The patient is given an explanation of the cause(s) of the pain, and when appropriate, reassurance, such as "your ongoing pain does not mean that there is ongoing damage to your body," or "ongoing pain is not due to serious pathology such as cancer." Unrealistic expectations are dispelled, such as the hope for total eradication of pain. The goals, treatment options, and prognosis are then discussed. Goals of treatment are often discussed in terms such as "we will aim to keep your pain at tolerable levels, but don't expect it to go away completely" or "we will aim to keep your current level of function into the future." Family members often benefit from an explanation of the relative contribution of pain to the level of function, in distinction to the impact of dementia or other comorbidities. Other issues identified during the CGA are also discussed.

All treatment programs are individual. The size of the clinic and heterogeneity of the clientele does not permit group programs. Management options include pharmacological, physical, and psychological approaches, together with advice about aerobic fitness, maintenance of function, and social interaction. To ensure patient safety, many of the strategies need to be supervised, for instance, to ensure adherence to prescribed medications or to ensure that a patient with dementia does not become lost on a walking program. Therapy is usually delivered in facilities close to the patient's residence, rather than in the clinic. The needs of the carers are taken into consideration. Supportive counseling is offered, either in the clinic or through other agencies. Advice is given about services to reduce the burden of

TABLE 23-1 Features of a Multidisciplinary Pain Clinic for Older People

Referrals	Referrals must come via the primary care physician who maintains responsibility for medication prescriptions and long-term follow-up.
Appointments	The patient is offered the option of one 3-h attendance for initial assessment and management plan, or scheduled over a number of shorter attendances. Most patients prefer, and are able to tolerate, one longer attendance.
	Patients are not required to complete questionnaires prior to first attendance, as this may be a barrier for attendance especially for people with dementia or limited English language skills.
	Patients are encouraged to bring a support person along at each attendance.
Facility	Easy access to public transport and parking
	Easy access to refreshment and bathroom facilities
	Large rooms to accommodate multiple people and mobility aids
Assessments	Slow pace to avoid fatigue, with scheduled breaks
	Therapists work in pairs to avoid the need for the patient to repeat the history and physical examinations.
	Comprehensive geriatric assessment and pain assessment protocols (see Table 23-2).
	Patients are assisted to complete psychometric instruments (see Table 23-3).
Case conference and feedback	Treatment goals are negotiated with the patient.
	Multifaceted approach includes psychoeducation, pharmacological therapy, physical therapies, aerobic fitness, cognitive–behavioral strategies, activities of daily living, social engagement, and living environment.
Adherence	The patient receives a written summary of the assessment and recommendations.
	The letter aids adherence to recommendations and helps families and carers understand the program and reinforce the message.
Support for carers	When appropriate, carers are offered counseling either in the clinic or referred to external agencies. Advice is given about personal and domiciliary support services, respite options, and social outlets. Pamphlets are available covering a range of topics relevant to this population.
Follow-up	Patients are offered the option of follow-up in the clinic or by the primary care physician, especially if access to the clinic is difficult.
	Telephone follow-up is made 3 months after the last attendance.

care, such as domiciliary and personal care assistance, social outlets, and respite programs. A report is sent to the primary care physician who implements the pain management plan. A separate letter is sent to the patient to enhance understanding and aid compliance. The letter helps family members who were not present at the assessment become involved in the implementation of the recommendations. This is particularly helpful for family members of patients with more advanced dementia and those with limited English language skills. Follow-up may be in the clinic, or by telephone, according to patient preference.

Most patients with dementia attending this clinic are capable of giving a pain history, and complete simple psychometric instruments such as the brief pain inventory (see Table 23-3). No questionnaires are sent to patients prior to the initial attendance, as this may be seen an indirect barrier for attendance, especially for people with dementia or limited English language skills. The staff assist patients with the psychometric instruments, using an interpreter when appropriate.

TABLE 23-2 Initial Comprehensive Assessment

Registration and demographic data	Age
	Living arrangements
	Relationships
	Carers
	Support structure—paid and unpaid
	Preferred language
Medical	Pain history
	Medical comorbidities
	Medications
	Current medications
	Previous analgesics—effectiveness
	Medication intolerances
	Medication adherence/delivery systems
	General physical examination with emphasis on the musculoskeletal and nervous systems
Hearing and vision	Vision, visual aids
	Hearing, use of hearing aids
Cognition	Dementia screen
Mood	Depression
	Anxiety
	Stress
	Frustration
Function	Activities of daily living
	Personal
	Domestic
Mobility	Mobility
	Mobility aids
	Falls
	Community access
	Transportation
Continence	Bladder
	Bowels
	Continence aids
Miscellaneous	Driving
	Smoking
	Alcohol
	Substance use
	Vaccination status
	Cultural and religious preferences
	Legal, for example, surrogate decision-makers, will

The mean age of the patients attending the clinic is 81.6 years (range 64–94), with 72% females. Patients tend to be frail; eighty five percent were rated vulnerable to severely frail on the clinical frailty scale [24]. Personal care assistance was being used by 34%, and 18% were living in residential care facilities. More than 50% reported back pain as the major pain site, with 85% reporting pain at more than one site. Pain had been present for ≥24 months in 66.2%, ranging up to 40 years. Cognitive assessment was undertaken with

TABLE 23-3 Psychometric Measures

Demographic data	Registration details
	Living arrangements
	Personal care
	Domestic care
Pain	Pain duration
	Pain sites—Manchester coding [16]
	Brief pain inventory [5]
Medication	Total number of medications
	Use of opioid analgesia, antidepressants, and anticonvulsants
Cognition	Mini-mental status examination [11]
	Clock drawing test [33]
	Occasionally used:
	Montreal cognitive assessment [22]
	Abbreviated mental test [15]
	Rowland Universal Dementia Assessment Scale (RUDAS) [28] (for patients with limited English language skills)
Medical comorbidities	Cumulative illness rating scale for geriatrics [21]
Frailty	Clinical frailty scale (Rockwood) [24]
Mood	Depression, anxiety, and stress scale [18]
	Occasionally used:
	Geriatric depression scale (short form) [26]
Function	Human activity profile [10]
Follow-up	Clinicians global impression of change
	Adherence to recommendations checklist

mini-mental status examination (MMSE), clock drawing test, and clinical assessment. Cognitive impairment using a cutoff on MMSE of ≤25 was present in 43.5% [11]. Moderate to severe cognitive impairment with MMSE scores of ≤20 was present in 20.6%. Cognitive impairment based on expert opinion was present in 43.1%. The average number of comorbid medical conditions was 7.2 of 14 possible categories, with 83.1% having at least one severe disability/health problem [21]. The average number of medications was 10.8 per person. At initial presentation 75.4% were taking opioid analgesia, 47.1% antidepressants, and 20.6% anticonvulsants.

The presence of cognitive impairment did not preclude patients showing an improvement during the multidisciplinary pain treatment program. Initial audit of treatment response revealed that the average pain score over 24 hours went from 5.97/10 at enrollment to 4.69 ($P < 0.005$) following treatment in the cognitively intact group, and in the cognitively impaired group from 6.43 to 4.64 ($P < 0.01$). Similarly, in the cognitively intact group interference in general activity went from 7.50 to 4.94 ($P < 0.001$), and in the cognitively impaired group from 7.15 to 4.96 ($P < 0.005$).

APPROACH TO PEOPLE WITH DEMENTIA

Routine screening for dementia should occur at initial health service contact, to avoid the possibility of missing a patient with dementia that has not yet be diagnosed. The approach

TABLE 23-4 Key Points for Communicating with People with Dementia

- Distraction-free environment.
- Ensure hearing aids are being worn and are working properly.
- Maintain eye contact.
- Avoid ignoring the individual by speaking only with the carer.
- Speak slowly, clearly and with short sentences.
- Avoid complex sentences.
- Use gestures and body language.
- Do not interrupt or pressure the patient.
- Be encouraging; do not show frustration.
- Avoid finishing the person's sentences.
- Do not patronize or ridicule by laughing at the person.

to a patient with dementia is determined by the severity, type of dementia, and the presence of other comorbid conditions such as hearing impairment. Individuals with dementia can often report their pain and complete pain scales, even in advanced stages of dementia [23]. Questions should be short, simple, and specific. It may be helpful to take the patient through provocative activities for pain such as walking, asking them along the way to report the pain. The conversation should not just be through the carer. Table 23-4 outlines key points in communication with people with dementia.

Two case studies of patients with dementia are presented to highlight the multidisciplinary approach to pain management. The first case focuses on a patient with early dementia, and how it affected pain report and management. In the setting of early dementia the individual is usually capable of reporting pain. The challenge is to identify the cognitive impairment and determine the impact that it is having on the pain report and to make appropriate modifications to the management plan. This stands in contrast to severe dementia when the individual may no longer be able to report pain. The diagnosis of dementia is not the challenge, but the identification of pain and its impact are.

Mrs. T, aged 84 years, presented to the Pain Clinic with a 2-year history of neck and lumbar back pain following a fall. She had a history of back surgery. The pain was considered secondary to lumbar canal stenosis with lumbar spine instability. Pain severity averaged 6/10 during the day, aggravated by physical activity and walking, when it became intolerable at 8/10 for up to 2 hours. She had previously attended an academic memory clinic. Alzheimer's disease was diagnosed, and she responded well to cognitive-enhancing therapy. On presentation at the pain clinic the features of dementia were subtle and could have been easily missed. Her MMSE score was 28/30. Her husband reported that her conversations were at times repetitive, that she was having difficulty with library books that she could previously follow, and he raised concern about her safety in the kitchen. Her pain management program comprised a combination of pharmacological and nonpharmacological treatments, including an exercise program and occupational therapy assessment of her safety in the kitchen.

Two months later Mrs. T reported that her pain had reduced by 50% and she was now more active. Her husband reported that pain was not having a significant impact on her function, but that her cognition was. She was keen to achieve even better pain control, requesting an increase in analgesic dose. The increased dose of opioid resulted in a deterioration in cognition, drowsiness, nighttime behavioral disturbance, and on one occasion not being able to find her way home following a walk. These symptoms improved once the dose was reduced. At the next clinic visit, she again requested an increase in medication dose. She had no recollection of the previous adverse response and subsequent conversations, but retained the capacity to work through the issues during the discussion, agreeing that a dose increase was not wise. The same conversation occurred on subsequent visits.

The management strategy was modified, with more emphasis being placed on supervised nonpharmacological strategies, such as an aerobic fitness program and support for her husband to help him manage her increasing care needs. Mrs. T was given a letter outlining the reasons why her medication dose should not be increased, and how to deal with exacerbations of pain. Her husband would refer her to the note when she requested additional medications at home.

This case highlights a number of important issues. Mrs. T's Alzheimer's disease could easily have been missed. She was well presented and articulate, with a normal MMSE score. When provided with facts, she retained the capacity to make decisions, but then forgot the discussion. The clues to her cognitive issues included her husband's report and the repetitive conversation. A normal score on MMSE does not exclude dementia. Failure to take her dementia into consideration may have resulted in more adverse treatment effects. It was important to confine her medical care to a limited number of physicians familiar with her case, who would not submit to her request to increase her medications. The multidisciplinary pain management was modified. As pharmacological options were limited, more emphasis was placed on nonpharmacological approaches for her pain, environmental modification, and memory aids. Her husband received counseling about pain and dementia, and was provided with information about domiciliary support services and respite.

The second case study is of a person with more advanced dementia. Mrs. O, aged 82 years, presented to the pain clinic with widespread pain secondary to generalized osteoarthritis, rotator cuff tendinopathy, and fibromyalgia. Osteoarthritis of the right knee resulted in severe pain and disability. To avoid aggravating the pain, she was spending up to 18 hours/day sitting or lying down. She was referred to the pain clinic after she had had been refused total knee joint replacement on the grounds of unacceptable operative risk. She had multiple comorbidities requiring frequent hospital visits for chronic obstructive pulmonary disease, together with obesity, profound visual and hearing impairments, anxiety, depression, and benzodiazepine abuse. She lived alone, supported by her children and a government-funded Home Care Package. A diagnosis of dementia was made in the pain clinic. Her MMSE was 17/30.

Mrs. O was very angry that she had been refused surgery, especially as her older brother had successfully undergone this operation 6 months earlier. She had come to the pain clinic in the hope that we would advocate on her behalf so that she could undergo surgery. She considered that surgery would relieve her pain and enable her to remain independent in her home. She feared nursing home admission. Mrs. O was preoccupied with undergoing surgery, and did not comprehend the contribution that her other comorbidities were having on her function.

As joint arthroplasty was not possible, other options were considered. Intra-articular steroids and oral opioid analgesia were not giving adequate relief and physical therapies were not likely to be effective because of the severity of her musculoskeletal disease and the limitations related to her comorbidities. Could cognitive–behavioral approaches be effective in the setting of dementia? Her anger, centered on the refusal of surgery, was considered most amenable to intervention. Counseling was undertaken. She was asked what risk she would consider acceptable with surgery. Initially the discussion focused on the risk of death. She did understand the discussion, and when given options to choose a 1-in-10 chance of death as acceptable. When the discussion shifted to the risk of unsuccessful surgery or rehabilitation resulting in the need for nursing home admission, Mrs. O was not prepared to accept any risk, no matter how small. She responded by saying that she would refuse surgery if she could not be given a guarantee that she would not end up in a nursing home. Following this discussion her anger waned. The focus of management shifted to optimizing her quality of life within the limits of her pain and disabilities. Negotiations were ensued with her Home Care Package case manager. Resources previously used to escort her to frequent medical appointments were redeployed to a focus on her quality of life. She received additional home support, companionship, and a scribe to write down her poetry, that she had been unable to do because of visual impairment.

This case highlights the role a biopsychosocial approach. A disease-centered approach had failed to identify what Mrs. O really wanted, that is to remain in her own home. In contrast, the multidisciplinary team managed to overcome barriers related to dementia and severe hearing impairment to deal with her anger and improve her quality of life. Dementia needed to be taken into consideration when counseling her. The discussion was taken slowly, engaging her by focusing on what was her major priority [2].

CONCLUSIONS

The aging of the population will result in a larger proportion of the population at risk of aged-related degenerative diseases. Given the high prevalence of both dementia and pain in older adults, they are likely to coexist in many. This poses additional challenges for management of pain and of dementia. There is a need for more research into the optimal treatments for older people with pain and dementia, but the inherent difficulties in undertaking these studies means that we are likely to continue to rely on the results of studies undertaken of each problem separately, or from studies involving younger healthier subjects.

Pharmacological approaches have been the mainstay of the treatment of pain in older people, despite the increased risk of adverse drug effects. A multidisciplinary approach reduces the reliance on pharmacological options, and offers other important physical and mental health benefits, with fewer adverse effects. Cost and accessibility remain important barriers.

There are relatively few Pain Management Clinics for Older People. They are resource intensive and manage a relatively small number of patients. Most people who could potentially benefit are unable to access these clinics. Apart from their service role, these clinics have the potential of playing an important role in developing models of care required for an aging population, and to provide an evidence base to inform therapeutic guidelines.

This chapter has described the features that have been incorporated into a multidisciplinary pain clinic designed to manage the special needs of frail older people with multiple comorbidities including dementia. Preliminary results indicate that patients with mild to moderate dementia respond similarly to cognitively intact patients to a multidisciplinary pain management program.

REFERENCES

1. Abdulla A, Adams N, Bone M, Elliott A, Gaffin J, Jones D, Knaggs R, Martin D, Sampson L, Schofield P. Guidance on the management of pain in older people. Age Ageing 2013;42:i1–57.
2. American Geriatrics Society Expert Panel on the Care of Older Adults with Multimorbidity. Patient-centered care for older adults with multiple chronic conditions: a stepwise approach from the American Geriatrics Society. J Am Geriatr Soc 2012;60:1957–68.

3. American Geriatrics Society Panel on Persistent Pain in Older Persons. The management of persistent pain in older persons. J Am Geriatr Soc 2002;50:S205–224.
4. Australian Institute of Health and Welfare. Dementia among aged care residents: first information from the Aged Care Funding Instrument. Aged care statistics Vol. 32. Canberra: Australian Institute of Health and Welfare; 2011. Accessed March 30, 2014 at https://www.aihw.gov.au/publication-detail/?id=10737419025
5. Cleeland C. Brief pain inventory. The University of Texas M. D. Anderson Cancer Center; 1991.
6. Corbett A, Husebo B, Malcangio M, Staniland A, Cohen-Mansfield J, Aarsland D, Ballard C. Assessment and treatment of pain in people with dementia. Nat Rev Neurol 2012;8:264–74.
7. Cutler RB, Fishbain DA, Rosomoff RS, Rosomoff H. Outcomes in treatment of pain in geriatric and younger age groups. Arch Phys Med Rehabil 1994;75:457–64.
8. Ellis G, Whitehead MA, O'Neill D, Langhorne P, Robinson D. Comprehensive geriatric assessment for older adults admitted to hospital. Cochrane Database of Syst Rev 2011;7:CD006211.
9. Ferri CP, Prince M, Brayne C, Brodaty H, Fratiglioni L, Ganguli M, Hall K, Hasegawa K, Hugh Hendrie, Huang Y, et al. Global prevalence of dementia: a Delphi consensus study. Lancet 2005;366:2112–7.
10. Fix A, Daughton D. Human activity profile professional manual. Psychological Assessment Resources; 1988.
11. Folstein MF, Folstein SE, McHugh PR. "Mini-mental state". A practical method for grading the cognitive state of patients for the clinician. J Psychiatr Res 1975;12:189–98.
12. Fransen M, McConnell S. Exercise for osteoarthritis of the knee. Cochrane Database of Syst Rev 2008;4:CD004376.
13. Guzman J, Esmail R, Karjalainen K, Malmivaara A, Irvin E, Bombardier C. Multidisciplinary rehabilitation for chronic low back pain: systematic review. BMJ 2001;322:1511–6.
14. Helme RD, Katz B, Neufeld M, Lachal S, Herbert J, Corran T. The establishment of a Geriatric Pain Clinic—a preliminary report of the first 100 patients. Australas J Ageing 1989;8:27–30.
15. Hodkinson HM. Evaluation of a Mental Test Score for assessment of mental impairment in the elderly. Age Ageing 1972;1:233–8.
16. Holliday KL, Nicholl BI, Macfarlane GJ, Thomson W, Davies KA, McBeth J. Genetic variation in the hypothalamic-pituitary-adrenal stress axis influences susceptibility to musculoskeletal pain: results from the EPIFUND study. Ann Rheum Dis 2010;69:556–60.
17. Katz B, Scherer S, Gibson SJ. Multidisciplinary pain management clinics for older adults. In: Gibson SJ, Weiner DK, editors. Pain in older persons, progress in pain research and management, Vol. 35. Seattle: IASP Press, 2005. p. 309–26.
18. Lovibond SH, Lovibond Pf. Manual for the depression anxiety stress scales, 2nd edition. Sydney: Psychology Foundation, 1995.
19. McQuay H, Moore R, Eccleston C, Morley S, de C Williams A. Systematic review of outpatient services for chronic patient control. Health Technol Assessment 1997;1:i–iv.
20. Middaugh SJ, Levin RB, Kee WG, Barchiesi FD, Roberts JM. Chronic pain: its treatment in geriatric and younger patients. Arch Phys Med Rehabil 1988;69:1021–6.
21. Miller MD, Towers A. A manual of guidelines for scoring the Cumulative Illness Rating Scale for Geriatrics (CIRS-G). Pittsburgh, PA: University of Pittsburgh; 1991.
22. Nasreddine Z, Phillips N, Bédirian V, Charbonneau S, Whitehead V, Collin I, Chertkow JCH. Montreal Cognitive Assessment (MoCA©): a brief screening tool for mild cognitive impairment. J Am Geriatr Soc 2005;53:695–9.
23. Pautex S, Michon A, Guedira M, Emond H, Le Lous P, Samaras D, Michel JP, Herrmann F, Giannakopoulos P, Gold G. Pain in severe dementia: self-assessment or observational scales? J Am Geriatr Soc 2006;54:1040–45.
24. Rockwood K, Song X, MacKnight C, Bergman H, Hogan DB, McDowell I, Mitnitski A. A global clinical measure of fitness and frailty in elderly people. CMAJ 2005;173:489–95. Instrument accessed March 30, 2014 at http://geriatricresearch.medicine.dal.ca/pdf/Clinical%20Faily%20Scale.pdf
25. The President's Council on Bioethics. Dilemmas of an Aging Society: taking care—ethical caregiving in our Aging Society. Washington, DC: The President's Council on Bioethics, 2005.
26. Sheikh JI, Yesavage JA. Geriatric Depression Scale (GDS): recent evidence and development of a shorter version. Clin Gerontol 1986:165–73.
27. St Sauver JL, Warner DO, Yawn BP, Jacobson DJ, McGree ME, Pankratz JJ, Melton LJ, Roger VL, Ebbert JO, Rocca WA. Why patients visit their doctors: assessing the most prevalent conditions in a defined American population. Mayo Clin Proc 2013;88:56–67.

28. Storey JE, Rowland JT, Basic D, Conforti DA, Dickson HG. The Rowland Universal Dementia Assessment Scale (RUDAS): a multicultural cognitive assessment scale. Int Psychogeriatr 2004;16:13–31.
29. Stuck AE, Siu A, Wieland G, Adams J, Rubenstein L. Comprehensive geriatric assessment: a meta-analysis of controlled trials. Lancet 1993;342:1032–36.
30. Taylor JS, DeMers SM, Vig EK, Borson S. The disappearing subject: exclusion of people with cognitive impairment and dementia from geriatrics research. J Am Geriatr Soc 2012;60:413–9.
31. Van Spall HG, Toren A, Kiss A, Fowler RA. Eligibility criteria of randomized controlled trials published in high-impact general medical journals: a systematic sampling review. JAMA 2007;297:1233–40.
32. WHO. Health topics—ageing. Accessed March 24, 2014 at http://www.who.int/topics/ageing/en/
33. Wolf-Klein GP, Silverstone FA, Levy AP, Brod MS. Screening for Alzheimer's disease by clock drawing. J Amer Geriatr Soc 1989;37:730–34.

CHAPTER 24

Ethical Issues in Research with Persons with Dementia: Potential and Restrictions

Colleen Doyle, Leslie Dowson, Gail Roberts, and Stephen J. Gibson

Informed consent is an essential ethical prerequisite for participant enrollment in any research activity, including the conduct of clinical trials. Randomized controlled trials (RCTs) require the consent of potentially being treated only by a placebo. It is questionable that patients with dementia are able to provide full consent when still living without a guardian. The consequences of these limitations for designing appropriate clinical trials will be discussed in this chapter. Furthermore, alternative strategies for research design and respecting the preferences of people with dementia will be presented.

People living with dementia have the same rights as others in the community to be involved in research if that is their preference, and to have their preferences respected if they change their mind during their involvement in research. However, cognitive impairment will interfere with the individual's ability to understand the complex concepts associated with research participation, and with the individual's ability to communicate their preferences to the researcher. Participation in research into pain and dementia may be particularly problematic from an ethical point of view.

This chapter outlines the main ethical issues to be considered when conducting pain research with people living with dementia. It outlines recent research into informed consent issues for people living with dementia, and summarizes research into assessment tools that can be used to identify capacity to given informed consent. A case study of a research project is presented to illustrate how ethical issues were addressed in one RCT of pain treatment in dementia. Alternative research strategies to RCTs and the role of advance care plans (ACPs) as an adjunct to immediate consent and assent procedures in supporting participants and their roles in future research are discussed.

WHY PEOPLE PARTICIPATE IN RESEARCH TRIALS

People who agree to participate in research trials are not representative of the entire population. Those who have tried to recruit participants into research will know that there is only a subgroup of the population who are willing to be involved in research, and this also applies to people living with dementia and their families or carers. Studies of recruitment and reasons for participation in research have indicated that most people agree to participate for altruistic reasons. According to Edwards et al. [19], over 60% of participants in seven studies participated for altruistic reasons, while in four other studies over 70% participated for self-interest. Bartlam et al. [2] found that of 402 people participating in an Alzheimer's disease (AD) trial, the main reasons for participating were altruism, personal benefit, and family history of AD.

Proxy decision-makers are often instructed to use substitute judgment when choosing to decide whether someone who lacks capacity to make an informed decision should participate in research. That is, they are asked to choose what the person with dementia would choose if they were able to make an informed choice. In practice, research has revealed that decisions on whether or not to participate in research made on behalf of someone with dementia will at least in part be influenced by factors valued by the proxy decision-maker [8, 15]. Direct benefit to the person with dementia has been found to be the most influential factor in proxy decision-making to participate in research. The possibility of serious side effects for the person with dementia is the second most influential consideration [8].

INFORMED CONSENT IN RESEARCH IN GENERAL AND SPECIFICALLY IN DEMENTIA RESEARCH

Informed Consent

Informed consent in research is the voluntary authorization given by a potential participant to participate in a research study. This authorization must be informed, meaning the significant details of the research study are disclosed by the researchers and the potential participant has the capacity to understand and make a voluntary decision after considering the information disclosed. The capacity to make a decision, known as decisional capacity, can be defined as the ability to (1) understand the relevant information, (2) appreciate the nature of the situation and its consequences, (3) reason by manipulating the information rationally, and (4) express a choice [5]. To provide informed consent potential participants in research should understand (1) the study's purpose, (2) what procedures they will undergo, (3) any risks, (4) any potential benefits, (5) voluntariness, (6) their rights to withdrawal, (7) confidentiality, and (8) the alternatives to participation [5].

Informed Consent in Dementia Research

Research involving people living with dementia is ethically challenging because of the effects of dementia on cognitive function. These effects will eventually make gaining informed consent for research impossible, and no clear-cut line exists between capacity and incapacity [30].

Capacity to provide informed consent is a relational determination [9]. That is, it is specific to the individual, the context of the situation, and the choice that is to be made. Many legal jurisdictions assume capacity for all adults, unless there is (1) evidence of cognitive impairment or disturbance and (2) that impairment or disturbance means the person is unable to make (or communicate) a specific informed decision when it is required [36, 38]. Therefore, a diagnosis of dementia does not necessarily exclude someone from providing informed consent for research. For people living with dementia, the determination of capacity ought to be made at the time of research enrollment and reaffirmed at every contact point throughout the study [30]. Every reasonable effort should be made to inform potential research participants with dementia about the research study. This may take more time than is usual to obtain informed consent, and it may involve building rapport, adapting the information provided or using an intermediary known to the potential participant. Capacity judgments vary considerably. They are inherently value-laden judgments incorporating risks-versus-benefits considerations [30].

When a potential participant does not have the capacity to provide informed consent, many jurisdictions allow for consent by proxy. A proxy decision-maker is often a family member or other trusted party. There may be a formal or legal appointment, but often it is an informal designation based on family or another trusted relationship [9].

Researchers are required to comply with the requirements of their local ethics review board and any legal requirements in their jurisdictions. In some cases, this will require a legally appointed proxy for research enrollment [23], while in others, if a legally appointed proxy does not exist, one's spouse may act as a proxy for research enrollment, and if there is no spouse, then various family members may act as a proxy, in accordance with a statutory list [41].

Proxy decision-makers are ethically obligated to act in the interests of the person, and should not be influenced by a conflict of interest when making a decision whether to enroll a potential participant in research. Proxies are often instructed to use substitute judgment when making decisions for a person with dementia. Because notions of autonomous decision-making when there is no longer a competent self are fraught with difficulty [30], and other factors often influence proxies' decisions [15], it is suggested that "authenticity" is a better guide for proxy decision-making. Authenticity is the moral authority of substitute judgment, and refers to the congruence between a person's values and a decision [30]. So a more accurate guide for proxies would be to consider whether or not participating in a specific research project is in accordance with the person's values.

Picking one's own proxy is ethically preferable because it expresses a value held by the person, and relationships are important to who we are as people [31]. Research shows that the capacity to appoint a proxy may remain even after someone is incapable of providing informed consent for research. This may be possible even in the middle to late stages of dementia [31, 41].

Respecting Assent and Dissent

In dementia a person may lack the capacity for informed consent but retain ethically relevant capabilities such as communicating a preference, maintaining relationships, and exercising some level of decision-making [30]. These ethically relevant capabilities ought to be respected. The World Medical Association Declaration of Helsinki [45] requires assent from potential participants even when informed consent from the proxy has been obtained. Assent generally means agreement to participate without full understanding [41]. People living with dementia may be able to provide assent to participate in research. This may be a clear verbal agreement or inferred if the person cooperates. Depending on the severity of a participant's dementia, it may be appropriate to judge assent by behavior [9].

If a person with dementia declines to participate during any research-related procedure, their dissent should be respected [45]. Dissent may be expressed directly as a verbal refusal or indirectly as frustration, discomfort, distress, unhappiness, or passivity [41]. Because passing fatigue and irritation in people with dementia may also cause expressions of dissent that have nothing to do with the research, it may be appropriate to immediately terminate the research procedure, but return later and try again [41]. Reasonable guidelines to assess assent and dissent in participants with middle- to late-stage dementia in a residential care facility have been published by Slaughter et al. [41]. The guidelines assume willingness to go along with the research protocol is assent, and where a participant expresses dissent, the researcher will immediately stop the protocol and (1) create a more comfortable environment and try again, (2) if the participant still shows dissent, return on a different day, (3) on a different day, if the participant still shows dissent, the person is withdrawn from the study.

THE ROLE OF ASSESSMENT TOOLS FOR IDENTIFYING CAPACITY TO GIVE INFORMED CONSENT

A number of assessment tools have been developed to assist in assessing decision-making capacity of cognitively impaired adults. While clinical judgment is still considered the "gold standard" for capacity determination, it can be unreliable, and there have been few empirical studies of interrater reliability of clinical capacity assessment. Instruments to give a more objective indication of capacity have been developed to supplement clinical judgment, with limited success. Most of the instruments to assist in assessing decision-making capacity have not established reliability and validity to date, and so a score on one of these instruments cannot supplant clinical judgment, but rather is best used as a supplement. There is a need for further research on reliability and validity of these instruments. According to Moye et al. [34], those studies where clinician rating has been compared with assessment instruments have found that despite a high concordance, a considerable proportion of patients are assessed as having capacity by clinical judgment but without capacity by instrument assessment. Moye et al. [35] compared three instruments to assess capacity to consent to treatment in older adults. They examined four areas of decisional capacity that are important in legally competent decision-making. Understanding was the ability to understand diagnostic- and treatment-related information and to demonstrate the understanding. Appreciation was the ability to understand the significance of treatment information relative to the person's own situation. Reasoning was the process of comparing alternatives with an awareness of the consequences of the decision. And finally, expressing a choice was the ability to communicate a decision about treatment.

For understanding, most individuals with mild dementia performed in the unimpaired range for the instruments, but reservations were made about how much information should be disclosed, and in what way. Appreciation was operationalized quite differently on the three instruments—the Capacity to Consent to Treatment Instrument (CCTI) did differentiate between people living with dementia and controls, but the other two scales, the MacArthur Competence Assessment Tool—Treatment (MacCAT-T) and the Hopemont Capacity Assessment Interview (HCAI) did not differentiate in performance. Adults with dementia had more difficulty with the CCTI appreciation, which involved foresight. Reasoning was again operationalized quite differently in the three scales assessed; however, people living with dementia performed more poorly on all three scales. It was also found that when the decision is complicated, people with memory impairments are likely to be at a disadvantage because capacity requires comprehension, encoding, and retrieval over time while coping with interference caused by comparing a first treatment choice with a second treatment choice. Finally, Moye et al. [35] found no difference in choice capacity between those with dementia and controls, except for individuals at the most advanced stages of dementia. The authors concluded that most people with mild dementia can participate in

TABLE 24-1 Summary of Instruments to Assess Capacity to Give Informed Consent (After [34])

Scale	Author	Description
Aid to capacity evaluation (ACE)	Etchells et al. [20]	Assesses seven facets of capacity of actual medical decision: the medical problem, the treatment, alternatives to treatment, option of refusing treatment, accepting treatment, refusing treatment, ability to make a decision
Capacity assessment tool (CAT)	Carney et al. [10]	Evaluates capacity based on six abilities: communication, understanding choices, comprehension of risks and benefits, insight, decision/choice process, judgment
Capacity to consent to treatment instrument (CCTI)	Marson et al. [32]	Based on two clinical vignettes, a neoplasm condition and a cardiac condition. Assesses decisional abilities in four areas: understanding, appreciation, reasoning, expression of choice
Competency interview schedule (CIS)	Bean et al. [3]	Assesses consent capacity for electroconvulsive therapy
Decision assessment measure	Wong et al. [44]	Assesses understanding, reasoning, and communicating a choice using a vignette to assess recall, verbal recognition, and nonverbal recognition
Hopemont capacity assessment interview (HCAI)	Edelstein [18]	Uses two clinical vignettes to assess general concepts of choice, risk, and benefit
MacArthur competence assessment tool—treatment (MacCAT-T)	Grisso and Appelbaum [26]	Uses a semi-structured interview to assess understanding, appreciation, reasoning, and expression
Perceptions of disorder (POD)	Appelbaum and Grisso [1]	Uses the patient's actual disorder to assess understanding of disorder and treatment potential
Thinking rationally about treatment (TRAT)	Grisso and Appelbaum [25]	Assesses functions relevant to decision-making and problem-solving: information seeking; consideration of treatment consequences; simultaneous processing of information about two treatments; complex thinking; consequences; probabilistic thinking
Understanding treatment disclosures (UTD)	Grisso and Appelbaum [24]	Assesses phrased recall and recognition using three vignettes about schizophrenia, depression, and ischemic heart disease

decision-making as defined by legal standards for competency and they should be encouraged to do so—perhaps with some help to compensate for problems with verbal recall, complex simultaneous processing, and intentional planning.

When selecting a capacity assessment instrument for research on a particular population, researchers should choose an instrument developed for use with that population, where possible. Of the instruments listed in Table 24-1, for dementia participants, the CCTI could be a useful supplement to clinical judgment, and the HCAI for more impaired participants in residential care settings. Participants with moderate to severe dementia are most likely to have problems understanding diagnostic or treatment information, but research indicates that diagnosis alone does not predict capacity impairment completely [34].

Whether using an instrument or clinical judgment or both, information needs to be presented in a way that is appropriate to the participant's education level, and is as simple and organized as possible using visual cues.

DESIGNING APPROPRIATE PAIN RESEARCH TRIALS FOR PEOPLE LIVING WITH DEMENTIA

It is unethical to exclude people living with dementia from taking part in pain research. Furthermore, there is a need for pain research in people living with dementia, as pain is a common phenomenon among people living with dementia [21, 22]. However, people with advanced dementia receive less pain treatment than people who are more cognitively intact [27]. Exactly why this occurs is unknown: does dementia change the brain such that people in the advanced stages are no longer as sensitive to pain, or is pain underrecognized and undertreated in this vulnerable population, and how effective are analgesics in someone with dementia given placebo efficiency reductions? Research has shown that people with mild to moderate AD are at least as sensitive to pain as aged-matched controls [11]. Presently, due to a lack of research in this area vulnerable people living with dementia may be suffering.

Ethical Guidelines

Many guidelines for conducting research on people who cannot consent require the risks of participating in the study to be minimal. Minimal risk is usually defined as "the probability and magnitude of harm or discomfort anticipated in the research are not greater in and of themselves than those ordinarily encountered in daily life or during the performance of routine physical or psychological examinations or tests" [43, Section 46.102]. Further it has been argued that "minor increase over minimal risk" and even "greater than a minor increase over minimal" risk (p. 1285) may be permissible with appropriate safeguards, if the potential benefits of such research exceed the risk of harm [33].

The International Association of the Study of Pain has set out ethical guidelines for pain research in humans [28]. Pain researchers must adhere to all of the guidelines, some of which are especially relevant to research design for people living with dementia:

- People who are unable to consent should not be used for research unless they are essential for the goals of the proposed research. The inclusion of people living with dementia in pain research is essential if the goal of the research is to improve pain understanding, recognition, or treatment in people living with dementia. In such cases, consent must be obtained from proxies.
- The pain stimuli should never exceed the participant's tolerance limit. Pain to tolerance trials are not permitted in some jurisdictions with participants who cannot themselves provide informed consent.
- The participant should be able to escape or terminate a painful stimulus at will. In the advanced stages of dementia this requirement will be challenging to meet and careful study design will be required.

- The minimum intensity of noxious stimulus necessary to achieve the goals of the research should be established, and not exceeded.
- In all circumstances, including placebo-controlled trials, an effective, accepted method of pain relief must be provided on request. The availability of alternative pain relief and options other than participating in the research should be made clear in the information disclosed before gaining consent and beginning the study [28]. In people living with dementia who cannot request pain relief, the study design must include safeguards to ensure participants receive pain relief if required, which is an ethical conundrum addressed in this chapter.

The standard of care needs to be very high and multiple safeguards must be in place for pain research in dementia to be ethical. Standard practices and safeguards include the following:

- Full disclosure of associated risks and benefits and study procedures—full disclosure is mandatory.
- Approval from an ethics review board which adheres to the Declaration of Helsinki for Ethical Principles of Medical Research Involving Human Subjects is necessary [45].
- Additional codes and statements of ethical conduct enacted and enforced by local jurisdictions must also be respected.
- Involvement of a medical doctor in the design and oversight of the research.
- Encouragement of proxies to consult with the participant's own medical doctor should they have any concerns.
- Research participation and any findings for individual participants should be reported to their medical doctor where possible and appropriate.
- Inclusion of proxies and any organizations which oversee the rights of disabled people in the research process. This may require having the proxies, a member of an ethics review board, and a person who safeguards the right of disabled people undergo the research procedures before proceeding [33].
- Inclusion of proxies and medical assessment during procedures to confirm participants with dementia are coping with the demands of the research.
- Usual care for comorbid medical conditions should continue during the person's research participation.

Types of Pain Trials

For ethical considerations in designing appropriate pain research trials that include people living with dementia, it is helpful to distinguish between pain treatment research and experiential pain research trials. As proxies generally consider the possible benefits to the person with dementia before enrolling them in research, it is likely research for pain treatment in people living with dementia would be more widely consented to by proxies than experiential research designed only to develop understanding of the pain experiences of people living with dementia. This makes the design of and recruitment for experiential pain trials with people with dementia more complicated.

Experiential Pain Research Trials

Prima facie, the idea of purposely inflicting pain on someone with dementia, who cannot consent, for the purpose of studying the experience sounds like gross ethical misconduct of the highest level. Designed without proper care, oversight and concern for the interests of the participants, research of this nature is unethical, but that does not mean all experiential pain research is unethical, even in people who cannot consent. This is why study design is important.

Pain attracts attention, and it is a normal response to avoid pain. When people living with dementia do not understand or remember they are participating in a research trial they may try to avoid noxious stimuli. Dissent may therefore be a normal reaction to experiential pain research. Dissent from people living with dementia should be respected. Use of normal procedural states may therefore be necessary when designing ethical experiential pain research trials in people living with dementia. Pain is an everyday experience. Pain of varying degrees is also associated with many routine physical tests, and is a known side effect of many necessary medical interventions in older people. For example, annual flu vaccinations, surgery after a fracture and assisting someone with osteoarthritis out of bed in the morning are known to produce pain, but are all considered usual and ethical care. Potential exists for the use of these experiences and other usual care experiences in designing ethical experiential pain research trials. By using pain that exists in everyday life, pain research can be ethically designed even with people who cannot themselves consent.

Case Study Summarizing Ethical Issues and How They Were Addressed in a Pain Treatment, Randomized Placebo-Controlled Trial in People Living with Dementia

A trial of analgesic interventions in people with dementia living in residential care facilities, to monitor the effects on pain and consequent changes in the frequency of behavioral and psychological symptoms of dementia (BPSD), demonstrates how an ethical randomized placebo-controlled pain treatment trial can be designed.

Study Design

Participants with dementia living in residential care facilities, who were not taking regular analgesics, had BPSD and were assessed by the researchers as also having pain, were randomized to one of three treatments: paracetamol or paracetamol plus codeine or placebo. (Australian New Zealand Clinical Trials Registry number RN12611000062921; Alfred Hospital Ethics Approval Project Number 35/11)

Recruitment of Participants

Undertaking this study with participants with dementia was essential to the goals of the research. Potential participants were initially selected based on the presence of marked cognitive impairment as reported by care staff. Their treating medical doctors were informed about the trial and informed consent was gained from their proxies and the participants themselves where it was possible. After obtaining consent to participate in the trial residents were medically screened to ensure they were medically stable and the treatments were not contraindicated.

Eligible participants were medically stable, not taking regular analgesics, had BPSD, and were assessed by the researchers as having pain.

Benefits

Participating in this research offered the possibility of direct benefits to the participants and to the wider community. BPSD may be considered a sign of unmet need in a person with dementia, and can indicate distress. Unrelieved pain is very common in older people in residential care facilities [21, 22] and is considered to be a particularly important target within the context of ameliorating BPSD. There are few studies that have examined the relationship between pain and BPSD and the evidence for a causal association between these conditions was lacking.

Screening for pain before and during the trial was itself an improvement on usual care. Regular screening for pain in dementia was not standard care in the residential care facilities participating in the research. Randomizing a participant identified with pain and not receiving pain treatment to a placebo group was in line with their usual care and appropriate safeguards were put in place to provide rescue analgesic medication and interventions for BPSD for participants, if they were required. The proxies and the treating doctors were informed the participants had been assessed as having pain. Alternatives to participation in the research were detailed, and the contact details of the research medical doctors were provided in an information letter. The proxies and care staff were asked to telephone one of the research doctors if they thought a participant was experiencing side effects related to their involvement in the research.

Safety and Risk Management

The possible known side effects of paracetamol and codeine were clearly explained to the proxies, care staff, and the participants where possible. This information was detailed in an information letter.

An adverse event log was maintained for all participants during the trial and completed daily by a researcher. All noted adverse events were monitored and managed according to standard clinical best practice. Adverse events included pain requiring a rescue analgesic and BPSD requiring rescue management.

If a rescue analgesic medication was required during the course of the trial, it was not possible to use paracetamol. As a result, either ibuprofen or oxycodone was administered, at the discretion of the participant's treating doctor.

In the case of BPSD management, it was not possible to specify a particular rescue medication as the type of intervention required depends upon the type of BPSD evident. Instead, a rescue assessment of the problematic BPSD was undertaken by a psychogeriatrician on the research team, and an appropriate course of treatment was tailored to the individual participant's needs.

AN ALTERNATIVE RESEARCH STRATEGY: SINGLE CASE EXPERIMENTAL DESIGN

Single-case research designs may be an alternative to conducting RCTs, particularly for people living with dementia, when issues of diagnosis and between subject variability may make within group effects difficult to control, and resources for determining capacity for informed consent for a large sample of participants are limited. Single-case research designs have been used in applied settings to evaluate the impact of psychological interventions. The participant also serves as a control rather than using another group of individuals [29]. For single-case experimental designs, the participant is measured or observed repeatedly over a period of time before, during and after the intervention takes place. This type of design allows the researcher or clinician to observe the effect of a treatment over time and to determine how consistently the outcome being observed occurs. Single-case designs highlight individual differences in response to treatment effects, but they can also be an effective method of accumulating evidence about the impact of a treatment on individuals [16]. Statistical methods for analyzing interrupted time series such as ITSACORR or alternatives can then be used to assess the overall impact of the treatment on a group of individuals who have all participated in the same single-case design.

ADVANCE CARE PLANS AND THEIR ROLE IN RESEARCH

Often "gatekeepers" will prevent people living with dementia from participating in research, with good intentions, but arguably due to an "over protective" response. This exclusion may impact on a person's right to choose to be involved in research. Second, excluding most people living with dementia from participating in research, including those with moderate to severe dementia, can seriously curtail the development of knowledge through research that can potentially help the many people who develop dementia. ACPs may be a way to help people living with dementia to maintain their rights to be involved in research, and continue to contribute to society once their cognitive functioning has declined.

ACP is an ongoing discussion between a person and their significant others, including health-care professionals, and can guide the future health and social care of the person. The planning process may help facilitate autonomous decision-making for a person with dementia, and can assist proxy decision-makers and health professionals to make decisions that accord with the person's values and stated preferences at a time when the person no longer has capacity to make such decisions. A person's preferred process for health and social care decision-making might also be ascertained in ACP [4] and this may include the formal appointment of a proxy decision-maker and formal documentation of health- and social care preferences.

Research Participation and ACP

There is some recognition of the potential value of ACP in recruiting people living with dementia as research participants [37], and of the likely willingness of people living with dementia to participate in (pharmacological) intervention studies [12]. However, a recent systematic review of ACP for people living with dementia cautioned that it may be hasty to draw conclusions about the "feasibility and acceptability" of ACPs without further evidence [14]. The implementation of ACP for people living with dementia also held "significant challenges" according to a comprehensive qualitative study, the findings of which may also have implications for recruiting people living with dementia for future research participation [39].

Applicability of ACP to Research Participation

Although an ACP may include a person's preferences about their future participation in research, this is not standard practice and evidence suggests it is rare [33, 40]. In fact, few studies consider the subject at all [6, 7, 17, 23, 42].

It is possible that an increasing proportion of people living with early dementia in the community may be introduced to and choose to participate in ACP, although the question of whether it is ethical and justified to influence people living with dementia to compose an ACP has been raised for further consideration [13]. In the early dementia process, people will most likely retain their capacity to indicate preferences about care, and possibly about their interest and willingness to participate in research. Crucially, an early diagnosis of dementia, where it is determined that the person still has capacity, is usually required to make formal legal arrangements about future decision-making, such as appointment of a proxy decision-maker and completion of other forms of advance directives such as a limitation or refusal of medical treatment.

We need to know more about the ethics of encouraging people living with dementia to engage with the ACP process, and to learn more about how best to identify when and how is the most ethical way of engaging people living with dementia and their families in ACP, if ACP is to become a more common way of supporting people to participate in research.

Adults living in the community who currently have legal capacity to make decisions and who do not have a dementia diagnosis may increasingly, through increased exposure to people and families living with dementia in the community, and in anticipation of the possibility of a dementia diagnosis, choose to appoint and instruct a future proxy decision-maker. Aware of their preferences, the proxy decision-maker could consent on their behalf to research participation. Currently, in some legal jurisdictions, a person who is a formally appointed proxy decision-maker may already be able to make such a decision about participation in research, although this aspect of decision-making remains largely unexplored (ironically) in research terms, and remains ethically contentious [15].

CONCLUSION

To avoid the unethical exclusion of people with dementia from participating in research, proxies, the general community, and people living with dementia require better understanding of the risks and benefits associated with participating in research. Health professionals and other gatekeepers, including ethics review boards, must be aware of their abilities to promote ethical research and advance dementia care. Conducting pain research with people living with dementia is necessary if we are to improve dementia care, and ethical pain research trials can be designed.

In the absence of accurate or efficient "gold-standard" measures of capacity to consent to research, clinical judgment continues to be the most common method of introducing participants with dementia into research studies, although there are increasing efforts to incorporate assessment tools into the process. Currently, ethics review boards and researchers continue to set their own criteria for best practice and may be unwittingly perpetuating the unethical exclusion of a group of people. The development of "gold standard" measures of capacity to consent to research, and ACPs may be strategies that can assist the promotion of ethical dementia research in the future.

REFERENCES

1. Appelbaum A, Grisso T. Manual for preceptions of disorder. Worcester, MA: University of Massachussetts Medical School; 1992.
2. Bartlam B, Lally F, Crome P. The PREDICT study: increasing the participation of the elderly in clinical trials. The opinions of patients and carers. Lay report. The PREDICT study: increasing the participation of the elderly in clinical trials. The opinions of patients and carers. Lay report. Staffordshire: Keele University; 2010.

3. Bean G, Nishisato S, Rector NA, Glancy G. The assessment of competence to make a treatment decision: an empirical approach. Can J Psychiat 1996;41:85–92.
4. Berger JT. What about process? Limitations in advance directives, care planning, and noncapacitated decision making. Am J Bioethics 2010;10:33–4.
5. Black BS, Kass NE, Fogarty LA, Rabins PV. Informed consent for dementia research: the study enrollment encounter. IRB 2007;29:7–14.
6. Bravo G, Arcand M, Blanchette D, Boire-Lavigne AM, Dubois MF, Guay M, Hottin P, Lane J, Lauzon J, Bellemare S. Promoting advance planning for health care and research among older adults: a randomized controlled trial. BMC Med Ethics 2012;13:1.
7. Bravo G, Dubois MF, Cohen C, Wildeman S, Graham J, Painter K, Bellemare S. Are Canadians providing advance directives about health care and research participation in the event of decisional incapacity? Can J Psychiatry 2011;56:209–18.
8. Bravo G, Kim SY, Dubois MF, Cohen CA, Wildeman SM, Graham JE. Surrogate consent for dementia research: factors influencing five stakeholder groups from the SCORES study. IRB 2013;35:1–11.
9. Cacchione PZ. People with dementia: capacity to consent to research pariticipation. Clin Nurs Res 2011;20:223–7.
10. Carney MT, Neugroschl J, Morrison RS, Marin D, Siu AL. The development and piloting of a capacity assessment tool. J Clin Ethics 2001;12:17–23.
11. Cole LJ, Farrell MJ, Duff EP, Barber JB, Egan GF, Gibson SJ. Pain sensitivity and fMRI pain-related brain activity in Alzheimer's disease. Brain 2006;129:2957–65.
12. Cooper C, Ketley D, Livingston G. Systematic review and meta-analysis to estimate potential recruitment to dementia intervention studies. Int J Geriatr Psychiatry 2014;29:515–25.
13. de Boer ME, Dröes R-M, Jonker C, Eefsting JA, Hertogh CMPM. Thoughts on the future: the perspectives of elderly people with early-stage Alzheimer's disease and the implications for advance care planning. AJOB Prim Res 2012;3:14–22.
14. Dening KH, Jones L, Sampson EL. Advance care planning for people with dementia: a review. Int Psychogeriatr 2011;23:1535–51.
15. Dowson L, Doyle C, Rayner V. Scoping the ethics of dementia research within an Australian human research context. J Law Med 2013;21:210–6.
16. Doyle C, Zapparoni T, O'Connor D, Runci S. Efficacy of psychosocial treatments for noisemaking associated with severe dementia. Int Psychogeriatr 1997;9:405–22.
17. Dubois MF, Bravo G, Graham J, Wildeman S, Cohen C, Painter K, Bellemare S. Comfort with proxy consent to research involving decisionally impaired older adults: do type of proxy and risk-benefit profile matter? Int Psychogeriatr 2011;23:1479–88.
18. Edelstein B. Hopemont capacity assessment interview manual and scoring guide. Morgantown, WV: West Virginia University; 1999.
19. Edwards SJL, Lilford RJ, Hewison J. The ethics of randomised controlled trials from the perspectives of patients, the public and health care professionals. Br Med J 1998;317:1209–12.
20. Etchells E, Darzins P, Silberfeld M, Singer PA, McKenny J, Nagle G, Katz M, Guyatt GH, Molloy DW, Strang D. Assessment of patient capacity to consent to treatment. J Gen Int Med 1999;14:27–34.
21. Ferrell BA, Ferrell BR, Osterweil D. Pain in the nursing home. J Am Geriatr Soc 1990;39:64–73.
22. Ferrell BA, Ferrell BR, Rivera L. Pain in cognitively impaired nursing home residents. J Pain Symptom Manag 1995;10:591–8.
23. Galeotti F, Vanacore N, Gainotti S, Izzicupo F, Menniti-Ippolito F, Petrini C, Chiarotti F, Chattat R, Raschetti R, AdCare Study Group. How legislation on decisional capacity can negatively affect the feasibility of clinical trials in patients with dementia. Drugs Aging 2012;29:607–14.
24. Grisso T, Appelbaum P. Manual for understanding treatment disclosures. Worcester, MA: University of Massachussetts Medical School; 1992.
25. Grisso T, Appelbaum P. Manual for thinking rationally about treatment. Worcester MA: University of Massachussetts Medical School; 1993.
26. Grisso T, Appelbaum P. Assessing competence to consent to treatment: a guide for physicians and other health professionals. New York: Oxford University Press; 1998.
27. Horgas AL, Tsai P-F. Analgesic drug prescription and use in cognitively impaired nursing home residents. Nurs Res 1998;47:235–42.
28. International Association of the Study of Pain. Ethical guidance for pain research in humans, Vol. 2014. Seattle: International Association of the Study of Pain; 2014.

29. Kazdin AE. Single-case research designs; methods for clinical and applied settings. Oxford: Oxford University Press; 2011.
30. Kim SY. The ethics of informed consent in Alzheimer disease research. Nat Rev Neurol 2011;7:410–4.
31. Kim SY, Karlawish JH, Kim HM, Wall IF, Bozoki AC, Appelbaum PS. Preservation of the capacity to appoint a proxy decision maker: implications for dementia research. Arch Gen Psychiatry 2011;68:214–20.
32. Marson DC, Ingram KK, Cody HA, Harrell LE. Assessing the competency of patients with Alzheimer's disease under different legal standards. A prototype instrument. Arch Neurol 1995;52:949–54.
33. Monroe TB, Herr KA, Mion LC, Cowan RL. Ethical and legal issues in pain research in cognitively impaired older adults. Int J Nurs Stud 2013;50:1283–7.
34. Moye J, Gurrera RJ, Marel MJ, Edelstein B, O'Connell C. Empirical advances in the assessment of the capacity to consent to medical treatment; clinical implications and research needs. Clin Psychol Rev 2006;26:1054–77.
35. Moye J, Karel MJ, Azar AR, Gurrera RJ. Capacity to consent to treatment: empirical comparison of three instruments in older adults with and without dementia. Gerontologist 2004;44:166–75.
36. Murray A. The mental capacity act and dementia research. Nurs Older People 2013;25:14–20.
37. Nuffield Council on Bioethics. Dementia: ethical issues. In: Nuffield Council on Bioethics, editor. Dementia: ethical issues. London: Nuffield Council on Bioethics; 2009.
38. Office of the Public Advocate. Mental Incapacity is decision specific. In: Office of the Public Advocate editor. Mental incapacity is decision specific, Vol. 2014. Office of the Public Advocate; 2014.
39. Robinson L, Dickinson C, Bamford C, Clark A, Hughes J, Exley C. A qualitative study: professionals' experiences of advance care planning in dementia and palliative care, 'a good idea in theory but . . .'. Palliat Med 2013;27:401–8.
40. Robinson L, Dickinson C, Rousseau N, Beyer F, Clark A, Hughes J, Howel D, Exley C. A systematic review of the effectiveness of advance care planning interventions for people with cognitive impairment and dementia. Age Ageing 2012;41:263–9.
41. Slaughter S, Cole D, Jennings E, Reimer MA. Consent and assent to participate in research from people with dementia. Nurs Ethics 2007;14:27–40.
42. Stocking CB, Hougham GW, Danner DD, Patterson MB, Whitehouse PJ, Sachs GA. Empirical assessment of a research advance directive for persons with dementia and their proxies. J Am Geriatr Soc 2007;55:1609–12.
43. US Department of Health and Human Services. Code of Federal Regulations Title 45: Public welfare. Part 46: protection of human subjects. In: Department of Health and Human Services, editor. Code of Federal Regulations Title 45 Public Welfare Part 46 Protection of Human Subjects. Washington, DC: US Department of Health and Human Services, 2005.
44. Wong JG, Clare ICH, Holland AJ, Watson PC, Gunn M. The capacity of people with a 'mental disability' to make a health care decision. Psychol Med 2000;30:295–306.
45. World Medical Association Declaration of Helsinki. Ethical principles of medical research involving human subjects. Ethical principles of medical research involving human subjects. Ferney-Voltaire: WMA General Assembly; 2008.

CHAPTER 25

Pain in Dementia: Cross-Cultural Considerations

Wilco P. Achterberg and Marjolein Gysels

Dementia has an enormous influence on the processing, assessment, and management of pain. Next to the biological problem due to changes in brain pathology affecting the pain matrix in dementia, cultural aspects of the person in pain play a role. Individuals with dementia and pain have different cultural backgrounds. Factors influencing the meaning and experience of both conditions in these cultural groups also influence the individual with pain and dementia. Next to the cultural context of the individual in pain, also the culture of those detecting and managing the pain influence the course of pain of the individual. Caregivers, nurses, family members, physicians, and researchers are members of social, cultural, and professional groups as well as of societies with different health-care systems.

Therefore, this chapter will review cultural differences in barriers and promoters for pain assessment, management, and research in patients with dementia.

APPROACHES TO CULTURE

The focus on culture has received modest attention due to the complexity of the concept of culture. Without taking account of the theoretical knowledge on culture, there is the risk that research reaches results which are at best simplistic and at worst careless or harmful to the people in question. Unfortunately, medical curricula in general lack sufficient input from other sciences, such as (medical) anthropology, making sound transdisciplinary approaches to the understanding of diseases difficult.

Studies inquiring about differences between populations or groups often use categories such as ethnicity and race, the latter especially in the USA. Race was used for the biological classification of people but is now viewed with apprehension due to its doubtful assumptions and questionable consequences. Intra-racial genetic variation is larger than between races, an argument which renders it into a useless concept. Race is not so much a natural category but rather a social construction [34]. Ethnicity is another concept which is frequently confused with cultural variation. It refers to the heritage that people share in a particular society, based on a common language or religion and leading to a sense of identity or group awareness [62]. People with the same ethnicity can however differ vastly in terms of worldview and values, and these are highly variable according to changing circumstances

[12]. In quantitative analyses ethnicity is often used as a demographic variable for the prediction of specific behavioral characteristics. However, culture is infinitely more complex. It occupied anthropologists for decades to develop different models.

Culture is defined by Holland and Quinn [22] as "presupposed, taken-for-granted models of the world, that are widely shared (although not necessarily to the exclusion of other, alternative models) by the members of a society, and that play an enormous role in their understanding of that world and their behavior in it." Cultural models are in other words systems of shared ideas, and rules and meanings, that underlie and are expressed in the ways that people live [30]. These shared meanings are learned and sustained through shared practice. They are internalized as they are learned through socialization and therefore underlie and guide people's actions. But what is important here is that we do not simply act routinely in everyday life, choosing between appropriate alternatives, but attach meaning to social interactions and interpret one another. Cultural meaning is negotiated, questioned, or confirmed in social processes, and it is shaped by specific circumstances and histories [15]. Understanding prevailing attitudes about illness, dying, and care and how that is distributed across time and place is an interpretive task.

CULTURE AND PAIN

There are many aspects of pain that are influenced by culture, and that have been described in literature. These are cultural differences in sources of pain, in pain experience, in the response to pain, and in pain management.

Differences in Sources of Pain

Sources of pain are not constant in different ethnic groups, because the distribution of painful conditions is variable. We will discuss a few examples:

- Insufficient vitamin D levels are associated with more pain, through various mechanisms (osteoporosis, muscle ache). Older people with a dark skin have a higher prevalence of vitamin D deficiency (especially those residing in long term care), because they need more sun exposure to produce vitamin D [52].
- Neuropathic pain, caused by diabetes mellitus, is an important source of pain in older people. Because there are huge differences in the prevalence of diabetes in different ethnic groups, this will lead to differences in prevalence and type of pain. For instance in the Amsterdam population, Turkish (5.6%) and Moroccan (8.0%) persons have a much higher prevalence of diabetes mellitus, compared to Dutch individuals (3.1%), and these differences are even larger after adjustment for age [58].
- Several ethnic groups from the Indian subcontinent (Gujarati, Punjabi, Bangladeshi, and Pakistani) have been shown to have a 50% higher prevalence of coronary heart disease than the autochthone English individuals [38].
- Osteoarthritis, one of the most important sources of pain in an aging population, is more prevalent in Europe than in Africa, and hip osteoarthritis more prevalent in Europe than in Asia [60].

The a priori chance of having a certain type of pain (neuropathic or nociceptive), caused by a certain disease (polyneuropathy, osteoarthritis, osteoporosis), is different according to the ethnic/racial background. Therefore, when assessing pain in a patient with dementia, these differences in the epidemiology of diseases should be taken into account. It is also apparent, that epidemiological studies have predominantly focused on ethnic differences, without taking other cultural aspects into account.

Differences in Pain Experience: Socio Cultural Factors

The International Association for the Study of Pain defines pain as "an unpleasant sensory and emotional experience associated with actual or potential tissue damage, or described in term of such damage" [Bonica JJ. The need of a taxonomy. Pain. 1979 Jun;6(3):247-8.]. Meaning and expression of pain may vary enormously in different cultures. In fact, "unpleasant experience" may well possess a completely different meaning in another culture.

In Europe, the word pain is derived from the Latin "poena," which means punishment. In Japan pain is called "itami," which means "extraordinary state of something," thus without the meaning of punishment. The cultural, religious, and historically grown philosophy of empathy and assimilation with nature has influenced this experience, and thereby influenced the expectations for its management. Pain is not necessarily something to overcome in Japan [21].

Also in Thailand pain experience and management expectations are heavily influenced by cultural and religious circumstance. For many Thai, influenced by Buddhism, doing good deeds is an important part of pain management [41].

Also the interpretation on how unpleasant pain is can be cultural different. Even when the rating of the intensity of pain is the same, African Americans rate the pain as more unpleasant than American Whites [44]. Searching the literature for empirical studies on racial and ethnic disparities in pain experience, it is apparent that it is mainly focused on differences between different groups in the USA, and that studies from other parts of the world are underrepresented.

Differences in Pain Response

There is enormous variability within individuals in the experience of pain, and some of these differences can be explained by ethnicity or racial differences. Experimental settings have the unique opportunity, to have a closer look at those differences. Rahim-Williams performed a systematic review of studies using experimental pain stimuli, and found 26 articles studying ethnic group differences [53]. Most (15) studies compared African Americans with non-Hispanic Whites, although also Asian, Alaskan Indians, and European population differences have been studied. The most prominent finding was that African Americans reported stronger perceptual responses to painful stimuli (the subjective dimension) and demonstrated a lower pain tolerance (the behavioral dimension). This was true for all kind of painful stimuli (ischemic, pressure, heat/cold). The reasons for this difference are multifactorial, and are thought to be a combination of several biological, psychological, and social factors. In Table 25-1, several factors that play a role in these cultural differences in pain response are listed [53].

Epidemiological research on different reactions to pain and biopsychosocial consequences of pain as mediated by culture has—just as the experimental studies—predominantly focused on differences between American white population and Afro Americans [44]. The latter group, besides having higher sensitivity to pain, suffers from more extensive physical limitations as a result of pain, especially greater limitations in activities and functional

TABLE 25-1 Factors Influencing Ethnic Group Differences in Pain Sensitivity [54]

Social cultural factors influencing pain sensitivity
    Beliefs
    Attitudes
    Language
    Expressiveness
    Gender/sex
    Medication practices and beliefs
    Spirituality
    Social roles and expectations
    Cultural group membership
    Socialization of pain expression
    Perceived discrimination
    Socio economic status
    Acculturation
    Age
    Environmental factors
Psychological factors influencing pain sensitivity
    Pain-coping strategies
    Mood
    Hypervigilance
Biological factors
    Alterations endogenous pain modulation
    Hormonal differences
    Genetic factors

capacities, anxiety, fear, and helplessness. Individuals from ethnic minority groups in general more often suffer more from mood disorders caused by pain and have a higher likelihood of experiencing a higher burden and a diminished quality of life as a result of (chronic) pain. Remarkably, although minority groups generally have a higher sensitivity to pain and more extensive burden, they tend to underreport their pain. Several factors may contribute to this like the felt status difference between physician and patient or cultural pressure to react "stoic" to pain. The way we talk about pain, the way we act when in pain: it is all part of our upbringing, and the implicit and explicit values of our society. Bearing your pain in dignity and silence may be one of those values, leading to the inclination to underreport pain [44].

Differences in Pain Management

For many years, there have been consistent reports of inadequate pain management in almost all populations. This has led to several initiatives from both professional organizations and politics in different countries to improve this situation. Examples are "The European Year against Pain" and "Decade of Pain Control and Research"[1]. Within the people with

---

[1] http://www.efic.org/index.asp?sub=F8AMLHLAP9216P http://lifeinpain.org/node/141

pain, several subgroups, including racial/ethnic minorities, have even a much higher prevalence of inadequate pain management [44]. What are the reasons for this inequity?

When pain ratings are compared between physicians and patients, physician ratings typically underestimate the individual report. This underestimation is however much larger for minorities like African Americans as patients, compared to non-African Americans. This is reflected in the prescription of analgesics, with Hispanic and African Americans being two to three times as likely as Whites not receiving any pain medication [57]. Interestingly, this difference is not accounted for by pain severity or other patient characteristics. Although later studies suggest the difference in analgesic prescription has become smaller, they do seem to persist in the prescription of opioids, with African American, Latino, and Asian Americans receiving less opioid prescriptions and lower opioid dosages. This has been found in perioperative pain, chronic nonmalignant pain and cancer pain, and both in children and adults [44].

Negative attitudes of physicians toward racial/ethnic minorities and prejudicial racial stereotyping probably play an important role in the explanation of the poorer pain management in ethnic minorities. This is a process that is often not intentional or conscious (based on explicit values) but rather associative and automatic (based on implicit values) [44].

Limited cultural competence of health-care workers has been suggested as an additional factor in sustaining the inequities in pain management in ethnic minorities. "Care delivery in a manner that is respectful of and sensitive to the patients (cultural) background and health beliefs" is the definition of cultural competence. It is needless to say that this has unfortunately not been the focus of medical schools, at least not in the past [6].

CULTURE AND DEMENTIA

If one wants to understand the cultural aspects of pain in dementia, it is necessary to introduce the cultural aspects of dementia and dementia care. Differences have been noted between populations in relation to perceptions, responses, and practices toward dementia. Most of this knowledge has been generated by studies that applied a focus on ethnicity, and despite the criticisms the concept of ethnicity has received, it has nevertheless produced some useful insights. This showed the specific meanings attributed to dementia by different ethnic groups, depending on whether the condition is understood as part of normal aging or whether it is seen as a mental illness and carrying stigma [20]. Diverse ways of caring for people with dementia have been identified in different ethnic minority groups. The study by Adamson and Donovan, for example, showed different reasons for considering caregiving as a valued and self-evident practice in two ethnic groups [1]. Among the South Asian sample this was related to cultural and religious views while for the African and Caribbean participants this was related to expectations for caregiving within the family and determined by more secular considerations. Such findings can point toward disparities between different populations regarding the estimated need for services. The finding that caregiving is often taken for granted by members of the extended family in ethnic minority groups does not mean that they prefer to "look after their own" and do not need support. Ethnic groups with strong filial piety (the feeling of obligation to provide care for older family members) may not be inclined to look for formal care options or they may even not be aware about services despite having high needs for support with caregiving [1].

These findings documenting differences between racial or ethnic groups and the resulting disparities regarding care reinforce the view of culture as ethnicity. Ethnicity is different from race (as explained above). Differences in ideas about dementia, perceptions regarding pain, and care needs are much more complex than just coinciding with different groups of people.

The idea of "cultural competence" in educational programs has been a response to the health professionals' wish to provide appropriate care, which aims at taking "cultural" differences into account [5]. Cultural competence refers to groups of people with homogeneous characteristics and clearly distinguishable boundaries. Such an approach provides clinicians with a well-delineated body of knowledge which they are required to become competent in. General knowledge about differences in understandings or care practices is undoubtedly useful. However, the attempt to classify ethnic beliefs and practices under the label of "culture"—also referred to as the "fact file" or "cookbook" approach—risks reinforcing stereotypes it purports to overcome [17, 25]. This entails the risk of reifying culture, and concretizing "it" as a thing whereby it is attributed an existence as an entity (for example, that it is a group that someone can belong to) or as a causal agent, (where a certain culture leads its members to undertake specific actions) which it cannot [51].

That inquiry into cultural issues has not been further developed in dementia research is related to the view that people with dementia were considered incapable of contributing to research [7], and only recently their views are elicited in research to get insight into their experiences of the illness, or their symptoms, such as pain to inform about their care needs [2]. Research has almost exclusively attended to what dementia is and how it needs to be perceived, rather than its lived experience. Those who typically raise their voice have middle-class backgrounds, are well educated, with early-stage dementia, have a supportive family, and have strong views about the way people with dementia are represented. Less is known about people from other backgrounds, such as ethnic minorities.

THE CULTURAL DIFFERENCES IN CARE SETTINGS

In the trajectory of dementia, the individual and his family gradually is involved with many different health-care workers, in many settings. Because of the complexity of the disease, pain is seldom the first priority.

Usually, the first complaints of cognitive (memory) impairment are discussed in primary care, with the family physician. Although, remarkably, often patients with minimal cognitive impairment or early stage dementia do not particularly complain of memory deficits, close family and friends are often very concerned of this deficit. Priorities are mostly on diagnosis, trials of treatment, for instance with acetylcholine inhibitors and getting help and home care in place. In the course of dementia a huge amount of disabling physical, behavioral, and psychiatric problems arise, and in many cases some form of long-term care is eventually needed. In this process, several visits to the emergency room usually take place, for instance, for the results of a fall like hip or wrist fracture. In the end, the patient is in need of palliative care.

What are some characteristics of these care settings that influence pain management in dementia?

Home/Community Care: "I Asked Him Didn't I?"

Most people with dementia live at home and their family are providing most of their care [46]. The experiences and burden of care by informal carers are well explored in the literature. Disabling pain and other symptoms have a major impact on independence and people's quality of life [56]. Where specialist palliative programs are less common in home settings, symptoms and pain are not recognized and are left untreated [54]. Home care traditionally has low status and the care workers who are employed in home care are generally not well trained, have little supervision, receive low wages, and get little recognition for their work. In general, the assessment of pain is at the most only asking the patient "are you in pain?" In people with dementia, this is certainly not adequate.

As home care workers are increasingly caring for the oldest old, their work is changing from providing domestic help to more personal care and specialized nursing activities [8]. The close contact of these frontline workers with people with dementia and their informal carers as well as families requires additional training and supervision. As they have to interact with people who have communication problems and cognitive impairment they need to be aware of ways of interpreting behavior as a mode of expression. These care workers could fulfill a key role in the identification, assessment, and management of symptoms that compromise patients' daily quality of life. Research and policy have so far paid little attention to this group of care workers [26]. The challenges and dynamics of this workforce in relation to their supervisors, the people they care for and the circumstances in which they work need to be studied in order to change the culture of home care for older people with dementia and more adequately address complex problems such as pain in dementia.

As a response to the increasing care needs which are presented by aging societies, many governments are restructuring their care systems by shifting the emphasis away from care in institutional settings toward home-based services [11]. Home is often also the preferred place of care and death for most people [16, 63]. However, a European study showed that a home death for people with dementia only occurred in a minority of cases (ranging from 3.3% in Wales to 16.4% in Belgium) [23]. Although home as the place to receive care at the end of life was still uncertain in Belgium, continued primary care and paid home care or specialist palliative home care were responsible for preventing transitions to the hospital [45, 54]. Home death is more common in the USA [54], where hospice programs are operating in the community. Specialist palliative care support was shown to enhance the chances of dying in a home environment [54]. In Germany, 42% of patients with dementia died at home. Although, it was the preferred place of death by both patients and family, a high symptom burden was reported in the last 2 days of life. Family members were generally more satisfied with the care provided at home, than in the hospital or nursing home [50].

Good home health care at the end of life in dementia requires improving informational strategies, care organization, symptom monitoring and treatment, and support for surviving relatives [14].

Acute Care: "No Time to Waste"

The emergency hospital setting is a very confusing place for a person with dementia. There are a lot of sounds, people walking in and out, and generally staff is focused on getting the right diagnosis as soon as possible, and making decisions on when and how and where to give curative treatment. Staff is generally extensively trained in traumatology, acute internal medicine, stroke management, with little or no training in geriatrics or psychiatry. In this setting, staff is not likely to pick up signals, such as agitated behavior or facial expressions of pain in dementia. This is how we can explain that people with dementia and a hip fracture receive less opioids before and after their surgery [43].

Long-Term Care: "We Are So Busy"

People with dementia are most likely to need institutional care at one point [27]. People with dementia impose a greater burden of care than people with somatic conditions [18, 61]. In the course of their illness, a change in their situation or a crisis will trigger their admission to a nursing home, although this is not always the wish of people with a diagnosis of dementia or the people caring for them [50]. It is estimated that about one third of people with dementia live in long-term care settings and this number increases with age [33].

Several studies have shown poor conditions of living and working in long-term care institutions and have provoked a general sense of indignation. As a response, an alternative model of care was developed by Kitwood [31, 32] with an emphasis on personhood, which is currently promoted as the ideal of care. Although, there is greater awareness about the conditions in long-term care and much has been done to raise the standards of care, there are important problems which remain unchanged. For example, the difficult working conditions of care workers such as the nurses and care assistants in institutions who provide the hands-on work have stayed the same [4]. These people work long shifts and have heavy workloads. They attend to difficult physical and emotional needs of patients which are worsened and less well perceived by communicative and behavioral problems. Care workers often have minimal training and earn very little money. Their working conditions reflect the carers' low societal status; they are often female migrant workers who take on these jobs because of necessity rather than of positive choice [37]. Therefore, they experience high levels of stress and little satisfaction or pride in their work which leads to desensitization and routinization. This has consequences for the quality of care that is available and leads to shortages in the workforce, low motivation, and high levels of burnout and turnover [3]. This is not a climate which stimulates attention for the individual. The emphasis is rather on physical care and on completing the range of tasks to meet people's most basic needs. This task-directed culture or what was called bed and body care [19], prevents an empathic approach which is required to sense discomfort or suffering of people who have communication problems [13]. The literature provides accounts of care workers who react in negative ways to people who do not conform to socially expected norms in care facilities [28]. In this way the underlying reasons for challenging behavior go unnoticed; pain and its causes are therefore missed and remain untreated [54].

Hospice Care: "Cancer is Our Thing"

A study investigated the place of death of people aged 65 and older, whose underlying cause of death was a dementia-related disease by using death certificates in five different countries, Belgium, the Netherlands, England, Scotland, and Wales [24]. The authors found that when standardized for age and sex and compared with deaths from cancer and other major diseases, deaths from dementia were less likely to occur at home, in a hospital, or (in England, Wales, and the Netherlands) in a hospice and more likely to take place in a nursing home. Nowhere did the number of deaths in a palliative care institution (hospices in England and Wales and mainly hospices in the Netherlands) exceed 1% [24]. Hospice is still the place where people with advanced malignant disease are cared for at the end of their lives. Admission of people with dementia to inpatient hospice facilities is rare, although a UK study found that this has recently slightly increased. An underlying cause of death of cancer and being married were strongly associated with this increase [55]. These differences are influenced by the way health services are organized in different countries. For example, the higher chance of nursing home death rather than hospital death in the Netherlands can be explained by the availability of nursing home beds and specialist care professionals. But also a myriad of other factors play a role, such as the low number of people with dementia who are referred to hospices in the UK, Scotland, and Wales, while these are the places where most of specialist end of life care is provided to people. Also, beside the low availability of nursing home beds, negative attitudes toward nursing homes as a place of care at the end of life may contribute to the higher likelihood of patients dying at home in Belgium.

That people with dementia are generally not cared for in hospice may be because they are not perceived to be terminally ill. However, although life expectancy is known to be longer for people with dementia than for people with cancer, this has shown to be much shorter at older ages (90 or older) [64]. Other studies found even shorter survival times in care home populations [39, 40]. Besides, people with dementia suffer from a comparable symptom load as patients with advanced cancer such as pain as well as dyspnea and have similar care needs [36]. There is growing awareness that the expertise regarding management of pain and other symptoms as well as the ethos of care which has developed in the hospice movement can also benefit those patients who have nonmalignant diagnoses, including people with dementia [59]. In turn, this can expand the knowledge base of palliation with dementia-specific strategies.

CULTURE AND PAIN ASSESSMENT INSTRUMENTS

Accurate assessment of pain and the (positive) impact as well as potential adverse effects of analgesic medications are major prerequisites for adequate pain management. Assessment of pain in people with dementia is particularly challenging due to the loss of communication ability inherent in the symptomology of the condition, which limits the subjective reporting of pain that would normally be expected with cognitively healthy adults (see also Chapters 9 and 10 on assessment of pain in dementia).

Self-Report Instruments

In the earlier stages of dementia, when cognitive impairment is limited and communication ability is mostly intact, self-report of pain is usually possible. There are several self-report scales, among which the visual analog scale (VAS), the numerical rating scale (NRS), and the faces pain scale (FPS) are the most frequently used. These instruments have a long history, and are usually available in many languages with an adequate global distribution.

Culture-related biases may be present in these instruments, derived from the culture-specific issues in the countries where they were developed. Therefore, before studies adopt such instruments, they tend to apply rigorous protocols of translation, back translation and consensus. However, such literal translations can be meaningless and still not grasp the cultural meanings attributed to specific terms. Interpretation and the involvement of people of the target culture in the testing of outcome measures are needed to ascertain cultural equivalence. Biases can be introduced on many levels such as gender, age, ethnicity of both the respondents as the interviewers, but also other factors are at play, such as low literacy levels, perceptions of appropriateness of measures (the preference of face-to-face communication whereas telephone interviewing may be experienced as insulting) or communication styles (with variations in readiness to disclose emotions and social desirability).

Specific Dementia Behavioral Assessment Instruments

Where self-report is not possible, observation and detection of pain-related behavior is a valuable approach to identify pain in dementia. A common conclusion of the current body of literature is that there is a number of promising pain assessment tools available but that most these require further validation in people with dementia and assessment of their utility in clinical settings (see also Chapter 10).

If we look at the roughly 35 observational pain instruments that have been developed, it is clear that there is—next to the observed flaws in psychometric evaluations—a major problem regarding global coverage. English is the dominant language, and most instruments have been developed in the USA or Europe. Also evaluation studies on feasibility and psychometric properties have almost exclusively been performed in the western affluent societies by White western researchers. In addition to that, most of these studies have used selected populations that can be described as White and western (mainly female) dementia patients. Therefore, it is very uncertain that the typical cultural issues in pain experience and expression that are described in this chapter are sufficiently addressed in these instruments.

Availability and Feasibility of Behavioral Assessment Instruments

Although the behavioral assessment instruments are available for many years now, implementation in clinical practice has proven to be very poor. Even in the countries where they have been developed, everyday use in acute, community, long-term, and palliative care is almost nonexisting. Although dissemination efforts have been taken (for instance City of Hope Pain & Palliative Care Resource Center: http://prc.coh.org/pain_assessment.asp), availability of observational pain scales for patients with dementia and communication problems in other languages than English is poor. If there are instruments available in the right language, hospitals, nursing homes, and primary caregivers seldom use them.

It has long been established that inaccurate beliefs, poor knowledge, and inadequate training of staff responsible for management in long-term care are important barriers for high quality care. Even experienced staff would still be expected to benefit from specific education and training in pain assessment and management. This chapter shows that cultural aspects should also be addressed in this education and training.

Next to training recommendations, it is of the utmost importance that a feasible and sound observational instrument becomes available for many languages. Valid translation protocols are essential, but also tests on the cultural validity should be performed. One of first steps of testing these cultural factors is the "think aloud test." In this test, the properly translated instrument is tested in practice, and the rater who is using this instrument explicitly tells all his thoughts on what he thinks of this item, and how and why he rates a specific behavior. In this way, implicit beliefs and values will be made explicit. Needless to say, that one also has to make sure to test these instruments in relevant cultural subgroups.

NONPHARMACOLOGICAL TREATMENT

Cultural Barriers to Nonpharmacological Treatment

In this chapter, several cultural barriers for pharmacological pain management have been discussed. However, there seems to be even more barriers for nonpharmacological treatment.

Due to the uncertainties and risks associated with the pharmacological treatment of symptoms occurring in dementia, nonpharmacological interventions are increasingly considered more appropriate. As it appears from various clinical guidelines there is now consensus that nonpharmacological therapies should be adopted as first-line treatment for behavioral symptoms, and that only in case these show to be ineffective, pharmacological alternatives should be introduced [35]. These behavior interventions have also been shown to reduce pain in dementia [48]. However, a study has shown multiple barriers to the use of these nonpharmacological therapies in a nursing home setting [10]. These were related to resident attribute barriers—such as explicit or passive refusal to participate—communication problems, and unresponsiveness, which cannot be changed and need to be accommodated. However, there were also many external impediments which were related to staff, relatives, and the culture of care in these institutions. The most frequent barrier related to staff was the failure to identify pain, while pain was found to be present when formally assessed with the use of an instrument or through observation. Other studies have attested broader forces that prevent the successful integration of nonpharmacological therapies despite the evidence of their effectiveness [9, 2]. Pharmacological interventions are still standard practice; their use is reimbursed while this is not the case for nonpharmacological therapies. The structural conditions are not provided for the latter in that professional support is lacking and there are unclear or inappropriate roles of physicians, medicine aides, pharmacies, monitoring, and quality control [10]. Also ideas based on prejudicial stereotypes add to misconceptions that there is nothing that can be done for people with dementia [29]. A wide range of conditions including cultural, organizational, social, legal, and regulatory factors still present considerable obstacles for the successful adoption of nonpharmacological therapies. Those therapies which were shown to effectively reduce symptoms such as aromatherapy and progressive muscle relaxation [47] could potentially be helpful strategies for informal carers at home, who are currently unaware of such remedies and resort for the most part to psychotropic medications [42]. In part, this is related to the more traditional culture in medicine, in which integrative medicine has difficulties finding its place.

CONCLUSIONS AND RECOMMENDATIONS

Cultural aspects play an important role in the causation of pain, the perception of pain, the reaction to pain, and also the management of pain. Health-care workers are usually poorly trained in addressing complex problem of pain in dementia and this certainly also applies to the cultural aspects. Behavioral observation instruments for the recognition of pain in dementia are predominantly developed by and for a white western population. Also the cultural aspects of health-care settings are important to consider when one tries to improve the situation of people with dementia in pain. However, this is an underresearched area and is therefore lacking empirical evidence.

REFERENCES

1. Adamson J, Donovan J. 'Normal disruption': South Asian and African/Caribbean relatives caring for an older family member in the UK. Soc Sci Med 2005;60:37–48.
2. Aggarwal N, Vass AA, Minardi HA, Ward R, Garfield C, Cybyk B. People with dementia and their relatives: personal experiences of Alzheimer's and of the provision of care. J Psychiatr Ment Health Nurs 2003;10:187–97.
3. Astrom S, Nilsson M, Norberg A, Sandman PO, Winblad B. Staff burnout in dementia care—relations to empathy and attitudes. Int J Nurs Stud 1991;28:65–75.
4. Beck C, Ortigara A, Mercer S, Shue V. Enabling and empowering certified nursing assistants for quality dementia care. Int J Geriatr Psychiatry 1999;14:197–211; discussion 211–212.
5. Betancourt JR. Cultural competence: marginal or mainstream movement? N Engl J Med 2004;351:953–5.
6. Boone S, Schwartzberg JG. 21st century medicine: a case for diversity, health literacy, cultural competence and health equity. In: CPPD report: continuing medical education, vol. 31; 2010. p. 1–3. Acessed at http://www.ama-ssn.org/amal/pub/upload/mm/455/cppd431.pdf
7. Clare L. Managing threats to self: awareness in early stage Alzheimer's disease. Soc Sci Med 2003;57:1017–29.
8. Cobban N. Improving domiciliary care for people with dementia and their carers: the raising the standard project. In: Innes A, Archibald C, Murphy C, editors. Dementia and social inclusion. London: Jessica Kingsley Publishers; 2004.
9. Cohen-Mansfield J, Jensen B. Nursing home physicians' knowledge of and attitudes toward nonpharmacological interventions for treatment of behavioral disturbances associated with dementia. J Am Med Dir Assoc 2008;9:491–8.
10. Cohen-Mansfield J, Thein K, Marx MS, Dakheel-Ali M. What are the barriers to performing nonpharmacological interventions for behavioral symptoms in the nursing home? J Am Med Dir Assoc 2012;13:400–5.
11. Colombo F, Llena-Nozal F, Mercier J, Tjadens F. Help wanted? Providing and paying for long-term care. In. OECD health policy studies. New York: OECD Publishing; 2011.
12. Cornell S, Hartmann D. Ethnicity and race: making identities in a changing world. London: Pine Forge Press; 1998.
13. English J, Morse JM. The 'difficult' elderly patient: adjustment or maladjustment? Int J Nurs Stud 1988;25:23–39.
14. Forstl H, Bickel H, Kurz A, Borasio GD. Versorgungssituation und palliativemedizinischer ausblick. Fortschr Neurol Psychiatr 2010;78:203–12.
15. Geertz C. The interpretation of cultures. New York: Basic Books; 1973.
16. Gomes B, Calanzani N, Gysels M, Hall S, Higginson IJ. Heterogeneity and changes in preferences for dying at home: a systematic review. BMC Palliat Care 2013, 12:7.
17. Good-DelVecchio MJ, Good JCB, Becker AE. The culture of medicine and racial, ethnic,and class disparities in health. In: Russell Sage Foundation Working Paper 199; 2002.
18. Grafstrom M, Fratiglioni L, Sandman PO, Winblad B. Health and social consequences for relatives of demented and non-demented elderly. A population-based study. J Clin Epidemiol 1992;45:861–70.
19. Gubrium J. Living and dying at Murray Manor. Charlottesville, VA: University of Virginia Press; 1997.
20. Hinton WL, Levkoff S. Constructing Alzheimer's: narratives of lost identities, confusion and loneliness in old age. Cult Med Psychiatry 1999;23:453–75.
21. Hoka S. Do Japanese express pain as Western people do? [in Japanese]. Masui: Jap J Anesthesiol 2004; 53:572–6.
22. Holland D, Quinn N. Culture and cognition. In: Holland D, Quinn N, editors. Cultural models in language and thought. Cambridge: Cambridge University Press; 1987.
23. Houttekier D, Cohen J, Bilsen J, Addington-Hall J, Onwuteaka-Philipsen B, Deliens L. Place of death in metropolitan regions: metropolitan versus non-metropolitan variation in place of death in Belgium, The Netherlands and England. Health Place 2010;16:132–9.
24. Houttekier D, Cohen J, Bilsen J, Addington-Hall J, Onwuteaka-Philipsen BD, Deliens L. Place of death of older persons with dementia. A study in five European countries. J Am Geriatr Soc 2010;58:751–6.
25. Hunt LM, de Voogd KB. Clinical myths of the cultural 'Other': implications for Latino patient care. Acad Med 2005;80.918–24.
26. Innes A. Towards an understanding of care assistants' constructions of residents as 'difficult'. Stirling: University of Stirling; 1997.
27. Jagger C, Andersen K, Breteler MM, Copeland JR, Helmer C, Baldereschi M, Fratiglioni L, Lobo A, Soininen H, Hofman A, et al. Prognosis with dementia in Europe: a collaborative study of population-based cohorts. Neurologic Diseases in the Elderly Research Group. Neurology 2000;54:S16–20.

28. Johnson M, Webb C. Rediscovering unpopular patients: the concept of social judgement. J Adv Nurs 1995;21:466-75.
29. Jones RW. Barriers to optimal intervention and care for people with dementia. Int J Clin Pract 2005;59:266-7.
30. Keesing RM, Strathern AJ. Cultural anthropology. A contemporary perspective. New York: Rinehart & Winston; 1998.
31. Kitwood T. Dementia reconsidered: the person comes first. Buckingham: The Open University Press; 1997.
32. Kitwood T. Towards a theory of dementia care: the interpersonal process. Ageing Soc 1993;13:51-67.
33. Knapp M, Comas-Herrera A, Somani A, Banerjee S. Dementia: international comparisons. In Summary report for the National Audit Office. London: Institute of Psychiatry at the Maudsley; 2007.
34. Lock M. The concept of race: an ideological construct. Transcult Psychiatr Res Rev 1993;30:203-27.
35. Lyketsos CG, Colenda CC, Beck C, Blank K, Doraiswamy MP, Kalunian DA, Yaffe K, Task Force of American Association for Geriatric Psychiatry. Position statement of the American Association for Geriatric Psychiatry regarding principles of care for patients with dementia resulting from Alzheimer disease. Am J Geriatr Psychiatry 2006;14:561-72.
36. McCarthy M, Addington-Hall J, Altmann D. The experience of dying with dementia: a retrospective study. Int J Geriatr Psychiatry 1997;12:404-9.
37. McElmurry BJ, Solheim K, Kishi R, Coffia MA, Woith W, Janepanish P. Ethical concerns in nurse migration. J Prof Nurs 2006;22:226-35.
38. McKeigue PM, Marmot MG. Mortality from coronary heart disease in Asian communities in London. BMJ 1988, 297:903.
39. Mitchell SL, Kiely DK, Hamel MB. Dying with advanced dementia in the nursing home. Arch Intern Med 2004;164:321-6.
40. Mitchell SL, Teno JM, Kiely DK, Shaffer ML, Jones RN, Prigerson HG, Volicer L, Givens JL, Hamel MB. The clinical course of advanced dementia. N Engl J Med 2009;361:1529-38.
41. Mongkhonthawornchai S, Sangchart B, Sornboon A, Chantarasiri J. Thai perspectives on pain. J Med Assoc Thai 2013;96:S91-97.
42. Moore K, Ozanne E, Ames D, Dow B. How do family carers respond to behavioral and psychological symptoms of dementia? Int Psychogeriatr 2013;25:743-53.
43. Morrison RS, Siu AL. A comparison of pain and its treatment in advanced dementia and cognitively intact patients with hip fracture. J Pain Symptom Manag 2000;19:240-8.
44. Mossey JM. Defining racial and ethnic disparities in pain management. Clin Orthop Relat Res 2011;469:1859-70.
45. Motiwala SS, Croxford R, Guerriere DN, Coyte PC. Predictors of place of death for seniors in Ontario: a population-based cohort analysis. Can J Aging 2006;25:363-71.
46. Nolan M, Grant G, Keady J. Understanding family care. Buckingham: Open University Press; 1996.
47. O'Connor DW, Ames D, Gardner B, King M. Psychosocial treatments of behavior symptoms in dementia: a systematic review of reports meeting quality standards. Int Psychogeriatr 2009;21:225-40.
48. Pieper MJ, van Dalen-Kok AH, Francke AL, van der Steen JT, Scherder EJ, Husebo BS, Achterberg WP. Interventions targeting pain or behaviour in dementia: a systematic review. Ageing Res Rev 2013;12:1042-55.
49. Pinzon LC, Claus M, Perrar KM, Zepf KI, LetzelS, Weber M. Dying with dementia: symptom burden, quality of care, and place of death. Dtsch Arztebl Int 2013;110:195-202.
50. Pointon B, Keady J. Dementia and long-term care: costs and compassion. Br J Nurs 2005, 14:426.
51. Pool R, Gessler W. Medical anthropology. Berkshire: Open University Press; 2005.
52. Prentice A. Vitamin D deficiency: a global perspective. Nutr Rev 2008;66:S153-64.
53. Rahim-Williams B, Riley JL, 3rd, Williams AK, Fillingim RB. A quantitative review of ethnic group differences in experimental pain response: do biology, psychology, and culture matter? Pain Med 2012;13:522-40.
54. Shega JW, Hougham GW, Stocking C, Cox-Hayley D, Sachs D. Management of non-cancer pain in community-dwelling persons with dementia. J Am Geriatr Soc 2006;54:1892-97.
55. Sleeman KE, Ho YK, Verne J, Gao W, Higginson IJ, project GUC. Reversal of English trend towards hospital death in dementia: a population-based study of place of death and associated individual and regional factors, 2001-2010. BMC Neurol 2014, 14:59.
56. Smith AK, Cenzer IS, Knight SJ, Puntillo KA, Widera E, Williams BA, Boscardin WJ, Covinsky KE. The epidemiology of pain during the last 2 years of life. Ann Intern Med 2010;153:563-9.
57. Todd KH, Deaton C, D'Adamo AP, Goe L. Ethnicity and analgesic practice. Ann Emerg Med 2000;35:11-6.
58. Ujcic-Voortman JK, Schram MT, Jacobs-van der Bruggen MA, Verhoeff AP, Baan CA. Diabetes prevalence and risk factors among ethnic minorities. Eur J Public Health 2009;19:511-5.

59. van der Steen JT, Radbruch L, Hertogh CM, de Boer ME, Hughes JC, Larkin P, Francke AL, Junger S, Gove D, Firth P, et al. White paper defining optimal palliative care in older people with dementia: a Delphi study and recommendations from the European Association for Palliative Care. Palliat Med 2014;28:197–209.
60. van Saase JL, van Romunde LK, Cats A, Vandenbroucke JP, Valkenburg HA. Epidemiology of osteoarthritis: Zoetermeer survey. Comparison of radiological osteoarthritis in a Dutch population with that in 10 other populations. Ann Rheum Dis 1989;48:271–80.
61. Wijeratne C. Review: pathways to morbidity in carers of dementia sufferers. Int Psychogeriatr 1997;9:69–79.
62. Wimmer A. The making and unmaking of ethnic boundaries: a multilevel process theory. Am J Sociol 2008;113:987–1022.
63. Wolff JL, Kasper JD, Shore AD. Long-term care preferences among older adults: a moving target? J Aging Soc Policy 2008;20:182–200.
64. Xie J, Brayne C, Matthews FE, Medical Research Council Cognitive Function, Ageing Study collaborators. Survival times in people with dementia: analysis from population based cohort study with 14 year follow-up. BMJ 2008;336:258–62.

CHAPTER 26

Pain Assessment in Cognitively Impaired Animals

Lydia Giménez-Llort and C. G. Pick

"Pain" is defined by the International Association for the Study of Pain (IASP) [76] as "an unpleasant sensory and emotional experience associated with actual or potential tissue damage or described in terms of such damage." Such a psycho-physiological experience is difficult to assess wholly in nonhuman animals, and it is still not exempt of speciesist discussions. Thus, some still consider that the conscious nature of the pain experience would not entitle other animal species to feel "pain" as it is conceptually understood in humans. Since nonhuman animals exhibit an aversive response to noxious stimulation, the pure physiological concept of "nociception" [133]—defined as "the neural processes of encoding and processing noxious stimuli"—was traditionally recommended to be used instead [102]. Nevertheless, the translational relevance of the study of pain in nonhuman animals provides new insights to this regard, and it is the focus of the present chapter.

TRANSLATIONAL RELEVANCE OF THE STUDY OF PAIN IN NONHUMAN ANIMALS

Like in humans, the primary goal of studying pain/nociception in the other animal species is to prevent, alleviate, and relief the subject from the perception of noxious stimuli as well as to improve anesthetic and analgesic management. These are issues that have classically received most attention for domestic and farm animals [101] but also apply for laboratory specimens [55, 68]. It is reflected by the increasing public and scientific concern regarding animal welfare [146], which leads to improved and refined ethical guidelines and regulatory imperatives in the investigations of "experimental pain" in conscious animals [3, 22, 30, 62, 100, 123, 124] and animal "pain" scales [115]. The other undeniable relevance of the study of pain in nonhuman animals is their significant contribution to the understanding of the fundamental neurobiological mechanisms of pain that we all have in common. Their role as models for developing new and better analgesic compounds and management strategies becomes critical [66]. For the current topic, the translational relevance of the study of pain in nonhuman animals originates from the option to easily study the impact of impaired cognition and dementia. These are clinical situations that render the concepts of perception, assessment, and management to be an exceptional challenge. In the following paragraphs, we will first briefly present two key examples of close fruitful scientific cooperation between basic and clinical sciences in the study of pain that empathize the relevance of complementary but also synergistic bidirectional translational efforts. They illustrate how the translational approach, with joint basic and clinical research, is contributing to the faster advancement of knowledge that is needed to improve pain relief in both humans and nonhuman animals. This fast progress in knowledge is even more important when our frail aging populations are considered.

Among scientists, clinicians, health-care providers, and policymakers devoted to the study of pain and the translation of basic knowledge into improved pain relief worldwide—as the mission of IASP is defined—there is a growing number of those who are interested in "pain and pain management in nonhuman species" [76]. The aims of this "special interest group" of IASP are (1) to encourage basic and clinical research on the recognition of pain in animals, mechanisms of pain in animals, and management of pain in animals; (2) to encourage the use of spontaneous animal disease as a model for studying mechanisms and alleviation of human pain; (3) to encourage cross-species collaboration in pain research; and, finally, (4) to promote interdisciplinary discussion of pain in nonhuman species. Each of these statements reveals the significance, new meaning, and vision that assessment of nociception in nonhuman animals has been achieved in the last decades. More importantly, they can be foreseen eventually guiding the future conceptual and ethical frames that will lead to a better scenario for the study of "pain" and "pain management" in animals as well as its translational output to pain relief in humans.

Similarly as translational approach, the "European Cooperation in the Field of Scientific and Technical Research" (COST), an intergovernmental framework for fostering collaboration between researchers in Europe in a bottom-up manner, has also brought together leading researchers from a wide range of scientific disciplines in a COST Action TD1005 for "Pain Assessment in Patients with Impaired Cognition, Especially Dementia," to which the authors of this chapter belong [51]. It is an effort to prompt the urgently needed improvement of pain management in dementia since evidences warn that pain is grossly undertreated in these patients [31]. The major aim of this COST Action is the development of a comprehensive and internationally agreed-on assessment toolkit for older adults targeting the various subtypes of dementia and various aspects of pain, including pain diagnostics, cognitive examination, and guidelines for proper assessment [1, 75]. It will have an obviously relevant application in the management of pain in palliative care [5, 46, 75]. For the validation of this toolkit, joint action of both basic and clinical sciences has been requested. For this purpose, neuroscientists, physiologists, pharmacologists, and neuropsychologists are participating and together providing experimental tests for the validity of the tools and physiological markers of pain, which do not solely rely on self-report. Experimental designs will be used to help testing the validity and pain specificity of the toolkit in development. To do this, different pain biomarkers (e.g., EEG, ERP, facial expression, autonomic responses [ECG, skin conductance]) are being assessed in individuals with different types of cognitive impairment (Alzheimer's, frontotemporal dementia [FTD], vascular dementia, mild cognitive impairment, mental retardation) using different types of experimental pain induction procedures [38]. Of course, the impact of cognitive impairment on pain processing is also investigated in murine models trying to reproduce the cognitive deficits of Alzheimer's disease (AD) [8]. Special attention is paid to study nociceptive behaviors at the different stages of the disease and how the neuropathological and neuropsychiatric-like symptoms affect perception and processing of noxious stimuli.

NOCICEPTION IN ANIMAL MODELS

Species [136] and even strains [45, 94, 110, 111, 116] may show different behaviors to a similar noxious stimulus. Nevertheless, the homology of "nociception" among animals and "pain experiences" in humans—including the conscious sensation of "pain"—has rendered some species, mainly rodents, a relevant model in basic and preclinical pain research [66]. Thus, tests and animal models of nociception in rats and mice [93] complement the use of molecular, biochemical, and cellular experimental approaches, which are limited by the absence of other factors known to drive and modulate pain in human individuals. These factors are the wide variety of external stimuli as well as those idiosyncratic factors such as the cognitive and emotional traits and states [11, 70] but also gender and age [15, 109]. Overall, the animal models have significantly contributed to our understanding of the physiology, pathophysiology, and pharmacology associated with experimentally induced or naturally occurring acute and chronic pain states [15, 109]. Still, controversies questioning the face and predictive validity of these models (mostly for chronic pain) arise, and basic and preclinical researchers are challenged to ensure the expected and necessary translational results [80, 109].

In a review of the actual progress and challenges of animal models of pain, Mogil [109] examined the factors that may underlie the slow translational progress in spite of the increasing availability of mutant animal models, assays that more closely resemble clinical pain states, and dependent measures beyond simple reflexive withdrawal. Although his critical analysis was done with regard to the effectiveness and safety of analgesic drugs, he took notice of the confusion that results from the different use of the term "animal model." Mogil claimed the existence of the following three types of concepts of "animal model" in the literature:

The Pain Test as the "Animal Model"

Classical studies of pain use the concept of "animal model" to refer to the "experimental procedure" or "laboratory method" by which the noxious stimulus is applied to the subject. A wide range of assays seeks to mimic human forms of clinical pain in hopes of gaining a better understanding of the etiology and pathophysiology of disease-related pain phenomena: nociceptive (thermal, mechanical, chemical, or electrical stimuli), inflammatory (algogen and sensitizing compounds, inflammatory mediators, polyarthritic, or monoarthritic agents), or neuropathic (mechanical or surgical lesions). The time point postinjury (acute, persistent, or chronic) and the part of the body studied (cutaneous, muscular, orofacial, visceral) are the other features that are chosen to define the experimental design. Examples of the most prominent pain induction methods are the hot-plate test, the pinch test, and the formalin test. All these models allow the experimenter various degrees of control over the parameters of pain stimulus: intensity, duration, location, and temporal patterning.

The Measures of Pain as the "Animal Model"

This concept of "model" may also refer to the wide range of responses that can be measured. The responses can be a simple spinal withdrawal reflex response to sudden mechanical or thermal (heat or cold) stimuli such as induced in the tail-flick nociception test but also an avoidance response requiring higher brain centers such as jumping up or raising or licking the forepaw as elicited in the hot plate nociception test. Thus, responses may also involve spontaneously emitted behaviors: the so-called directed behaviors such as biting, flinching, guarding, licking, lifting, and shaking or—as the most severe behavioral expression—autotomy. Gait, walking, sitting, standing, and posture are also possible measures. Finally, nociception measures may consist in the choice the animal takes to avoid noxious stimulus in operant behaviors such as learned escape, place aversion, or reinforcement conflict. Indirect measures of nociception can be pain-affected complex behaviors such as anxiety, disability, changes in attention, sociability, or sleep. However, they are not preserved from being confounding factors, too.

The Subject as the "Animal Model"

The animal "model" may refer to the "experimental subject." That is a species or strain that spontaneously develops a painful disease or that is sensitive or resistant to pain. Mutant animals such as transgenic mice and rats, knockout and knock-in mice have become experimental subjects with a target mutation that modifies the pain phenotype. The idiosyncratic factors of the subject that will influence the study of pain are the genetic background (of the mutation), the gender, and the age. The husbandry (cage density, diet, social factors) and the context of the testing procedures (arousal, communication, handling, and restraint) are the most important environmental factors that must be controlled for as well.

PAIN-RELATED COMORBIDITY AND PAIN IN DEMENTIA

In the last two decades, the modeling of neurological and psychiatric diseases [56] in spontaneously mutant or genetically engineered rodents, in parallel to classical neuropsychopharmacological approaches, has provided new chances to study pain comorbidity [17, 99]. Analgesia is one of the behavioral items included in standardized protocols that screen for comprehensive phenotypes of animal models of disease prior to further functional analysis [33, 79, 121]. However, a limited number of experimental studies have yet examined the comorbidity of pain in cognitively impaired rodents or in naturally occurring canine and feline "cognitive dysfunction syndrome" (CDS) [89, 90]. A recent review [99] covers this important gap—but still from an opposite perspective—because it focuses on the negative impact that chronic pain has on affective disorders and cognitive dysfunctions as pain-related comorbidities. The question about pain perception and assessment in animal models of cognitive impairment or dementia is, for several reasons, still scarcely addressed and request the best endeavor undertakings. Some of the key questions are (1) how these diseases compromise the characteristics of pain, (2) how the validity of the models is to replicate pain in mild to moderate AD [78], or (3) what can we learn from these animal models whose shorter generation cycles and life spans imply a substantial advantage for longitudinal studies.

The first obvious limitation for the translational assessment and quantification of human pain is that self-report of the aversive nociception requiring verbal expression is not possible in nonhuman animals. Instead, pain must be estimated from the measurement of a range of responses, from simple avoidance reflexes to more complex behavioral responses of the animal to the nociceptive stimuli, as detailed before [93]. This is to the extent that some authors advice to rather refer to them as "tests and animal models of nociception" [11, 102].

Interestingly, this scenario resembles the difficulties that neurologists and psychiatrists face when they assess pain in patients with poor or absent verbal communicative abilities, cognitive impairment, or even dementia [4, 29], including patients in palliative care [5, 75]. Most authors agree that the combination of pain and dementia makes pain recognition in humans much more difficult, resulting in major diagnostic challenges [104]. Interestingly, preclinical pain research has gained interest because of its experience with the restrictive frames set by behavioral pain assessment tools that rely on nonverbal communications or behavioral responses. Since the first descriptions of nociception tests in the 1940s [34, 143], the perception of experimental pain has been measured with standardized methods that assess nociception by means of reliable and objective scores. Best example is the latency of appearance of an avoidance behavior, usually a nocifensive withdrawal reflex of the paw or tail exposed to the thermal (heat or cold), mechanical (von Frey filaments) but also electrical or chemical stimuli [93]. As mentioned before, the measurable behavioral changes may also be spontaneously emitted behaviors (autotomy, goal-directed oral or body movements, gait or posture), operant behaviors (learned escape, place aversion, reinforcement conflict) and changes induced by pain in complex cognitive (attention, memory), emotional (freezing, neophobia, anxiety-like behaviors, behavioral despair), physical (e.g., disability), physiological (e.g., sleep), or social behaviors [71, 109]. Some other authors also consider the traditional observer assessments of the body appearance (i.e., coat condition, piloerection, anorexia), posture/gait (i.e., hunched posture, abnormal gait), demeanor (i.e., aggression, hiding) but also objective assessments of locomotion and motor activity, food and water intake or changes in body weight and physiological measures (respiratory rate, heart rate, and blood pressure). Still, some authors warn that the relative high basal heart and respiratory rates of small mammals present technical difficulties in their use as physiological indices. Therefore, alternatives such as food and water intake and weight loss have been used for the evaluation of chronic pain, without perfect confidence in the precision of these measures [101]. Systematic evaluation of simultaneous behaviors in complex ethograms can also be done, although their sensitivity to analgesics as well as their specificity, reliability, and frequency are not considered to be completely satisfactory [109].

ON THE RELEVANCE OF NONVERBAL COMMUNICATION IN THE STUDY OF PAIN IN DEMENTIA

Most of the observational pain behavior rating scales that have been developed to assess pain in patients with dementia include classical nonverbal communication categories such as facial expression with furrowed brow, narrowed eyes, closed eyes known as "facial action units" (FAU), body movement (e.g., freezing, crouching, limping), and vocalization (e.g., groaning, mumbling, sighing) [29]. These behavioral indicators of pain are considered relevant for guiding the management of pain in dementia [1] and their translational relevance and applicability have started to be considered. Especially, the facial indicators assessed by the Facial Action Coding System (FACS), which seem to specifically encode the experience of pain and do only change little in the course of dementia [72, 92], have been successfully translated in the so-called grimace scale (GS) [91]. In rats (RGS) and mice (MGS) the GS comprises 4 or 5 FAU, respectively. The GS shows a high reliability (ICC: 0.9) and accuracy (72–97%) in mice [91] but is even more accurate in rats (accuracy >81%, ICC also 0.9) [135]. Besides, the scale showed a high correlation with other behavioral pain scores and can effectively assess pain associated with routine procedures [91]. In contrast, contradictory opinions exist on the utility of other spontaneously emitted pain behaviors such as the audible and ultrasonic vocalizations [19]. Their fine computerized recording has allowed the standardization of the measure in rats [65], and they have been found also useful to assess acute pain in laboratory mice [142]. However, other authors argue that they are not specific for the pain status [81] and do not correlate with behavioral measures of persistent pain [141]. Further studies using other experimental settings together with the improvement of our methodological skills to discriminate different vocalization registers, as achieved in cats [21] and in rats [65], will provide new insights in the vocal expression of pain in nonhuman animals that may closely resemble human verbal and paralanguage pain expression.

LIMITATIONS AND CONFOUNDING FACTORS IN THE STUDY OF PAIN IN DEMENTIA

The criticisms of the poor predictive validity of the animal models for chronic pain [13] may also apply to animal models for dementia when studied with experimental pain. That is in part due to the interspecies gaps in terms of pharmacodynamics and pharmacokinetics [14]. Furthermore, the background factor "aging" has strong implications and differs from one species to the other. The short life-span of small animals is an obvious advantage to answer questions that otherwise require too much time to be answered by the only means of human studies. However, this idiosyncrasy may also turn into a limiting factor as the life-span of small animals may be too short to perfectly mimic the time-depending modifications of the "neuromatrix" [6] that are involved in the processing of the noxious stimuli in the elderly patients. Here, those large animals, which mostly develop pain spontaneously [70], are likely to be the more successful models of pain in aging. However, Livingston [101] drew attention to the situation that, in contrast to humans, many large species show much less overt behaviors during noxious stimulation as a survival strategy to avoid showing signs of pain and weakness that may increase the chances to become a prey. Similarly, small rodents show specific pain-related behaviors, which are not always noticeable during casual observations [122, 123]. Among the limiting factors, the ethical considerations as regards the study of large animals are the most sensitive issues that restrict research on them [100], while studies on pain and pain management are very welcome as soon as these animals were seen as domestic or farm animals [101]. Interestingly, the "CDS" is a naturally emerging disease of the aging canine and feline brains [89] that is also considered useful from a translational perspective as a canine model of human brain aging and AD [69]. Yet, second-generation models (transgenic rodents harboring the human familial Alzheimer's disease [FAD] mutations) that closely mimic the temporal, neuroanatomical, and behavioral patterns of the human disease have greatest advantages due to their shorter time requirements [60].

Cognitive impairment or intellectual disability in humans have historically raised the question to which extent the influence of pain-modulatory factors differs from patients with other conditions [107], in spite of the apparent methodological limitations due to the doubtful level of understanding of the pain tests and the poor reliability of self-report in consequence of the limited ability to communicate. In nonhuman animals, the individual cognitive and emotional traits and states as well as prior experiences of the animal but also external influences such as the interaction with the researcher, the novel context and the restrain procedures are considered important—sometimes stress-related—confounders. These problems are counteracted by procedures including handling, preparatory experiences, or habituation in order to control and stabilize the influence of the confounding factors [16] as well as to establish a basal line of background noise. Such experimental problem solutions are not always available in clinical care settings. Moreover, each animal model (test, measure, or subject) has its strengths and weaknesses, and therefore, special precautions dependent on the model are strongly recommended to be taken [82, 83]. Whenever possible, a battery of several nociceptive assays is also advised in order to confirm the findings by different tests. Even in this case, important factor interactions effects with gender, tester, and cohort are needed to be controlled to avoid confounding results [112].

ANIMAL MODELS OF AGING, COGNITIVE IMPAIRMENT, AND DEMENTIA

During the last two decades, the neurobiology of aging has emerged as one of the scientific disciplines with a vast and quick expansion and its future looks promising. The major methodological advances in recent years offer a unique scientific capacity to study aging. However, the dramatically increasing prevalence of neurodegenerative diseases in the elderly, in parallel with the increase of life expectancy and social aging, makes such an historical success both a challenge and obligation.

Most scientific research efforts have focused on the understanding of the genetic basis and the brain mechanisms (neuronal and glial) related to changes in the nervous system that occur during aging and may underlie neurodegenerative diseases. To support these efforts from the side of animal research, we could make use of three tremendously valuable principles: (1) the similarity in the basic biological mechanisms of the various animal species, (2) the difference in longevity between them and (3) their different complexity. Thus, those species, which are simpler, produce easier "biological" scenarios for a better understanding of crucial etiological processes. For example, a 18-month-old mouse, a 30-day-old *Drosophila melanogaster* (fruit fly), or the small nematode *Caenorhabditis elegans*, which has only 1099 genes and lives only for about 3 weeks, all of them have the equivalent biological age of an octogenarian human. This higher pace in animal research allows us to ask, seek, and answer pressing questions for humans and in particular for the sick and their families, which would otherwise take years to be addressed or are even totally inaccessible.

A wide variety of animal models of cognitive impairment has been established based on genetic, lesion, and pharmacological approaches or naturally occurring aging-related cognitive impairments [95]. The scientific background of the classical studies on learning and memory allowed that already the first animal models for cognitive impairment and dementia addressed key questions, that is, what anatomical regions and neurotransmitter systems are affected and associated with memory loss. Thus, the neurobiological starting points were based on the loss of integrity of the basal forebrain cholinergic neurons in Alzheimer's disease and the ability of anticholinergic drugs to reproduce the cognitive deficits [20, 35]. Nowadays, these models based on cholinergic lesions in areas critical to learning and memory (such as the hippocampus and the basal nucleus of Meynert, among others) are far from being considered just traditional methodological approaches. Thus, cortical cholinergic deafferentation by selective immunotoxins in rodents leads to the development of β-amyloid deposits that render this biochemical lesion an animal model for "sporadic AD" and human cerebral amyloid angiopathy [12, 128]. Currently, important issues and tools of interest for researchers are other models of cognitive impairment–induced pharmacologically (i.e., muscarinic, nicotinic, and NMDA receptor antagonists; ethanol), models of the cognitive deficits of Parkinsonism (by chronic-low-dose MPTP) and the toxicologic models reproducing the teratological or ontogenic cognitive impairments induced by exposure to ambient toxicants (i.e., to lead, polychlorinated biphenyls (PCBs), or methylmercury) [95].

Advances in biotechnology, which have allowed to genetically manipulate animals by cancellation (knockout), substitution (knockout—knock in), or incorporation (transgenes) of genes have catapulted these manipulations to become one of the most promising strategies to create more valid animal models for human diseases. In the case of AD, the determination of the genetic basis of the forms of early-onset FAD and genetic risk factors implicated in sporadic patients (i.e., ApoE) have been instrumental in establishing animal models useful for knowledge and study of this disease [131, 132], even though the "natural" animal models such as the CDS in dogs and cats, are also providing promising findings [18, 69, 90]. In fact, only 5–10% of patients of AD have a known genetic cause (gene mutations APP, PS1, or PS2 in the FAD and trisomy 21 in Down syndrome [DS]) or are due to an identifiable risk factor other than age (i.e., genetic susceptibility due to ApoE) [132]. However, the basic disease mechanisms seem to be the same for sporadic patients. Thus, at the neurochemical level, cholinergic dysfunction and glutamatergic hyperfunctionality with associated oxidative stress are claimed by the other two hypotheses that together with the β-amyloid cascade hypothesis (suggesting proinflammatory and neurotoxic effects) attempt to explain the biological basis of this disease. Although no identifiable mutations in the tau gene have yet been found in AD, tau filament formations are characteristic in other neurodegenerative diseases such as FTD with parkinsonism linked to chromosome 17 (FTDP-17). There, mutations in the tau gene have been detected and allowed generating different animal models for tauopathies. Another successful strategy has been the one employed in the BACE1 knockout mice, which demonstrated that the BACE type 1 is the responsible for the improper proteolysis of APP, the latter being a key element for forming β-amyloid plaques.

Despite these advances, assessments at the behavioral level have not always received enough attention. Thus, the validity of some models to reproduce the whole array of symptoms of the disease, including the "behavioral and psychological symptoms associated with dementia" (BPSD), has been limited [60]. In fact, the last reference guides that attempt to define the criteria to improve current and future animal models for AD [77] postulate that the models should show, at least, (1) progressive AD-like neuropathology, (2) cognitive deficits, and (3) replications in other laboratories (to show interlaboratory reliability). The guidelines also emphasize the importance of selecting suitable strains of animals with cognitive–behavioral profiles of the same genetic background. Also, they remind on the relevance of the longitudinal studies since, as already proven in humans, they are critical in determining the actual timing of the cognitive deficits associated with aging. The most recent animal models do fulfill these criteria and have shown, with varying success, the expected clinical-like profile, that is, deficits in learning and memory tasks but also BPSD-like symptoms [60, 126].

The mouse model Tg2576 has been by far the most used so far [7, 74]. Other models such as PDAPP (PDGF-hAPP) mice [57], APP23Tg mice, CRND8Tg mice,

Tg2576+TgPS1-A246E mice, 3xTg-AD mice, TASTPM mice, APPswe/PS1DE9 mice are listed among those currently available that integrate the knowledge of extensive neurobiological research on AD in recent years [126]. Remarkably, the literature has shown as probably the three most interesting mouse models: (1) The triple transgenic mice overexpressing mutated tau and conditional GSK-3β [103], which is a protein kinase that is related to many of the elements involved in the neuropathology of AD (APP, PS1, β-amyloid, tau, and neuronal death), and presenting with tauopathies such as FTDP-17; (2) the triple transgenic mice 3xTg-AD [114] showing synaptic dysfunctions and cognitive deficits, when still only immunoreactivity β-amyloid is found, and thereafter developing β-amyloid plaques and tangles tau in a neuroanatomical and temporal pattern parallel to that of humans; (3) APPSLPS1KI mice [25] presenting the first time with massive neuronal death, which is independent of the presence of extracellular plaques, in a topographic distribution similar to that of humans with AD.

Despite the undeniable power of the models in rodents [60, 126], today there are many research projects that incorporate in their experimental panel other animal models with great scientific value. These additional animal models have complementary advantages, even though they do not meet some of those requirements that the validation guides ask for [77]. Among them, we find the *Caenorhabditis elegans* worm or the *Drosophila* fly with simple, familiar and easy to study genetic maps but also the *Danio rerio*, zebrafish, whose physical transparency allows seeing the neuropathological changes in the tau protein. Also, yeasts have been very useful to study easily the mechanisms and cellular signals related to the pathophysiology of disease. Moreover, in the nature itself there are "natural" models of AD such as the chick embryo that has been proven to be very useful for studying and testing drugs that regulate the metabolism of the precursor protein of β-amyloid. Also some breeds of dogs (i.e., the dachshund, the poodle, or the Yorkshire) are prone to suffer from sporadic diseases with cognitive impairment. Furthermore, "CDS" is an established neurodegenerative disorder of senior dogs—and now also recognized in cats—characterized by progressive decline and increasing brain pathology [18, 63, 90, 108]. Finally, the stranding of cetaceans is postulated as a result of dementia in the old male leader, and nonhuman primates, as the closest phylogenetic species to us, are also considered to be prone to neurodegeneration processes during their aging process [127].

PAIN IN ANIMAL MODELS OF COGNITIVE IMPAIRMENT AND DEMENTIA

The Pain Genes Database gives access to all published pain-related phenotypes of mutant mice [87], providing valuable information about genotype–phenotype relationships for pain. However, compared to all the other neurophysiological and behavioral aspects covered in these models, the number of studies that include pain is very small considering the global burden that pain causes. Thus, only a limited number of experimental studies have examined the comorbidity of pain in cognitively impaired rodents, and even less have considered critical factors such as aging, the standard background in dementia. Aging is usually accompanied by an increase of painful disorders among other disease comorbidities. Some studies in the Pain Genes Database do also omit the consideration of gender, which determines not only differences in pain perception and sensitivity but plays also a key role in determining the incidence of diseases, their comorbidity as well as the associated levels of burden and disability. Here, we will report on some of the studies that have considered pain in animals with induced or naturally occurring cognitive impairment.

For instance, changes in behavior across the life span (4–28 months of age) have been studied in C57BL/6J mice, the gold-standard murine strain, and usual genetic background in mutant mice. The results showed that in both genders certain aspects of basic behavior, mostly that related to the drive to explore, and locomotor activities are modulated by aging in a continuous manner. In these animals, advanced age encompasses impairment of motor skills acquisition and memory consolidation, but noxious threshold and working memory were well preserved [52, 53]. We have described a gender-dependent impairment of the neuroimmunoendocrine system [59] and an advanced biological/chronological age [62] in 3xTg-AD mice. Filali et al. [54] have found that at advanced stages of disease male 3xTg-AD mice show pain thresholds in the hot-plate test equivalent to those of controls. Recently, we have also described that, both at early and advanced stages of disease, tail-flick responses of 3xTg-AD mice to cold water are similar to that exhibited by age-matched controls and depend on age [8]. In the case of TASTPM mice for AD, the mutant animals showed altered sensitivity depending on the noxious stimuli, with paw withdrawal responses similar to the ones in control mice when tested with mechanical stimuli but different when tested with thermal stimuli: lower nociceptive sensitivity in the tail-flick test with hot water but increased one in the hot-plate test [31]. It remains to be studied how the progress of the disease affects the different dimensions of pain, and how the neuropathology of AD has an impact on pain processing and perception. Here, mild cognitive impairment, which has emerged as an identifiable clinical condition and is in many patients the transitional state preceding diagnosable AD, can be studied as one of the steps from premorbid/prodromal to advanced stages of AD disease, as shown in the P301S mutant human tau transgenic mice [137] and more recently in the 3xTg-AD mice [62].

The clinical features of AD as the German physician Alois Alzheimer described for just over a hundred years ago in his patient Augusta and its disease processes are complex and, for now, its diagnosis is neuropathological, based on the presence of exacerbated amyloid β and tau protein accumulation. These neuropathological features follow a fairly broad regional pattern of neurodegeneration in which the regions involved in cognitive processes as well as learning and memory are most affected; the pattern also explains why some patients display serious behavioral disorders in the more advanced stages of the disease [118]. Depression, anxiety, aggression, apathy, aberrant and stereotyped behaviors, sun downing behavior, restlessness, and hallucinations are some of the symptoms associated with dementia, commonly referred as BPSD. Some animal models have become able to model the presence of BPSD [9, 60, 61]. It is especially relevant for the present chapter to note that clinicians are also aware that BSPD such as, for example, agitation and irritability may reflect pain in patients with dementia [10, 71]. Supporting such an association, rats with different pain thresholds are also characterized by a different sensitivity to emotional stimuli, probably reflecting altered activation thresholds of some brain structures controlling anxiety [94]. Interestingly, the classic signs of CDS in ancient dogs and cats are summarized by the acronym DISHAAL or DISHA, which refers to disorientation/confusion (awareness, spatial orientation), alterations in interactions with owners, other pets, and the environment, sleep–wake cycle disturbances or reversed day/night schedule, house soiling, and changes in activity (hyperactivity, stereotypes, apathy or depressed, smaller grooming), and anxiety (vocalizations, agitation and signs of fear, phobias, agitation, and anxiety) that are associated with learning and memory cognitive impairment [90]. On the other hand, pain and discomfort associated with arthritis and other medical conditions (i.e., dental, gastrointestinal, bladder) can cause behavioral signs such as altered response to stimuli, decreased activity, restless/unsettled state, vocalization, house soiling, aggression/irritability, self-trauma, and walking at night. In sum, "DISHA and similar signs" might be due to CDS but also pain or sensory deficits need to be considered and ruled out.

Overall both clinical and preclinical data suggests that, at advanced stages of the disease, when verbal communication is already missing in the patients, a proper assessment of these symptoms that overlap with indicators of pain may be critical to control them as confounding factors. Besides, the neuropsychiatric symptoms per se may interfere with the experience of pain or worsen the pain induced by other comorbid diseases naturally occurring in the aged subject.

Some evidence suggests that the affective–motivational pain dimension dependent on the medial pain pathway in the brain is most affected in dementia. This can be a critical issue for some experimental models since operant and conditioned tests for learning and memory use aversive stimuli as negative reinforcement strategy and, thus, might be affected by changes in emotional processing. For instance, we have found that in APP_{Ind}, $APP_{Sw,Ind}$ and triple-transgenic mice 3xTg-AD for AD, contextual and conditioned neophobic response (freezing) in a fear conditioning test was paradoxically remembered and enhanced while spatial learning and memory in the water maze was impaired. The results were related to intraneuronal accumulation of β-amyloid in the basolateral amygdala and reversed after treatment with classical anxiolytics and valproate [50], which are adjuvant analgesics as well [105].

Several neurodegenerative diseases including FTD, Alzheimer disease, Pick Disease, argyrophilic grain disease, progressive supranuclear palsy and cortico-basal degeneration have abnormal filamentous tau deposits as a pathological characteristic. Mutations in the gene encoding tau (MAPT) identified in patients diagnosed with FTD and parkinsonism linked to chromosome 17 (FTD–PD17) are known to disrupt the normal binding of tau to tubulin resulting in these pathological deposits of hyperphosphorylated tau. Still, scarce number of animal models for FTD and related tauopathies based on these mutations are available and only in a few of them the study of pain has been taking into consideration. This was the case in the Parkin-null, human tau overexpressing (PK−/−/TauVLW) mice, a model of complex FTD, parkinsonism and lower motor neuron disease, which has been recently described [120]. The model combines cerebral and peripheral deposition of amyloid with lesions of the hippocampus, substantia nigra and lower motor neurons resembling a multisystemic neurological disease such as FTD with parkinsonism and amyotrophy. In the FTDs, the degeneration of orbito-frontal and anterior temporal areas, which are responsible of the emotional aspects in pain, led to a reduction in pain perception and expressivity [129]. The few studies of pain perception and tolerance in clinically diagnosed FTD patients with SPECT cerebral hypoperfusion [23] suggest differences in pain processing between distinct types of dementia and pain perception to depend on the exact diagnosis of dementia.

From animal research, no reports of altered pain perception have been obtained, except for the work in Progranuline (PGRN)-deficient mice, another animal model for FTD, which is currently used to study pain defense after nerve injury and the development or maintenance of neuropathic pain. Loss-of-function mutations of PGRN have been discovered as the cause of familial ubiquitin-positive FTD [97]. A reduction of PGRN by traumatic brain injury (TBI) may also increase the risk for FTD. Besides for FTD, the plasma level of PGRN has been suggested to serve as a marker for other neurodegenerative diseases including AD [47, 58]. In mice, progranulin haploinsufficiency leads to exaggerated inflammation in the brain, with greater activation of microglia and astrocytes than their wild-type counterparts. The PGRN-deficient mice show behavioral deficits, progressive neuropathology, and signs of premature aging. This animal model develops intense nociceptive hypersensitivity after spared nerve injury, which worsens with aging [97].

The partial trisomic Ts(17^{16})65Dn mice (Ts65Dn mice) [36] are widely used as a model of DS [42]. The distal region of the chromosome 16 of these mice is homologous to the "critical region" of human chromosome 21 that contains APP, Girk1, and SOD1 genes among others, in a series of genes relevant for the disease. In contrast to previous exiting DS models, the Ts65Dn mice survive, reaching adulthood [73, 85]. This model shows developmental abnormalities and age-related neurodegeneration [73] that results in spatial memory deficits [40, 41] with impaired short- and long-term memory [49], anxiety-like behaviors [32], hyperactivity [48, 117] as well as difficulties in habituating or inhibiting behavior [32]. When the pain responsiveness of the Ts65Dn mice was studied, these mice presented with an overall depressed responsiveness to nociceptive stimulation compared to that in their control littermates, [106]. Reduction of sensitivity was shown by the nociceptive threshold in the tail-flick test but sensitivity to morphine assessed in this test was similar to the control mice. In the formalin test, all mice displayed the known biphasic curve of licking behavior of the injured paw, but reduced sensitivity of Ts65Dn mice was shown in both the early and late phases of the test. Alterations in the second messenger systems involved in the postreceptoral response of noradrenergic neurotransmission related to pain have also been described in the Ts65Dn mice [43]. Besides, in vitro studies in normal and trisomic human samples have shown altered synaptic transmission with spike shortening that alters the timing of neural activity in the dorsal root ganglion [26, 113]. However, the study in Ts65Dn mice did not allow to ascertain whether the reduced sensitivity was due to diminished peripheral nociceptor responsiveness or less effective processing of the nociceptive signals. Finally, it is noteworthy that the same experimental set of animals failed to exhibit differences in nociception in the hot-plate test compared to their control littermates. They even showed a faster escape response in subsequent sessions, a result that could be explained by the presence of altered emotional patterns and increased activity acting as confounding factors. Overall, the Ts65Dn model allowed concluding that the overexpression of genes leads to disrupted transmission and/or processing of painful stimuli. Another model of DS, the single-minded 2 gene [Sim2] shows phenotypes similar to some of those present in the Ts65Dn mice including anxiety-related reduced exploratory behavior and sensitivity to pain [28]. The double transgenic mice, overexpressing both amyloid precursor protein (APP) and Cu/Zn superoxide dismutase (SOD1) genes, were also used as mouse model of DS. They showed increased neuroma formation and decreased autotomy after peripheral nerve injury; or in other words, APP/SOD1 overexpressing mice are less sensitive for neuropathic pain associated with neuroma [86]. SOD1 mice showed mild deficits in sensorimotor responsiveness at various body sites but were not different in motor activity and anxiety [88]. In a different transgenic mice model for mental retardation, the FMR1 knockout mice, which is a murine model for fragile X mental retardation 1, acute responses to noxious stimuli assessed in the hot-plate and tail-flick tests were found to be normal [145]. A comparative microarray analysis of the trisomic genes in the human [67] and mice [125] chromosomes identified six possible candidate genes (ADAMTS5, Girk1, S100B, RUNX1, KCNJ6, KCNE1) related to the pain phenotype in the DS [87].Their respective mutant mice show more (Kcnj6) or less (Grik1, Runx1) nociceptive sensitivity, less hypersensitivity (ADAMTS5, S100B, Runx1) or even analgesia (Kcnj6) [139]. Overall, the studies just reported as well as further translational research [106] and the studies of pain management in intellectually disabled children [39] suggest that there is a pain genotype. However, it will be very difficult to distinguish the effects from the pain phenotype on the pain expression from those of the intellectual disability per se [139].

Among the long-term disabilities resulting from TBI, posttraumatic headache (PTH) disorders [98, 130] represent the most common chronic pain syndrome within this TBI patient population [144]. The neurobiological sequelae of mild TBI includes anxiety, depression, and cognitive complains [2, 134]. The somatic and neuropsychiatric problems after TBI unravel what the clinicians call "the silent epidemic" [138] characterized by deficits in attention, memory, and executive functions but also by primary psychiatric disorders (e.g., mood and anxiety disorders), personality disorders, and others [119]. Quantitative somatosensory testing has shown that chronic PTH (CPTHA) may be a form of central pain. The cranial mechanical hyperalgesia may originate from peripheral tissue damage accompanying the TBI and psychological factors may contribute to the development and maintenance of CPTHA in susceptible individuals [38]. These questions have also been addressed in animal models of head trauma, that is, the fluid percussion (FP) method and the controlled cortical impact (CCI) injury, two well-known animal models of TBI [27, 96, 140]. Also some other studies have reported that the injury to the somatosensory cortex results in persistent periorbital allodynia and increase in brain stem nociceptive neuropeptides [44].

CONCLUSION

Although the studies of pain in induced or naturally occurring animal models of cognitive impairment and dementia needs best endeavors, important advances have been achieved in recent years. Aging is a physiological condition accompanied by much comorbidity, often including pain disorders. Traditionally, most of research has focused on the impact and the way how pain interferes with the cognitive abilities as well as with the emotional traits and states of an individual. However, the opposite direction of consideration such as how cognitive impairment affects the nociceptive sensitivity and the experience of pain has only started to be successfully addressed. The lessons learned from the non-verbal expression of pain in the nonhuman animals are useful to advance our knowledge of pain assessment in the no longer perfectly communicative patient with cognitive impairment or dementia. Many of the assessment tools used in these patients, which were tailored to the lack of communicative abilities, find their parallel in the usual methods, and techniques of basic nonhuman animal research. In this context, it is important to warn about the confounding factors and limitations. They are due to the multiple etiological natures of cognitive impairment and the complexity of the mental disorders, which include behavioral and psychological symptoms that interact or overlap with those associated with acute and chronic pain. It is encouraging that recent translational efforts bridge the gap between basic experimental nociception studies in nonhuman animals and clinical pain studies in humans. This helps to provide the scientific resources that are necessary to deal with the limits of human studies and, thus, allows for faster answering the pressing questions as regards pain in dementia.

REFERENCES

1. Achterberg WP, Pieper MJC, van Dalen-Kok AH, de Waal MWM, Husebo BS, Lautenbacher S, Kunz M, Scherder EJA, Corbett A. Pain assessment in patients with dementia. Clin Interv Aging 2013;8:1471–82.
2. Alexander MP. The evidence for brain injury in whiplash injuries. Pain Res Manag 2003;8:19–23.

3. Alkire MT, Hudetz AG, Tononi G. Consciousness and anesthesia. Science 2008;322:876–80.
4. Álvaro González LC. The neurologist facing pain in dementia. Neurología 2012;30:574–85.
5. Anderson CM. Pain relief at the end-of-life: a clinical guide. Mo Med 2002;99:556–9.
6. Apkarian AV, Baliki MN, Geha PY. Towards a theory of chronic pain. Prog Neurobiol 2009;87:81–97.
7. Ashe KH. Molecular basis of memory loss in the Tg2576 mouse model of Alzheimer disease. J Alzheimer Dis 2006;9:123–6.
8. Baeta-Corral R, Defrin R, Pick CG, Giménez-Llort L. Tail-flick test response in 3xTg-AD mice at early and advanced stages of disease. Neurosci Lett 2015;600:158–63.
9. Baeta-Corral R, Giménez-Llort L. Bizarre behaviors and risk assessment in 3xTg-AD mice at early stages of the disease. Behav Brain Res 2014;258:97–105.
10. Ballard C, Smith J, Husebo BS, Aarsland D, Corbett A. The role of pain treatment in managing the behavioural and psychological symptoms of dementia (BPSD). Int J Palliat Nurs 2011;17:420–3.
11. Barrot M. Tests and models of nociception and pain in rodents. Neuroscience 2012;211:39–50.
12. Beach TG, Potter PE, Kuo YM, Emmerling MR, Durham RA, Webster SD, Walker DG, Sue LI, Scott S, Layne KJ, Roher AE. Cholinergic deafferentation of the rabbit cortex: a new animal model of Abeta deposition. Neurosci Lett 2000;283:9–12.
13. Berge O-G. Predictive validity of behavioral animal models for chronic pain. Br J Pharmacol 2011;164:1195–206.
14. Berge O-G. Behavioral pharmacology of pain. Berlin: Springer; 2014.
15. Berkley KJ. Sex differences in pain. Brain Sci 1997;20:371–80.
16. Boix F, Fernández-Teruel A, Escorihuela RM, Tobeña A. Handling-habituation prevents the effects of diazepam and alprazolam on brain serotonin levels in rats. Behav Brain Res 1990;36:209–15.
17. Borsook D. Neurological diseases and pain. Brain 2012;135:320–44.
18. Bosch MN, Pugliese M, Gimeno-Bayón J, Rodríguez MJ, Mahy N. Dogs with cognitive dysfunction syndrome: a natural model of Alzheimer's disease. Curr Alzheimer Res 2012;9:298–314.
19. Calvino B, Besson JM, Boehrer A, Depaulis A. Ultrasonic vocalizations (22–28 kHz) in a model of chronic pain, the arthritic rat: effects of analgesic drugs. Neuroreport 1996;7:581–4.
20. Camps P, Muñoz-Torrero D. Cholinergic drugs in pharmacotherapy of Alzheimer's disease. Mini Rev Med Chem 2002;2:11–25.
21. Carballo SG. The language of the cats [El lenguage de los gatos]. Madrid: Atele; 2003.
22. Carbone L. Pain in laboratory animals: the ethical and regulatory imperatives. PLoS One 2011;6:e21578
23. Carlino E, Benedetti F, Rainero I, Asteggiano G, Cappa G, Tarenzi L, Vighetti S, Pollo A. Pain perception and tolerance in patients with frontotemporal dementia. Pain 2010;151:783–9.
24. Carstens E, Moberg GP. Recognizing pain and distress in laboratory animals. ILAR J 2000;41:62–71.
25. Casas C, Sergeant N, Sergeant N, Itier JM, Blanchard V, Wirths O, van der Kolk N, Vingtdeux V, van de Steeg E, Ret G, et al. Massive CA1/2 neuronal loss with intraneuronal and N-terminal truncated Abeta42 accumulation in a novel Alzheimer transgenic model. Am J Pathol 2004;165:1289–300.
26. Caviedes P, Ault B, Rapoport SI. The role of altered sodium currents in action potential abnormalities of cultured dorsal root ganglion neurons from trisomy 21 (Down syndrome) human fetuses. Brain Res 1990;510:229–36.
27. Cernak I. Animal models of head trauma. Neuro Rx 2005;2:410–22.
28. Chrast R, Scott HS, Madani R, Huber L, Wolfer DP, Prinz M, Aguzzi A, Lipp H-P, Antonarakis SE. Mice trisomic for a bacterial artificial chromosome with the single-minded 2 gene (sim2) show phenotypes similar to some of those present in the partial trisomy 16 mouse models of Down syndrome. Hum Mol Genetics 2000;9:1853–64.
29. Cohens-Mansfield J. Pain assessment in noncommunicative elderly persons—PAINE. Clin J Pain 2006;22:569–75.
30. Committee on Guidelines for the Use of Animals in Neuroscience and Behavioral Research. Guidelines for the care and use of mammals in neuroscience and behavioral research. National Academy of Sciences, editor. Washington: National Academies Press; 2003.
31. Corbett A, Husebo B, Malcangio M, Staniland A, Cohen-Mansfield J, Aarsland D, Ballard C. Assessment and treatment of pain in people with dementia. Nat Rev Neurol 2012;8:264–74.
32. Coussons-Read ME, Crnic LS. Behavioral assessment of the Ts65Dn mouse, a model for Down syndrome: altered behavior in the elevated plus maze and open field. Behav Genet 1996;26:7–13.
33. Crawley JN. Behavioral phenotyping of transgenic and knock out mice: experimental design and evaluation of general health, sensory functions, motor abilities, and specific behavioral tests. Brain Res 1999;835:18–26.

34. D'Amour FE, Smith DL. A method for determining the loss of pain sensation. J Pharmacol Exp Ther 1941;72:74–9.
35. Davis KL, Mohs RC, Marin D, Purohit DP, Perl DP, Lantz M, Austin G, Haroutunian V. Cholinergic markers in elderly patients with early signs of Alzheimer disease. JAMA 1999;281:1401–6.
36. Davisson MT, Schmidt C, Reeves RH, Irving NG, Akeson EC, Harris BS, Bronson RT. Segmental trisomy as a mouse model for Down syndrome. Prog Clin Biol Res 1993;384:117–33.
37. Defrin R, Amanzio M, Dimova V, Filipovic S, Finn D, Giménez-Llort L, Jensen-Dahm C, Lautenbacher S, Oosterman J, Petrini L, et al. Experimental pain processing in individuals with cognitive impairment: state of the art. Pain 2015. doi:10.1097/j.pain.0000000000000195.
38. Defrin R, Gruener H, Schreiber S, Pick CG. Quantitative somatosensory testing of subjects with chronic post-traumatic headache: implications on its mechanisms. Eur J Pain 2010;14:924–31.
39. Defrin R, Pick CG, Peretz C, Carmeli E. A quantitative somatosensory testing of pain threshold in individuals with mental retardation. Pain 2004;108:58–66.
40. Demas GE, Nelson RJ, Krueger BK, Yarowsky PJ. Spatial memory deficits in segmental trisomic Ts65Dn mice. Behav Brain Res 1996;82:85–92.
41. Demas GE, Nelson RJ, Krueger BK, Yarowsky PJ. Impaired spatial working and reference memory in segmental trisomy (Ts65Dn) mice. Behav Brain Res 1998;90:199–201.
42. Dierssen M. Down syndrome: the brain in trisomic mode. Nat Rev Neurosci 2012;13:844–58.
43. Dierssen M, Vallina IF, Baamonde C, García-Calatayud S, Lumbreras MA, Flórez J. Alterations of central noradrenergic transmission in Ts65Dn mouse, a model for Down syndrome. Brain Res 1997;749:238–44.
44. Elliott MB, Oshinsky ML, Amenta PS, Awe OO, Jallo JI. Nociceptive neuropeptide increases and periorbital allodynia in a model of traumatic brain injury. Headache 2012;52:966–84.
45. Elmer GI, Pieper JO, Negus SS, Woods JH. Genetic variance in nociception and its relationship to the potency of morphine-induced analgesia in thermal and chemical tests. Pain 1998;75:129–40.
46. Emmons KR, Dale B, Crouch C. Palliative wound care, part 2: application of principles. Home Healthc Nurse 2014;32:210–2.
47. Eriksen JL, Mackenzie IR. Progranulin: normal function and role in neurodegeneration. J Neurochem 2008;104:287–97.
48. Escorihuela RM, Fernández-Teruel A, Vallina IF, Baamonde C, Lumbreras MA, Dierssen M, Tobeña A, Flórez J. A behavioral assessment of Ts65Dn mice: a putative Down syndrome model. Neurosci Lett 1995;199:143–6.
49. Escorihuela RM, Vallina IF, Martínez-Cué C, Baamonte C, Dierssen M, Tobeña A, Flórez A. Impaired short- and long-term memory in Ts65Dn mice, a model for Down syndrome. Neurosci Lett 1998;247:171–4.
50. España J, Giménez-Llort L, Valero J, Miñano A, Rábano A, Rodríguez-Álvarez J, LaFerla FM, Saura CA. Intraneuronal B-amyloid accumulation in the amygdala enhances fear and anxiety in Alzheimer's disease transgenic mice. Biol Psychiatry 2010;67:513–21.
51. European Cooperation in Science and Technology (COST). Action TD1005: pain assessment in patients with impaired cognition, especially dementia [web page on the Internet]. Brussels: European Cooperation in Science and Technology. Accessed at http://www.cost-td1005.net/
52. Fahlström A, Qian Yu, Ulfhake B. Behavioral changes in aging females C57BL/6 mice. Neurobiol Aging 2011;32:1868–80.
53. Fahlström A, Zeberg H, Ulfhake B. Changes in behaviors of male C57BL/6J mice across adult life span and effects of dietary restriction. Age (Dordr) 2012;34:1435–52.
54. Filiali M, Lalonde R, Theriault P, Julien C, Calon F, Planel E. Cognitive and non-cognitive behaviors in the triple-transgenic mouse model of Alzheimer's disease expressing mutated APP, PS1 and Papt (3xTg-AD). Behav Brain Res 2012;234:334–42.
55. Flecknell PA. The relief of pain in laboratory animals. Lab Anim 1984;18:147–60.
56. Flint J, Shifman S. Animal models of psychiatric disease. Curr Opin Genet Dev 2008;18:235–40.
57. Games D, Adams D, Alessandrini R, Barbour R, Berthelette P, Blackwell C, Carr T, Clemens J, Donaldson T, Gillespie F, et al. Alzheimer-type neuropathology in transgenic mice overexpressing V717F beta-amyloid precursor protein. Nature 1995;373:523–7.
58. Ghidoni R, Paterlini A, Benussi L. Circulating progranulin as a biomarker for neurodegenerative diseases. Am J Neurodegener Dis 2012;1:180–90.
59. Giménez-Llort L, Arranz L, Maté I, De la Fuente M. Gender-specific neuroimmunoendocrine aging in a triple-transgenic 3xTg-AD mouse model for Alzheimer's disease and its relation with longevity. Neuroimmunomodulation 2008;15:331–43.

60. Giménez-Llort L, Blázquez G, Cañete T, Johansson B, Oddo S, Tobena A, LaFerla FM, Fernández-Teruel A. Modeling behavioral and neuronal symptoms of Alzheimer's disease in mice: a role for intraneuronal amyloid. Neurosci Biobehav Rev 2007;1:125–47.
61. Giménez-Llort L, Blázquez G, Cañete T, Rosa R, Vivo M, Oddo S, Navarro X, LaFerla FM, Johansson B, Tobeña A, Fernández-Teruel A. Modeling neuropsychiatric symptoms of Alzheimer's disease dementia in 3xTg-AD mice. In: Iqbal K., Winblad B, Avila J, editors. Alzheimer's disease: new advances. Englewood, NJ: Medimond; 2006. p. 513–6.
62. Giménez-Llort L, Torres-Lista V, De la Fuente, M. Crosstalk between behavior and immune system during the prodromal stage of Alzheimer's disease. Curr Pharm Des 2014;20:4723–32.
63. González-Martínez Å, Rosado B, Pesini P, Suárez ML, Santamarina G, García-Belenguer S, Villegas A, Monleón I, Sarasa M. Plasma beta-amyloid peptides in canine aging and cognitive dysfunction as a model of Alzheimer's disease. Exp Gerontol 2011;46:590–6.
64. Gross DR, Tranquilli WJ, Greene SA, Grimm KA. Critical anthropomorphic evaluation and treatment of postoperative pain in rats and mice. J Am Vet Med Assoc 2003;222:1505–10.
65. Han JS, Bird GC, Li W, Jones J, Neugebauer V. Computerized analysis of audible and ultrasonic vocalizations of rats as a standardized measure of pain-related behavior. J Neurosci Methods 2005;141:261–9.
66. Handwerker HO, Arendt-Nielsen L, editors. Pain models: translational relevance and applications. Washington, DC: International Association for the Study of Pain/IASP Press; 2013.
67. Hattori M, Fujiyama A, Taylor TD, Watanabe H, Yada T, Park HS, Toyoda A, Ishii K, Totoki Y, Choi DK, et al. The DNA sequence of human chromosome 21. Nature 2000;18:405:311–9. Erratum in: Nature 2000;407:110.
68. Hawkins P. Recognizing and assessing pain, suffering and distress in laboratory animals: a survey of current practice in the UK with recommendations. Lab Anim 2002;36:378–95.
69. Head E. A canine model of human aging and Alzheimer's disease. Biochim Biophys Acta 2013;1832:1384–9.
70. Henze DA, Urban MO. Large animal models for pain therapeutic development (Chapter 17). In: Kruger L, Light AR, editors. Translational pain research: from mouse to man. Boca Raton, FL: CRC Press; 2010.
71. Herr K, Bjoro K, Decker S. Tools for assessment of pain in nonverbal older adults in dementia: A state-of-the-science review. J Pain Symptom Manag 2006; 31:170–92.
72. Hjortsjö CH. Man's face and mimic language. Lund, Sweden: Student Litteratur; 1969.
73. Holtzman DM, Santucci D, Kilbridge J, Chua-Couzens J, Fontana DJ, Daniels SE, Johnson RM, Chen K, Sun Y, Carlson E, et al. Developmental abnormalities and age-related neurodegeneration in a mouse model of Down syndrome. Proc Natl Acad Sci USA 1996;93:13333–8.
74. Hsiao K, Chapman P, Nilsen S, Eckman C, Harigaya Y, Younkin S, Yang F, Cole G. Correlative memory deficits, Abeta elevation, and amyloid plaques in transgenic mice. Science 1996;274:99–102.
75. Husebo B, Achterberg WP, Lobbezoo F, Kunz M, Lautenbacher S, Kappesser J, Tudose C, Strand LI. Pain in patients with dementia: a review of pain assessment and treatment challenges. Nor Epidemiol 2012;22:243–51.
76. International Association for the Study of Pain (IASP). [Web page on the Internet]. Washington: IASP. Accessed at http://www.iasp-pain.org/
77. Janus C, Westaway D. Transgenic mouse models of Alzheimer's disease. Physiol Behav 2001;73:873–86.
78. Jensen-Dahm C, Werner MU, Dahl JB, Jensen TS, Ballegaard M, Hejl AM, Waldemar G. Quantitative sensory testing and pain tolerance in patients with mild to moderate Alzheimer's disease compared to healthy control subjects. Pain 2014;155:1439–46. doi:10.1016/j.pain.2013.12.031
79. Johansson B, Halldner L, Dunwiddie TV, Masino SA, Poelchen W, Giménez-Llort L, Escorihuela RM, Fernández-Teruel A, Wiesenfeld-Hallin Z, Xu XJ, et al. Hyperalgesia, anxiety, and decreased hypoxic neuroprotection in mice lacking the adenosine A1 receptor. Proc Natl Acad Sci USA. 2001;98:9407–12.
80. Joshi SK, Honore P. Animal models of pain for drug discovery. Expert Opin Drug Discov 2006;1:323–34.
81. Jourdan D, Ardid D, Eschalier A. Analysis of ultrasonic vocalization does not allow chronic pain to be evaluated in rats. Pain 2002;95:165–73.
82. Keefe FJ, Fillingim RB, Williams DA. Behavioral assessment of pain: nonverbal measures in animals and humans. ILAR 1991;33:3–13.
83. Kilkenny C, Browne WJ, Cuthill IC, Emerson M, Altman DG. Improving bioscience research reporting: The ARRIVE guidelines for reporting animal research. PLoS Biol 2010;8:e1000412.
84. Kleschevnikov AM, Belichenko PV, Salehi A, Wu C. Discoveries in Down syndrome: moving basic science to clinical care. Prog Brain Res 2012;197:199–221.
85. Korenberg JR. Mental modeling, Nat Genet 1995;11:109–11.
86. Kotulska K, Larysz-brysz M, LePecheur M, Marcol W, Olakowska E, Lewin-Kowalik J, London J. APP/SOD1 overexpressing mice present reduced neuropathic pain sensitivity. Brain Res Bull 2011; 85:321–8.

87. LaCroix-Fralish ML, Austin JS, Zheng FY, Levitin DJ, Mogil JS. Patterns of pain: meta-analysis of microarray studies of pain. Pain 2011;152:1888–98.
88. Lalonde R, Dumont M, Paly E, London J, Strazielle C. Characterization of hemizygous SOD1/wild-type transgenic mice with the SHIRPA primary screen and tests of sensorimotor function and anxiety. Brain Res Bull 2004;64:251–8.
89. Landsberg GM, Denenberg S, Araujo J. Cognitive dysfunction in cats. A syndrome we used to dismiss as old age. J Fel Med Surg 2010;12:837–48.
90. Landsberg GM, Nichol J, Araujo JA. Cognitive dysfunction syndrome: a disease of canine and feline brain aging. Vet Clin North Am Small Anim Pract 2012;42:749–68
91. Langford DJ, Bailey AL, Chanda ML, Clarke SE, Drummond TE, Echols S, Glick S, Ingrao J, Klassen-Ross T, Lacroix-Fralish ML, et al. Coding of facial expressions of pain in the laboratory mouse. Nat Methods 2010;7:447–9.
92. Lautenbacher S, Niewelt BG, Kunz M. Decoding pain from the facial display of patients with dementia: a comparison of professional and nonprofessional observers. Pain Med 2013;14:469–77.
93. Le Bars D, Gozariu M, Cadden SW. Animal models of nociception. Pharmacol Rev 2001;59:597–652.
94. Lehner M, Taracha E, Skórzweska A, Maciejak P, Wislowska-Stanek A, Zienowicz M, Szyndler J, Bidzinski A, Plaznik A. Behavioral, immunocytochemical and biochemical studies in rats differing in their sensitivity to pain. Behav Brain Res 2006;171:189–98.
95. Levin ED, Buccafussco JJ. Animal models of cognitive impairment. Boca Raton, FL: CRC Press, 2006.
96. Lighthall JW, Dixon CE, Anderson TE. Experimental models of brain injury. J Neurotrauma 1989;6:83–97.
97. Lim Hy, Albuquerque B, Häussler A, Myrczek T, Ding A, Tegeder I. Progranulin contributes to endogenous mechanisms of pain defence after nerve injury in mice. J Cell Mol Med 2012;16:708–21.
98. Linder SL. Post-traumatic headache. Curr Pain Headache Rep 2007;11:396–400.
99. Liu M-G, Chen J. Preclinical research on pain comorbidity with affective disorders and cognitive deficits: challenges and perspectives. Prog Neurobiol 2014;116:13–32. doi:10.1016/j.neurobio.2014.01.003.
100. Livingston A. Ethical issues regarding pain in animals. J Am Vet Med Assoc. 2002;221:229–33.
101. Livingston A. Pain and analgesia in domestic animals. Comparative and veterinary pharmacology, In: Cunningham F, editor. Handbook of experimental pharmacology, Vol. 199. Berlin: Springer-Verlag; 2010. p. 159–89.
102. Loeser JD, Treede RD. The Kyoto protocol of IASP basic pain terminology. 2008;137:473–7.
103. Lucas JJ, Hernández F, Gómez-Ramos P, Morán MA, Hen R, Avila J. Decreased nuclear beta-catenin, tau hiperphosphorylation and neurodegeneration in GSK-3beta conditional transgenic mice. EMBO J 2001;20:27–39.
104. Lukas A, Schuler M, Fischer TW, Gibson SJ, Savvas SM, Nikolaus T, Denkinger M. Pain and dementia: a diagnostic challenge. Z Gerontol Geriat 2012; 45:45–9.
105. Martin WJ. Pain processing: paradoxes and predictions. Pain Pract 2001;1:2–10.
106. Martínez-Clue C, Baamonde C, Lumbreras MA, Vallina IF, Dierssen M, Flórez J. A murine model for Down síndrome shows reduced responsiveness to pain. Neuro Rep 1999;10:1119–22.
107. McGuire BE, Kennedy S. Pain in people with an intellectual disability. Curr Opin Psychiatry 2013; 26:270–5.
108. Milgram NW, Head E, Weiner E, Thomas E. Cognitive functions and aging in the dog: acquisition of nonspatial visual tasks. Behav Neurosci 1994;108:57–68.
109. Mogil JS. Animal models of pain: progress and challenges. Nat Rev 2009;10:283–94.
110. Mogil JS, Grisel JE. Transgenic studies of pain. Pain 1998;77:107–28.
111. Mogil JS, Lichtensteiger CA, Wilson SG. The effect of genotype on sensitivity to inflammatory nociception: characterization of resistant (A/J) and sensitive (C57BL/6J) inbred mouse strains. Pain 1998;76:115–25.
112. Mogil JS, Ritchie J, Sotocinal SG, Smith SB, Croteau S, Levitin DJ, Naumova AK. Screening for pain phenotypes: analysis of three congenic mouse strains on a battery of nine nociceptive assays. Pain 2006;126:24–34.
113. Nieminen K, Suarez-Isla BA, Rapoport SI. Electrical properties of cultured dorsal root ganglion neurons from normal and trisomy 21 human fetal tissue. Brain Res 1988;474:246–54.
114. Oddo S, Caccamo A, Shepherd JD, Murphy MP, Golde TE, Kayed R, Metherate R, Mattson MP, Akbari Y, LaFerla FM. Triple-transgenic model of Alzheimer's disease with plaques and tangles: intracellular Abeta and synaptic dysfunction. Neuron 2003;39:409–21.
115. Orlans FB. Animal pain scales in public policy. ATLA Abstr 1990;18:41–50.
116. Pick CG, Cheng J, Paul D, Pasternak GW. Genetic influences in opioid analgesic sensitivity in mice. Brain Res 1991;566:295–8.

117. Reeves RH, Irving NG, Moran TH, Wohn A, Kitt C, Sisodia SS, Schmidt C, Bronson RT, Davisson MT. A mouse model for Down syndrome exhibits learning and behaviour deficits. Nat Genet 1995;11:177–84.
118. Reisberg b, Borenstein J, Salb SP, Ferris SH, Franssen E, Georgotas A. Behavioral symptoms in Alzheimer's disease phenomenology and treatment. J Clin Psychiatry 1987;48:9–15.
119. Riggio S, Wong M. Neurobehavioral sequelae of traumatic brain injury. Mt Sinai J Med 2009; 76:163–72.
120. Rodríguez-Navarro JA, Gómez A, Rodal I, Perucho J, Martínez A, Furio V, Ampuero I, Casarejos MJ, Solano RM, de Yebenes JG, Mena MA. Parkin deletion causes cerebral and systemic amyloidosis in human mutated tau overexpressing mice. Hum Mol Genet 2008;17:3128–43.
121. Rogers DC, Fisher EMC, Brown SDM, Peters J, Hunter AJ, Martin JE. Behavioral and functional analysis of mouse phenotype: SHIRPA, a proposed protocol for comprehensive phenotype assessment. Mamm Genome 1997;8:711–3.
122. Roughan JV, Flecknell PA. Effects of surgery and analgesic administration on spontaneous behaviour in singly housed rats. Res Vet Sci 2000;69:283–8.
123. Roughan JV, Flecknell PA. Pain assessment and control in laboratory animals. Lab Anim 2003;37:172.
124. Ryder RD. Experiments on Animals. In: Godlovitch S, Godlovitch R, Harris J, editors. Animals, men and morals. London: Victor Gollanz; 1971. p. 41–82.
125. Salehi A, Faizi M, Belichenko PV, Mobley WC. Using mouse models to explore genotype-phenotype relationship in Down syndrome. Ment Retard Dev Disabil Res Rev 2007;13:207–14.
126. Saraceno C, Musardo S, Marcello E, Pelucchi S, Luca MD. Modeling Alzheimer's disease: from past to future. Front Pharmacol 2013;4:77. doi:10.3389/fphar.2013.00077
127. Sarasa M. Experimental animal models for Alzheimer's disease. Rev Neurol 2006;42:297–301.
128. Schliebs R, Rossner S, Bigl V. Immunolesion by 192IgG-saporin of rat basal forebrain cholinergic system: a useful tool to produce cortical cholinergic dysfunction. Prog Brain Res 1996;109:253–64.
129. Schroeter ML, Raczka K, Neumann J, von Cramon DY. Neural networks infrontotemporal dementia—a meta-analysis. Neurobiol Aging 2008;29:418–26.
130. Seifert TD, Evans RW. Posttraumatic headache: a review. Curr Pain Headache Rep 2010;14:292–8.
131. Selkoe DJ. The deposition of amyloid proteins in the aging mammalian brain: implications for Alzheimer's disease. Ann Med 1989;21:73–6.
132. Selkoe DJ. Alzheimer's disease: genes, proteins and therapy. Physiol Rev 2001;81:741–66.
133. Sherrington CS. The integrative action of the nervous system. New Haven: Yale University Press; 1906.
134. Silver JM, McAllister TW, Arciniegas DB. Depression and cognitive complaints following mild traumatic brain injury. Am J Psychiatry 2009;166:653–61.
135. Sotocinal SG, Sorge RE, Zaloum A, Tuttle AH, Martin LJ, Wieskopf JS, Mapplebeck JC, Wei P, Zhan S, Zhang S, et al. The Rat Grimace Scale: a partially automated method for quantifying pain in the laboratory rat via facial expressions. Mol Pain 2011;7:55. doi:10.1186/1744-8069-7-55.
136. Stasiak KL, Maul D, French E, Hellyer P, Vandewoude S. Species-specific assessment of pain in laboratory animals. Contemp Top Lab Anim Sci 2003;42:13–20.
137. Takeuchi H, Iba M, Inoue H, Higuchi M, Takao K, Tsukita K, Karatsu Y, Iwamoto Y, Miyakawa T, Suhara T, et al. P301S mutant human tau transgenic mice manifest early symptoms of human taupathies with dementia and altered sensorimotor gating. PLoS One 2011;6:1–14, e21050.
138. Vaishnavi S, Rao V, Fann JR. Neuropsychiatric problems after traumatic brain injury: unraveling the silent epidemic. Psychosomatics 2009;50:198–205.
139. Valkenburg AJ, van Dijk M, de Klein A, van den Anker JN, Tibboel D. Pain management in intellectually disabled children. Dev Disabil Res Rev 2010;16:248–57.
140. Vink R, van den Heuvel C. Substance P antagonists as a therapeutic approach to improving outcome following brain injury. Neurotherapeutics 2010;7:74–80.
141. Wallace VCJ, Norbury TA, Rice ASC. Ultrasound vocalization by rodents does not correlate with behavioural measures of persistent pain. Eur J Pain 2005;9:445–52.
142. Williams WO, Riskin DK, Mott KM. Ultrasonic sound as an indicator of acute pain in laboratory mice. J Am Assoc Lab Anim Sci 2008;47:8–10.
143. Woolfe G, MacDonald AD. The evaluation of the analgesic action of pethidine hydrochloride Demerol. J Pharmacol Exp Ther 1944;80:300–7.
144. Zaloshnja E, Miller T, Langlois JA, Selassie AW. Prevalence of long-term disability from traumatic brain injury in the civilian population of the United States, 2005. J Head Trauma Rehabil 2008;23:394–400.
145. Zhao M-G, Toyoda J, Ko SW, Ding H-K, Wu L-J, Zhuo M. Deficits in trace fear memory and long-term potentiation in a mouse model for Fragile X Syndrome. Neurobiol Dis 2005;25:7385–92.
146. Zimmermann M. Ethical guidelines for investigations of experimental pain in conscious animals. Pain 1983;16:109–10.

CHAPTER 27

Future Direction of Research

Stefan Lautenbacher, Wilco P. Achterberg, Elizabeth L. Sampson, and Miriam Kunz

After a book of many chapters about pain in dementia, it might appear redundant to highlight special directions of development of future research because the authors have all made educated guesses about future directions for their respective fields. However, a shortlist of hot topics may not be comprehensive and may even appear biased but is in its special form definitive thought-provoking and communication-promoting. Therefore, the present authors have intensively discussed and compiled some ideas they found especially relevant for future directions of research on pain in dementia. They hope to hereby elicit active formation of opinions and (re)start scientific dialogues.

NEW PERSPECTIVES ON PAIN MANAGEMENT IN DEMENTIA

Over the years, many reports have been on the undertreatment of pain in persons with dementia, and this is reflected in many chapters of this book. After the study by Ferrell et al. [12], many other scholars have showed lower rates of pharmacological pain treatment in people with cognitive impairment. This holds for studies in the community, in residential settings and nursing homes, and also in acute and postoperative hospital patients [7, 28, 29].

Several factors are thought to contribute to this undertreatment [1]. First, older patients might complain less about their pain to their doctors because they want to be "a good patient," or because they have many other ailments to complain about, or because they believe that pain is a normal part of aging. Second, they may not be able to complain about pain because of cognitive impairment or aphasia, hampering their ability to communicate about pain with their doctor. Third, doctors may be unwilling to treat pain rigorously because they also believe that pain is associated with normal aging (a form of ageism). Some might be willing to treat, but have difficulty in making an accurate pain diagnosis because of the cognitive and communicative barriers; moreover, they may be reluctant to add yet another medication for a patient with a vulnerable body and brain that already suffers from polypharmacy. In addition, worldwide, long-term care has suffered from a lack of good medical care and sound implementation of knowledge regarding adequate pain assessment and pain management.

Recent literature however seems to contradict the fact that persons with dementia suffer from pain undertreatment. For instance, analgesic prescription in Norwegian nursing homes increased by 65%, with paracetamol prescription increasing by 113% between 2000 and 2011 [33]. The greatest change was seen in the use of strong opioids: an increase from

1.9% in 2000 to 17.9% in 2011. Interestingly, patients with dementia no longer had lower levels of analgesic prescription. Therefore, one might conclude that, after all those years of poor pain management in people with dementia or long-term care, treatment is finally at a satisfactory level. Several other recent studies also showed higher levels of pharmacological pain management in older people and people with dementia [14, 26].

In the United Kingdom, the prescription of strong opioids has risen substantially, especially in noncancer patients, women, and those aged 66–80 years [40]. However, we should be cautious about being too enthusiastic about this—at first sight—marked improvement. Having higher aggregate prescription rates does not tell us anything about the appropriateness of the prescriptions. Several trials on short-term pharmacological pain management in patients with dementia have pointed out the beneficial effects on their emotional well-being, agitation, and mood [6, 19, 20]. Although short-term pharmacological pain interventions (also with stronger opioids) after proper assessment and including adequate evaluation are without doubt desirable, there is no evidence for the efficacy of long-term use without proper assessment and evaluation. Especially the introduction of fentanyl and buprenorphine patches seems to have accelerated long-term opioid use in vulnerable older patients. In Denmark, 41% of nursing home residents and 27.5% of the dementia community-based population now use an opioid, which definitely raises questions about appropriateness and safety [22]. Sound pain management is surely not just supplying patches for many years as a panacea for all problems of people with dementia [1]. We have a long way to go because, for instance, studies on the pharmacodynamics and pharmacokinetics of pain medication in persons with cognitive impairment are almost completely missing in action (see Chapter 18). We do not know how the potential lack of placebo effect (see Chapter 21) relates to preferred dosage of pain medication in patients with advanced Alzheimer's disease. We also have controversies about the potential side effects of opioids in patients with dementia: are they more prone for delirium? Although we see in practice that this is one of the reasons why opioids are withheld in acute care settings, there is little evidence that opioids in dementia will indeed lead to delirium [15].

Good assessment and evaluation of pain treatment is still considered poorly implemented in all sectors of care. Adequate pain measurement instruments for people with dementia are rarely used properly [10]. Stepped-treatment approaches to address pain, with a full medical review and personalized nonpharmacological "comfort" approaches before escalating to pharmacological treatment, are recommended, but are often not put into practice [2]:

To date, there is no pain management protocol for persons with impaired cognition that takes into account the many aspects that are covered in this book, such as valid assessment, evaluation, biological, psychological and cultural influences, relation to correlates of pain (such as neuropsychiatric symptoms and functional impairment), and benefits as well as harms of both pharmacological and psychosocial interventions. Also the practical aspects of pain management in different settings, such as acute hospital care, community care, palliative care and long-term care, have not been established.

International research on pain in persons with impaired cognition from the last 15 years definitively has had impact on clinical practice: in some countries and settings the awareness of potential undertreatment has risen. However, we have little evidence that this is based on thorough assessment and evaluation. *The message from some of the recent studies mentioned is hopeful, but we need more longitudinal and in-depth studies on the indications and duration as well as the beneficial and harmful effects of pain management (also nonpharmacological) in persons with impaired cognition.*

QUEST FOR A GENERALLY ACCEPTED TOOL FOR PAIN ASSESSMENT IN PEOPLE WITH DEMENTIA

A number of observational and informant-based assessment tools have been developed over the last 20 years based on identification of specific behaviors, many of which align closely with the AGS guidelines [3]. The tools are applied by a proxy rater, usually a caregiver (health professional or family carer) who is familiar with the individual, and combines observation of behaviors, emotions, interactions, and facial expressions. A number of systematic reviews have examined the range of tools currently available for use in dementia. One recent review concludes that there are 12 promising pain assessment tools available, but most of these require further validation in people with dementia and for day-to-day use in clinical settings [11]. While many of the available tools have been developed through robust methodology, including intensive observation in the clinic, consultation with users and patients, and refinement of items, the existing tools are disparate and there is no one universal tool. In particular, while there is large agreement between existing tools on the concepts for pain assessment, there is great disparity in the methods by which they are operationalized. Importantly, existing tools frequently lack comprehensive data on face and construct validity, reliability, and responsiveness (see Chapter 10). Few specify the specific situation in which assessment should take place, for example during rest, guided movement, or during daily activities, nor have the majority been developed for ease of use in clinical settings and clinical utility. As a result, no truly universal tool for pain detection in dementia exists. There remains an urgent need to draw on the currently available resources and to develop an easy-to-use assessment tool which has utility in both research and clinical settings, and robust validation data to support its implementation.

To address this, the EU-COST[1] Action "Pain in impaired cognition, especially dementia" decided to develop a meta-tool based on the best of the available tools for pain assessment in dementia [10]. The decision to create a meta-tool based on existing instruments was informed by a thorough review of the literature and current clinical practice which revealed the absence of a single tool for use in all settings which is embedded in the practicalities of clinical practice and user-based design. *The initiative aims to develop a truly unique meta-tool which, instead of being developed from patient observations, is based on the scrutiny and inclusion of items from existing assessment tools based on empirical evaluation of each item.* This innovative approach ensures that the best, most informative items are used. Furthermore, the meta-tool will form part of a more comprehensive toolkit which will provide supporting resources and guidance to capture the nuances of pain in dementia including the specific needs of assessing pain in different locations and settings, and to support decision-making regarding the most suitable treatment.

Since this approach requires joint forces of many experts and may fail, it remains favorable to back up such approaches by further validation and improvements attempts of the existing tools. The glut of preexisting pain assessment tools favor strict criteria for the development of further tools without urgent necessity. One acceptable reason may be specific scopes of application as detailed in the present chapter.

---

[1]European Cooperation in Science and Research

ADDING TOOLS FOR SPECIFIC PAINS

The commonest causes of pain in people with dementia are musculoskeletal, gastrointestinal and cardiac conditions, genitourinary infections, pressure ulcers, and oral pain [10]. Neuropathic pain is also common and likely to be undertreated compared with other types of pain [35]. *Thus, to give a comprehensive picture of the pain a person with dementia is suffering from, tools should facilitate the assessment of the location of pain.* Chronic pain is particularly difficult to detect, and therefore, there is increasing interest in developing tools which detect pain of specific parts of the body or etiologies. Back pain is one such area, and an observational scale for back pain in people with dementia is currently in development [25]. This approach takes into account the need to assess specific features of musculoskeletal back pain, for example, body positions and postures, muscle stiffness and changes in movement patterns, and intensification of paratonia.

Another example of this developing field of "assessments" for specific pain is oral pain. Poor dentition and mouth care is very common in older people with dementia, particularly care home residents, yet none of the currently available tools for the assessment of pain in nonverbal individuals are designed to specifically assess orofacial or dental pain (see Chapter 12). Specific items, which may prove more reliable in detecting orofacial pain include the patient holding or rubbing the orofacial area, limiting their mandibular movements and lack of cooperation or resistance to oral care. Thus, an advantage of developing a comprehensive, multidisciplinary "toolkit" for the assessment of pain in dementia is that specific pain tools such as an Orofacial Pain Scale for Nonverbal Individuals can be included (see Chapter 12).

DIFFERENTIATING PAIN AND DISCOMFORT FROM A PALLIATIVE CARE PERSPECTIVE

Pain tools assume the source of observed discomfort is pain; however, as person with dementia approaches the end of life, a palliative care approach may be more appropriate and then wider concepts such as discomfort are important. Discomfort can be caused by factors other than "nociceptive" stimuli such as feeling too hot or cold, psychological distress, boredom or poor positioning. *The future development of tools to be used at the end of life in dementia requires reference to theoretical frameworks, and the selection of items in the development process, with consideration of similar tools, to provide an optimal item pool representing probable pain or probable discomfort in patients with severe dementia or at the end of life* [37]. To improve the (re)development and testing of pain and (dis)comfort tools for people with advanced dementia or those who may be dying, we should evaluate separate items and consider the dual constructs of pain and discomfort in parallel (see Chapter 22). Moreover, validity testing of pain tools should include patients at the end of life, where assessment of pain and discomfort can be very challenging.

THE FUTURE OF AUTOMATIC PAIN ASSESSMENT WITH VIDEO SYSTEMS

Despite promising developments, pain assessment in people with dementia is still challenging and often erroneous (see Chapters 9 and 10). Some of the reasons for this are time constraints of care takers, difficulty of observing patients pain behavior while simultaneously providing care, the subtle and transitory indicators of some pain behaviors (e.g., facial expressions), the difficulty of differentiating pain from other causes of distress, and observer biases that might hinder correct pain assessment.

New developments in automatic pain detection systems hold the promise that such systems might help to overcome some of the aforementioned problems. Although automatic pain detection systems can never fully substitute a human observer or caregiver, they could be used as a complementary instrument supporting the human caregiver [16]. Thus, such systems could unburden nurses and caregivers and give them more time for the psychosocial and empathic side of human care. Most attempts to develop automatic pain detection systems have focused on the automatic analysis of facial expressions, although other indicators like physiological signals such as skin conductance, pupil dilatation, and electrocardiogram (ECG) may be useful and added [36]. However, the facial expression promises best discriminative validity and, thus, better pain specificity compared to these other indicators, which often cannot differentiate the specific type of distress.

The video-based automatic pain detection systems would especially be feasible for patients with dementia who are immobile and are lying in bed. Given the technical solutions available at the moment, the reliable capture of the face will be possible only when the range of motions of the face is limited. Patients with dementia lying in bed (e.g., postsurgery, palliative care stage) can be expected to present enough facial aspects in frontal and lateral views to allow video systems to detect the relevant facial expressions of pain.

In the last decade, several preliminary systems have been developed with different aims of assessment. These aims were differentiate pain versus no pain [27], genuine versus faked pain [4], pain versus other emotions [18], and differentiation of different pain intensity [17]. So far, none of these systems focused on pain in people with dementia but focused more on pain detection in young or middle aged individuals. In the context of pain assessment in people with dementia, the first objective of an automatic pain detection system should be to correctly answer the question: Is that person in pain or is the facial expression due to other forms of distress? The second objective to be achieved will be to grade the intensity of pain.

The automatic detection of pain and intensity of pain from facial expressions is usually performed as a single or a two-level detection process. In a single detection process, image sequences are processed and based on changes in predefined facial feature characteristics, the systems tries to detect pain [21, 39]. In the two-level detection process, image sequences are first processed for detecting single facial motions and coding them in terms of the Facial Action Coding System (FACS) (namely as AUs) (see Chapter 11). Then (in a second step), the detected AUs and their intensities are processed to determine the likelihood of the presence and intensity of pain according to some thumb rules based on the available literature [4]. All automatic pain detection systems define numerical features describing the geometric shape or textural appearance of the face. In order to assess dynamic facial expressions, the defined features are extracted over multiple images within a certain time interval [21] and these extracted features are processed using various machine learning methods in order to detect pain.

Although the process in the development of automatic pain detection system is very impressive, there are still several obstacles that need to be overcome in order to be able to use these automatic pain detection systems for pain assessment in people with dementia. First of all, most of these systems have been developed using video recordings of facial expressions of pain in young or middle aged individuals. Given the enormous age-related changes in facial appearance, especially due to wrinkles, it is questionable whether the systems and their defined features are able to correctly detect facial movements in elderly faces. Especially those systems that rely mostly on texture information (wrinkles are interpreted to be a result of facial muscle movements) will lead to many false-positive errors in people with dementia. Second, most automatic pain detection systems were trained with video recordings of facial expressions during painful situations but not with facial expressions occurring during other types of negative emotions. Thus, the systems will not be able to validly differentiate between pain and other types of distress. Third, most systems were developed to find characteristic facial features indicative for pain in a large sample of individuals but did not undertake a more individualized approach. Given that we know that facial responses to pain vary between individuals [23] (see Chapter 11), it would be advisable to develop automatic pain detection systems that are also able to learn individual-specific characteristics indicative of pain.

In summary, the development of automatic pain detection systems holds great promises for a better detection of pain in people with dementia. Although several groups have started to develop such systems—relying mostly on video recordings of facial expressions—these systems are not yet ready to be used for clinical pain detection in patients with dementia. But given the fast development in this area, one can surely expect such systems to be available within the next decade.

BETTER USE OF NEUROPSYCHOLOGICAL TESTS

The question has remained which types of neuropathological changes and cognitive impairments associated with different forms of dementia are of particular relevance when changes in nociception and pain processing are under investigation. Several routes exist in order to answer these questions.

Definitely, studying subtypes of dementia is a necessity. Studies investigating the prevalence of pain in dementia subtypes have yet been rare (see Chapter 3). There seems to be a high prevalence of pain in dementia without significant differences between the dementia subtypes [38]. However, minor differences between subgroups may exist with potentially meaningful associations to brain pathology. For example, Fletcher et al. [13] found patients with frontotemporal lobe degeneration to be most affected by alterations in pain processing. From the experimental perspective, Carlino et al. [5] also reported findings suggestive of some differences between dementia subgroups. A lot of work has to be done following this line of reasoning, including large-scale multicenter studies, which guarantee the appropriate number of patients for epidemiologic research.

A tool, which has promised new insights into the association between dementia-related neurodegeneration and pain for many years, is of course magnet resonance imaging (MRI) in its structural and functional versions. Studies using this tool are still scarce (see Chapter 5). As just mentioned, Fletcher et al. [13] reported on a structural link between affection of the frontotemporal lobes and major changes in pain processing studying patients with dementia. Oosterman et al. [31] could demonstrate that white matter lesions (mainly periventricular hyperintensities) are associated with enhancement of affective pain processing. Cole et al. [8, 9] showed more single-area and network-related brain activity during noxious stimulation in patients with Alzheimer disease. These findings—although promising—represent at the moment more patchwork than systematic research. A likely excuse is that studying patients with cognitive impairment in the scanner is a major stress to the individuals, who do not understand the reasons for staying in a restricted and uncomfortable environment for an unforeseeable time. Thus, such ethical and methodological problems may limit this type of studies also in the future.

Such negative expectations as regards future use do not apply for better and more frequent application of neuropsychological tests. Evidence has accumulated that especially deterioration of forebrain-based processes indicated by neuropsychological tests of executive functions is associated with pathological changes in pain processing [24, 30, 34]. Thus, screening for dysexecutive syndromes may help to identify those patients, who are especially vulnerable for the development of pain problems. Furthermore, tests of explicit memory may help to grade the type and severity of dementia. The same tests in addition to tests of attention inform the investigators what quality of results can be expected when performing neuropsychological tests and self-report surveys. *Therefore, short test batteries of executive functions, memory, and attention are helpful for a better understanding of patients with increased pain vulnerability, their type and severity of dementia, as well as their testability and thus ought to be compiled on the basis of established tests for this purpose.*

INNOVATION MANAGEMENT

Despite the fact that we have some valid and reliable pain and discomfort tools and increased clinical interest in pain detection and management in people with dementia, studies show that pain remains poorly managed in this population [32]. Data on the feasibility of pain tools ("applicability in daily practice," including aspects such as ease of use and time to administer it) and clinical utility ("the usefulness of the measure for decision making," i.e., to inform further action, such as the administration of analgesics) are very limited. Research on how tools can be most effectively implemented in practice is lacking and requires more work in future to fully ensure that better assessment of pain and discomfort leads to better treatment and improved outcomes for people with dementia. *Research projects identifying the implementation barriers against new diagnostics and therapies in institutions and societies as well as developing strategies of how to remove these barriers are required to prepare innovation management.*

REFERENCES

1. Achterberg, WP. Pain management in long-term care: are we finally on the right track?. Age Ageing 2016; 45:7–8.
2. Achterberg WP, Pieper MJ, van Dalen-Kok AH, de Waal MW, Husebø BS, Lautenbacher S, Kunz M, Scherder EJ, Corbett A. Pain management in patients with dementia. Clin Interv Aging 2013;8:1471–82.
3. AGS Panel on Persistent Pain in Older Persons. The management of persistent pain in older persons. J Am Geriatr Soc 2002;50:S205–224.
4. Bartlett MS, Littlewort GC, Frank MG, Lee K. Automatic decoding of facial movements reveals deceptive pain expressions. Curr Biol 2014;24:738–43.
5. Carlino E, Benedetti F, Rainero I, Asteggiano G, Cappa G, Tarenzi L, Vighetti S, Pollo A. Pain perception and tolerance in patients with frontotemporal dementia. Pain 2010;151:783–9.
6. Chibnall JT, Tait RC, Harman B, Luebbert RA. Effect of acetaminophen on behavior, well-being, and psychotropic medication use in nursing home residents with moderate-to-severe dementia. J Am Geriatr Soc 2005;53:1921–9.
7. Closs SJ, Barr B, Briggs M. Cognitive status and analgesic provision in nursing home residents. Br J Gen Pract 2004;54: 919–21.

8. Cole LJ, Farrell MJ, Duff EP, Barber JB, Egan GF, Gibson SJ. Pain sensitivity and fMRI pain-related brain activity in Alzheimer's disease. Brain 2006;129:2957–65.
9. Cole LJ, Gavrilescu M, Johnston LA, Gibson SJ, Farrell MJ, Egan GF. The impact of Alzheimer's disease on the functional connectivity between brain regions underlying pain perception. Eur J Pain 2011;15:568.e1–11.
10. Corbett A, Achterberg W, Husebo B, Lobbezoo F, de Vet H, Kunz M, Strand L, Constantinou M, Tudose C, Kappesser J, et al. An international road map to improve pain assessment in people with impaired cognition: the development of the Pain Assessment in Impaired Cognition (PAIC) meta-tool. BMC Neurol 2014;14:229.
11. Corbett A, Husebo B, Malcangio M, Staniland A, Cohen-Mansfield J, Aarsland D, Ballard C. Assessment and treatment of pain in people with dementia. Nat Rev Neurol 2012;8:264–74.
12. Ferrell BA, Ferrell BR, Rivera L. Pain in cognitively impaired nursing home patients. J Pain Symptom Manag 1995;10:591–8.
13. Fletcher PD, Downey LE, Golden HL, Clark CN, Slattery CF, Paterson RW, Rohrer JD, Schott JM, Rossor MN, Warren JD. Pain and temperature processing in dementia: a clinical and neuroanatomical analysis. Brain 2015;138:3360–72.
14. Haasum Y, Fastbom J, Fratiglioni L, Kareholt I, Johnell K. Pain treatment in elderly persons with and without dementia: a population-based study of institutionalized and home-dwelling elderly. Drugs Aging 2011;28:283–93.
15. Habiger TF, Flo E, Achterberg WP, Husebo BS. The interactive relationship between pain, psychosis, and agitation in people with dementia: Results from a cluster-randomised clinical trial. Behav Neurol 2016;2016:7036415.
16. Hadjistavropoulos T, Herr K, Prkachin KM, Craig KD, Gibson SJ, Lukas A, Smith JH. Pain assessment in elderly adults with dementia. Lancet Neurol 2014;13:1216–27.
17. Hammal Z, Cohn JF. Automatic detection of pain intensity. In: Proceedings of the 14th ACM International Conference on Multimodal Interaction (ICMI); 2012. p. 47–52.
18. Hammal Z, Kunz M. Pain monitoring: a dynamic and context-sensitive system. Pattern Recognit 2012;45:1265–80.
19. Husebo BS, Ballard C, Fritze F, Sandvik RK, Aarsland D. Efficacy of pain treatment on mood syndrome in patients with dementia: a randomized clinical trial. Int J Geriatr Psychiatry 2014;29:828–36.
20. Husebo BS, Ballard C, Sandvik R, Nilsen OB, Aarsland D. Efficacy of treating pain to reduce behavioural disturbances in residents of nursing homes with dementia: cluster randomised clinical trial. BMJ 2011;343:d4065.
21. Irani R, Nasrollahi K, Simon MO, Corneanu CA, Escalera S, Bahnsen C, Lundtoft D, Moeslund TB, Pedersen T, Klitgaa ML, Petrini L. Spatiotemporal analysis of RGB-DT facial images for multimodal pain level recognition. In IEEE Conference on Computer Vision and Pattern Recognition Workshop (CVPRW). Washington, DC: IEEE Computer Society Press; 2015. p. 89–95.
22. Jensen-Dahm C, Gasse C, Astrup A, Mortensen PB, Waldemar G. Frequent use of opioids in patients with dementia and nursing home residents: a study of the entire elderly population of Denmark. Alzheimers Dement 2015;11:691–9.
23. Kunz M, Lautenbacher S. The faces of pain: a cluster analysis of individual differences in facial activity patterns of pain. Eur J Pain 2014;18:813–23.
24. Kunz M, Mylius V, Schepelmann K, Lautenbacher S. Loss in executive functioning best explains changes in pain responsiveness in patients with dementia-related cognitive decline. Behav Neurol 2015;2015:878157.
25. Laekeman M, Bartholomeyczik S, Lautenbacher S. Development of an observational back pain scale for persons with cognitive impairment. In: Conference Paper: EFIC*—9th "Pain in Europe IX" Congress, September; 2015.
26. Lovheim H, Karlsson S, Gustafson Y. The use of central nervous system drugs and analgesics among very old people with and without dementia. Pharmacoepidemiol Drug Saf 2008;17:912–8.
27. Lucey P, Cohn JF, Matthews I, Lucey S, Sridharan S, Howlett J, Prkachin KM. Automatically detecting pain in video through facial action units. IEEE Trans Syst Man Cybern B Cybern 2011;41:664–74.
28. Mäntyselkä P, Hartikainen S, Louhivuori-Laako K, Sulkava R. Effects of dementia on perceived daily pain in home-dwelling elderly people: a population-based study. Age Ageing 2004;33:496–9.
29. Morrison RS, Siu AL. A comparison of pain and its treatment in advanced dementia and cognitively intact patients with hip fracture. J Pain Symptom Manag 2000;19:240–8.
30. Oosterman JM, Traxler J, Kunz M. The influence of executive functioning on facial and subjective pain responses in older adults. Behav Neurol 2016;2016:1984827.
31. Oosterman JM, van Harten B, Weinstein HC, Scheltens P, Scherder EJ. Pain intensity and pain affect in relation to white matter changes. Pain 2006;125:74–81.
32. Sampson EL, White N, Lord K, Leurent B, Vickerstaff V, Scott S, Jones L. Pain, agitation, and behavioural problems in people with dementia admitted to general hospital wards: a longitudinal cohort study. Pain 2015;156:675–83.

33. Sandvik R, Selbaek G, Kirkevold O, Aarsland D, Husebo BS. Analgesic prescribing patterns in Norwegian nursing homes from 2000 to 2011: trend analyses of four data samples. Age Ageing 2016;45:54–60.
34. Scherder EJ, Eggermont L, Plooij B, Oudshoorn J, Vuijk PJ, Pickering G, Lautenbacher S, Achterberg W, Oosterman J. Relationship between chronic pain and cognition in cognitively intact older persons and in patients with Alzheimer's disease. The need to control for mood. Gerontology 2008;54:50–58.
35. Scherder EJ, Plooij B. Assessment and management of pain, with particular emphasis on central neuropathic pain, in moderate to severe dementia. Drugs Aging 2012;29:701–6.
36. Temitayo A, Olugbade MS, Aung H, Bianchi-Berthouze N, Marquardt N, Williams AC. Bimodal detection of painful reaching for chronic pain rehabilitation systems. In: Proceedings of the 16th International Conference on Multimodal Interaction (ICMI); 2014. p. 455–8.
37. van der Steen JT, Sampson EL, Van den Block L, Lord K, Vankova H, Pautex S, Vandervoort A, Radbruch L, Shvartzman P, Sacchi V, et al. Tools to assess pain or lack of comfort in dementia: a content analysis. J Pain Symptom Manag 2015;50:659–75.
38. van Kooten J, Binnekade TT, van der Wouden JC, Stek ML, Scherder EJ, Husebo BS, Smalbrugge M, Hertogh CM. A review of pain prevalence in Alzheimer's, vascular, frontotemporal and Lewy body dementias. Dement Geriatr Cogn Disord 2016;41:220–32.
39. Werner P, Al-Hamadi A, Niese R. Pain recognition and intensity rating based on comparative learning. In:19th IEEE International Conference on Image Processing (ICIP); 2012. p. 2313–6.
40. Zin CS, Chen LC, Knaggs RD. Changes in trends and pattern of strong opioid prescribing in primary care. Eur J Pain 2014;18:1343–51.

INDEX

Page numbers followed by *f* indicate figures; by *t* indicate tables.

A

Abbreviated Mental Test Score (AMTS), 214
Absorption, 245
Advance care planning, dementia and, 4–5
AES. *See* Apathy Evaluation Scale (AES)
Agitation, 79–80
AGS. *See* American Geriatrics Society (AGS)
AMDA pain management guideline. *See* American Medical Directors' Association (AMDA) Pain Management Guideline
American Geriatrics Society (AGS), 181
American Medical Directors' Association (AMDA) Pain Management Guideline, 182
AMTS. *See* Abbreviated Mental Test Score (AMTS)
Animals, cognitively impaired, 345–357
   comorbidity, 348–349
   limitations and confounding factors, 350–351
   models, 351–357
   noiception in models, 347–348
   nonverbal communication in studies, 349–350
   translational relevance of study, 345–346
Apathy Evaluation Scale (AES), 199
ASD. *See* Autism spectrum disorders (ASD)
Australian and New Zealand Society for Geriatric Medicine, 181
Australian Pain Society, 181
Autism spectrum disorders (ASD), 99–100
Autonomic responses, 78–79

B

Barthel index scoring form, 220*t*
BEHAVE-AD. *See* Behavioral Pathology in Alzheimer Disease Rating Scale (BEHAVE-AD)
Behavioral Pathology in Alzheimer Disease Rating Scale (BEHAVE-AD), 195
Behavioral responses, 155–163
   body movements, 161–162
   facial responses, 156–161, 158*f*
   vocalization, 162–163
Behavioral symptoms, assessment of, 194–196, 197*t*, 201*f*
   BEHAVE-AD, 195
   CMAI, 196
   neuropsychiatric inventory, 195

   NOSGER, 195–196
   PAS, 196
Behavioral variant frontotemporal dementia (bvFTD), 23
Behavioral and psychological symptoms of dementia (BPSD), 86, 248–249
Body movements (pain), 161–162
BPI-SF. *See* Brief pain inventory (BPI-SF)
BPSD. *See* Behavioral and psychological symptoms of dementia (BPSD)
Brain
   dementia related brain changes, 59–62
   neuroimaging of Alzheimer disease, 56–57
Brief pain inventory (BPI-SF), 124–125
The British National Guideline for Assessment of Pain in Older People, 183

C

CDR Scale. *See* Clinical Dementia Rating (CDR) Scale
Cerebral palsy, 100
CGA. *See* Comprehensive Geriatric Assessment (CGA)
Chochinov, H., 2
Chronic pain, definition, 46, 47*t*
Clinical Dementia Rating (CDR) Scale, 225
CMAI. *See* Cohen-Mansfield Agitation Inventory (CMAI)
Cognitive assessment tools, 209–216
Cognitive function, exercise and, 258–261
   cross-sectional and longitudinal studies, 258
   practical considerations, 260–261
   program selection, 260–261
   trials, randomized controlled, 259–260
Cognitive screening, dementia, 209–216
   biomedical examination, 212, 212*t*
   domains measured by tools, 213*t*
   history, 209–211
   management, 215–216
   mental state examination, 211
   neuropsychological assessment, 215
   physical examination, 211
Cohen-Mansfield Agitation Inventory (CMAI), 196
Comprehensive Geriatric Assessment (CGA), 306
Cornell Scale for Depression in Dementia (CSDD), 198

Cross-cultural considerations, 331–341
  approaches, 331–332
  care settings, difference in, 336–339
  dementia and, 335–336
  nonpharmacological treatment, 341
  pain assessment instruments, 339–340
    behavioral assessment instruments, 340
    self-report, 339–340
CSDD. *See* Cornell Scale for Depression in Dementia (CSDD)
Culture. *See also* Cross-cultural considerations
  defined, 332
  and dementia, 335–336
  and pain, 332–335

D
Dementia
  advance care planning, 9
  Alzheimer's disease, 16–19
    diagnosis, 17–18
    genetic risk factors, 17
    pathology, 17
    treatment, 18–19
  in animals, cognitively impaired, 345–357
    comorbidity, 348–349
    limitations and confounding factors, 350–351
    models, 351–357
    noiception in models, 347–348
    nonverbal communication in studies, 349–350
    translational relevance of study, 345–346
  causes of, 16–19, 18f, 19f
  central pathophysiology of, 55–66
  cognitive assessment tools, 15
  cognitive screening, 209–216
    biomedical examination, 212, 212t
    domains measured by tools, 213t
    history, 209–211
    management, 215–216
    mental state examination, 211
    neuropsychological assessment, 215
    physical examination, 211
  culture and. *See* Cross-cultural considerations
  Down's syndrome (DS), 24–25
    diagnosis, 25
    pathology, 24–25
    risk factors, 25
    treatment, 25
  epidemiology of, 44–45, 44t, 45t
  frontotemporal, 23–24
    diagnosis, 23–24
    genetic risk factors, 23
    pathology, 23
    treatment, 23–24
  functional impairment, pain -related, 219–232
  human rights and, 9
  Lewy Body Dementia (LBD), 21–23
  multidisciplinary and multiprofessional treatments, 310–313, 311t
  pain management and, 3–4, 31–39. *See also individual entry*
  palliative care. *See* Palliative care (dementia and pain)
  Parkinson's Disease Dementia (PDD), 21–23
    diagnosis, 22
    genetic risk factors, 22
    pathology, 21–22
    treatment, 22–23
  placebo analgesia, 285–290
    absence of prefrontal control, 288–289
    clinical implications, 289–290
    future directions, 290
    prefrontal areas in, 286–288
  psychological interventions, 267–281. *See also individual entry*
  research ethical issues. *See* Ethical issues (research)
  scope of, 11–26, 12t, 14t
  suffering and, 3
  symptoms and progression of, 12–14, 13f
  treatment of, 14–16
  vascular, 20–21
    diagnosis, 20–21
    pathology, 20
    risk factors, 20
    treatment, 21
Dementia Mood Assessment Scale (DMAS), 198–199
Developmental disability
  clinical implications, 113–114
  definitions, 99–100
  etiology and prevalence, 100–101
  pain
    behavioral indices, 108–111, 110f, 111f
    challenges and biases, 111–112
    exposure to, 101–102
    scaling abilities, 107–108
    sensitivity, 103–107, 104t, 105f, 106f
    undertreatment, 102–103
  self-injurious behavior, 112–113
Dignity
  autonomy, with lack of, 2–3
  cognitive failure, patients with, 5–7
  description, 1–2
DMAS. *See* Dementia Mood Assessment Scale (DMAS)
Down's syndrome (DS), 24–25
  diagnosis, 25
  pathology, 24–25
  risk factors, 25
  treatment, 25

E
Ethical issues (research), 317–327
  assent and dissent, 319–320

INDEX 375

informed consent, 318–319, 321t
　role of assessment tools, 320–322
pain research trials, designing, 322–325
　benefits, 324–325
　experiential pain trials, 323–324
　guidelines, 322–323
　recruitment of participants, 324
　safety and management, 325
　study design, 324
　types of trials, 323
research trials, 317–318
Exercise
　and cognitive function, 258–261
　　cross-sectional and longitudinal studies, 258
　　practical considerations, 260–261
　　program selection, 260–261
　　trials, randomized controlled, 259–260
　and pain management (in dementia), 253–261
　　introduction, 253–254
　　multifactorial chronic pain frameworks, 254
　　outcomes, pain-related, 256–257
　　perception, 255
　　physical activity treatment, considerations of, 257
　　physical therapies, barriers to, 255

F
Facial action coding system (FACS), 108, 155-158, 160
Facial responses (pain), 108–111, 110f, 156–161, 158f
FACS. *See* Facial action coding system (FACS)
FAST. *See* Functional Assessment Staging Test (FAST)
FD. *See* Frontotemporal dementia (FD)
Frontotemporal dementia (FD), 23–24
　diagnosis, 23–24
　genetic risk factors, 23
　lateral pain, 77
　medial pain, 77
　pathology, 23
　treatment, 23–24
Functional Assessment Staging Test (FAST), 225t

G
Geriatric pain measure (GPM), 125
Grimace scale (GS), 349

H
Hope, dementia and, 5
Human rights, dementia and, 9

I
Instrumental Activities of Daily Living scale, 222t
International Classification of Functioning, Disability and Health model, 221–223
Informant Questionnaire on Cognitive Decline in the Elderly (IQCODE), 214, 215t
Informed consent, 7–9

Instrumental Activities of Daily Living (IADL) scale. *See* IADL scale
Intellectual disability (ID), 100
International Interdisciplinary Consensus Statement on Pain Assessment in Older Persons, 182
International Classification of Functioning Disability and Health (ICF) model. *See* ICF model
IQCODE. *See* Informant Questionnaire on Cognitive Decline in the Elderly (IQCODE)

L
LBD. *See* Lewy Body Dementia (LBD)
Lewy Body Dementia (LBD), 21–23

M
MoCA. *See* Montreal Cognitive Assessment (MoCA)
Montreal Cognitive Assessment (MoCA), 214
Mood symptoms, assessment of
　AES, 199
　characteristics of, 201t
　CSDD, 198
　DMAS, 198–199
Multidisciplinary and multiprofessional treatments, 305–313, 308, 309t, 310t, 311t
　approaches, 310–313, 311t
　pain management clinic, 306–310, 308t
　publication bias, 305–306
　　geriatric medicine, 306
　　pain management, 306
Multiple sclerosis
　lateral pain, 78
　medial pain, 78
Multivoxel pattern analysis (MVPA), 65
MVPA. *See* Multivoxel pattern analysis (MVPA)

N
National Nursing Home Pain Collaborative, 182–183
Neuroimaging
　pain, measuring with, 63–66
Neuropathic pain treatment, 247–248
Neuropsychiatric inventory (NPI), 88, 93, 195
Neuropsychiatric symptoms, pain and, 90–92
Neuropsychology, 368–369
Nociception, 345
NOSGER. *See* Nurses' Observation Scale for Geriatric Patients (NOSGER)
NPI. *See* Neuropsychiatric inventory (NPI)
Non-Steroidal Anti-Inflammatory Drugs (NSAIDs), 247
Neuropsychiatry Unit Cognitive Assessment Tool (NUCOG), 214
Nurses' Observation Scale for Geriatric Patients (NOSGER), 195–196

Nursing care, pain management (in dementia), 235–241
    assessment, 237–238
    background and significance, 235
    management, 238
    nonpharmacological treatment, 239–240
    pharmacological treatment, 238–239

O

Observational tools
    assessment of pain, reviews on, 134, 135*t*
    background, 133–134
    practical approaches for pain assessment, 186–187
    specific information, 137*t*–147*t*
Opioid analgesics, 247
Orofacial pain, 167–174, 171*t*, 172*t*
    assessment of, 169–171, 172*t*
    in healthy older persons, 168
    impaired chewing and, 173–174
    new developments in, 172
    in older persons with dementia, 168–169

P

Pain intensity scales, 122–124
Pain assessment
    agitation, relationship to, 79–80
    Alzheimer disease and, 34–36
    in animals, cognitively impaired, 345–357
    autonomic responses, 78–79
    behavioral responses, 155–163
    behavioral symptoms, assessment of, 194–196, 201*f*
    brain and, 55–62
    central pathophysiology of, 55–66
    clinical, in persons with dementia, 33–34, 33*f*
    concept of, 3–4
    culture and. *See* Cross-cultural considerations
    dementia and, 38–39, 92–93. *See also individual entry*
    in developmental disability, 99–114. *See also individual entry*
    epidemiology of, 43–52
    guidelines and practical approaches, 178–186, 179*t*–180*t*
        frameworks for, 177–178
    lateral, 74–78
    management cycle, 94*f*
    medial, 73–78
    mood symptoms, assessment of, 198–199, 201*t*
    neuroimaging, measuring with, 63–66
    neuropathology, with dementia, 71–80
    neuropsychiatric and, 85–95, 90*t*
    observational pain tools, 133–149
    orofacial pain, 167–174, 172*t*
    psychophysics, 163–164
    research, future directions of, 363–369
    risk factors, 50
    self-assessment, 119–128
    undetected, impact of, 50

Pain management (in dementia)
    exercise and, 253–261
    multidisciplinary and multiprofessional treatments, 306
    nursing care of, 235–241
        assessment, 237–238
        background and significance, 235
        management, 238
        nonpharmacological treatment, 239–240
        pharmacological treatment, 238–239
    observational tools. *See individual entry*
    palliative care. *See* Palliative care (dementia and pain)
    pharmacological treatment, 245–250
        analgesics for elderly, 246–248
        behavioral symptoms, 248–249
        neuropathic pain, 247–248
        pharmacodynamic changes, 246
        pharmacokinetic changes, 245–246
        psychological symptoms, 248–249
    psychological interventions of, 34–36, 267–281. *See also individual entry*
        in cognitively impaired populations, 274–278, 277*t*
        in elder persons, 272–274
        evaluation of, 272
        implications of, 278–280
Palliative care (dementia and pain), 293–302
    clinical assessment and practical approaches, 298–300
        nutrition and hydration, 299–300
        pain, 298
        pressure sores, 299
        shortness of breath, 298–299
    complexities and potential controversies, 301–302
    discomforts, 300–301
    end of life and, 297–298
    holistic approaches, 296–297
    introduction of, 293–294
    role in dementia, 295–296, 296*f*
Paracetamol, 247
Parkinson disease
    lateral pain, 77–78
    medial pain, 77–78
Parkinson's Disease Dementia (PDD), 21–23
    diagnosis, 22
    genetic risk factors, 22
    pathology, 21–22
    treatment, 22–23
Pharmacological treatment, 245–250
    analgesics for elderly, 246–248
    behavioral symptoms, 248–249
    pharmacodynamic changes, 246
    pharmacokinetic changes, 245–246
    psychological symptoms, 248–249
Pick's disease, 23

Pittsburgh Agitation Scale (PAS), 196
Placebo analgesia (and dementia), 285–290
   absence of prefrontal control, 288–289
   clinical implications, 289–290
   future directions, 290
   prefrontal areas in, 286–288
Pseudodementia, 210
Psychological intervention (of pain), 268–272
   cognitive behavioral therapy, 269–270
   in cognitively impaired populations, 274–278, 277t
   dementia and, 268
   in elder persons, 272–274
   evaluation of, 272
   implications, 278–280
   mindfulness approaches, 270–271
   self-regulatory approaches, 271–272
Psychological and behavioral symptoms of dementia (BPSD), 14, 86
Psychophysics (of pain), 163–164

R

Research
   ethical issues in. *See* Ethical issues (research)
   future directions of (dementia and pain), 363–369
      adding tools, 366
      automatic pain assessment, 366–368
      innovation management, 369
      neuropsychological tests, use of, 368–369
      new perspectives of, 363–364
      palliative care perspective, differentiation, 366
      quests, generally accepted, 365
Rowland Universal Dementia Assessment Scale (RUDAS), 214

S

Self-assessment (pain)
   cognitive impairment, barriers and prerequisites, 120
   consequences of pain, 122
   disability scale, 124
   exacerbating and alleviating factors, 121
   guidelines for caregivers, 121
   importance of, 119–120
   intensity scales, 122–124
   location of pain, 122
   multidimensional tools, 124–125
   observer rating, divergence between, 126–127
   onset, duration, variations, 121
   in pain management, uses of, 125–126
   practical approaches, 186
   qualitative description of pain, 121–122
   recommendations, 127–128
   sensory impairment, barriers and prerequisites, 120
Self-injurious behavior, 112–113
Self-report assessment. *See* Self-assessment (pain)
Short-Form McGill Pain Questionnaire (SF-MPQ), 124
Short Portable Mental Status Questionnaire (SPMSQ), 214

T

Task Force of the American Society for Pain Management Nursing, 183–185
Transforming Long-Term Care Pain Management in North America Guidelines, 185–186

V

Vascular dementia (VD), 20–21
   diagnosis, 20–21
   lateral pain, 76–77
   medial pain, 76–77
   pathology, 20
   risk factors, 20
   treatment, 21
Vocalization (pain), 162–163
Voxel-wise analyses, 64–65